Imaging Strategies in Oncology

Imaging Strategies in Oncology

Edited by

Daniel Vanel, MD

Chairman of the Department of Radiology, Institut Gustave Roussy, Villejuif, France

David Stark, MD

Professor of Radiology, Director of MRI, Department of Radiology
University of Massachusetts Medical Center, Worcester, Massachusetts, USA

Martin Dunitz

First published in the United Kingdom in 1993
by Martin Dunitz Ltd, The Livery House, 7–9
Pratt Street, London NW1 0AE

A CIP catalogue record for this book is available
from the British Library.

ISBN 1 85317 052 6

Composition by Scribe Design, Gillingham, Kent,
United Kingdom
Origination by Imago Publishing Ltd
Manufactured by Imago Publishing Ltd
Printed and bound in Singapore

Foreword

The imaging needs of the patient with cancer are complex challenges and the physician's response must be based upon an understanding of the specific neoplasm, its biological characteristics and its response to treatment.

This text, organized by major anatomic sites, is a practical working guide to the application of radiology to oncologic patients. Decision trees and illustrations will serve as procedural guidelines to assist the reader in understanding the proper applications and limitations of our technology. Although the text is addressed primarily to a radiologic audience, it will also serve to guide the oncologic clinician responsible for patient management.

The authors have been selected from Europe and the United States to balance the oncologic experience presented. Some variation may exist in the various protocols used to treat cancer among the authors' institutions and countries, but the editors have ensured a cohesive presentation. The TNM staging language is now virtually uniform worldwide. Some tumor sites do not, admittedly, lend themselves to the TNM classification system for cancer staging (for example, gynecologic, prostatic and urologic neoplasms and the lymphomas). Nevertheless, tremendous strides have been made in the recent past in unifying the staging language and systems of the American Joint Committee with those of the Union Internationale Contre le Cancer; the resulting TNM system should be used whenever possible in our reports.

I am pleased to have been a participant in this text and look forward to its integration in our daily oncologic practice.

David G. Bragg

Preface

This book attempts to provide a cohesive approach toward oncologic imaging. A group of distinguished authors from the United States and Europe discusses the appropriate timing and sequence of imaging studies in oncologic diagnosis. Extensive illustration and decision trees guide the practical application of these recommendations.

In these days of cost-containment, efficient diagnostic algorithms must be defined and adopted as the standard of care. Understanding the specific value of each imaging modality can conserve resources, save time, and help radiologists and clinicians interact to provide optimal care.

We would like to thank the associate editors and our distinguished contributors for their helpful advice and expertise in describing the diagnostic approach to various oncologic conditions.

We hope that our readers will enjoy and learn as much from this book as we did in editing it.

In dedicating this book to our patients and colleagues, we acknowledge the support of our familes: Christine, David, Stephane, Lila, Maïa and Zoë; and Susan and Elizabeth.

Daniel Vanel
David Stark

1

The brain

Danielle Balériaux, William O. Bank and Celso Matos

Introduction

In this chapter we discuss an imaging strategy that can be used whenever a cerebral neoplasm is suspected. Since most extra-axial intracranial tumors are benign (meningioma, schwannoma, etc.), they will not be considered here, although malignant tumors can exist in this location. The 20% of all childhood cancers that involve the brain are also excluded here; they are discussed separately in Chapter 3.

Intracerebral tumors are rare in adults. They are slightly more frequent in men than in women. The global incidence reported in the literature varies from 4.5 to 15.0 per 100 000. The variations are a function of the methodology used by the investigators and variations in their patient populations.[1–3]

Sixty per cent of brain tumors in adults are hemispheric lesions. Histologic differences will be addressed later, but it is important to note here that the type of neoplasm encountered most frequently in a given population varies with the age of that population. In like manner, the frequency and malignancy of the tumors encountered both increase with the age of the population studied, up to an age of 62 years, at which point both decrease abruptly.

A list of brain neoplasms is given in Table 1.1.

Although it is clear that the prognosis in brain tumors is poor, it is closely related to the histologic type of the tumor and the treatment chosen. While age plays a role, that role is variable. Supratentorial low-grade astrocytomas exhibit a potentially long period of latency during which time the patient remains asymptomatic or has minimal symptoms that can be controlled medically. The median survival is 7 years, with malignant transformation occurring in half of the patients during the first 6 years. In oligodendrogliomas, median survival falls to 5 years.[4]

Anaplastic astrocytomas (Figure 1.1) fall into a category on which age, surgical debulking and irradiation have a definite effect on longevity.[5,6] In patients under the age of 50, the 2-year survival is about 50%, with median survival of 100 weeks. In patients over the age of 50, the median survival falls to 48 weeks, with 2-year survival of only 10%, almost identical to that of the glioblastomas. While gross total resection is associated with longer and better-quality survival in glioblastomas,[5,7] 1-year survival falls to 15%, with patients less than 50 years old having a 1-month longer median survival. Nevertheless, if reoperation with extensive tumor resection is feasible, the patient may enjoy a good-quality prolongation of life of 10 weeks with a glioblastoma and 83 weeks with an anaplastic astrocytoma.[6,8]

The supratentorial low-grade astrocytomas (Figure 1.2) are the tumors in which imaging makes the biggest impact. Newer non-invasive techniques are providing conclusive diagnosis of these lesions at an earlier time in their development. The median interval until malignant transformation is now 56 months from radiologic diagnosis.[9] This apparent lengthening of the quiescent period before transformation may be related to earlier diagnosis, implying that the low-grade gliomas in previous studies may already have been in or close to malignant transformation at the time of diagnosis. It has been shown recently that biopsy and treatment regimens during the quiescent period make no difference in the eventual outcome, and their use in this period is thus controversial.[9] Imaging follow up remains

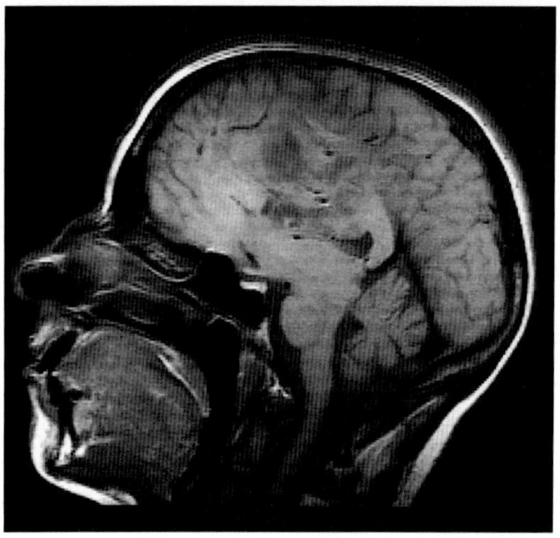

A

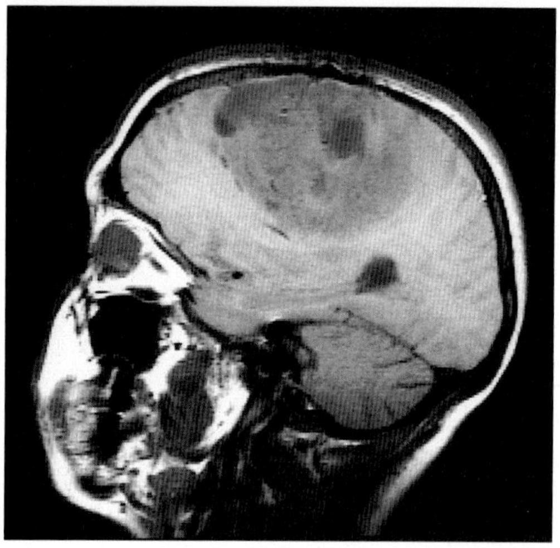

B

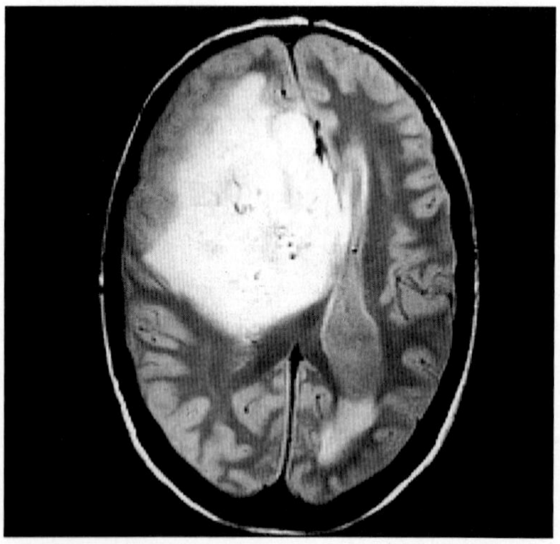

C

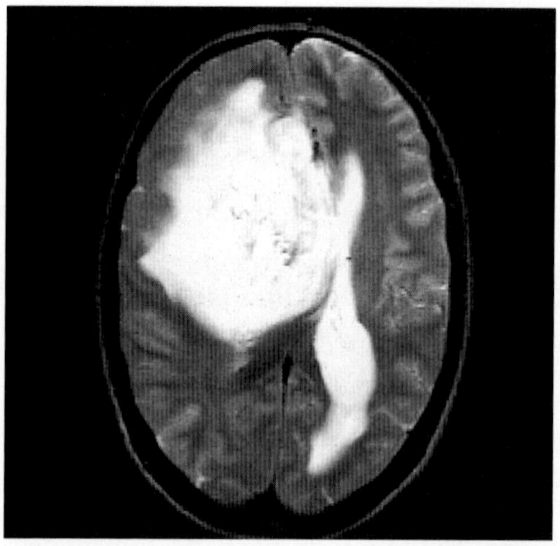

D

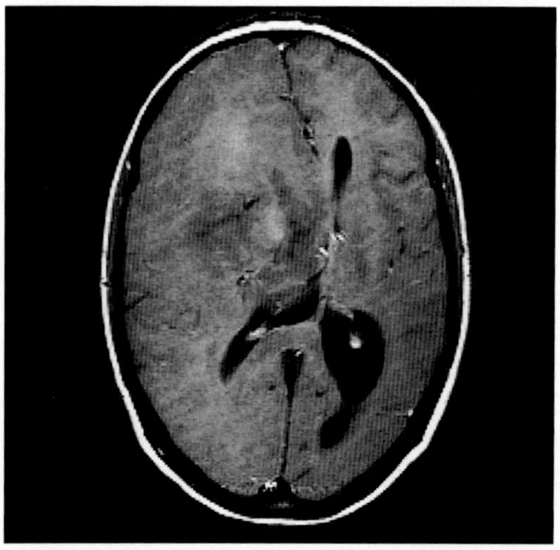

E

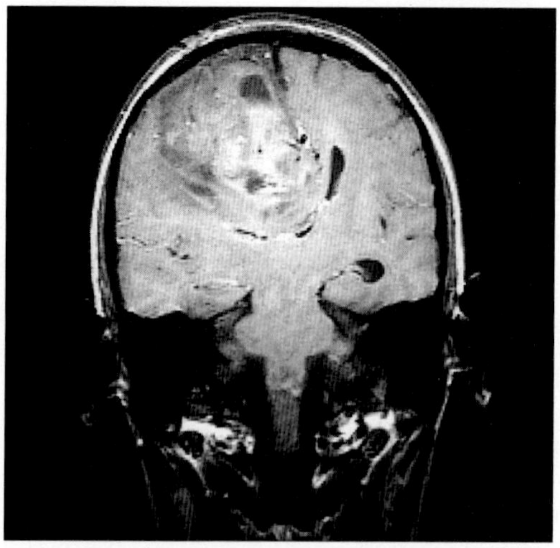

F

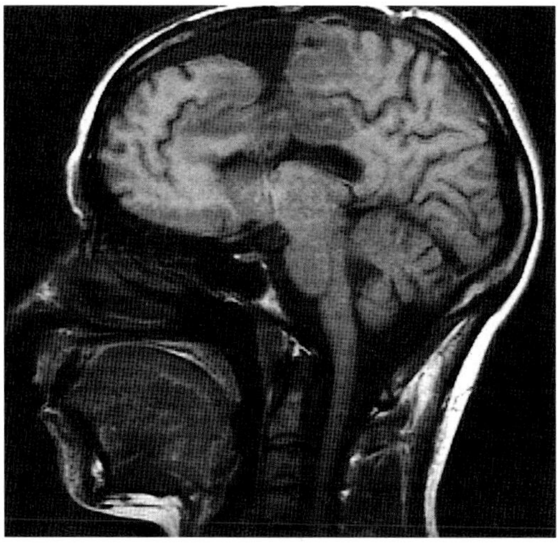

G

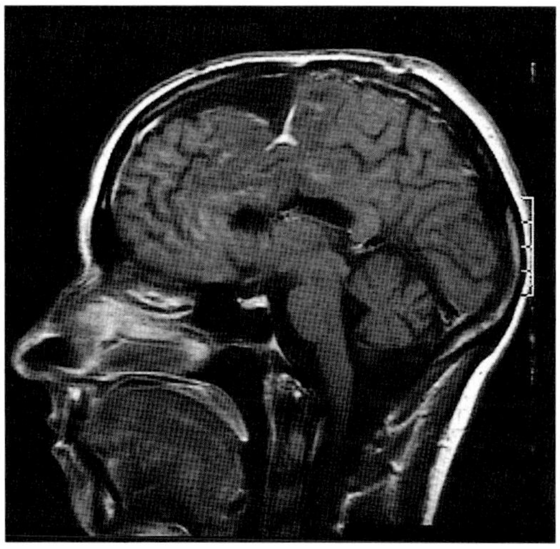

H

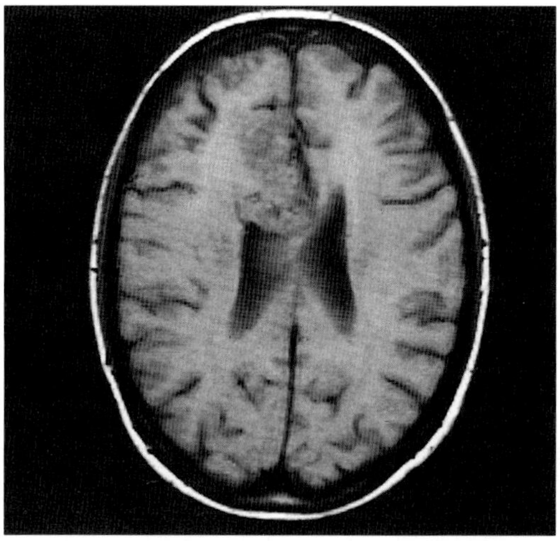

I

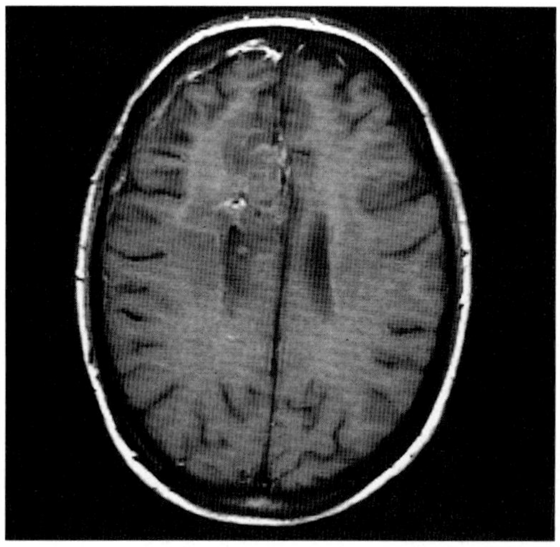

J

Figure 1.1

Frontal anaplastic astrocytoma with involvement of the corpus callosum pre and post partial resection. The images demonstrate the large amount of tumor that can be resected and the appearance of meningeal and intracerebral contrast enhancement following surgery.

A and **B** Sagittal T1-weighted images from the initial MR evaluation.

C and **D** Axial proton density (**C**) and T2-weighted (**D**) images.

E and **F** Axial **E** and coronal (**F**) T1-weighted images after gadolinium injection.

Although one might be tempted to call this tumor inoperable, armed with the multiplanar depiction of the large frontal tumor, the neurosurgeon can make preoperative preparations for an extensive debulking of clinically silent areas while preserving adjacent eloquent areas. In this case the sagittal images suggest that the rolandic sulcus is displaced posteriorly, allowing a more complete resection than might be attempted otherwise. Rapidity of regrowth is a function of the amount of tumor 'left behind'.

G and **H** Sagittal T1-weighted images before (**G**) and after (**H**) gadolinium injection obtained 5 months after extensive partial resection.

I and **J** Axial T1-weighted images before (**I**) and after (**J**) gadolinium injection.

5-month follow-up MR demonstrates the striking amount of tumor that could be removed without producing significant neurologic deficit. Note the enhancement at the margins of tumor resection. Only by repetitive follow-up examinations will we be able to identify the tumor progression.

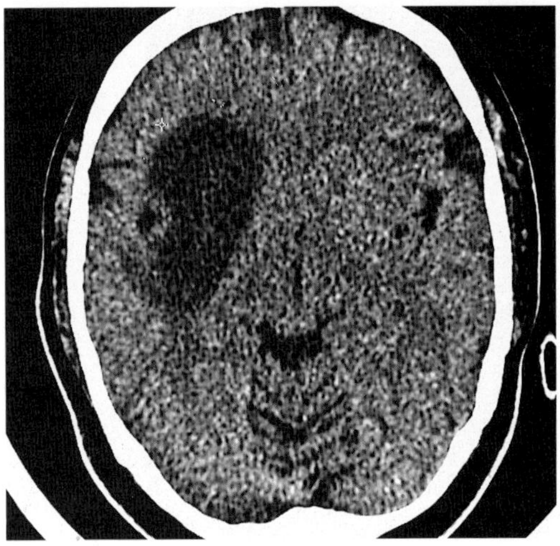
A

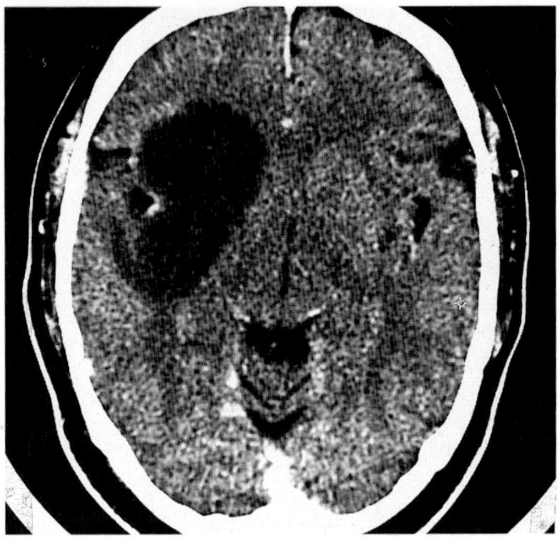
B

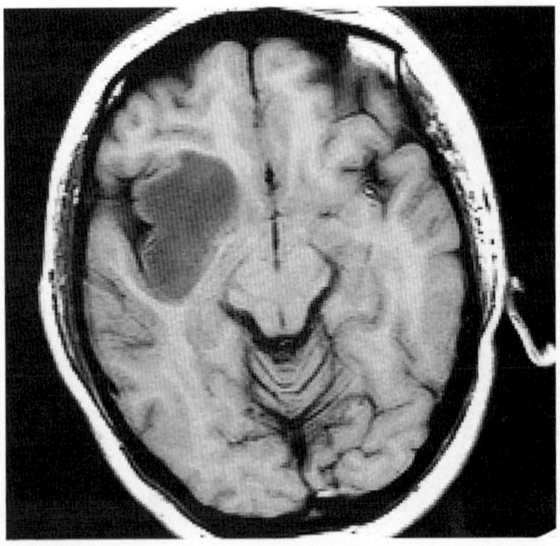
C

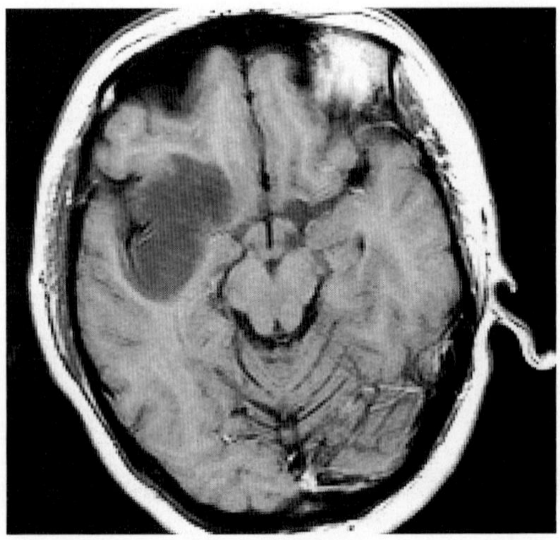
D

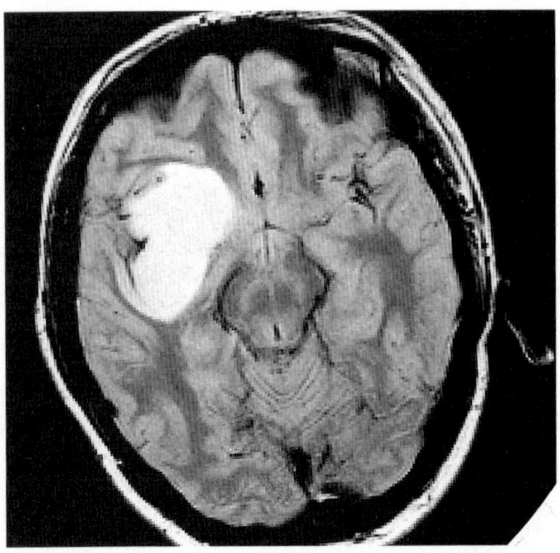
E

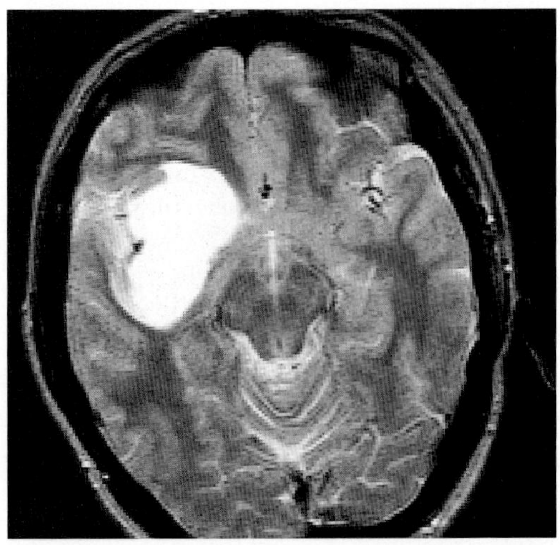
F

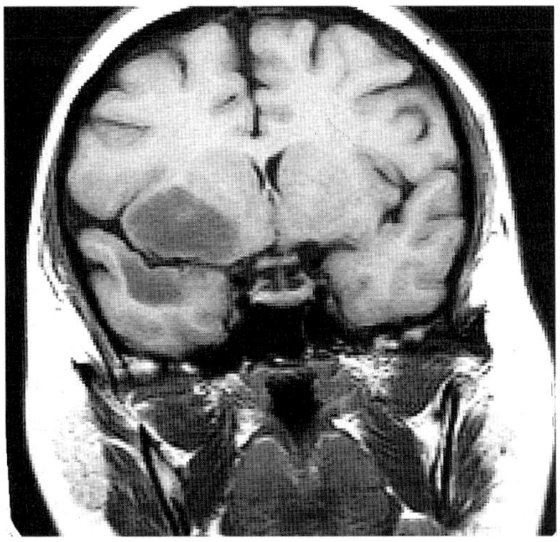

G

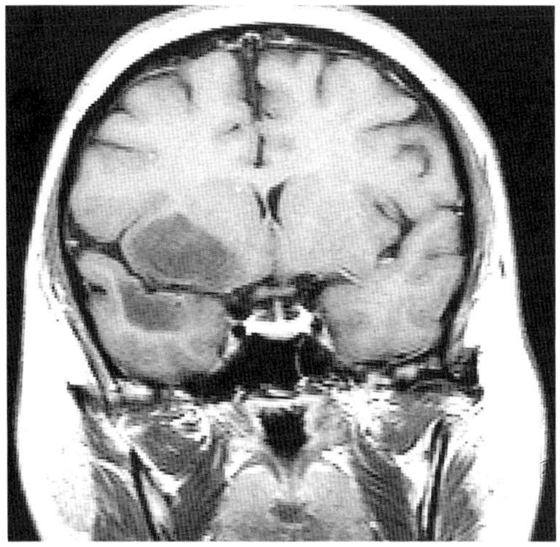

H

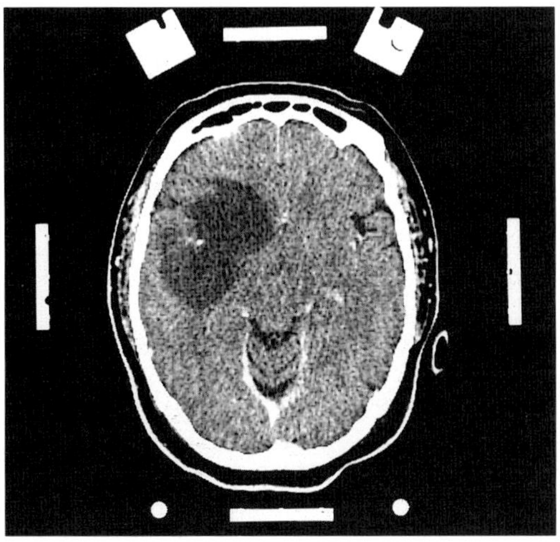

I

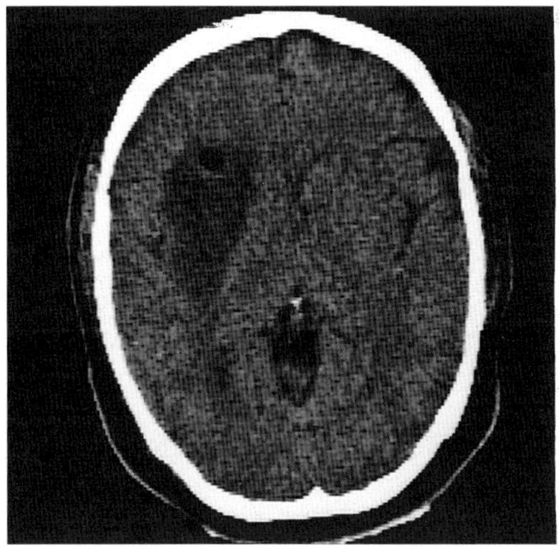

J

Figure 1.2

Low-grade frontotemporal astrocytoma. The images demonstrate the typical presentation of low-grade gliomas.

A and **B** CT scan before (**A**) and after (**B**), contrast administration obtained as part of an evaluation for a clinically suspected pituitary adenoma, reveals a vast well-defined low-density lesion with minimal mass effect that exhibits no contrast enhancement.

C and **D** Axial T1-weighted images before (**C**) and after (**D**) gadolinium injection demonstrate a homogeneous, hypointense, well-delimited mass with no contrast enhancement.

E and **F** Axial proton density (**E**) and T2-weighted (**F**) images show hyperintensity (T2 prolongation) in the region of the tumor without surrounding edema.

G and **H** Coronal T1-weighted images before (**G**) and after (**H**) gadolinium injection show the extension of the tumor into the frontal and temporal opercula.

The tumor remained static for three years before onset of symptoms necessitated biopsy.

I and **J** Enhanced CT performed in the stereotactic frame (**I**) immediately prior to biopsy and 24 hours post biopsy (**J**) shows no hemorrhagic complications, but the presence of an intentionally injected small bubble of air confirms the site of the tumor biopsy.

The localization of this tumor in the frontotemporal region, its incidental discovery in a young asymptomatic patient, and its slow evolution are fairly typical of low-grade gliomas.

Table 1.1 Histologic classification of neuroepithelial cerebral neoplasms.

ASTROCYTIC TUMORS
- Astrocytoma
  - Fibrillary
  - Protoplasmic
  - Gemistiocytotic
- Pilocytic astrocytoma
- Subependymal giant-cell astrocytoma (the ventricular tumor of tuberous sclerosis)
- Astroblastoma
- Anaplastic

OLIGODENDROGLIAL TUMORS
- Oligodendroglioma
- Mixed oligoastrocytoma
- Anaplastic oligodendroglioma

EPENDYMAL AND CHOROID PLEXUS TUMORS
- Ependymoma
  - Myxopapillary ependymoma
  - Papillary ependymoma
  - Subependymoma
- Anaplastic ependymoma
- Choroid plexus papilloma
- Anaplastic choroid plexus papilloma

PINEAL GLAND TUMORS
- Pineocytoma
- Pineoblastoma
- Pineal germinoma
- Embryonal carcinoma

NEURONAL TUMORS
- Gangliocytoma
- Ganglioglioma
- Ganglioneuroblastoma
- Gangliocytoma and anaplastic ganglioglioma
- Neuroblastoma
- Primitive neuroectodermal tumors

POORLY DIFFERENTIATED AND EMBRYONAL TUMORS
- Glioblastoma
  - Sarcomatous glioblastoma
  - Giant-cell glioblastoma
- Medulloblastoma
  - Desmoplastic medulloblastoma
  - Medullomyoblastoma
- Medulloepithelioma
- Primitive polar spongioblastoma
- Cerebral gliomatosis

important for early identification of the onset of malignant transformation.

In view of the relative rarity of primary brain neoplasms, routine screening of the general population for these lesions has not been performed or even advocated to our knowledge. However, as soon as a patient falls into a category at high risk of having an intracranial tumor, sensitive screening methods must be employed. For example, screening techniques become appropriate in a patient with a primary neoplasm that has a known potential to metastasize to the brain, or in a patient with a rare condition associated with intracranial tumors, such as phacomatomatoses. The strategies for screening in these cases is discussed later.

Clinical presentation of cerebral neoplasm

The symptoms and signs caused by brain tumors can be classified as follows.

- *Direct focal effects* related to focal tumor invasion and destruction of cerebral parenchyma.
- *Indirect focal effects* due to displacement and/or compression of normal brain by the tumor itself, and displacement and/or compression of normal brain by surrounding edema.
- *Remote or generalized effects* due to:

(1) Impairment of the vascular supply or drainage of otherwise normal brain by direct tumor invasion or compression of the feeding arteries or draining veins of the involved vascular territory.

(2) Secondary hydrocephalus caused by cerebrospinal fluid (CSF) overproduction, obstruction of CSF pathways by the tumor itself, or obstruction caused by tumor compression or displacement of these same pathways.

(3) Increased intracranial pressure caused by the volume of the mass itself and/or any of its secondary effects.

Although it appears at the end of the list, this etiological category is in fact the most frequently encountered.

The rate of tumor growth is an important factor in determining the clinical manifestations observed in brain tumors. Slowly growing tumors become symptomatic at larger volumes, while rapidly growing tumors do not allow the brain time to compensate for their presence and become symptomatic sooner. On the average, malignant tumors become symptomatic when they attain a volume of approximately 100 ml. In certain critical locations such as the brainstem, however, much smaller tumors can produce neurologic deficits. Hemorrhage into a pre-existent but previously asymptomatic tumor, or obstruction of the CSF pathways with sudden onset of obstructive hydrocephalus, may produce an abrupt onset of neurologic symptoms. Since the cranial vault cannot expand in adults, intracranial hypertension develops when anything within the confines of the calvarium expands too much or too rapidly.

Headache is the most common symptom in patients with brain tumors. It was found to be the initial manifestation of supratentorial malignant gliomas in over 50% of the patients included in the EORTC (European Organization for Research and Treatment of Cancer) brain tumor group studies. Typically these headaches are generalized but often predominate at the site of the tumor. They are aggravated by coughing and Valsalva maneuvers.

Bilateral papilledema is a common fundoscopic sign in older children and adults with intracranial hypertension. Arterial hypertension, bradycardia and depressed respiratory rate tend to be found during advanced stages of cerebral neoplastic diseases, but seldom at the time of diagnosis. Another clinical feature seen in late stages is tentorial herniation which initially produces ipsilateral mydriasis due to the compression of the 3rd cranial nerve, followed by a typical sequence of events leading to coma and death.[10]

The effects of intracranial hypertension and remote mass largely account for the rather poor correlation of clinical presentation and tumor location in comparison with cerebral infarcts. One of the best examples of a misleading focal sign is paralysis of the 6th cranial nerve; this sign has no localizing value whatsoever.

In most cases, the neurologic deficit caused by tumors is slowly progressive. An abrupt, stroke-like onset is not uncommon, however, in malignant gliomas and metastatic tumors. Intratumoral hemorrhage and acute peritumoral edema best explain such rapid clinical course (Figure 1.3). Intermittent symptoms may be caused by a pedunculated intraventricular tumor that intermittently produces an acute obstructive hydrocephalus. Seizures may occur either as an early or late manifestation in about a third of patients with brain tumors.[11,12] These seizures are usually focal, although they may generalize rapidly. A careful history may allow localization of the tumor, especially when seizures are an early manifestation of the neoplastic process.

Behavioral changes and cognitive disorders, such as aphasia, apraxia and memory deficits, are common in various types of brain tumors. Slowly growing tumors, especially in the frontal region, may lead to dementia.

In search of an imaging strategy

Whenever a brain neoplasm is clinically suspected, the neuroradiologist is expected to answer fundamental questions. These questions guide the subsequent strategic decisions and fall into five categories as follows.

- *Sensitivity*: Are the patient's clinical signs and symptoms caused by an intracranial expansile lesion?
- *Specificity*: With what kind of lesion are we dealing? Is it a neoplasm? Is it benign or is it malignant? Can we suggest a histopathologic diagnosis?
- *Location*: If a tumor is found, where is it located exactly, is it solitary or multiple, and what are its precise limits?
- *Treatment*: What kind of useful information may be provided in order to give appropriate treatment? Is this tumor resectable? What approach should the surgeon use? Where are the ideal locations from which to take an open or a stereotactic biopsy? What are the limits of the area to be irradiated?
- *Monitoring*: How can the neuroradiologist monitor and evaluate the efficacy of the treatment?

Answering these questions will lead us to the establishment of the most effective strategic approach to these diagnostic problems. Different neuroradiologic imaging modalities are presently available and are discussed here; they include primarily CT and/or MR, as well as cerebral angiography.

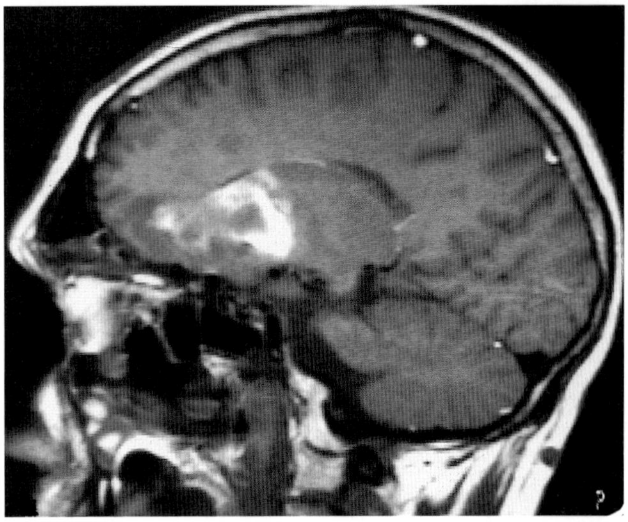

A

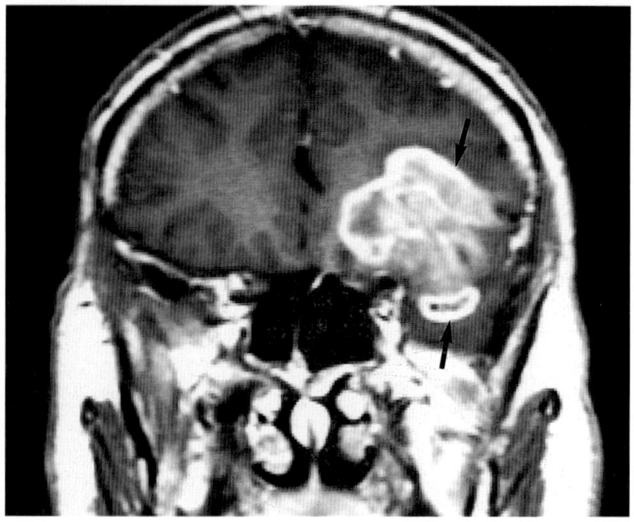

C

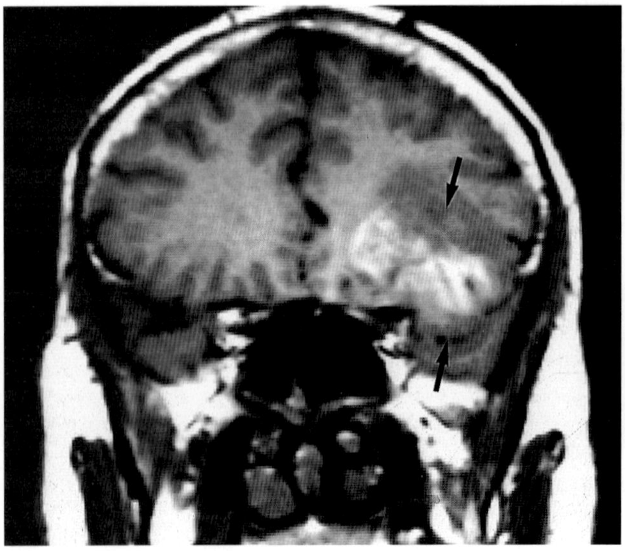

B

Figure 1.3

Hemorrhagic frontal glioblastoma. The images demonstrate a frontal hemorrhage with underlying neoplasm.

A Sagittal unenhanced MR.

B and **C** Coronal MR before (**B**) and after (**C**) gadolinium injection.

The location of the hemorrhage in this part of the frontal pole and the nodular non-homogeneity strongly suggest the presence of an underlying tumor. Enhancement of the large hypointense areas above and below the zones of hemorrhage (arrows, **B** and **C**) confirm this suspicion.

Standard radiography and tomography

Standard radiographs and standard tomographic images of the skull are known to be of little value in the detection of intracranial tumors and cannot be considered as a screening procedure. Brain neoplasms almost never invade the bony elements of the skull. Erosion of the clinoids or displacement of a calcified pineal gland, while classical indirect radiologic signs of intracranial expansive lesions, are not early signs of tumor and they are only occasionally recognized nowadays. Tumor calcifications may be seen on plain tomographs mainly in slow growing tumors such as oligodendrogliomas, subependymal giant-cell astrocytomas or choroid plexus papillomas (Figure 1.4), but are usually seen long after the tumor is clinically apparent and readily evident on CT and MR.

Pneumoencephalography, ventriculography and ultrasonography

Pneumoencephalography is no longer used, whereas ventriculography (positive contrast) is still performed exceptionally, usually when purely cystic intraventricular lesions are suspected. The use of ultrasonography in adults is usually limit 1 to intra-operative localization of small tumors situated close to the cortex. Ultrasonography has also been used to follow tumors post-operatively through the 'acoustic window' of the craniotomy burr holes,[13] but cannot be considered to represent a standard imaging tool for adult brain neoplasms.

Positron emission tomography and magnetic resonance spectroscopy

Positron emission tomography (PET) and magnetic resonance spectroscopy (MRS),[14–17] are valuable diagnostic imaging procedures but remain experimental for the most part. In our own clinical setting, PET is routinely used for certain specific diagnostic problems: differentiation between tumor recurrence and radiation necrosis, and choice of the most appropriate region within a tumor to be biopsied stereotactically[18] (Figure 1.5).

Computed tomography and magnetic resonance imaging

CT and MR currently provide the best visualization of the brain, its cerebrospinal fluid pathways and its surrounding bony enclosure. As MR is not readily available in all locations (mainly for economic reasons), and as CT is widely accessible, we will consider both as valuable imaging modalities to be used in a strategic approach to brain neoplasms (Figure 1.6).

CT, introduced to clinical practice in 1974, is nowadays a well-accepted and well-codified imaging modality. Examinations should include plain and iodinated contrast-enhanced series whenever one is looking for brain neoplasm. Enhancement patterns enrich the information provided by plain CT. Different injection techniques have been advocated, including bolus 'angio-CT' and delayed CT.[19] In clinical practice, however, the usefulness of angio-CT has not been generally accepted for tumor characterization. In contrast, the usefulness of double-dose delayed scanning has been clearly demonstrated for the detection of metastatic lesions.[20–23]

When available, MR should be the first imaging modality to be performed whenever an intracranial neoplasm is suspected clinically.[24] Routinely used in clinical practice for more than 8 years, it rapidly established itself as the imaging modality of choice as far as cerebral neoplasms are concerned. The great sensitivity of the method, its capacity for multiplanar imaging, the exquisite anatomic depiction of normal brain and pathologic conditions, the high contrast resolution, the sensitivity to flow and the ability to detect vascular elements have been documented extensively[25–29] (Figure 1.7).

When both CT and MR are used, it is not unusual to encounter lesions that produce little or no mass effect and exhibit only equivocal contrast enhancement on CT, but are more evident on MR. In like manner, calcified lesions can present a diagnostic problem on CT because the density of the calcium overwhelms the relatively subtle increase in density caused by the iodinated CT contrast agent. As calcium is of low signal intensity on T1-weighted MR images, it is easy to identify enhancement of the neoplastic matrix within even densely calcified tumors.

Another strong case for the preference for MR as the neuro-imaging modality of choice can be found in cases of multiple tumors. Glioblastomas not infrequently arise in multicentric fashion and must be differentiated from metastases, especially if there is no known primary. Many solitary intracranial metastases have a good prognosis following resection that degrades significantly in the presence of a second lesion. The critical additional lesion may lie close to bone in one of the CT blind spots, or its small size and pattern of enhancement may render it easy to miss on CT. MR proves its value in these cases (see Figure 1.8).

It must be emphasized that MR continues to evolve rapidly and, even today, new technical refinements appear in the literature at a high rate. Technical improvements tend to provide better contrast and spatial resolution, to shorten the examination time, to yield better tissue characterization and to give a more precise evaluation of vascular elements. Fast imaging techniques, three-dimensional techniques, and techniques of MR angiography are the most useful recent technical improvements to MR.[30,31]

From a 'strategic' point of view, we recommend routine performance of an initial series of sagittal T1-weighted images, followed by a multi-echo sequence with proton density and T2-weighted

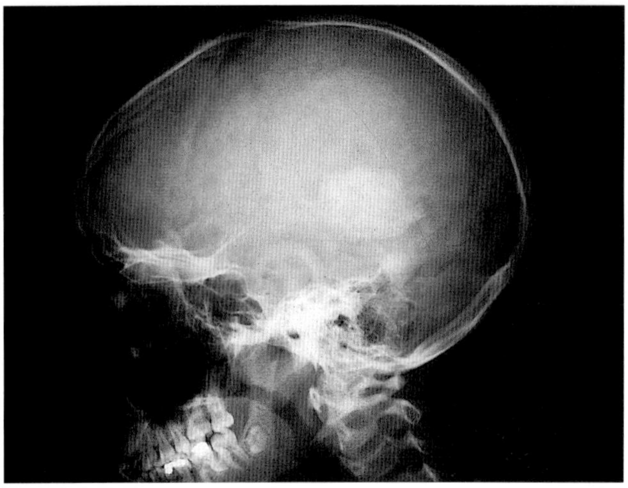

A

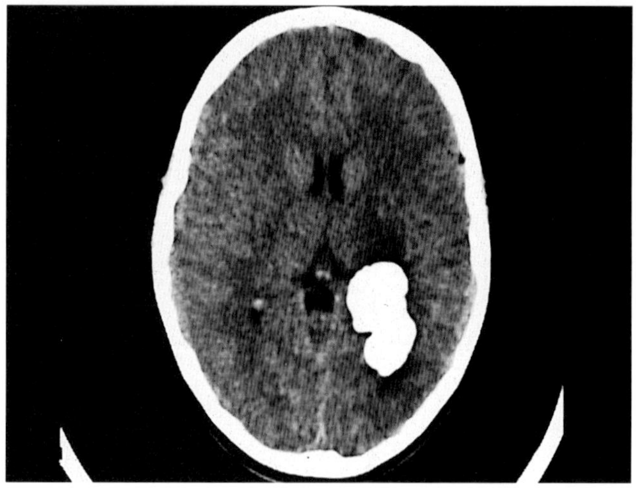

B

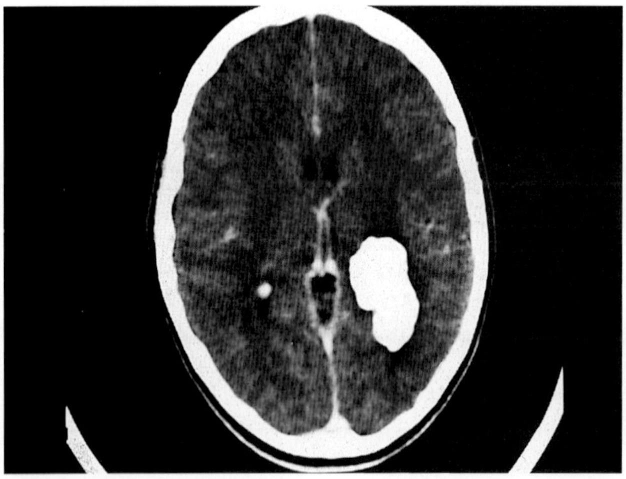

C

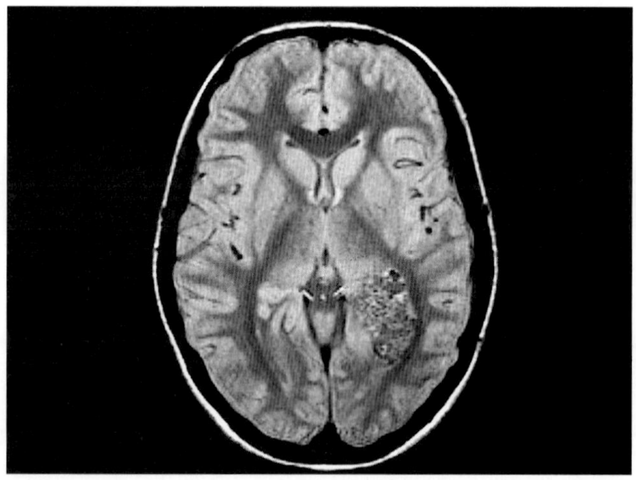

D

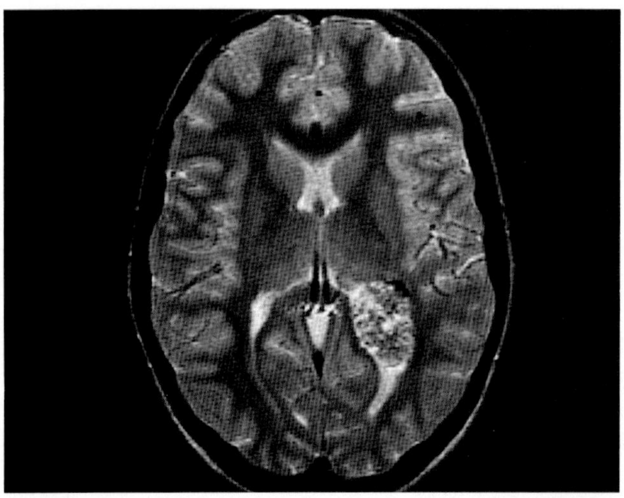

E

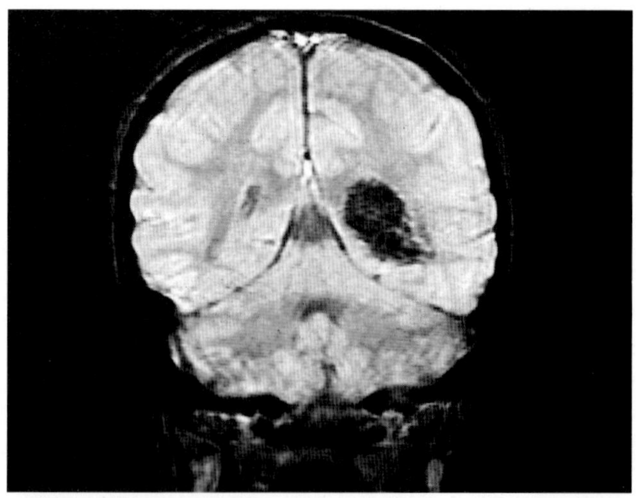

F

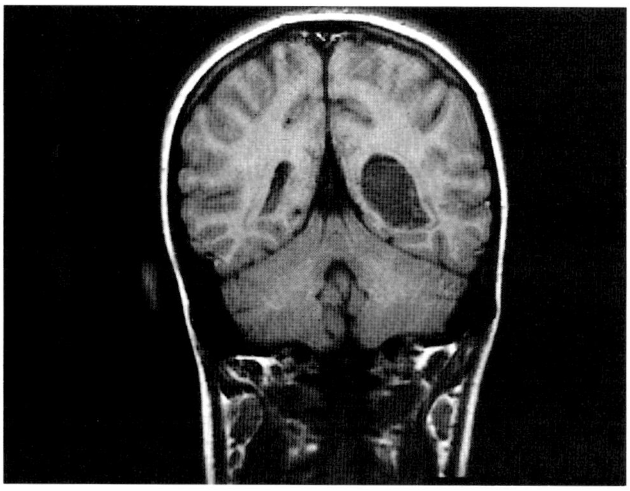

G

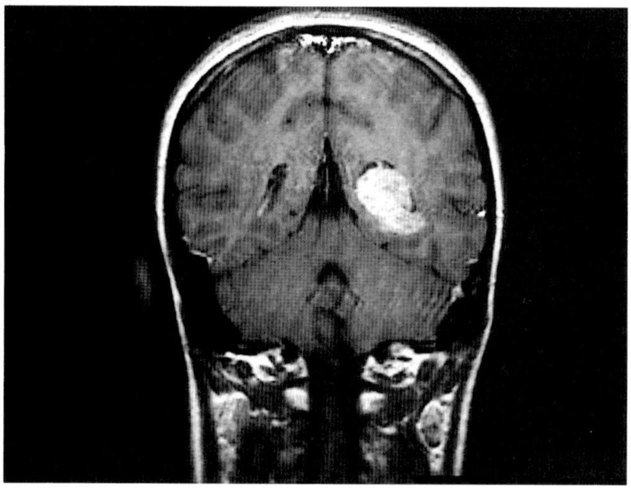

H

Figure 1.4

Choroid plexus papilloma, highly calcified, The images demonstrate the sensitivity of MR to contrast enhancement in the presence of calcifications.

A Lateral skull radiograph obtained in the emergency room after minor head trauma. Note the large calcification in the region of the atrium of the lateral ventricles.

B Unenhanced CT scan confirms the presence of a large calcified lesion in the temporo-occipital region, partially filling the atrium of the right lateral ventricle.

C No discernable modification of the CT appearance of the lesion after contrast injection.

D and **E** Axial proton density (**D**) and T2-weighted (**E**) images showing an inhomogeneous well-delineated mass. Neither edema nor secondary hydrocephalus are present, and associated mass effect is minimal.

F Coronal gradient-echo image best demonstrates the calcified component of the tumor.

G and **H** Intense contrast enhancement of the neoplasm, masked on the CT by the density of the calcium (**C**), shows clearly on the T1-weighted obtained before (**G**) and after (**H**) gadolinium injection.

images in the axial or coronal plane. If no abnormalities are found on these two sets of images, the examination may be stopped at this point unless specific clinical signs demand continuation. Although rarely the case, some tumors may only be visible after contrast administration. If any tumoral process is suspected to be shown, further acquisitions should be obtained, such as T1- or T2-weighted images in other planes for better localization purposes. We routinely inject paramagnetic contrast agents, gaining valuable information about the integrity of the blood–brain barrier.[32,33]

The enhancement pattern provides additional and more specific information. Although it is a very rare occurrence, one should nevertheless be concerned about the potential for allergic reaction to gadolinium, since it has been reported.[34,35]

For evaluating patients with suspected intracranial metastases the strategy depends upon the imaging modalities available. When limited to CT scanning, one can proceed immediately to double-dose delayed scanning .[21–23] Unenhanced scanning can be reserved for cases in which it is necessary to resolve questions on the enhanced study.

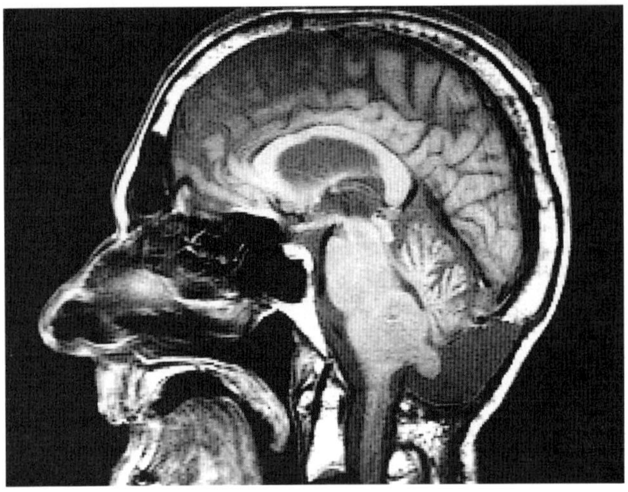

A

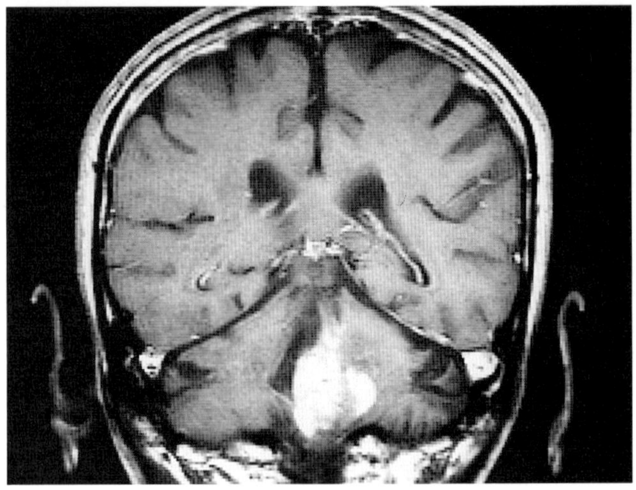

B

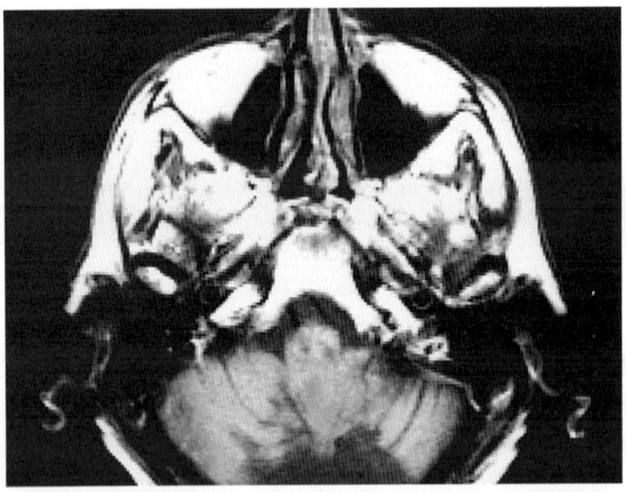

C

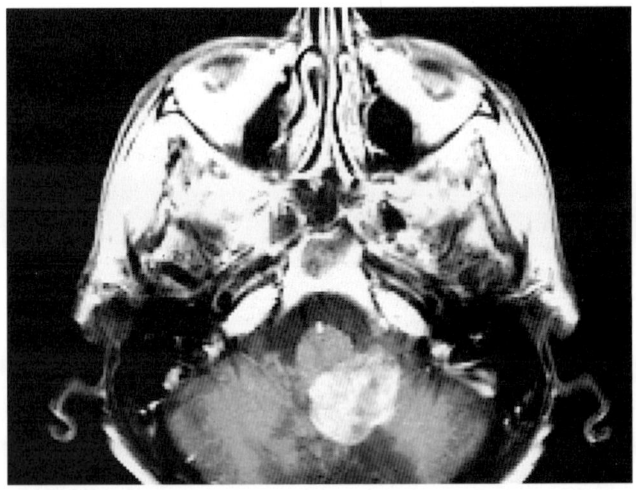

D

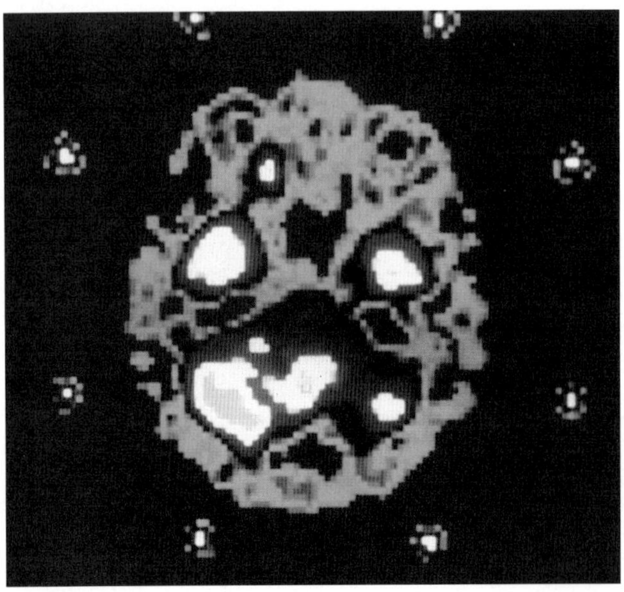

E

Figure 1.5

Brainstem astrocytoma (grade II) operated upon and then irradiated 7 years earlier. The images illustrate the value of PET scanning to distinguish between tumor recurrence and radiation necrosis.

A Sagittal unenhanced T1-weighted image.

B Coronal T1-weighted image after gadolinium injection.

C and **D** Axial T1-weighted images before (**C**) and after (**D**) gadolinium injection.

E Axial PET scan obtained at the same level with the patient in the stereotactic frame, after injection of [^{18}F]fluorodeoxyglucose (FDG) (courtesy of Dr S Goldman, Université Libre de Bruxelles, Hôpital Erasme).

Deep to the changes of the suboccipital craniectomy, the MR demonstrates a nodular, non-homogeneously enhancing mass in the right side of the medulla oblongata. The hyperintense appearance of the bodies of C1, C2, and the clivus delineate the radiation field. The PET scan reveals a hypermetabolic area of FDG uptake that was biopsied stereotactically (by Dr M Levivier) to reveal several malignant foci within a low-grade astrocytoma.

When MR availability is no problem, it is best to proceed immediately to this modality since it has been demonstrated to be superior to CT in this domain.[20] While double-dose delayed T1-weighted images are the most sensitive to the presence of metastases, the debate as to the usefulness of T2-weighted images persists. The T2-weighted sequences take more time, but are very sensitive to small foci of edema that may surround small metastases, and they may also help in the differential diagnosis between metastasis and ischemia in the older patient.[22,36,37] If patient throughput is a critical factor in MR system utilization, the T2-weighted sequences can be reserved for problem cases.

Digital intra-arterial angiography is still performed routinely as a pre-operative study in most tumor cases. Surgeons prefer an evaluation of vascular displacement and anomalies, a knowledge of the degree of tumor vascularization and a depiction of the cortical veins to serve as anatomic landmarks during their surgery (Figure 1.9).

Magnetic resonance angiography (MRA) continues to improve in the quality of information it provides in comparison with conventional angiography, and it is already a routine procedure in certain centers.[31,38,39] MRA is mainly performed to give anatomic details that are not obtained by standard MR. Vascular elements such as the middle cerebral artery and the internal cerebral vein can be identified routinely on current standard MR acquisitions, and tumor vascularity and perfusion may also be evaluated by standard MR.[40] The venous phase of conventional angiograms, often indispensable to neurosurgeons because of the essential surgical landmarks, can now be easily and clearly depicted on MRA. Sinus compression and invasion are also demonstrated on MRA in a manner comparable to conventional angiography, without the need of invasive procedures such as vascular catheterization and injection of iodinated contrast media.[39] Evaluating venous invasion is the main reason for using MRA.

The strategy for the choice of imaging modalities is summarized in Diagram 1.1.

Strategy of neuroradiologic diagnosis of brain cancer

Careful interpretation of CT and MR images should be done systematically in search of clues to the appropriate diagnosis. The morphologic abnormalities that suggest the presence of a brain tumor are structural changes of the brain and/or spinal fluid pathways; these are consequently similar on both CT and MR.

- *Indirect signs*: 'anatomic changes' (better seen on MR) include alteration of normal structures, mass effect, displacement, deformation of the ventricular system, sulcal effacement, cisternal distortion or filling.
- *Direct signs*: the lesion will exhibit abnormal density on CT or abnormal signal intensity on MR in comparison with normal brain on non-enhanced examinations, and may possibly vary in appearance after administration of an appropriate contrast agent (iodinated for CT, and gadolinium-chelate for MR). The enhancement patterns should carefully be observed and codified as far as homogeneity or non-homogeneity, ring-like appearance with regular or irregular wall-thickness, enhancement rapidity, delayed enhancement, and so forth.

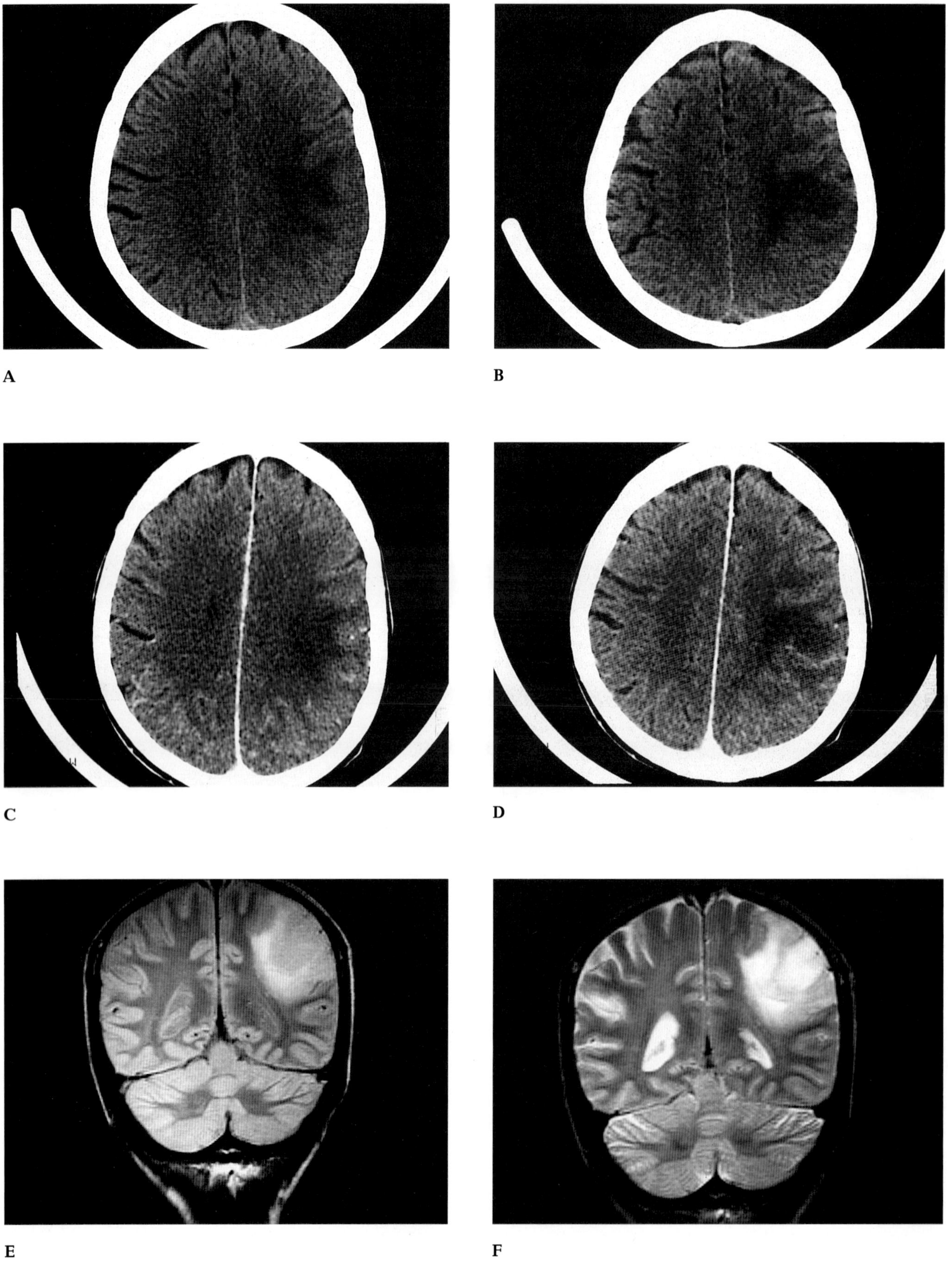

A B C D E F

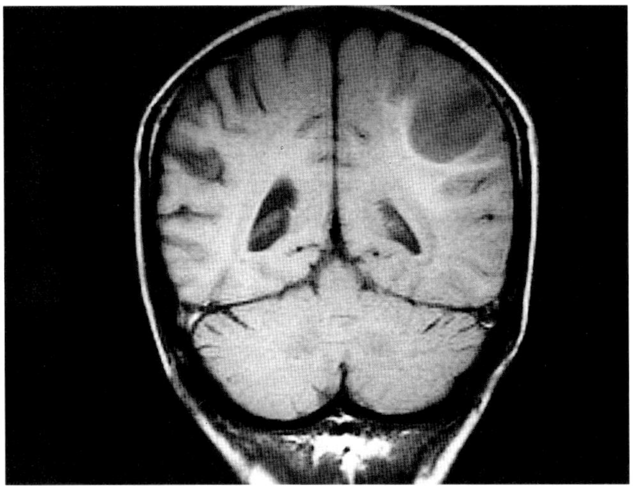

G

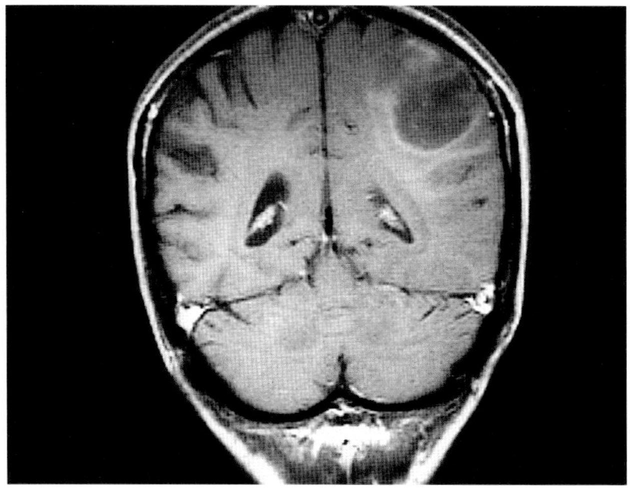

H

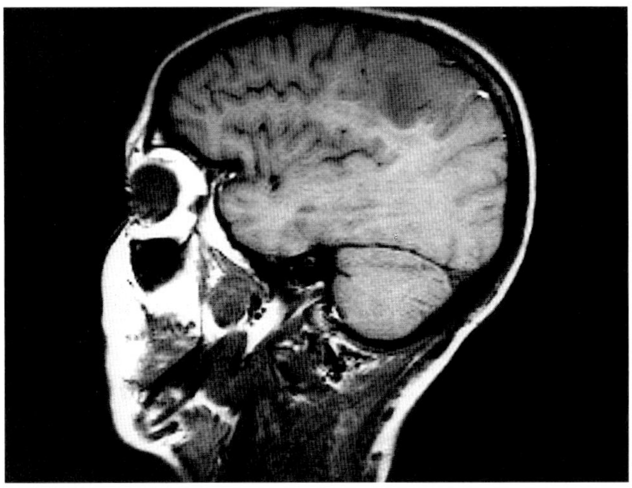

I

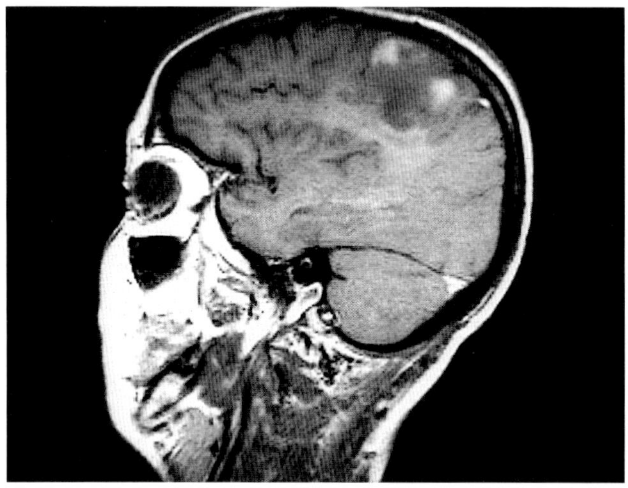

J

Figure 1.6

Astrocytoma (grade II). The images illustrate the respective usefulness of CT and MR.

A and **B** Unenhanced CT scan reveals an ill-defined hypodense mass at the left frontoparietal junction with effacement of adjacent cortical sulci.

C and **D** After contrast injection the same axial cuts demonstrate equivocal inhomogeneous enhancement in the parietal cortex.

E and **F** Proton density (**E**) and T2-weighted (**F**) images in the coronal plane clearly show the zone of edema surrounding the tumor.

G and **H** Coronal T1-weighted images obtained before contrast injection (**G**) reveals the tumor to be an inhomogeneous, predominantly hypointense lesion partly surrounded by zones in which spontaneous hyperintensity can be observed, and others in which definite enhancement can be seen after contrast injection (**H**.)

I and **J** Sagittal T1-weighted images before (**I**) and after contrast injection (**J**) help to confirm the frontoparietal, intra-axial location of this tumor. Note that the enhancing components of this tumor are better seen on the MR (**H** and **J**) than on CT (**C** and **D**) performed 5 days earlier.

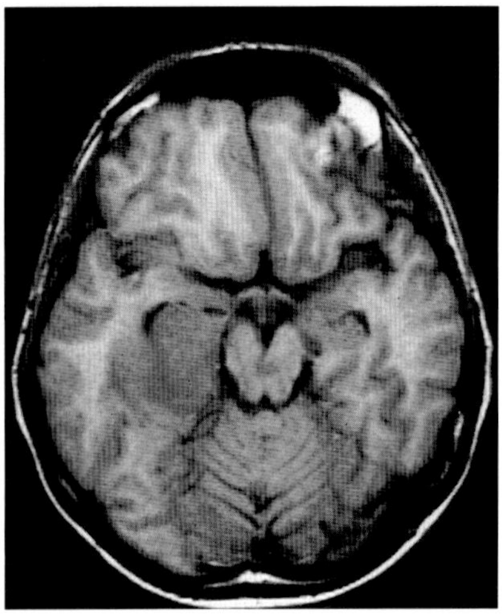
A

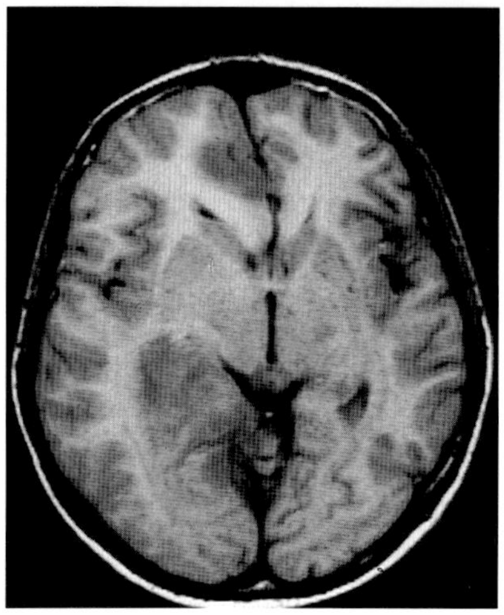
B

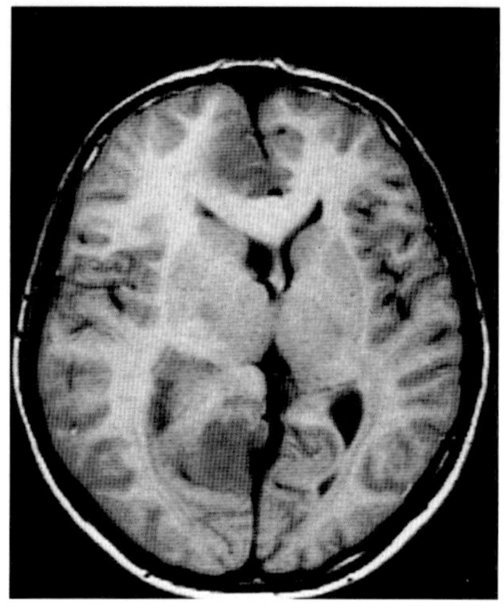
C

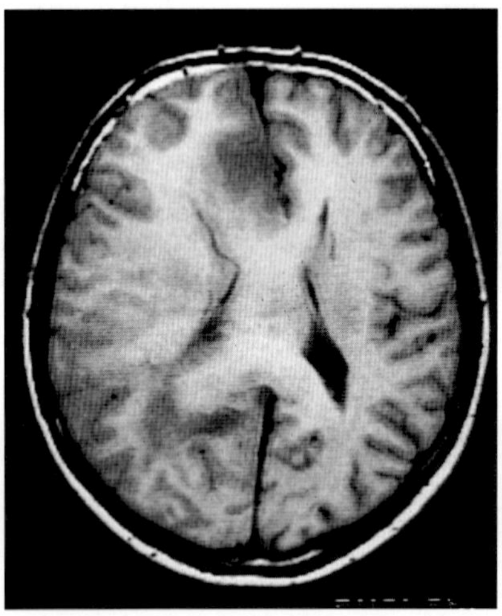
D

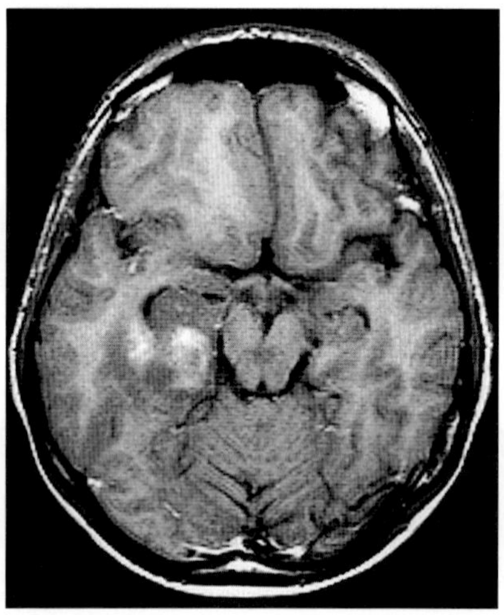
E

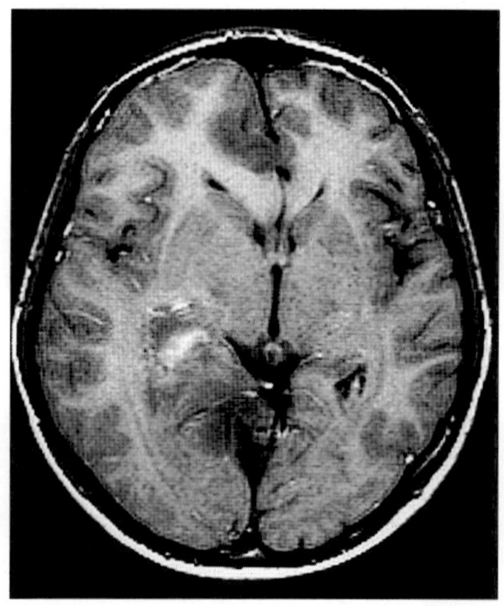
F

Figure 1.7

Multifocal astrocytoma (grade II). The images illustrate the superiority of MR in demonstrating extensive multifocal tumor infiltration and point out a limitation of contrast media: enhancement does not disclose all areas of tumor infiltration, nor does the lack of enhancement correspond to normal brain. The first 16 images compare the MR (**A–I**) and the CT obtained 4 months later (**M–P**) at similar levels.

A,E,I,M The brainstem and inferior temporal lobes;

B,F,J,N the 3rd ventricle and upper temporal lobes;

C,G,K,O the thalamus, atria and frontal horns; and

D,H,L,P the corpus callosum, frontal and parietal lobes.

A–D T1-weighted images without contrast;

E–H gadolinium-enhanced T1-weighted images;

I–L proton density images;

M–P enhanced CT;

Q–T axial MR images at a higher level with unenhanced T1- (**Q**), enhanced T1- (**R**), proton density (**S**) and T2-weighted (**T**) images;

U–X coronal enhanced T1-weighted images. Note how poorly the right temporal portion of the tumor is seen on the CT when compared with any of the comparable MR images, note the differences in distribution of the enhancement as seen on CT and MR, and note that not all areas containing tumor enhance.

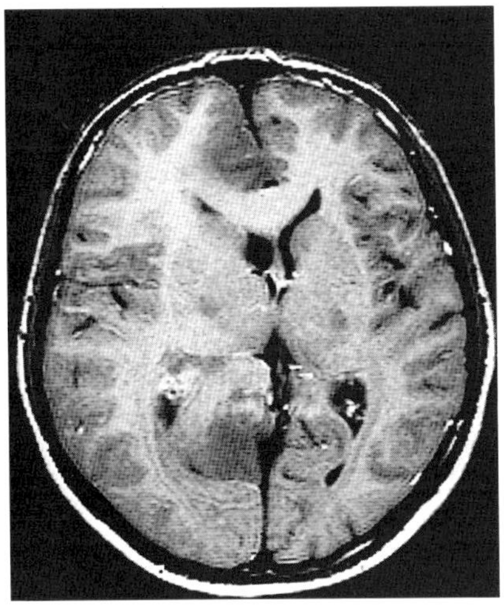

G

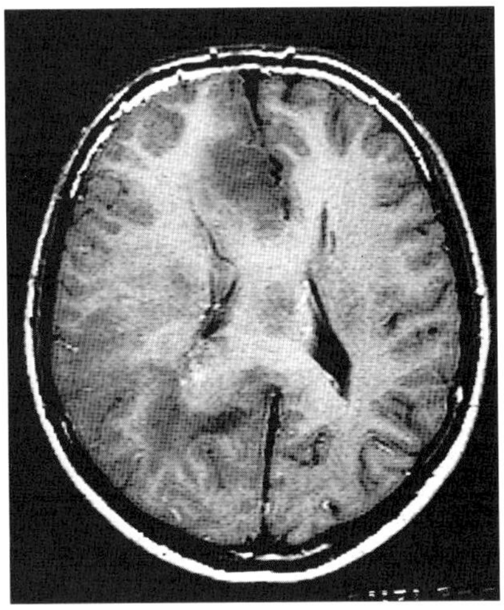

H

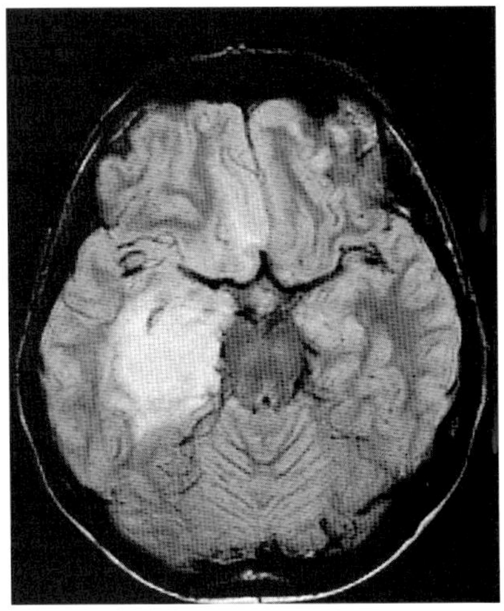

I

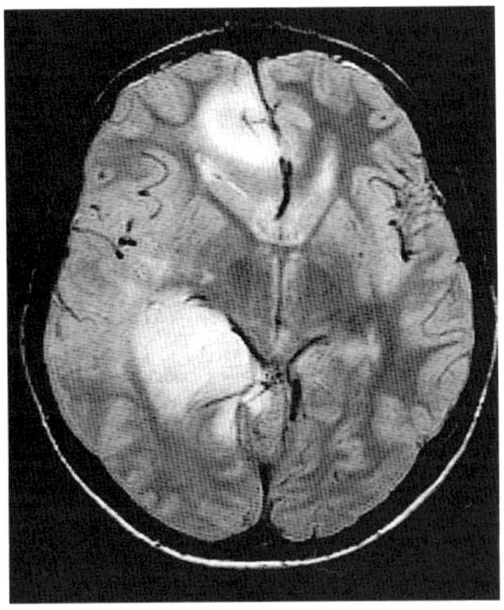

J

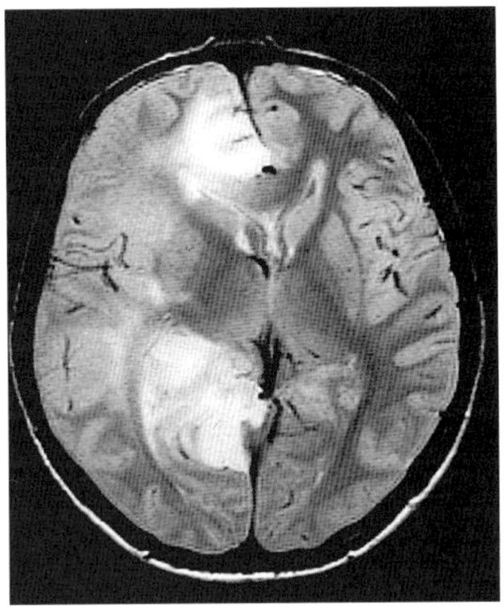

K

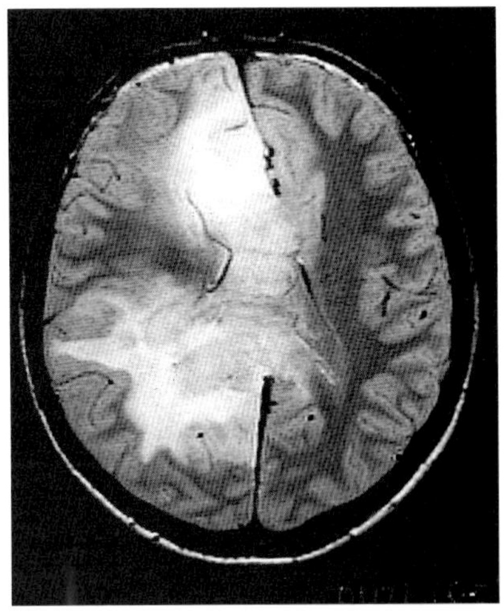

L

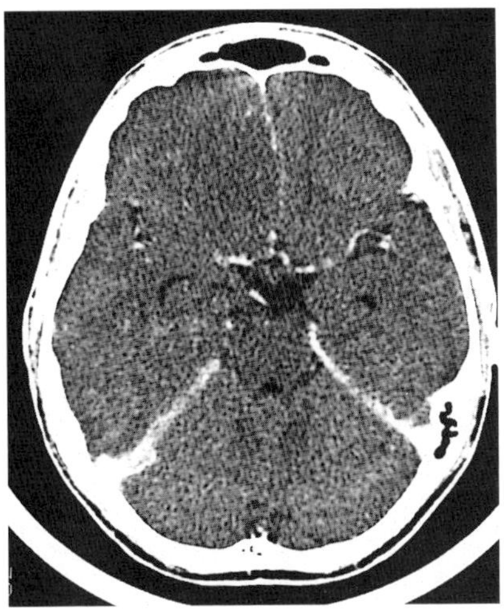

M

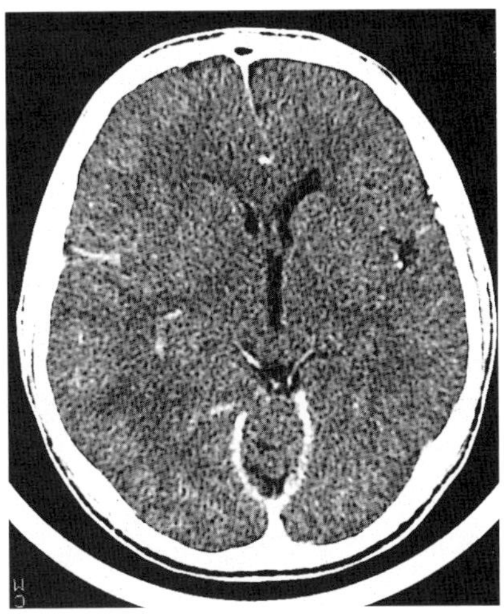

N

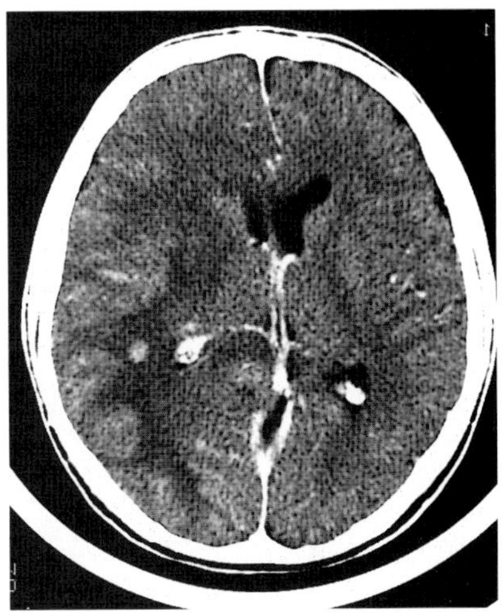

O

continued overleaf

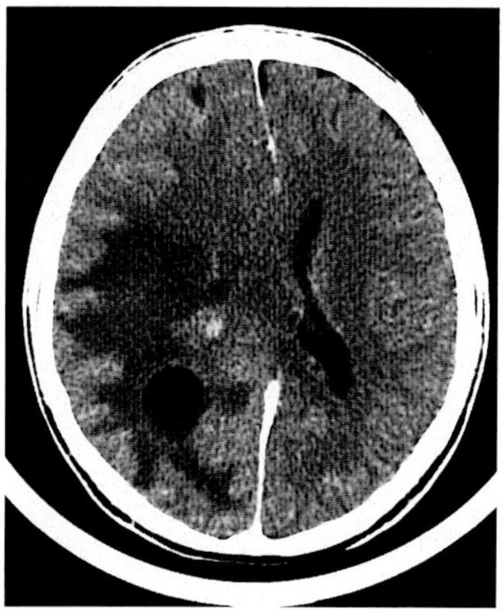
P

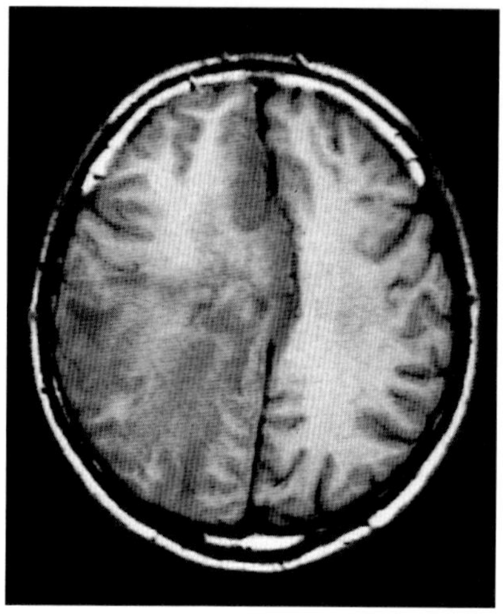
Q

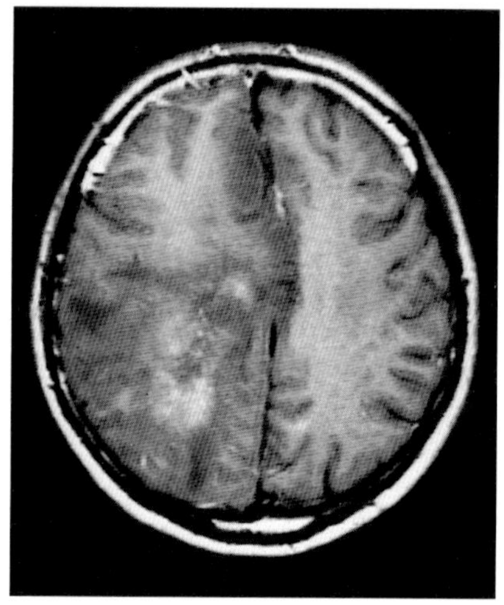
R

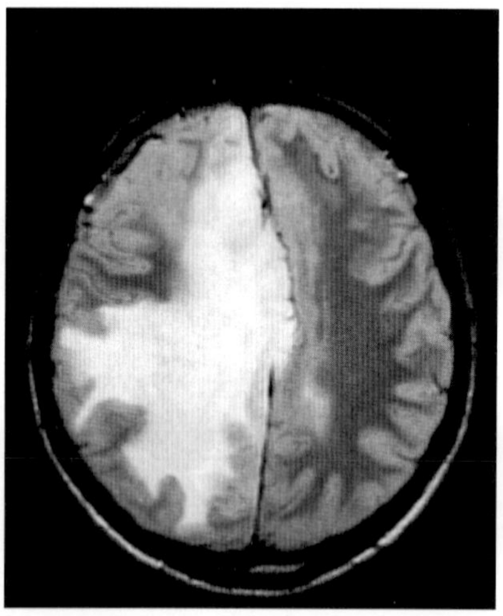
S

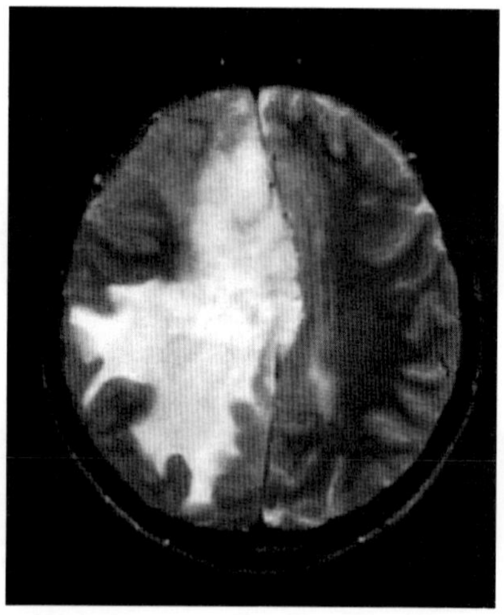
T

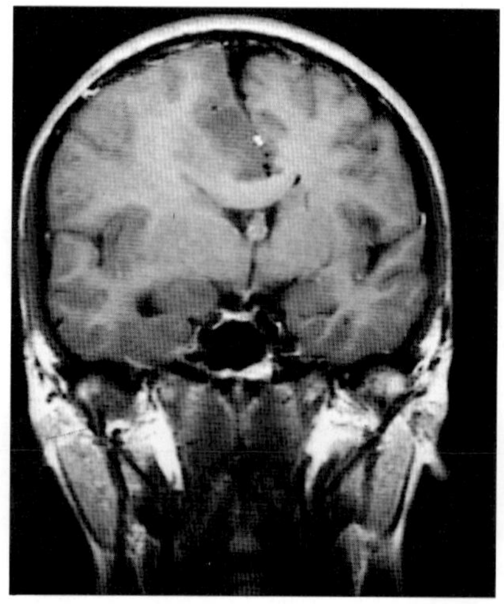
U

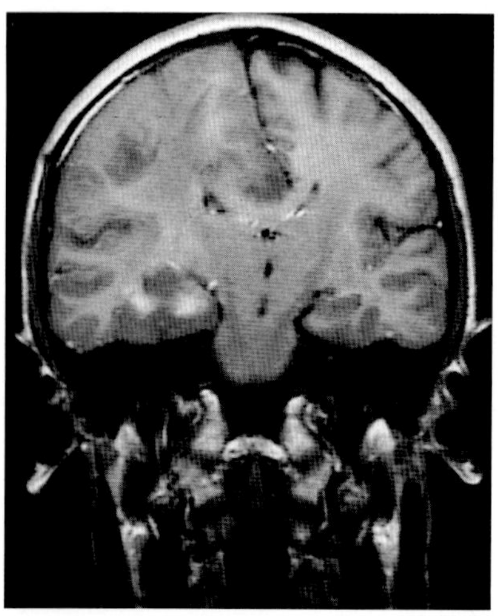
V

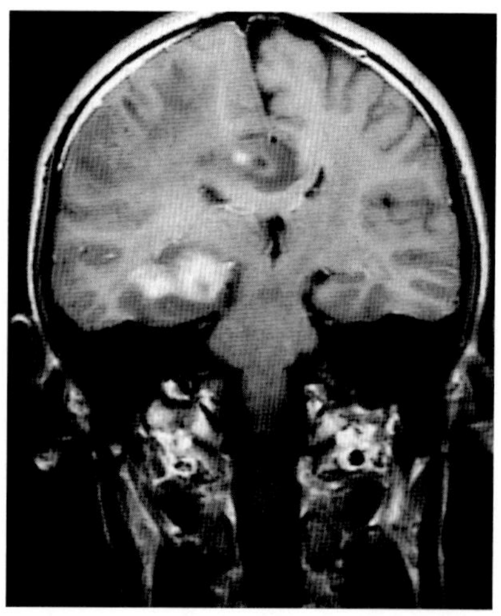
W

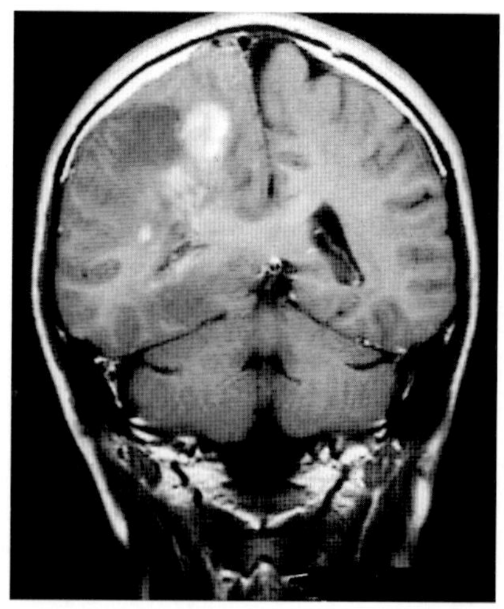
X

Figure 1.7 continued

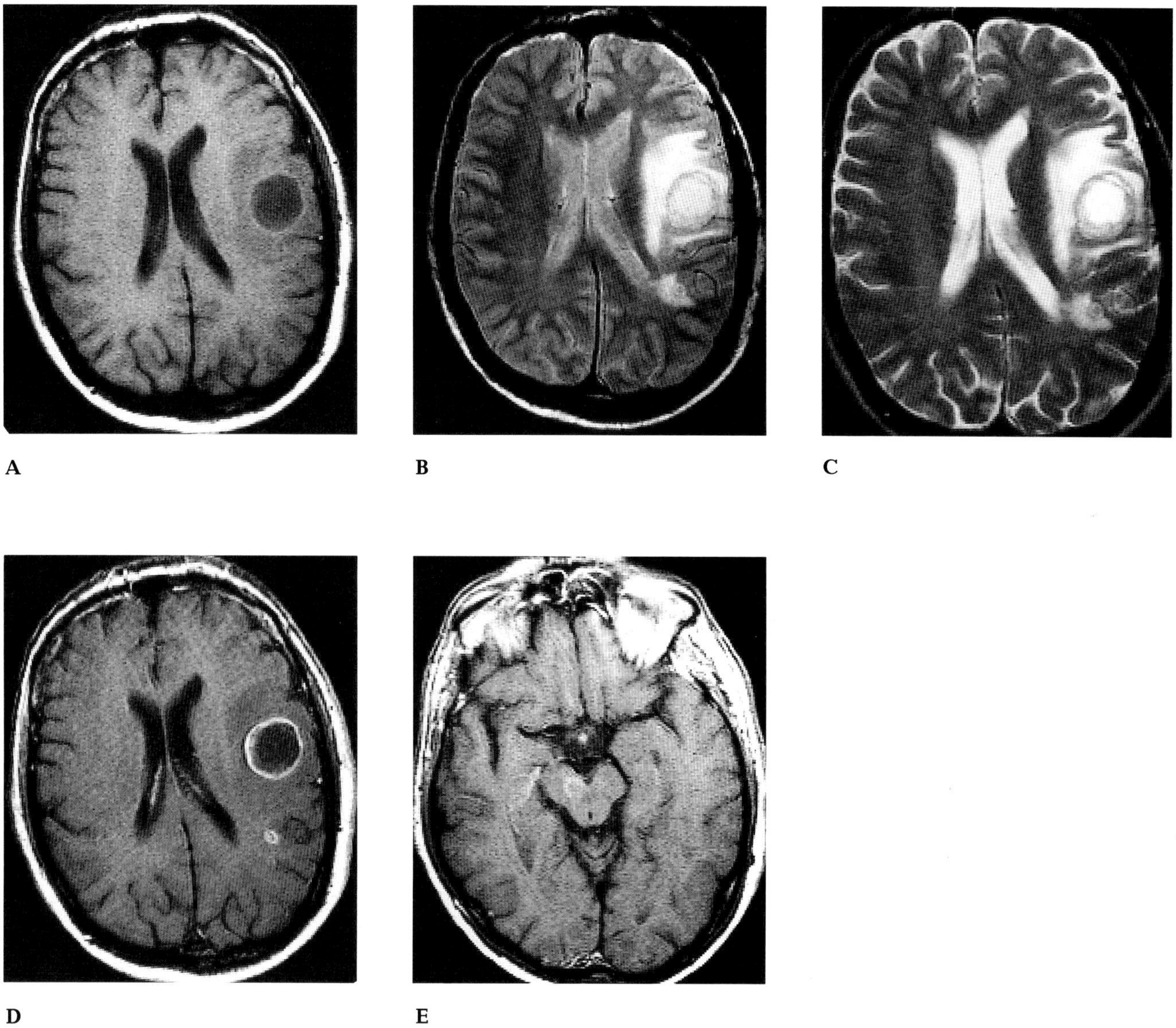

Figure 1.8

Brain metastasis from bronchial carcinoma. The images illustrate the role of MR in evaluating 'solitary' metastases.

A Axial T1-weighted image showing a left frontal lesion, previously diagnosed on CT as a solitary metastasis.

B and **C** Axial proton density (**B**) and T2-weighted (**C**) images demonstrate the tumor and the surrounding zone of edema. A suspicious area is seen posteriorly at the periphery of this region.

D Axial T1-weighted image after gadolinium injection confirms the large lesion in the left hemisphere, and a second small metastasis is clearly visible within the posterior aspect of the vast edematous region that surrounds the larger metastasis.

E A third lesion is clearly seen as a small focus of enhancement in the right part of the upper midbrain on a T1-weighted image after gadolinium injection.

Before surgery for a 'solitary' metastasis, MR should be performed to exclude small lesions which can be missed on CT.

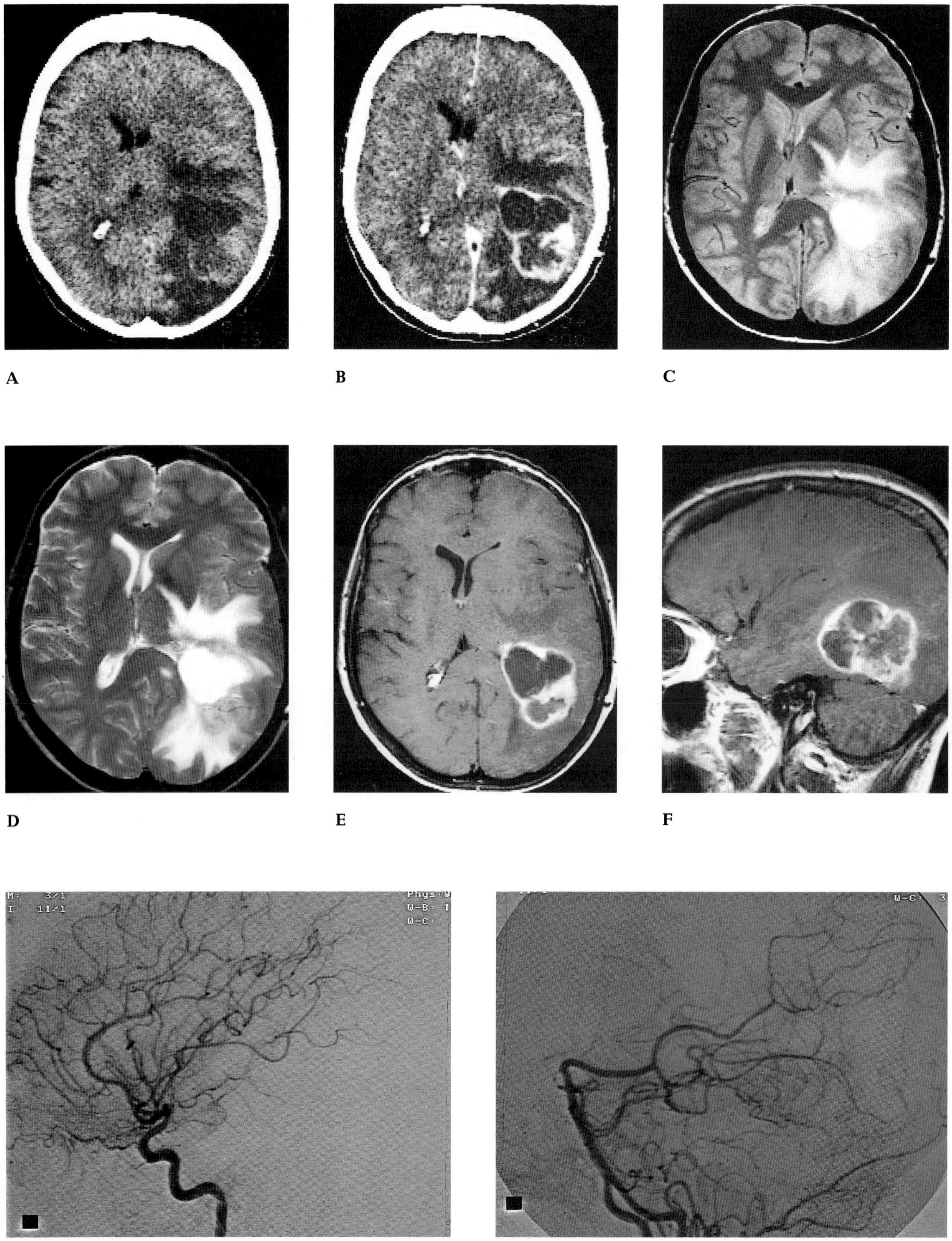

A B C D E F G H

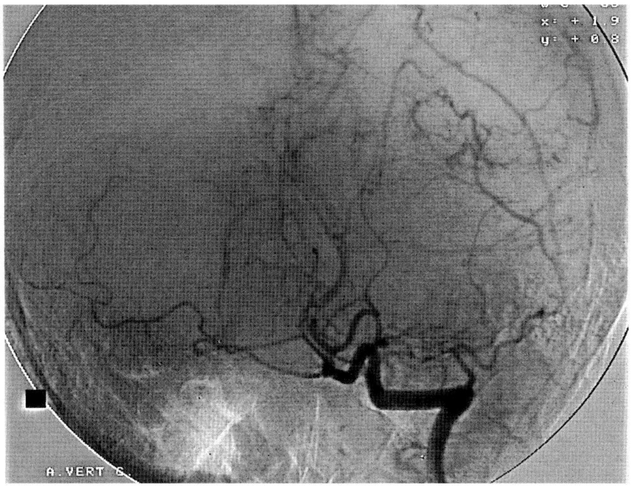

I

Figure 1.9

Glioblastoma multiforme of the left posterior temporal lobe extending to the temporo-occipital junction. The images demonstrate the complementary aspects of the neuroradiologists' tools.

A and **B** CT before (**A**) and after (**B**) contrast administration.

C–E Axial proton density (**C**), T2- (**D**) and T1-weighted (**E**) images after gadolinium injection.

F Parasagittal T1-weighted image following gadolinium injection.

G Lateral left internal carotid arteriogram.

H and **I** Left vertebral arteriogram in the lateral (**H**) and Towne's (**I**) projections.

The multicompartmented tumor and its surrounding zone of edema are well seen on the axial CT and MR images, but the parasagittal image (**F**) best localizes this tumor to the posterior part of the middle and inferior temporal gyri. As we could expect, the left internal carotid angiogram shows little more than a mass effect when the posterior temporal branches of the middle cerebral artery are splayed as they reach the region of the tumor. The inferior temporal branches of the left posterior cerebral artery better demonstrate the tumor vascularity and the early draining vein, strongly suggesting the surgically confirmed diagnosis of glioblastoma.

On both imaging modalities, certain tumor characteristics will be sought systematically: lesion border definition, homogeneous or non-homogeneous appearance, presence of associated hemorrhage, cystic elements, intratumoral necrosis, calcifications, associated edema and extension across the midline. To facilitate taking these different characteristics into account, we recommend comparison of results with the synoptic table adapted from a previous work.[41] (Table 1.2).

Adding the clinical information to the radiographic data, a statistically accurate diagnosis may be obtained. Nevertheless, it must always be kept in mind that *histologic confirmation of the diagnosis is required in all cases of suspected brain malignancies* regardless of their more or less 'specific' appearance on CT or MRI. Appropriate therapy can only be determined and prognosis can only be predicted in the light of a definite pathologic diagnosis. (Figure 1.10).

In the preceding section, a number of questions were raised with respect to sensitivity, specificity, location, treatment and monitoring of brain neoplasms. The answers to these are addressed below.

Sensitivity

Are the patient's clinical signs and symptoms caused by intracranial expansile lesion?

The higher sensitivity of MR in comparison with CT explains why MR usually provides a better delineation of cerebral tumor infiltration.[26,42,43] The absence of bone artifacts and the possibility of differentiating between tumor enhancement and adjacent bone enables MR to demonstrate better than CT those tumors located in the posterior fossa,[25,44] the temporal fossa, and the subfrontal regions. Meningeal infiltration may be observed in cases of malignant astrocytomas and is also best shown on MR. Thus the 'tail-sign' is non-specific and not exclusively observed in cases of primary meningeal tumors classically represented by meningiomas.[45]

Midline tumors are demonstrated best in the coronal and/or sagittal planes and therefore lend themselves to MR. Differential diagnosis is illustrated by Figures 1.11 to 1.14. Meningeal tumor infiltration is also shown better by MR, as it occurs close to bone and is often more apparent in a plane other than that of the axial plane to which CT is limited. Although CT is often not negative and frequently contributes additional information, tumor depiction by MR is usually superior to that by CT.

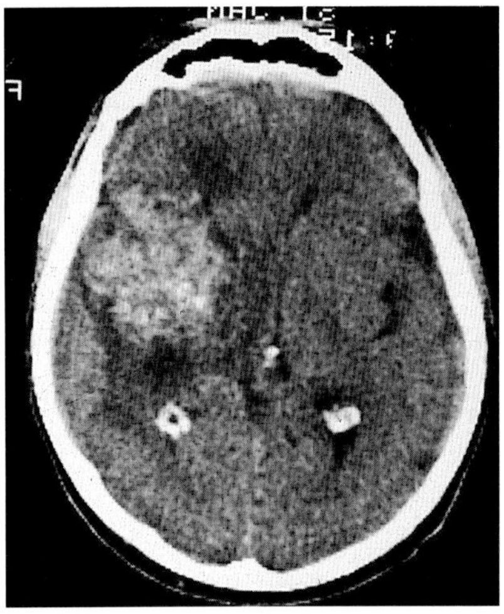

A

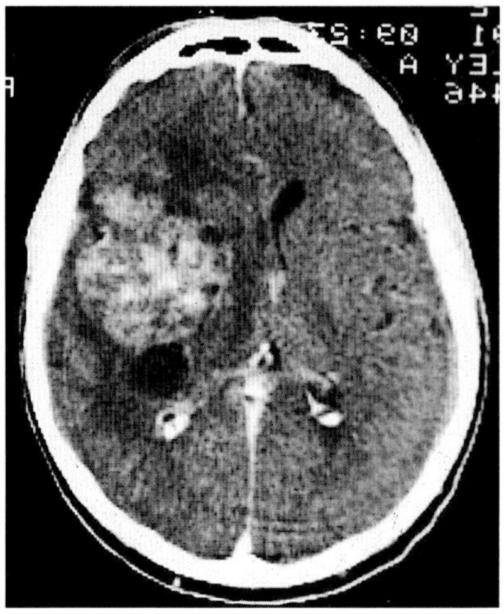

B

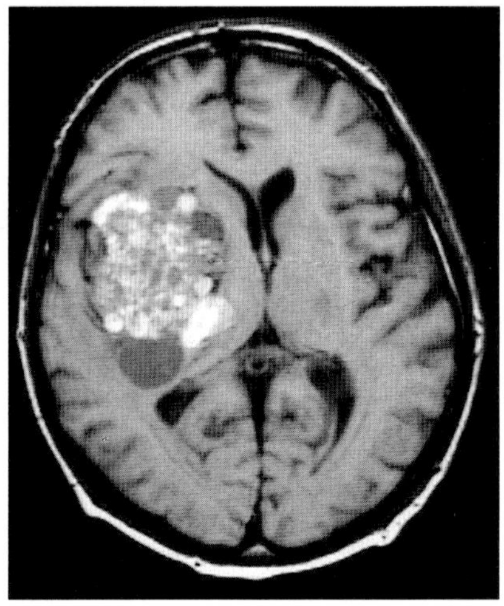

C

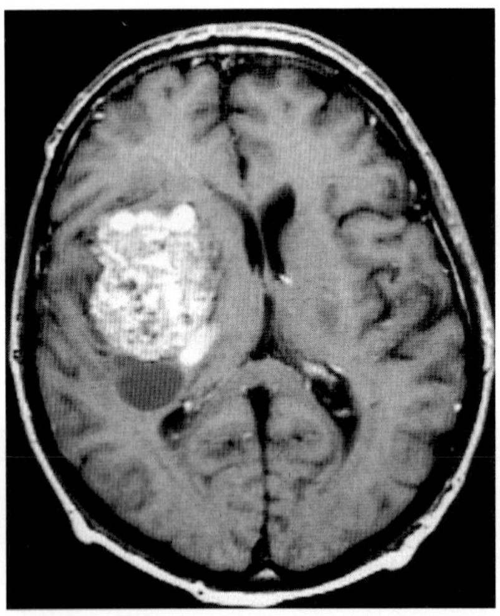

D

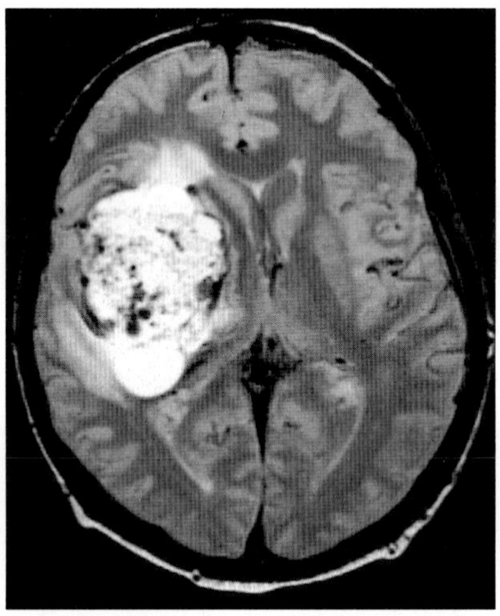

E

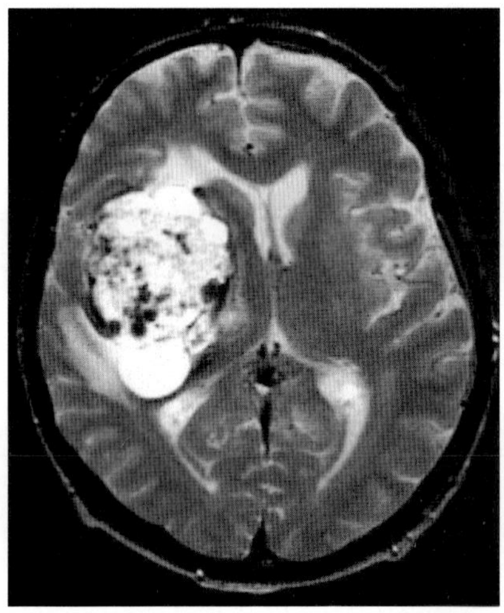

F

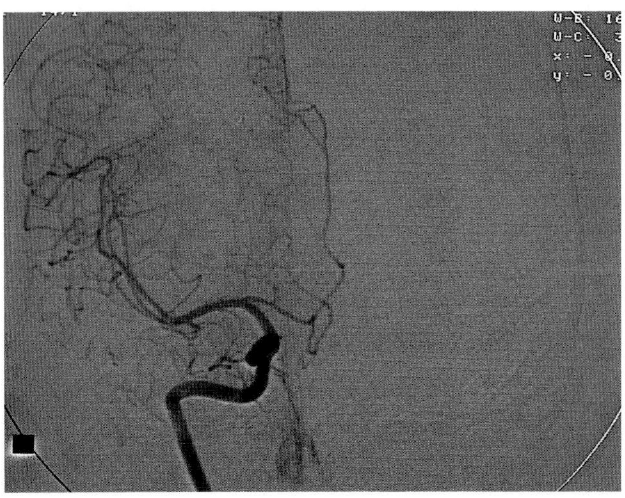

G

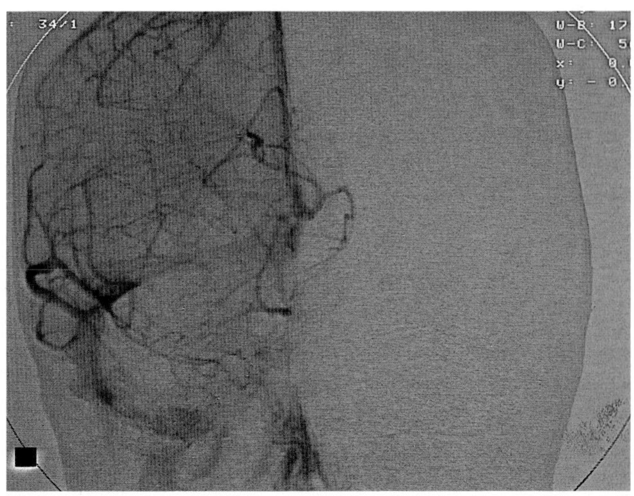

H

Figure 1.10

Giant cavernous hemangioma. The images stress the dangers in making a histologic diagnosis from images alone.

A and **B** CT scan before (**A**) and after (**B**) contrast administration, demonstrating an ill-defined heterogeneous tumor, predominantly hyperdense that exhibits inhomogeneous enhancement. This lesion was erroneously diagnosed as a glioblastoma on the basis of this CT, and then irradiated 'blindly' (without biopsy).

C and **D** MR obtained 8 months later at the time of a consultation for second opinion: T1-weighted images before (**C**) and after (**D**) gadolinium injection.

E and **F** Proton density (**E**) and T2-weighted (**F**) images.

G and **H** Arterial (**G**) and venous (**H**) phases of a selective right internal carotid angiogram.

This mass is a mosaic of hyper-, iso- and hypointense elements, zones of contrast enhancement, cysts and surrounding edema. The relatively minimal edema is unusual for a glioblastoma. The absence of both tumor vascularity and early drainage on the angiogram, the hemorrhagic nature of the lesion, the suspicion of calcifications on the outside CT, and the suspicion of hemosiderin deposits on the MR raised the possibility of cavernous hemangioma, subsequently confirmed at time of total excision.

Specificity

With what kind of lesion are we dealing? Is it a neoplasm? It is benign or is it malignant? Can we suggest a histopathologic diagnosis?

In assessing the malignant nature of a lesion, MR and CT have comparable capabilities, although in certain precise circumstances one of these modalities may be superior to the other (see later; Figure 1.15).

Numerous reports exist in the current literature describing the MR and CT characteristics of cerebral neoplasms as they relate to histopathologic findings.[46–48] Diagnoses based on MR data are more accurate if we know that calcifications and/or associated bony erosions (better shown on CT) are present.[49] The histopathologic predictive value of MR versus CT has been reported divergently, and is related to many factors, including experience and optimism.[50,51] While the various signs reported to be useful (density measurements in CT;[52] signal characteristics in MR;[52] behavior following administration of intravenous contrast agents;[48] border definition; hemorrhagic,[53] cystic, or necrotic components; mass effect; crossing of the midline; etc.) will provide statistically useful data to *predict* the histopathologic diagnosis, it will neither provide 100% accuracy nor replace the neuropathologist.[54–59]

Location

If a tumor is found, where is it located exactly, is it solitary or multiple, and what are its precise limits?

Due to the better anatomic detail provided by MR images, MR is usually equal to or superior to CT in the evaluation of tumor borders and the exact location of a tumor. Not only can we distinguish between intra- and extra-axial neoplasms, but we can often specify the exact gyri in which the tumor can be found. Regardless of these facts, three important points must be emphasized.

- Even on histopathologic specimens, precise limits of tumor infiltration are often impossible to delineate.[55,60,61]
- Differentiation between tumor infiltration and edema is often impossible on MR when we are dealing with certain malignant, infiltrating neoplasms, even when gadolinium-enhanced images are available (see Figure 1.7). On the other hand, MR provides better distinction between tumor and edema in some well-defined intra-axial tumors – metastases, hemangioblastomas,[62] medulloblastomas, etc. – as well as extra-axial tumors such as meningiomas.
- Infiltrating tumors can exhibit clear-cut borders on MR that will not correlate with surgical or histopathologic findings, while on CT these same lesions can exhibit ill-defined borders.

Treatment

What kind of useful information may be provided in order to guide appropriate treatment? Is this tumor resectable? What approach should the

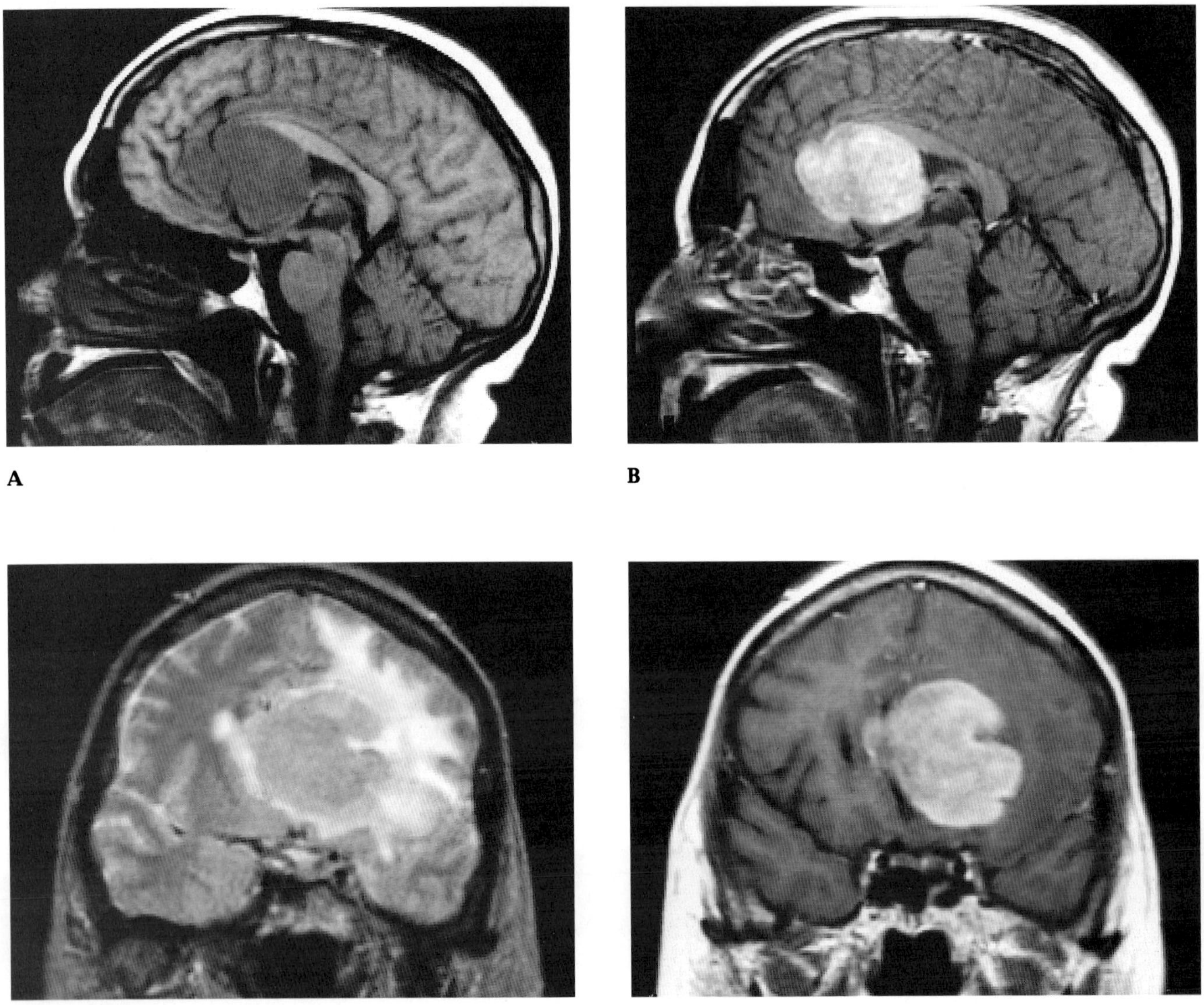

A

B

C

D

Figure 1.11

Primary intracerebral lymphoma. The images illustrate the differential diagnosis of midline intracerebral tumors.

A and **B** Sagittal T1-weighted images before (**A**) and after (**B**) gadolinium injection.

C and **D** Coronal T2-weighted image (**C**) and gadolinium-enhanced T1-weighted image (**D**).

The almost homogeneous enhancement of this sharply demarcated intracerebral lesion, its lobular margins, its position close to the midline, the small zone of surrounding edema, and its slightly hyperdense appearance on CT (not shown) suggest the diagnosis of lymphoma. Early tissue diagnosis is critical in these lesions, as they are extremely sensitive to irradiation, and mean survival changes from 3–4 months without irradiation to 12–24 months if irradiated. Nevertheless 3-year survival is only 8%,

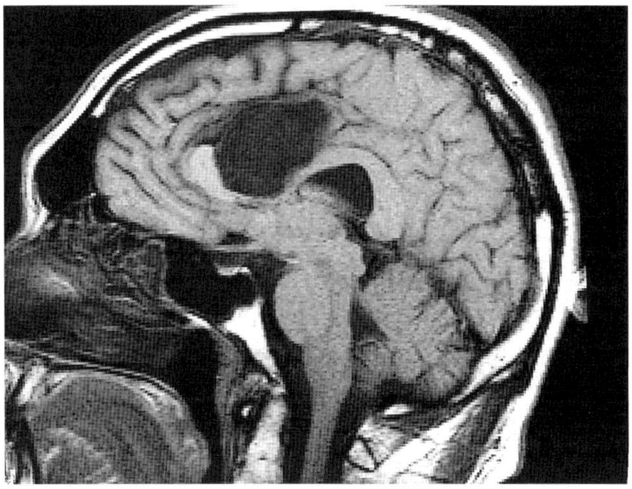

A

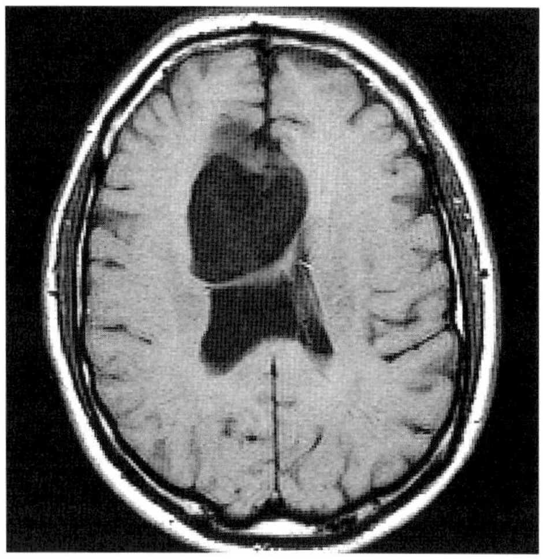

B

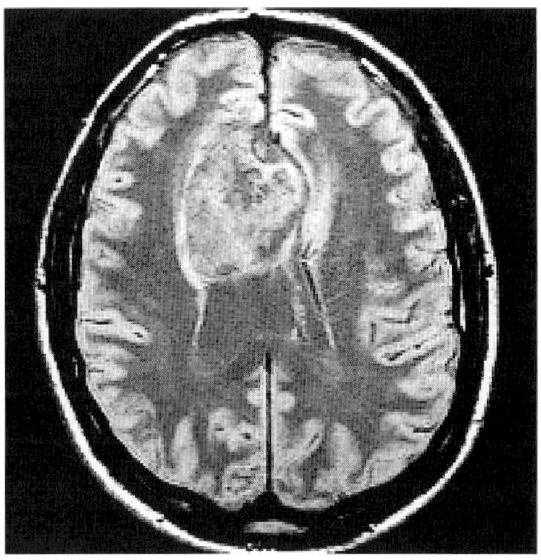

C

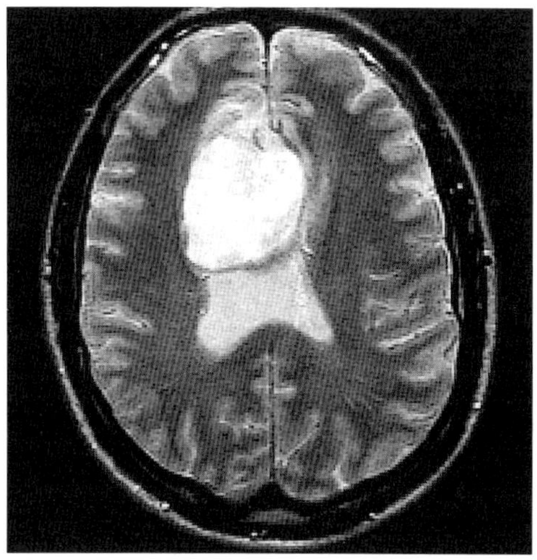

D

Figure 1.12

Epidermoid tumor. The images illustrate the differential diagnosis of midline intracerebral tumors.

A Unenhanced sagittal T1-weighted images.

B–D Unenhanced axial T1-weighted (**B**), proton density (**C**) and T2-weighted (**D**) images.

The sharp demarcation of this slightly lobular lesion, its midline position, its hypointensity on T1-weighted images and non-homogeneous appearance on proton density images, and the absence of significant edema, are the hallmarks of the epidermoid tumor. Confronted with this picture, injection of gadolinium is unnecessary.

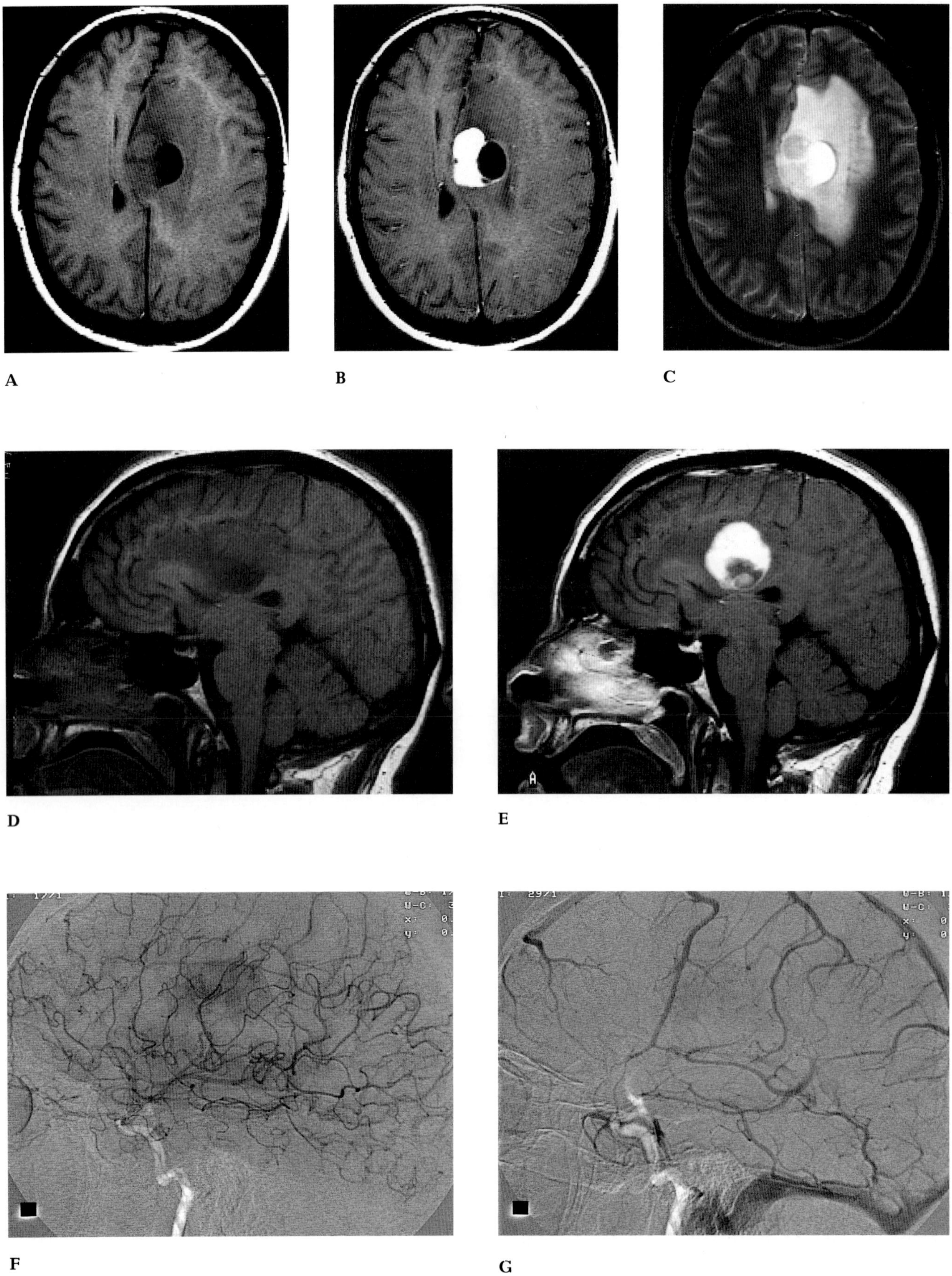
A
B
C
D
E
F
G

Figure 1.13

Glioma of the callosal region. The images illustrate the differential diagnosis of midline intracerebral tumors.

A–C Unenhanced axial T1-weighted images before (**A**) and after (**B**) gadolinium injection, and T2-weighted image (**C**).

D and **E** Sagittal T1-weighted images before (**D**) and after (**E**) gadolinium injection.

F and **G** Late arterial phase (**F**) and venous phase (**G**) of a selective left internal carotid angiogram in the lateral projection.

A sharply demarcated polymorphic lesion of the midline with invasion of the corpus callosum and a striking corona of edema suggests the diagnosis of glioblastoma on the MR. The angioarchitecture of the tumor blush and the presence of early venous filling corroborate this diagnosis.

surgeon use? Where are the ideal locations from which to take an open or a stereotactic biopsy? What are the limits of the area to be irradiated?

MR provides most of the information required for the planning of radiation therapy and/or stereotactic procedures. It is, therefore, the accepted primary imaging modality, replacing CT and angiography for the reasons mentioned above.[18] The known limitations concerning precise tumor margins and tissue characterization, however, must be kept in mind, and are the reasons why we are not always able to predict the ease or completeness with which a tumor can be resected.

In our experience, ideal biopsy sites are those in which contrast enhancement occurs, usually correlating well with the hypermetabolic regions observed within the tumor seen on PET scanning (see Figure 1.5).

Monitoring

How can the neuroradiologist monitor and evaluate the efficacy of the treatment?

MR appears to be superior to CT and angiography in evaluating both immediate and late post-operative changes, as well as demonstrating the efficacy of embolization. MR is also sensitive in the depiction of the secondary effects of irradiation and chemotherapy, especially compared with CT. Demonstration of calcifications remains the one domain in which CT is clearly superior to MR.

Hemorrhage into a pre-existent tumor presents a difficult problem in differential diagnosis (see Figure 1.3), as its high density on CT and hyperintensity on MR can obscure the causative tumor.[53] In early phases, contrast enhancement has little to offer to either CT or MR, as it too can be masked. It should be remembered that peripheral ring-enhancement can be seen on CT and MR as part of the normal evolution of uncomplicated hematomas.[63] When confronted with a hemorrhagic lesion, five factors should be carefully evaluated to help us confirm or exclude the presence of an underlying tumor.[53]

- *Location*: aneurysms and hypertensive intracerebral hemorrhages have preferred locations. An atypical hemorrhage location should always evoke the diagnosis of underlying neoplasm.
- *Edema*: while edema can occur in the presence of an acute hematoma, the presence of exuberant edema or persistent edema is indicative of underlying tumor.
- *Heterogeneity*: uncomplicated hematomas tend towards homogeneity. It is sometimes possible to identify a tumor nodule within a heterogeneous hematoma on CT or MR, and in these cases contrast enhancement can be useful.
- *Hemosiderin*: absent, diminished or irregular hemosiderin deposits within a hematoma have been associated with brain tumors.
- *Evolution*: a delay in the normal evolution of a hematoma strongly suggests the diagnosis of underlying tumor.

In most cases in which hemorrhage is encountered, the tumor will only be revealed by follow-up examinations. We recommend that (clinical conditions permitting) the initial follow-up study be obtained after 6 weeks.

MR is superior to CT in the evaluation of the post-operative patient for the possibility of recurrent or residual tumor, but this remains a

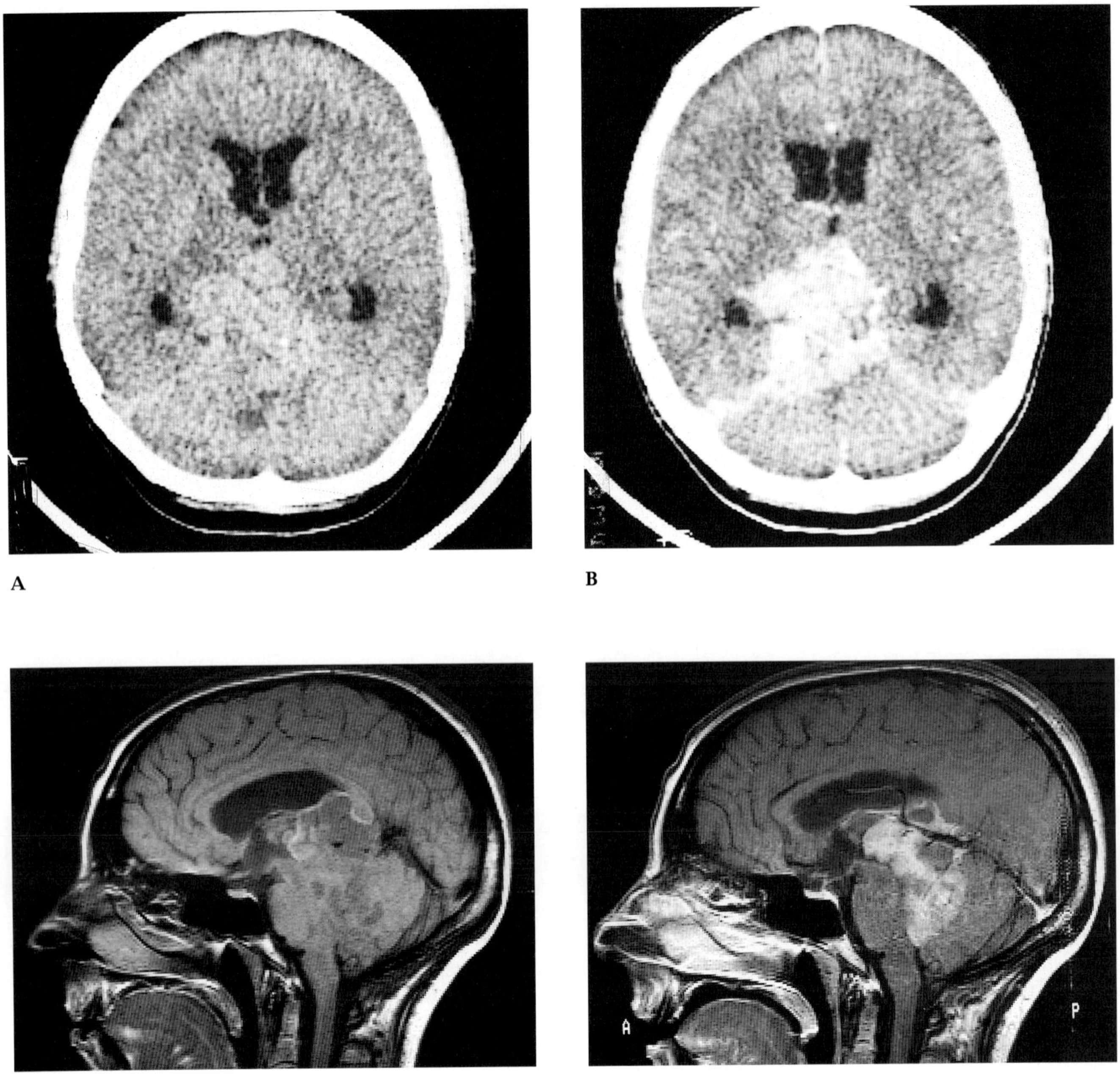

A B

C D

Figure 1.14

Pineoblastoma with a posterior fossa metastasis. The images illustrate the differential diagnosis of midline intracerebral tumors.

A and **B** CT before (**A**) and after (**B**) injection of intravenous contrast.

C and **D** Sagittal T1-weighted images before (**C**) and after (**D**) injection of gadolinium.

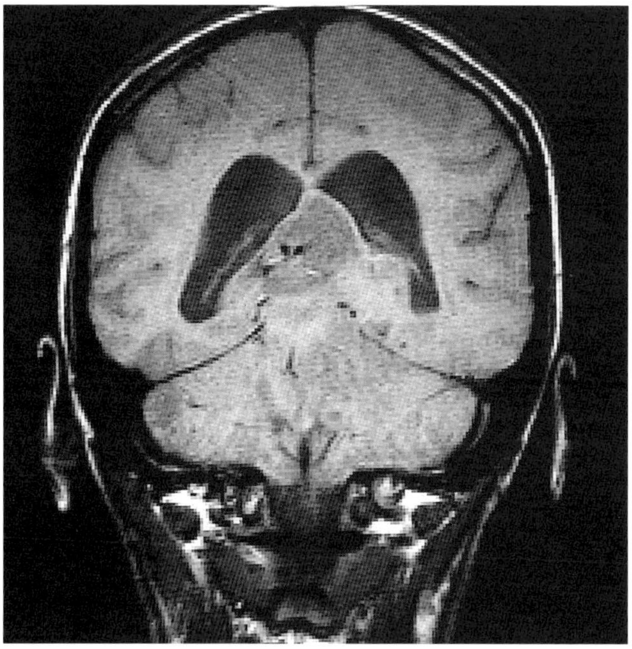

E

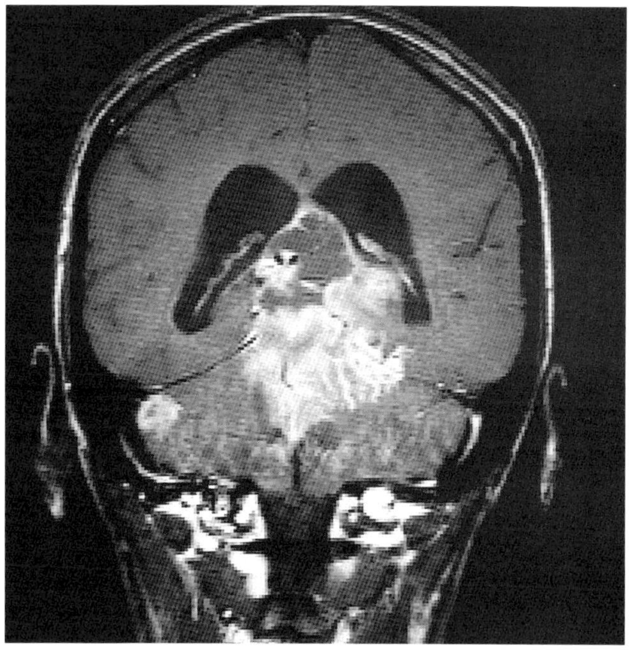

F

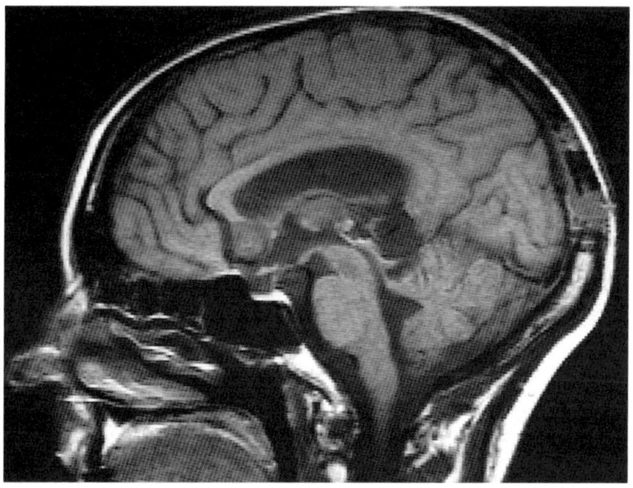

G

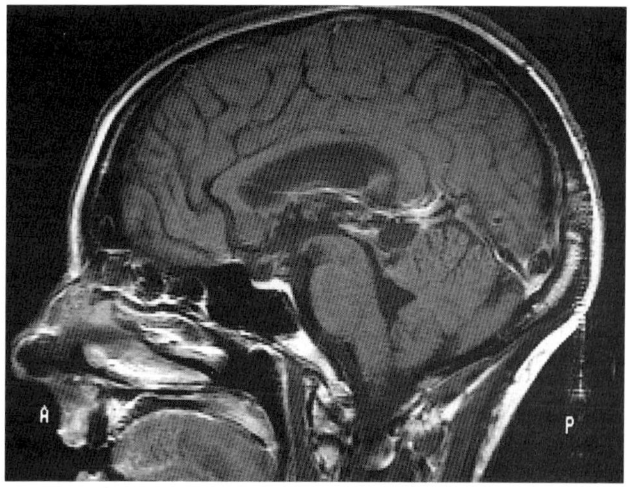

H

E and **F** Coronal T1-weighted images before (**E**) and after (**F**) injection of gadolinium.

G and **H** Follow-up sagittal T1-weighted images before (**G**) and after (**H**) injection of gadolinium.

A pineal region tumor with extension in multiple directions, evidence of hemorrhage on the unenhanced images, and the metastasis in the right cerebellopontine angle (**F**), direct our diagnosis towards pineoblastoma. Early tissue diagnosis is important since these lesions may be sensitive to irradiation, as seen on the follow-up MR (**G** and **H**).

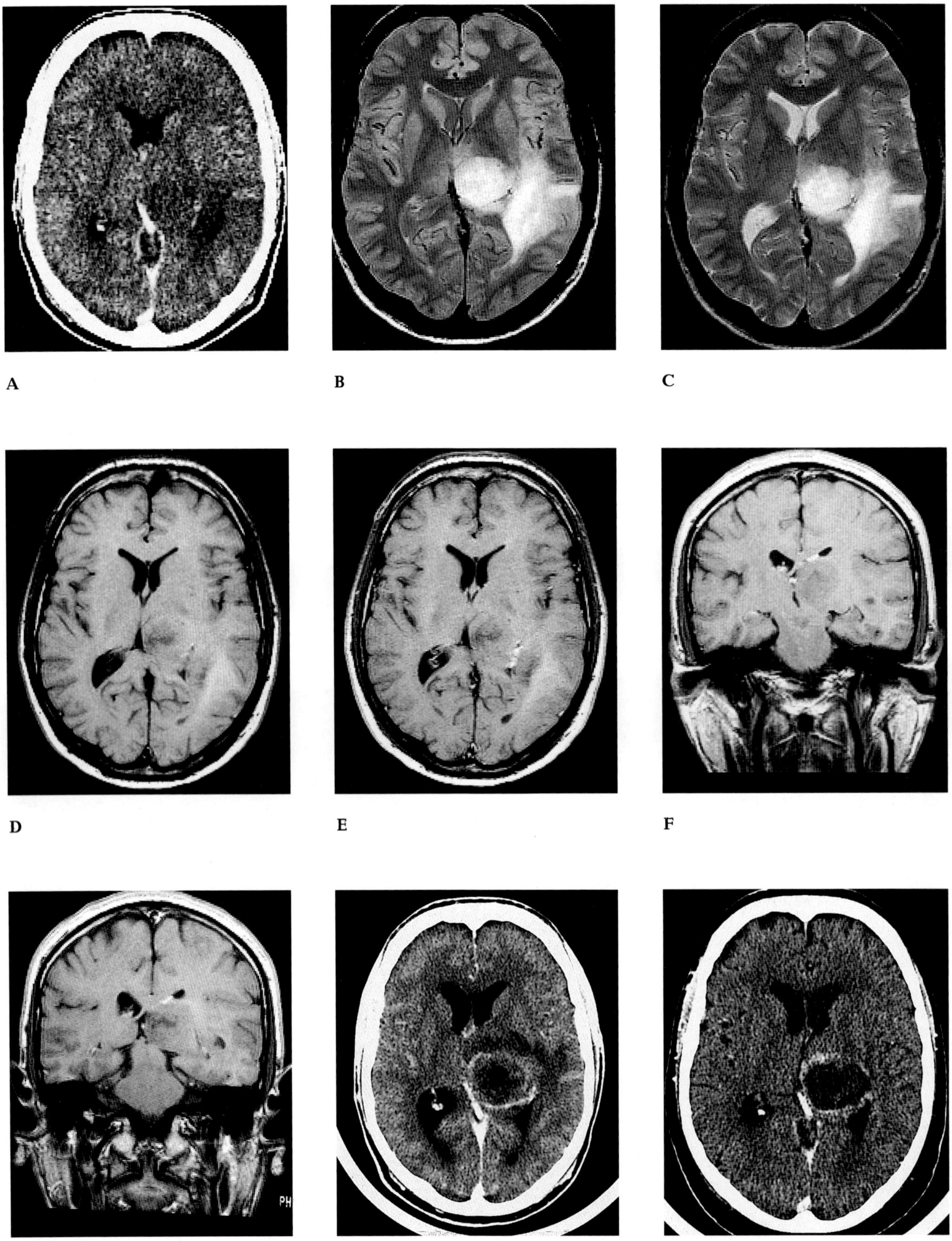
A
B
C
D
E
F
G
H
I
PH

Figure 1.15

Grade III left thalamic astrocytoma. The images illustrate the follow-up of tumor evolution.

A Initial CT revealed an ill-defined slightly hypodense lesion, extending from the right thalamus to the periatrial white matter with no significant enhancement, strongly favoring the diagnosis of a low-grade glioma. Precise tumor margins cannot be defined.

B and **C** Axial proton density (**B**) and T2-weighted (**C**) images.

D and **E** Axial T1-weighted images before (**D**) and after (**E**) contrast administration.

F and **G** Coronal T1-weighted images before (**F**) and after (**G**) contrast administration.

The MR (**B–G**) was performed 2 days after the CT. The rounded left thalamic component of the tumor, its zone of central necrosis, the mass effects on the third ventricle, the atrium of the lateral ventricle and the adjacent cisterns, the zone of surrounding edema, and the absence of enhancement are well seen. The central necrosis suggested the diagnosis of a more malignant tumor. Stereotactic biopsy at multiple levels confirmed the presence of the most malignant tissue in the thalamic region.

H Enhanced CT at the completion of irradiation (3 months after the diagnosis of this grade III astrocytoma) demonstrate rapid growth of the infiltrating tumor with progression of the central necrosis and development of rim enhancement.

I Follow-up enhanced CT performed 9 months after irradiation and three series of chemotherapy demonstrate regression of the peritumoral edema, diminution of mass effect, and stability of tumor size.

complex problem. Meningeal enhancement is a normal post-operative finding, and enhancement within the site of resection can also occur.[64] Whenever tumor resection is known to be incomplete, an immediately post-operative contrast-enhanced CT or MR should be obtained as soon as possible within the first 24 hours. The subsequent follow-up study should occur after a 6–8 week interval. The diagnosis of tumor recurrence or progression can only be made on the basis of the evolution of findings on the follow-up examinations. Caution must always be exercised, especially in those patients who undergo post-operative irradiation.

Both CT and MR are equally *ineffective* in the differentiation between radiation necrosis and tumor recurrence. For this particular problem, PET is superior to both of these modalities because it depicts actual metabolic activity[16] (Figure 1.16).

Conclusions

MR remains the imaging modality of choice, to be used as a screening method for unexplained neurologic signs and symptoms, and to be advocated as the definitive method for the detection and depiction of neoplastic infiltration, for the precise localization of a tumor and for the characterization of that tumor. None the less, CT maintains certain advantages over MR and provides additional, complementary information in an estimated 5–10% of tumor cases.

Amongst the new state-of-the-art MR techniques, three-dimensional acquisitions and MRA are the most useful techniques to be added as soon as feasible to the routines of the standard T1- and T2-weighted images and gadolinium-enhanced T1-weighted images required for a thorough MR evaluation of neoplastic conditions within the brain.

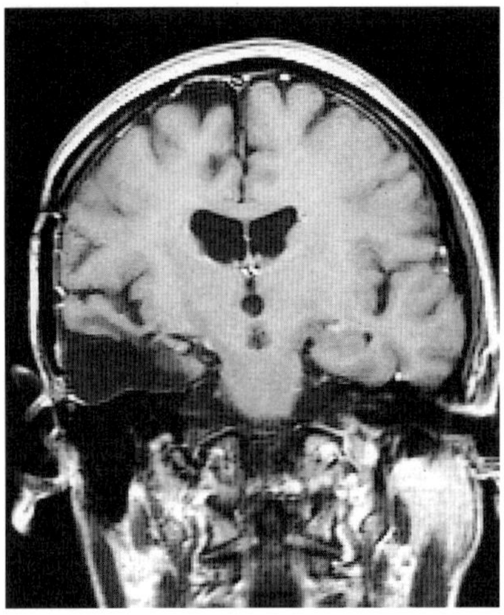

A

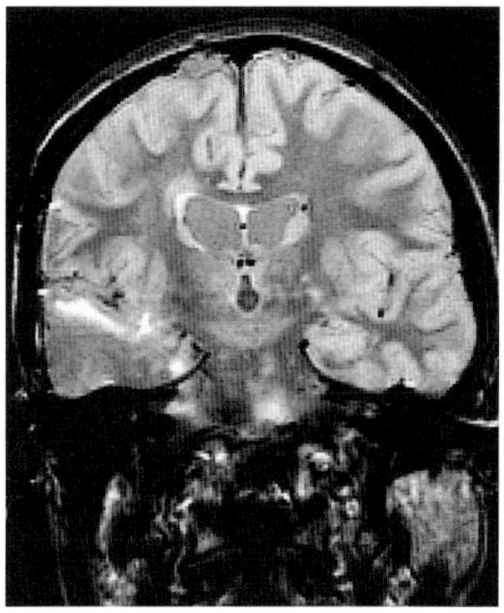

B

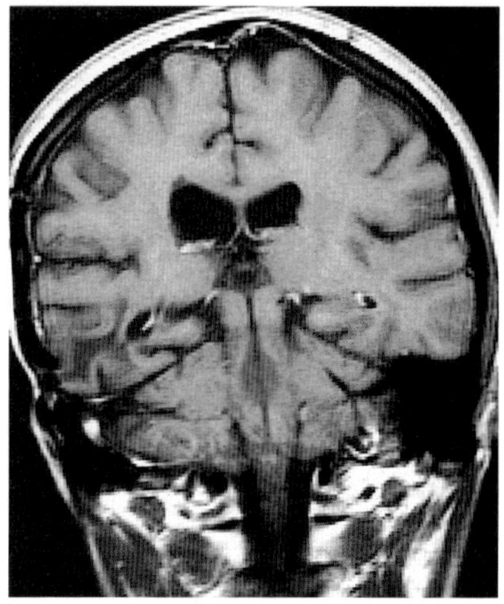

C

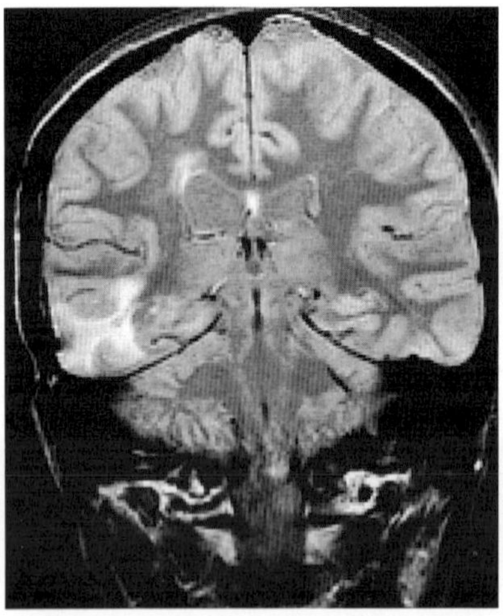

D

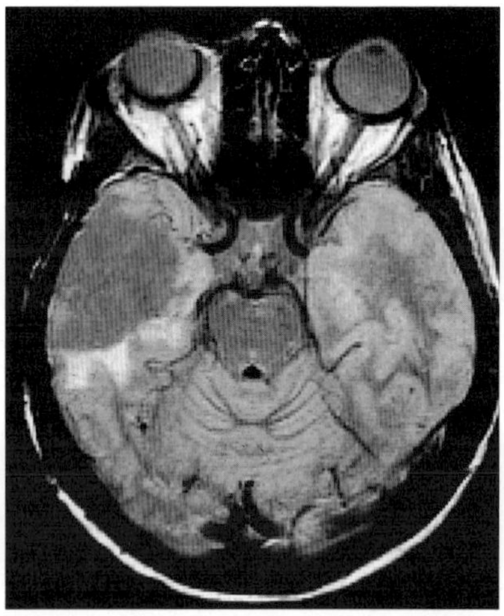

E

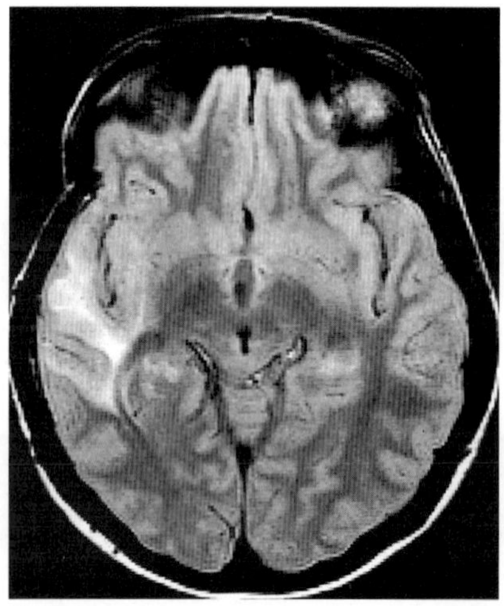

F

Figure 1.16

Astrocytoma (grade II/III) with post-irradiation changes (stable over a course of 3 years) in a tumor twice operated and subsequently irradiated. The images demonstrate the value of regular follow-up examinations, signs of associated atrophy, and absence of enhancement.

A and **B** Coronal T1-weighted images after gadolinium injection show the right temporal site of tumor resection without evident enhancement.

C and **D** Coronal proton density images slightly posterior demonstrate the irregular hyperintense rim superiorly, with 'digital' prolongations extending into the white matter and another small zone of hyperintensity in the white matter adjacent to the right frontal horn.

E and **F** On the axial proton density images the circumferential distribution of these lesions is clearly seen.

These foci of abnormal signal intensity are considered to present post-irradiation change because they appeared 6 months after irradiation and neither enhanced nor changed on subsequent MRs performed over a period of 3 years. Note the passive enlargement of the adjacent frontal horn of the lateral ventricle. When confronted with a clinical necessity for differentiation between radiation necrosis and tumor recurrence PET scans (or biopsy) would be necessary.

Table 1.2 Tumor characteristics on CT and MR.

Histopathology	*CT findings*		*MR findings*			*Edema*	*Cyst*	*Ca²⁺*	*Hemorrhage*	*Mass*
	–C	*+C*	*T1-weighted image*	*T2-weighted image*	*Gadolinium contrast*					
Pilocytic astrocytoma	iso/hypo	++	hypo	hyper	++	+	+++	+/–	–	+/–
Cerebellar astrocytoma	iso/hypo	+	hypo	hyper	+	+/–	+++	+/–	–	+/–
Astrocytoma grade I	hypo	–(+)	hypo	hyper	–/(+)	+/–	–(+)	–	–	+/–
Subependymal astrocytoma	iso/hyper	+++	hypo/iso	hypo/hyper	+++	+	–	+++	–	+
Astrocytoma grade II	hypo	+/–	hypo	hyper	+/–	+/–	+/–	–	–	+/–
Astrocytoma grade III	hypo/iso	++	hypo	hyper	++	+	+	–	+/–	+
Glioblastoma	hypo/iso/hyper	++/+++	hypo/iso	hyper	++	+++	+	–	++	++
Oligodendroglioma I and II	hypo/iso/hyper	–/+	hypo	hyper	–/+	+/–	+	+++	++	+/–
Oligodendroglioma III and IV	hypo/iso/hyper	++	hypo/iso	hyper	++	++	+++	+/–	+++	++
Ependymoma	iso/hyper	+	iso/hypo	hyper	+/++	++	+/–	++	+/–	++
Medulloblastoma	hyper	++	iso/hypo	iso/hyper	++	+	+/–	+/–	++	+
Primary lymphoma	hyper	+++	hypo	hyper	++	+++	–	–	–	++
Pineal tumors	iso/hyper	+++	iso	hyper	+++	+/–	–	+/–	+/–	+/–
Choroid plexus papilloma	iso/hyper	+++	iso/hypo	iso/hypo	+++	+/–	–	++	–	++
Epidermoid	hypo	–	iso/hyper	iso/hyper	–	–	–	+	–	+/–
Dermoid	hypo/hyper	–	hypo/hyper	hypo/iso/hyper	–	–	+/–	++	–	+
Teratoma	iso/hyper	–(+)	hypo/hyper	hypo/iso/hyper	–(+)	–	+/–	++	–	+
Lipoma	hypo	–	hyper	iso/hyper	–	–	–	+/–	–	+/–
Metastases	hypo/iso/hyper	+/++	hypo	hyper	+/++	++/+++	+	+/–	+	+/++

+, present; –, absent; iso, isodense or isointense; hypo, hypodense or hypointense; hyper, hyperdense or hyperintense.

References

1. Annegers JF, Schoenberg BS, Okasaki H et al., Epidemiologic study of primary intracranial neoplasms, *Arch Neurol* (1981) **38**:217–19.
2. Schoenberg BS, The epidemiology of central nervous system tumors. In: Walker MD, ed, *Oncology of the nervous system* (Martinus Nijhoff: Amsterdam, 1983) 1–29.
3. Peers JH, Occurrence of tumors of central nervous system in routine autopsies, *Am J Pathol* (1936) **12**:911–32.
4. Lindegaard KF, Mork SJ, Eide GE et al., Statistical analysis of clinicopathological features, radiotherapy, and survival in 170 cases of oligodendroglioma, *J Neurosurg* (1987) **67**:224–30.
5. Ammirati M, Vick N, Liao Y et al., Effect of the extent of surgical resection on survival and quality of life in patients with supratentorial glioblastomas and anaplastic astrocytomas, *Neurosurgery* (1987) **21**:201–6.
6. Harsh GR, Levin VA, Gutin PH et al., Reoperation for recurrent glioblastoma and anaplastic astrocytoma, *Neurosurgery* (1987) **21**:615–21.
7. Winger MJ, MacDonald DR, Cairncross JG, Supratentorial anaplastic gliomas in adults, *J Neurosurg* (1989) **71**:487–93.
8. Ammirati M, Galicich J, Arbit E et al., Reoperation in the treatment of recurrent intracranial malignant gliomas, *Neurosurgery* (1987) **21**:607–14.
9. Recht LD, Lew R, Smith TW, Suspected low-grade glioma: is deferring treatment safe? *Ann Neurol* (1992) **31**:431–6.
10. Plum F, Posner JB, *The diagnosis of stupor and coma*, 3rd edn (FA Davis: Philadelphia, 1982).
11. Bergen D, Bleck T, Ramsey R et al., Magnetic resonance imaging as a sensitive and specific predictor of neoplasms removed for intractable epilepsy, *Epilepsia* (1989) **30**:318–21.
12. Cascino GD, Hirschorn KA, Jack CR et al., Gadolinium-DTPA-enhanced magnetic resonance imaging in intractable partial epilepsy, *Neurology* (1989) **39**:1115–18.
13. Gooding GA, Boggan JE, Bank WO et al., Sonography of the adult brain through surgical defects, *AJNR* (1981) **2**:449–52.
14. Segebarth C, Balériaux D, Luyten PR et al., Detection of metabolic heterogeneity of human intracranial tumors in vivo by ^{1}H NMR spectroscopic imaging, *Magn Reson Med* (1990) **13**:62–76.
15. Alger JR, Frank JA, Bizzi A et al., Metabolism of human gliomas: assessment with H-1 spectroscopy and F-18 fluorodeoxyglucose PET, *Radiology* (1990) **177**:633–41.
16. Di Chiro G, Positron emission tomography using ^{18}F fluorodeoxyglucose in brain tumors. A powerful diagnostic tool, *Invest Radiol* (1987) **22**:360–71.
17. Heiss W, Hiendel W, Hernholz K et al., Positron emission tomography of fluorine 18 deoxyglucose and image guided phosphorus 31 magnetic resonance spectroscopy in brain tumors, *J Nucl Med* (1990) **31**:302–9.
18. Earnest F, Kelly PJ, Scheithauer BW et al., Cerebral astrocytomas: histopathologic correlation of MR and CT contrast enhancement with stereotactic biopsy, *Radiology* (1988) **166**:823–7.
19. Takeda N, Taaka R, Nakai O et al, Dynamics of contrast enhancement in delayed computed tomography of brain tumors: tissue–blood ratio and differential diagnosis, *Radiology* (1980) **136**:677–84.
20. Davis PC, Hudgins PA, Peterman SB et al., Diagnosis of cerebral metastases: double-dose delayed CT vs contrast-enhanced MR imaging, *AJNR* (1991) **12**:293–300.
21. Shalen PR, Hayman LA, Wallace S et al., Protocol for delayed contrast enhancement in computed tomography of cerebral neoplasia, *Radiology* (1981) **139**:397–401.
22. Hayman LA, Evans RA, Hinck VC, Delayed high iodine dose contrast computed tomography: a preliminary report, *Radiology* (1980) **136**:677–84.
23. Davis JM, Davis KR, Newhouse J et al., Expanded high iodine dose in computed cranial tomography: a preliminary report, *Radiology* (1979) **131**:373–80.
24. Dillon WP, Tumors in and adjacent to the brain, *Curr Opinion Neurol Neurosurg* (1990) **12**:266–74.
25. Balériaux D, Michelozzi G, Tumors of the posterior fossa: In: Huk WJ, Gademann G, Friedmann G, eds, *MRI of central nervous system diseases* (Springer-Verlag: Berlin, 1990) 277–96.
26. Brant-Zawadzki M, Badami JP, Mills CM et al., Primary intracranial tumor imaging: a comparison of magnetic resonance and CT, *Radiology* (1984) **150**:435–40.
27. Cohadon F, *Tumeurs du système nerveux et de ses enveloppes* (Flammarion Médecine-Sciences: Paris, 1989).
28. Higer HP, Just M, *MR-Atlas der Hirntumoren. Diagnostik und Nachsorge* (Thieme: Stuttgart, 1989).
29. Huk WJ, Heindel W, Intracranial tumors. In: Huk WJ, Gademann G, Friedmann G, eds, *MRI of central nervous system diseases* (Springer-Verlag: Berlin, 1990) 229–75.
30. Brant-Zawadzki M, Gillan GD, Nitz WR, MP RAGE: A three-dimensional, T1-weighted, gradient-echo sequence initial experience in the brain, *Radiology* (1992) **182**:769–75.
31. El Gammal T, Brooks BS, Conventional MR neuroangiography, *AJR* (1991) **156**:1075–80.
32. Elster AD, Moody DM, Ball MR et al., Is Gd-DTPA required for routine cranial MR imaging? *Radiology* (1989) **173**:231–8.
33. Schwaighofer BW, Kijen MV, Wesbey G et al., Clinical experience with routine GD-DTPA administration for imaging the brain, *J Comput Assist Tomogr* (1990) **14**:11–17.
34. Katayama H, Yamagushi K, Kosuka T et al., Adverse reactions to ionic and nonionic contrast media, *Radiology* (1990) **175**:621–8.
35. Niendorf HP, Haustein J, Cornelius I et al., Safety

of gadolinium-DTPA: extended clinical experience, *Magn Res Med* (1991) **22**:222–8.

36. Sze G, Milano E, Johnson C et al., Detection of brain metastases: comparison of contrast-enhanced MR with unenhanced MR and enhanced CT, *AJNR* (1990) **11**:785–91.

37. Sze G, Shin J, Crol G et al., Intraparenchymal brain metastases: MR imaging versus contrast-enhanced CT, *Radiology* (1988) **168**:187–94.

38. Masaryk TJ, Modic MT, Ross JS et al., Intracranial circulation: preliminary clinical results with three-dimensional (volume) MR angiography, *Radiology* (1989) **171**:793–9.

39. Poncelet B, Balériaux D, Grand C et al., MR inflow angiography for the evaluation of dural sinus patency, *Radiology* (1990) **177**:257 (abstr).

40. Le Bihan D, Breton E, Lallemand D et al., Separation of diffusion and perfusion in intravoxel incoherent motion MR imaging, *Radiology* (1988) **168**:497–505.

41. Balériaux D, Hildebrand J, Pathologie tumorale encéphalique. In: Buthiau D, ed, *TDM et IRM cliniques: indications et sémiologie de la tomodensitométrie et de l'imagerie par résonance magnétique* (Frison Roche: Paris, 1991) 208.

42. Kazner E, Wende S, Grumme T et al., *Computed tomography and magnetic resonance tomography of intracranial tumors. A clinical perspective* (Springer-Verlag: Berlin, 1989).

43. Keith E, Kortman E, Bradley WG Jr, Supratentorial neoplasms. In: Stark DD, Bradley WG Jr, eds, *Magnetic resonance imaging* (Mosby: St Louis, 1988) 375–422.

44. Hasso AN, Fahmy JL, Hinshaw DB, Tumors of the posterior fossa. In: Stark DD, Bradley WG Jr, eds, *Magnetic resonance imaging* (Mosby: St Louis, 1988) 425–50.

45. Wilms G, Lammens M, Marchal G et al., Prominent dural enhancement adjacent to nonmeningiomatous malignant lesions on contrast-enhanced MR images, *AJNR* (1991) **12**:761–4.

46. Lee Y, Van Tassel P, Intracranial oligodendrogliomas: imaging findings in 35 untreated cases, *AJNR* (1989) **10**:119–27.

47. Lee Y, Van Tassel P, Bruner JM et al., Juvenile pilocytic astrocytomas: CT and MR characteristics, *AJNR* (1989) **10**:363–70.

48. Schorner W, Laniado M, Kornmesser W et al., Comparison of multi-echo and contrast-enhanced MR scans: image contrast and delineation of intracranial tumors, *Neuroradiology* (1989) **31**:140–7.

49. Boulin A, Tumeurs intracrâniennes. In: Vignaud J, Boulin A, eds, *Tomodensitométrie crânio-encéphalique* (Vigot: Paris, 1988) 266–367.

50. Dean BL, Drayer BP, Bird CR, et al., Gliomas: classification with MR imaging, *Radiology* (1990) **174**: 411–15.

51. Komiyama M, Yagura H, Baba M et al., MR imaging: possibility of tissue characterization of brain tumors using T1 and T2 values, *AJNR* (1987) **8**:65–70.

52. Weill A, Tampieri D, Melançon D et al., Kyste épidermoide sus-calleux: à propos d'un cas, *J Radiol* (1990) **71**:373–6.

53. Atlas SW, Grossman RI, Gomori JM et al., Hemorrhagic intracranial malignant neoplasms: spin-echo MR imaging, *Radiology* (1987) **164**:71–7.

54. Chamberlain MC, Murovic JA, Levin VA, Absence of contrast enhancement on CT brain scans of patients with supratentorial malignant gliomas, *Neurology* (1988) **38**:1371–4.

55. Kernohan JW, Sayre GP, *Tumors of the central nervous system. Atlas of tumor pathology,* section 10, fascicle 35 (Armed Forces Institute of Pathology: Washington DC, 1972).

56. Pomeranz SJ, Posterior fossa, skull base, craniocervical junction. In: Pomeranz SJ, ed, *Craniospinal magnetic resonance imaging* (WB Saunders: Philadelphia, 1989) 248–74.

57. Rubinstein LJ, Tumors of the central nervous system. In: Rubinstein LJ, ed, *Atlas of tumor pathology,* 2nd series, fascicle 6 (Armed Forces Institute of Pathology: Washington DC, 1972) 160–98.

58. Russell DS, Rubinstein LJ, *Pathology of tumors of the nervous system,* 5th edn (Edward Arnold: London, 1989).

59. Zülch KJ, *Brain tumors: their histology and pathology, 3rd edn* (Springer-Verlag: Berlin, 1986).

60. Daumas-Duport C, Scheithauer BW, Kelly P, A histologic and cytologic method for the spatial definition of gliomas, *Mayo Clin Proc* (1987) **62**:435–49.

61. Johnson PC, Hunt SJ, Drayer BP, Human cerebral gliomas: correlation of postmortem MR imaging and neuropathologic findings, *Radiology* (1989) **170**:211–17.

62. Lee SR, Sanches J, Mark AS et al., Posterior fossa hemangioblastomas: MR imaging, *Radiology* (1989) **171**:463–8.

63. Zimmerman RD, Leeds NE, Naidich TP, Ring blush associated with intracerebral hematoma, *Radiology* (1977) **122**:707–11.

64. Elster AD, DiPersio DA, Cranial postoperative site: assessment with contrast-enhanced MR imaging, *Radiology* (1990) **174**:93–8.

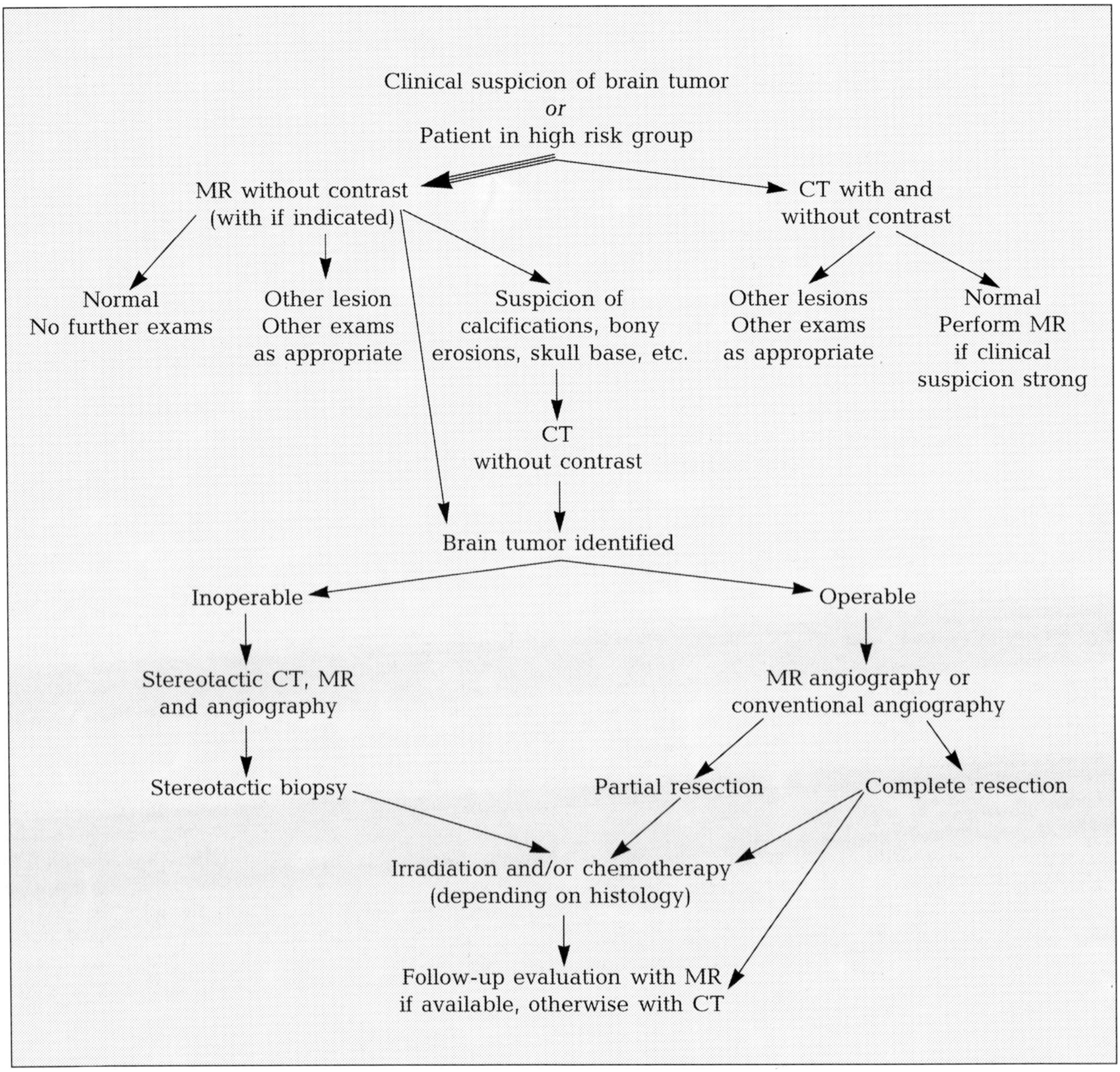

Diagram 1.1

The strategy for the choice of imaging modalities in suspected brain tumors. Note that MR is the modality of choice, but sometimes only CT is initially available.

2

The spine

Robert Sigal and Philippe Halimi

Introduction

Magnetic resonance imaging (MR) represents the sole imaging strategy in the diagnosis and follow up of intramedullary neoplasms, because it is the only diagnostic modality which allows a direct, multiplanar and non-invasive visualization of the entire spinal cord and its environment. All the other imaging techniques (plain films, myelography, computed tomography and angiography) are obsolete.

Gadolinium-MR has proved to be a method of choice in the imaging of leptomeningeal tumors. However, myelography and intrathecally enhanced computed tomography (CT) should be considered in the imaging strategy if MR findings are negative.

Intramedullary tumors

Primary intramedullary tumors (astrocytomas and ependymomas)

Intramedullary tumors are rare by comparison with tumors of the brain.[1] In adults, approximately 65% of these tumors are ependymomas and 30% are astrocytomas;[1,2] in children, more than 50% are astrocytomas.[3,4] Most patients with astrocytomas present in their thirties and forties; the peak incidence of ependymomas is the fourth and fifth decade. Clinical presentation is non-specific, with neck or back pain, radicular pain, motor and sensory disturbances, constipation and urinary incontinence. In children, back pain should raise suspicion, especially if associated with scoliosis.

Astrocytomas are distributed uniformly in the spinal cord, with 80% of lesions at the cervical and thoracic levels.[2] Ependymomas are most commonly located in the caudal spinal cord: 60% are found in the conus medullaris, filum terminale and cauda equina (myxopapillary type).[1,5]

The prognosis of these tumors depends primarily on the histopathologic grade.[6] Both astrocytomas and ependymomas are less malignant in the cord than they are in the brain. Grades I and II represent 75–92% of astrocytomas;[1,7,8] grades III or IV are rare.[2] In a series of 14 astrocytomas there was found to be a 5-year survival rate of 89% in low-grade tumors, and 0% in high-grade malignancies.[9] Almost all ependymomas are benign tumors.

The slow growth characteristic of benign astrocytomas and ependymomas underlies their gross appearance.[3,10–12] These lesions induce cord enlargement. They present a solid portion, limited to one or two vertebral segments, which usually is purely intramedullary. Rarely, the solid portion may be exophytic with an extramedullary intradural portion.[13] Small hemorrhagic areas are frequent. Associated cysts extend along a variable portion of the spinal cord, but the cystic portions of a given lesion are usually more important than the solid one. The entire spinal cord may be involved by cysts, in particular in child astrocytomas (holocord tumors). Three types of cysts may be described:

- Necrotic cysts result from a cystic degeneration of a portion of the tumor. They may contain cellular debris.

- Tumoral cysts are similar to the previous ones, but the walls of the cysts are made of active tumor. These cysts are most often contiguous to or included within the solid portion, but they may be also separated from the solid portion by an apparently intact spinal cord. This particular type of cyst is located at the craniocervical junction and it may be hypothesized that it results from a colonization by tumor cells of the central canal which ends at the C1 level. These cysts may be called craniocervical sentinel cysts, because when visualized they indicate the need to search the solid portion of the tumor.[14]
- Syrinx-like cysts are the results of abnormal cerebrospinal fluid (CSF) circulation. The solid portion of the tumor hampers normal CSF pulsations and generates a pressure gradient between the cranial and the medullary subarachnoid spaces, with the result that cerebrospinal fluid passes into the neural tissue. The mechanism is close to that described by Aboulker to explain syrinx formation.[15] However, abnormal pulsatile motions within the cyst has not been reported, in contradistinction to genuine syrinx cysts. Cysts are uncommon in high-grade tumors, which are rapidly-growing lesions.

The mechanism of formation of the various types of cysts remains to be completely elucidated.[14,16,17] Nevertheless, from a practical point of view, it is essential to differentiate the solid portion of the lesion from the associated cysts, because the solid portion requires complete excision, whereas there is no need to treat the necrotic and syrinx-like cysts.[6] Following resection of the solid portion, the cysts spontaneously reduce or disappear. Tumoral cysts are more problematic, however, because it is surgically difficult, if not impossible, to remove tumoral cyst walls. These particular lesions probably account for most tumor relapses.

Three factors combine to improve survival statistics for both astrocytomas and ependymomas:

- Most of these tumors are benign lesions.
- Progress in neurosurgical techniques (Cavitron™, laser, intraoperative registration of somatosensory evoked potentials) allows for total resection of the solid portion, with complete preservation of the underlying spinal cord.[4,10,18]
- Accurate delineation of the solid portion is feasible with MR, allowing limited laminectomy (or laminotomy in children).

Treatment consists essentially of radical resection of the solid portion. Postsurgical radiation therapy is recommended in high-grade malignancies.[7,10]

Magnetic resonance imaging

MR imaging is the only diagnostic examination that should be performed when there is a clinical suspicion of spinal cord lesion.[8,11,16,19–21] MR makes the diagnosis of intramedullary tumor, guides the surgical workup, and allows accurate follow up. Examinations should be performed with short repetition time (TR), short echo time (TE) sequences (T1-weighted sequences) and long TR, long TE sequences (T2-weighted sequences). The use of cardiac gating and/or gradient-moment nulling techniques significantly reduces artifacts and improves lesion conspicuity. Long TR, short TE images (proton density-weighted sequences) are less useful. Injection of a gadolinium compound, such as Gd-DTPA or Gd-DOTA, is mandatory because it allows clear recognition of the various parts of the tumor.[8,19,20]

T1-weighted sequences

Intramedullary tumors are responsible for a spinal-cord enlargement. Mass effect on the spinal canal may be seen, particularly in low-grade, slow-growing tumors. Most often, tumors involve multiple levels. Distinction between the solid portion and the associated cysts is difficult because they have similar signal intensities, lower than those of the cord.[8,12,20] Heterogeneous signal intensity may be seen, in particular within the cystic components);[22] isointensity with the spinal cord is frequent and suggests high protein content due to the presence of cellular debris. Cysts of high signal intensity are filled with hemorrhage. Craniocervical sentinel cysts are easily recognized: they present as rounded lesions, extending above the foramen magnum (Figure 2.1). This allows distinction with syringomyelic cysts which have a superior pointed expansion and end at the C1 level, below the foramen magnum. The CSF may show abnormal, high signal intensity, particularly in the thecal sac, due to an increased protein content.

T2-weighted sequences

The signal intensity of the solid portion depends on the magnetic field strength. At mid-field (0.5 T), the solid portion is displayed with high signal intensity characteristics due to increased water content.[11] At high-field (1.5 T), the solid portion may also show high signal intensity patterns (same mechanisms as at 0.5 T). However, tumors of low signal intensity are frequent (Figure 2.2).[8]

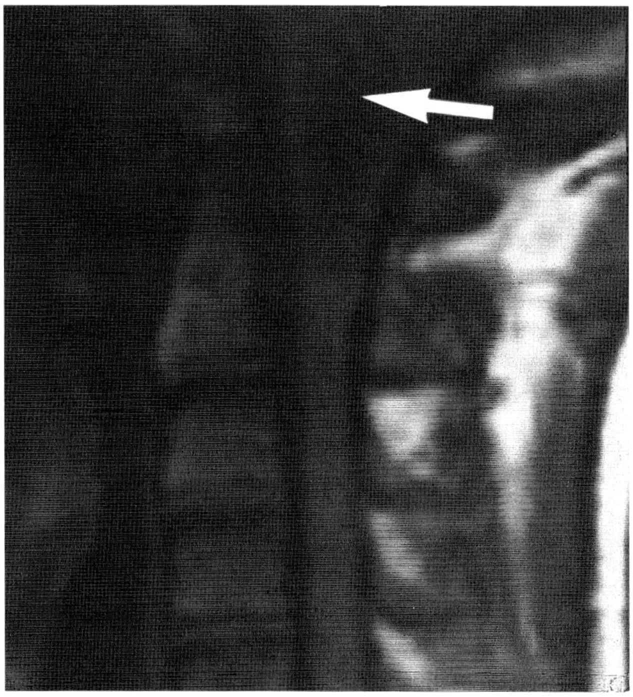

Figure 2.1

Sentinel cyst. T1-weighted sagittal view shows a round-shaped cyst (arrow) extending above the craniocervical junction. The solid portion of the astrocytoma was located at the mid-thoracic level. From Sigal et al.[16] with permission.

Hypointensity areas are either distributed throughout the entire solid portion, or located at the caudal and cranial extremities. Ferritin and hemosiderin staining is responsible for these low signal intensity zones. Slowly growing tumors are prone to chronic bleeding: ferritin and hemosiderin, final hemoglobin breakdown products, accumulate in the tumor, particularly at its front. Due to magnetic susceptibility differences from surrounding tissues, ferritin and hemosiderin are visualized at 1.5 T on T2-weighted images with low signal intensity.[23] Because magnetic susceptibility effects are proportional to the square of the external magnetic field, B_0, the same tumor may appear with high signal intensity characteristics at 0.5 T, or lower and low signal intensity at 1.5 T or higher.

The cysts are always displayed with high signal intensity. However, high signal intensity areas may correspond not only to true cysts but also to areas of edema or, at mid-field, to the solid portion itself. Areas of low signal intensity are not found, because of the absence of pulsatile motion.

Gadolinium

Both astrocytomas (Figures 2.3–2.5) and ependymomas (Figure 2.6) exhibit enhancement on T1-weighted images after gadolinium injection.[8,19,20,24] Although absence of contrast enhancement has been described,[20] most tumors have been reported to enhance, whatever their grade.[8] The fact that almost all intramedullary gliomas enhance probably reflects the fact that the blood–cord barrier does not have the same characteristics as the blood–brain barrier. In the brain, enhancement is primarily noticed in high-grade malignancies. The contrast enhancement pattern may help differentiate between ependymomas and astrocytomas. In high-grade astrocytomas, the margins may be irregular or poorly defined,[25,26] whereas ependymomas typically exhibit well-circumscribed, homogeneous areas of high signal enhancement.[19,20,25,27] However, enhancement patterns are non-specific and cannot ensure a pathologic diagnosis.

Follow-up studies

MR is the method of choice for detecting postoperative complications and relapses. Postoperative complications are mainly represented by hematomas. They are easily recognized after the first 48 h because of the presence of blood degradation products (deoxyhemoglobin and methemoglobin).

Obtaining evidence of relapse can be difficult. In most cases, the resection of the lesion has been satisfactory, and there is no need to search for relapses during the first few months following intervention. Moreover, surgically induced changes are confusing: T1-weighted low signal intensity and T2-weighted high signal intensity areas may represent postsurgical myelomalacia or residual tumor. Gadolinium enhancement may correspond to benign postsurgical inflammatory changes.

In fact, a new baseline for postsurgical follow up may be set at 4–6 months after surgery. In follow-up images, two major signs should be monitored: spinal cord enlargement and contrast enhancement.

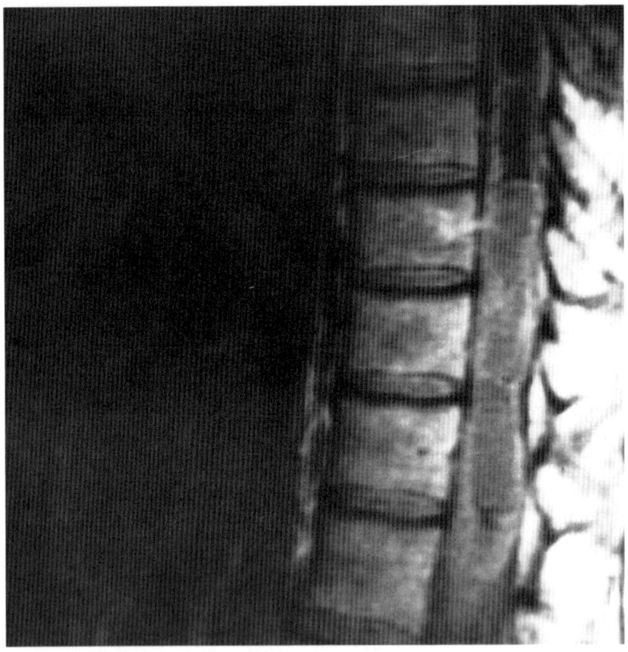

A

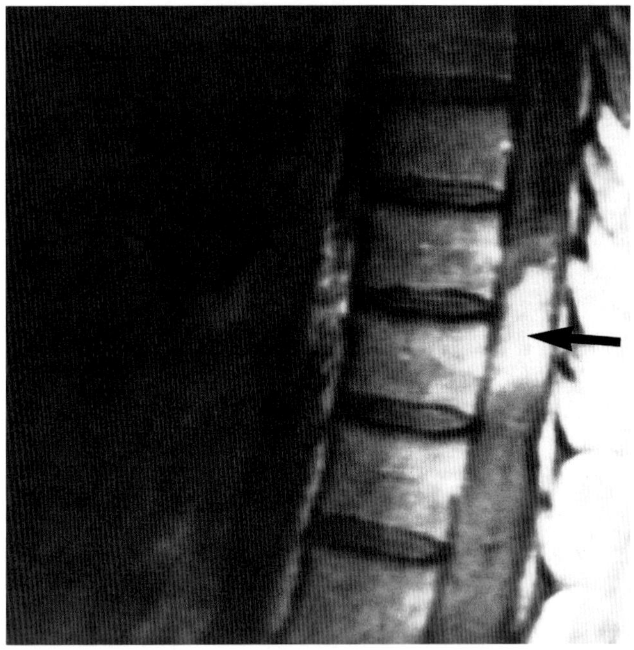

C

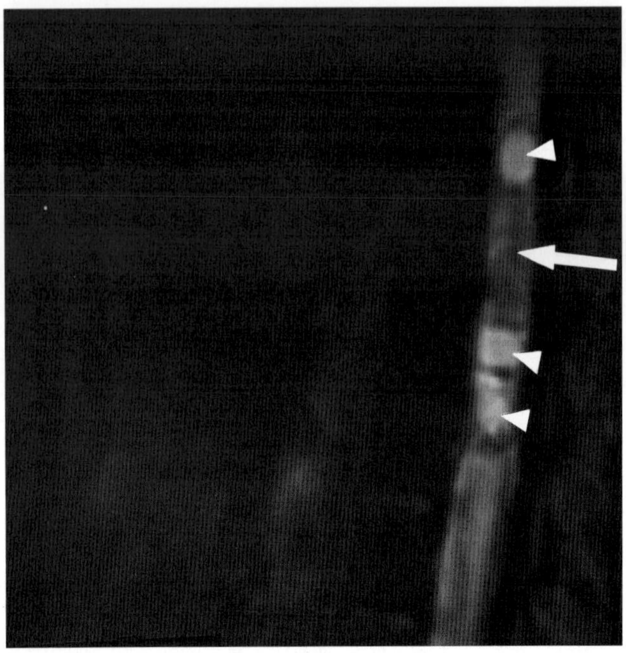

B

Figure 2.2

Glial tumor, inferior thoracic level.

A Sagittal T1-weighted image shows a heterogeneous lesion.

B On the T2-weighted view, the solid portion appears with low signal intensity (arrow), the inferior and superior cysts with high signal intensity (arrowheads).

C Post-gadolinium T1-weighted image clearly delineates the solid portion (arrow) which enhances with contrast. (From Sigal et al,[16] with permission.)

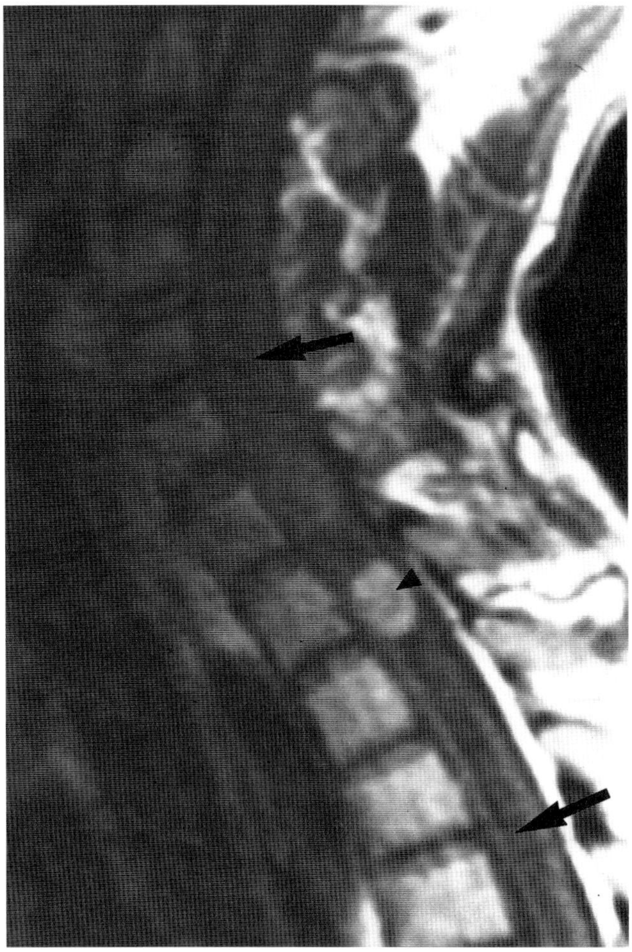

Figure 2.3

Upper dorsal astrocytoma. Sagittal, post-gadolinium, T1-weighted image shows a limited enhancing solid portion, at the T1 level (arrowhead), with extensive low-intensity adjacent cysts (arrows).

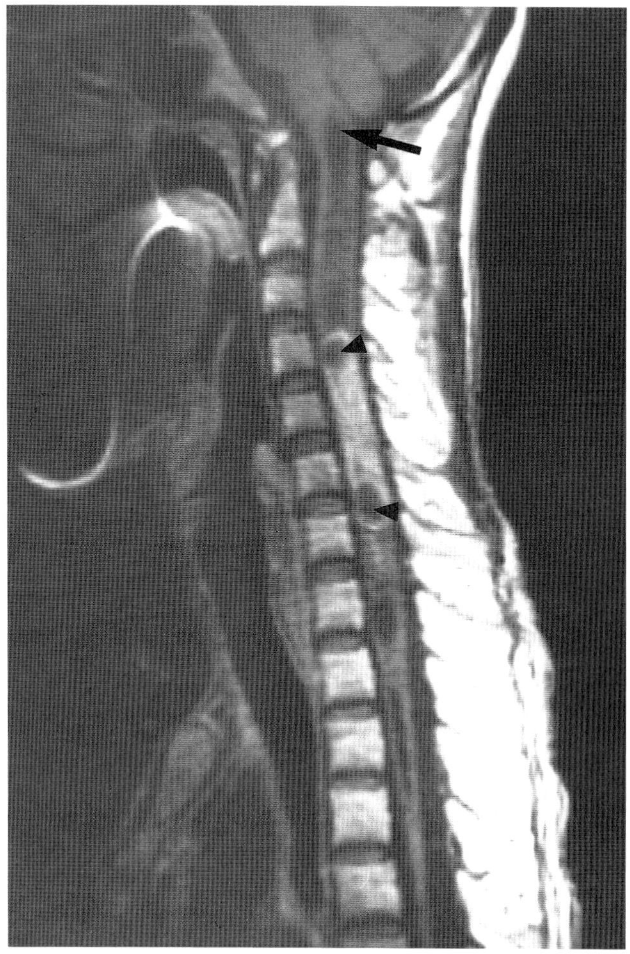

A

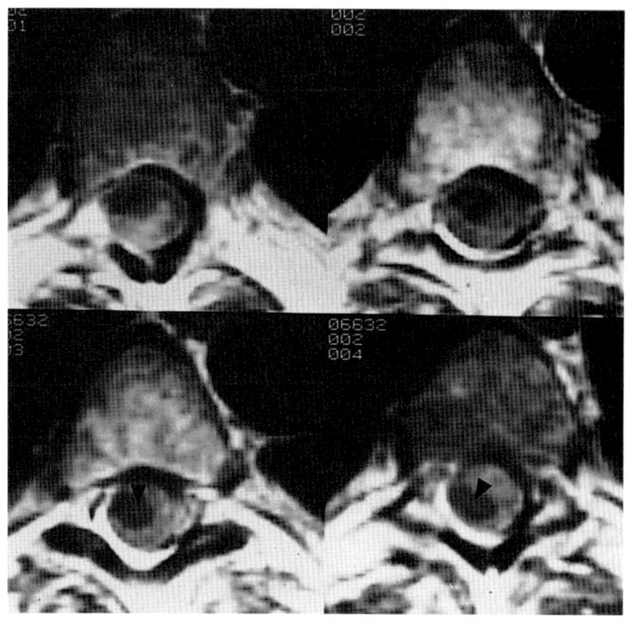

B

Figure 2.4

Cervical cystic astrocytoma.

A Sagittal post-gadolinium T1-weighted image shows a C4–C7 mass enhancing with contrast, with limited areas of low intensity, probably corresponding to tumor necrosis (arrowheads). Extensive low intensity cysts extend cranially and caudally. At its upper end in the posterior fossa, the superior cyst presents a round-shaped configuration (arrow).

B Axial view confirms partial necrosis of the solid portion (arrowheads).

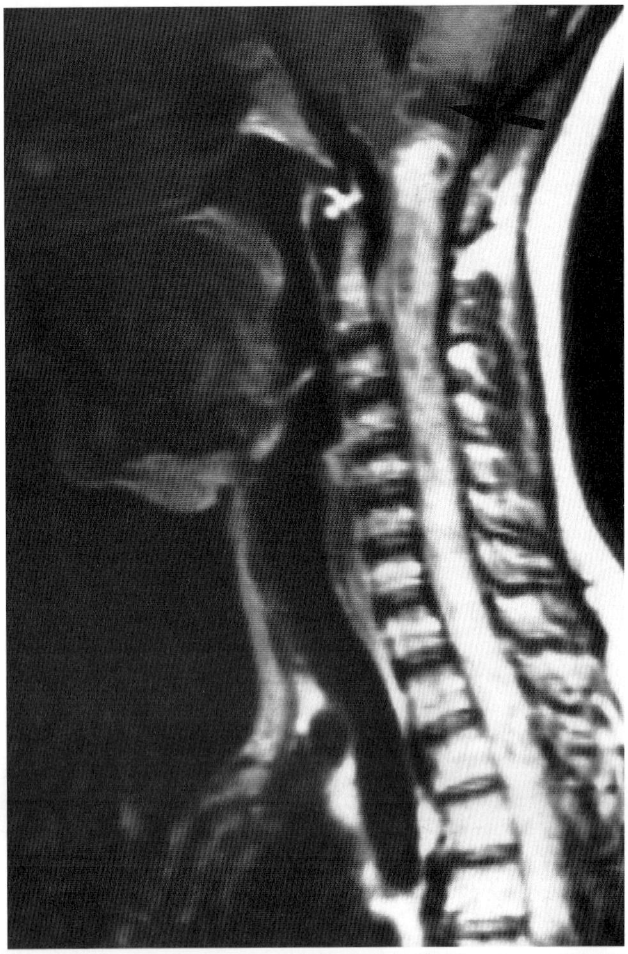

Figure 2.5

Astrocytoma. Post-gadolinium T1-weighted image shows a large enhancing solid portion. The upper part extends in the superior fossa, with a limited round-shaped, low-intensity cyst (arrow).

Other imaging modalities

Plain films and CT may show bony erosion, widening of the spinal canal[28] and, in children, scoliosis. With CT, the visualization of the cord is partial and accuracy is poor. While CT may find incidentally a cord enlargement (for instance in patient referred for cervical radicular pain), it no longer has a place in imaging strategies for intramedullary neoplasms.

Myelography, an invasive examination, should be restricted to patients in whom MR is not feasible (pacemakers, foreign metallic bodies, etc.). It almost invariably shows a fusiform regular enlargement of the cord. An exophytic portion of a tumor may simulate an intradural extramedullary lesion.

Angiography is still recommended by some neurosurgeons in order to visualize the spinal anterior medullary artery before surgical resection of the tumor.

Intraoperative ultrasonography is used by some neurosurgical teams to localize the solid portion when MR is not available.[17]

Differential diagnosis

Most astrocytomas and ependymomas share common characteristics and therefore MR findings are essentially non-specific. Other intramedullary tumors are exceptionally rare: oligodendroglioma,[29] intramedullary neurofibroma,[30] ganglioglioma,[31] hamartoma[21] and melanoma.[32] Hemangioblastoma, however, deserves specific comments: it is found primarily in the cerebellum, and represents only 2–4% of intramedullary tumors.[33,34] It is a small, benign and single or multicentric tumor. When multicentric, it is usually associated with von Hippel–Lindau disease, a familial disorder with cerebellar hemangioblastoma, retinal angiomatosis and renal and pancreatic cysts.[35,36] At MR, the lesion appears as small nodule that enhances strongly and homogeneously with gadolinium.[37] In more than 50% of cases, the lesion is associated to extensive non-tumoral cysts.[8,20] A relatively characteristic feature, seen in approximately 50% of patients, is the association with abnormal vasculature, usually on the dorsal surface of the cord. Angiography is still recommended before radical resection[38] because it allows recognition of small multicentric nodules (in the order of millimeters) that can be missed with MR.

Differentiation between intramedullary tumors and other lesions is usually easy. Syrinx cysts exhibit low signal intensity on T1-weighted images. On T2-weighted images, turbulent flow generates low signal intensity areas. If doubt remains, gadolinium should be injected. Acute myelitis may simulate high grade malignancies.[8] Cord is enlarged and presents low signal intensity on T1-weighted images and high signal intensity on T2-weighted images. Irregular contrast

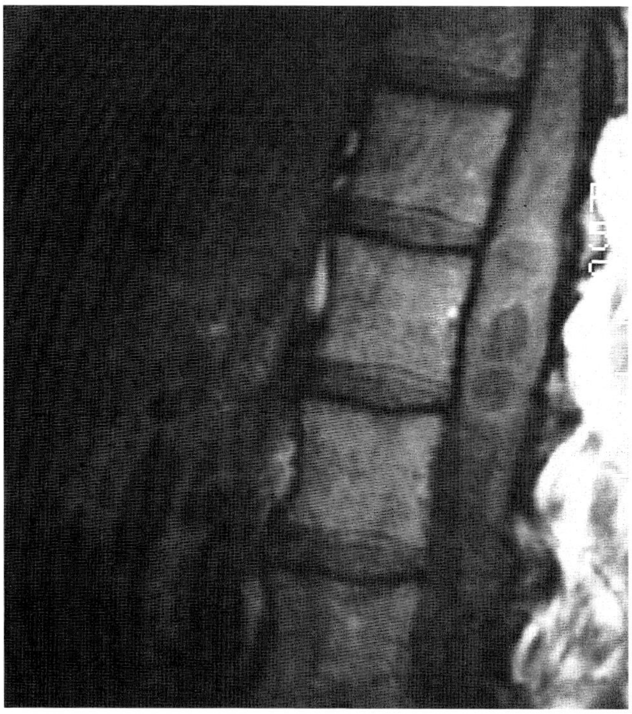

A

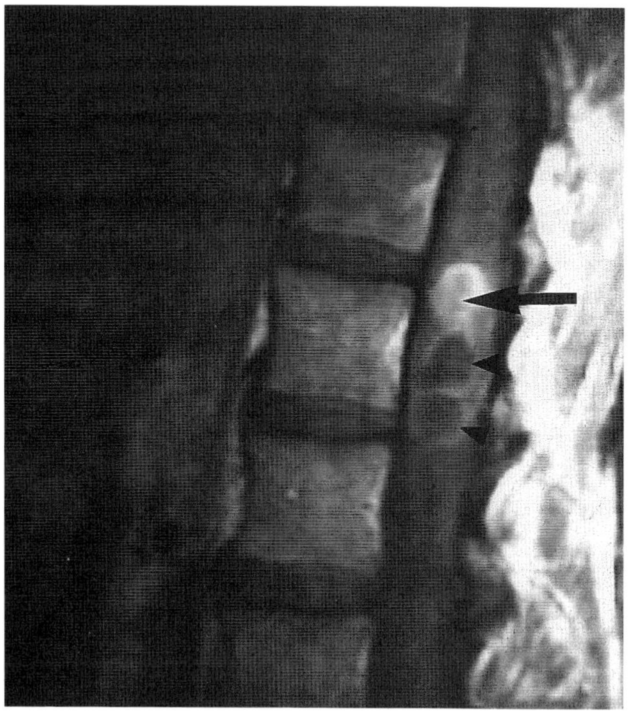

B

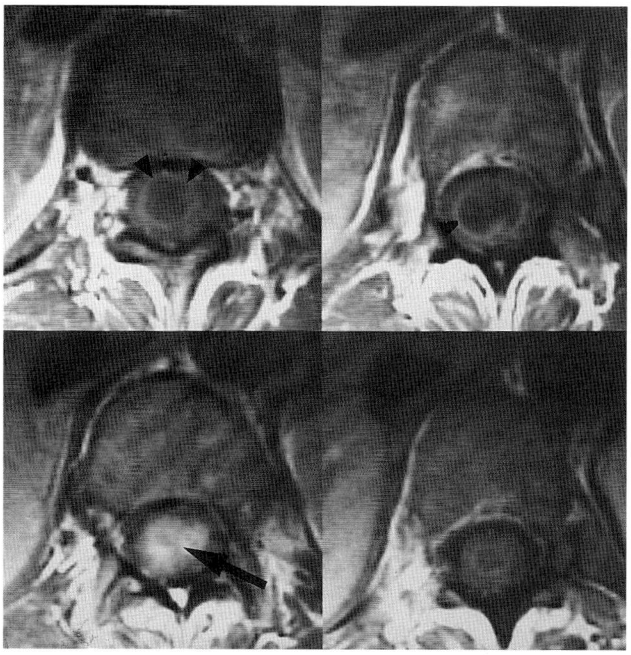

C

Figure 2.6

Cystic ependymoma of the conus medullaris.

A Sagittal T1-weighted image shows a heterogeneous lesion enlarging the spinal cord.

B After gadolinium injection, contrast enhancement is seen in the solid portion (arrow) but also in the wall of an adjacent cyst (arrowheads).

C Axial T1-weighted gadolinium view confirms that the tumor is made of a solid portion (arrow) with adjacent tumoral cysts (arrowheads). From Sigal et al,[16] with permission.

enhancement is noticed, similar to that seen in high-grade astrocytomas (or metastases). Follow-up examinations allow differentiation: at the chronic stage, myelitis is depicted with cord atrophy and absence of contrast enhancement.

Secondary intramedullary tumors (spinal cord metastases)

Metastatic intramedullary tumors are rare. In a retrospective autopsy series, 8.5% of patients with systemic neoplasms had cord metastases.[39] However, in living patients the figure is lower because of asymptomatic lesions. Carcinoma of the lung (small cell anaplastic carcinoma) accounts for more than 50% of the total. Other non-central nervous system (CNS) tumors are breast and renal carcinoma, melanoma and non-Hodgkin's lymphoma.[39,40] Spread to the cord may be due to hematogenous seeding (arterial or venous), or to direct penetration via CSF or nerve roots. In the latter case, leptomeningeal tumor coexists with cord metastasis. Such findings are also present when metastases arise from primary CNS tumor (medulloblastoma, glioblastoma and ependymoma).[20] The lesions are most commonly located in the thoracic spinal cord. When the lesion is purely intramedullary, it does not induce cord enlargement. The lesion is well circumscribed and there are no associated cysts, as it is a rapidly growing tumor. When it is associated to leptomeningeal seeding, cord enlargement is observed on multiple levels.[20]

The clinical presentation of secondary intramedullary tumors is not specific, although clinical progression is rapid, in contrast with primary tumors. The prognosis is poor.

Imaging strategy

Myelography is normal in approximately 50% of cases, because there is no cord enlargement.[40] MR is the examination of choice.[8,20,41]

When the metastasis is confined to the cord, it appears as a low signal intensity lesion on T1-weighted images, with a normal or minimally increased cord diameter. The high signal intensity area displayed on T2-weighted images represents the metastasis and the surrounding edema. After gadolinium injection, strong and homogeneous enhancement is noticed.[19,42]

When multiple levels are involved, cord enlargement is seen, with extensive high signal intensity areas, representing edema, on T2-weighted images. The metastases enhance with gadolinium. MR also allows recognition of leptomeningeal tumor. Epidural and vertebral metastases can be assessed.

Differential diagnosis

Differentiation from post-radiation myelitis may be difficult in patients with prophylactic irradiation of the spinal cord. Radiation-induced acute chronic progressive myelopathy may present as a swelling cord with extensive signal intensity areas on T2-weighted MR images. Contrast enhancement may be seen. In fact, follow-up scans will make the diagnosis: cord atrophy, a striking characteristic of chronic myelitis, is never observed in metastases.

Intradural neoplastic tumors

Neoplasms that metastasize to the intradural space and leptomeninges include both primary non-CNS and CNS tumors. Primary intracranial neoplasms are the most frequent, especially in children.[43,44] Medulloblastoma is the most common source of leptomeningeal tumor spread, followed by glioblastoma, ependymoma, oligodendroglioma, astrocytoma, retinoblastoma and pineal tumors.[45] Non-CNS tumors include lung carcinoma, breast carcinoma and melanoma.[1,29] Diffuse neoplasm such as non-Hodgkin's lymphoma and acute leukemia may also metastasize to the meninges.[46]

Pathologically, sheets of tumor cells coat the leptomeninges and form either a thin layer or large nodules. The underlying meninges become thickened.[20] Lesions can form at any level of the spinal canal, but the predominant site is the lombosacral level, probably due to the effects of gravity.[8,47]

Patients may be asymptomatic or present with non-specific symptoms, including intracranial symptoms due to diffusion of tumor cells through the entire CNS.

The final diagnosis is made by CSF cytology.[48] However, even serial lumbar punctures may be negative. In such cases, imaging can ensure the diagnosis, although the proportion of patients with negative cytology and positive imaging findings is not documented. Conversely, gadolinium-enhanced MR is positive in no more than 15–20% of patients with proved leptomeningeal carcinomatosis (Figure 2.7).[8] It is of primary importance to diagnose spinal leptomeningeal tumor because such findings require localized or whole spinal axis radiation therapy with or without intrathecal chemotherapy.

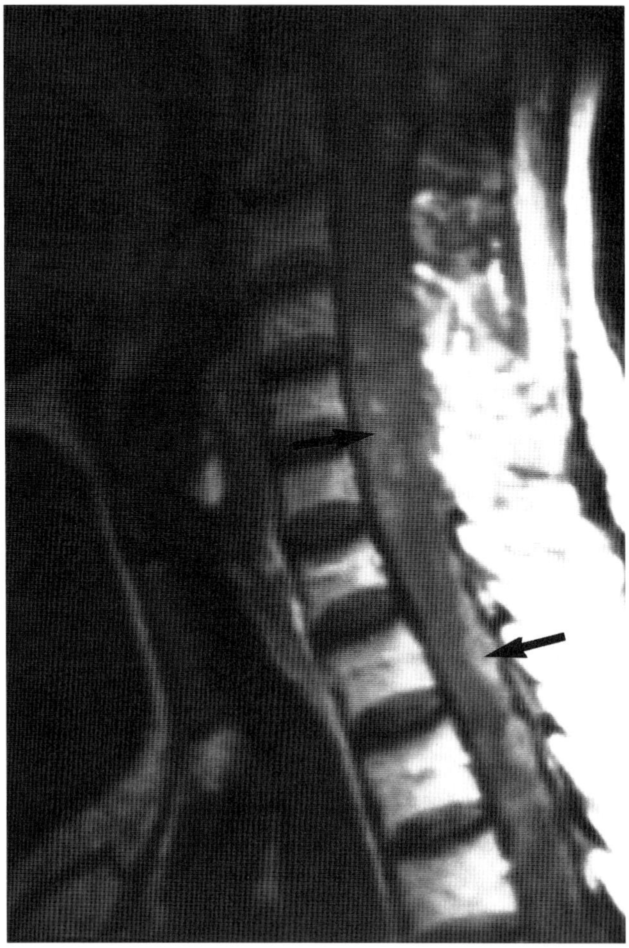

Figure 2.7

Leptomeningeal metastasis, cervical level. Sagittal post-gadolinium T1-weighted image shows multiple, enhanced, ill-defined nodules in the anterior and posterior subarachnoid spaces (arrows). The margins of the spinal cord are not clearly depicted.

Imaging strategy

Myelography may show single or multiple nodular filling defects in the subarachnoid space, irregularity or adhesion of nerve roots. Intrathecally enhanced CT should be performed in the supine and prone position to document loss of mobility of the cauda equina.

MR without gadolinium has low sensitivity, with a false-negative rate around 40%.[43,49] Use of gadolinium is mandatory to make the diagnosis.[42,46,50] On T1-weighted images, tumor spread may have different patterns: a thin layer along the cord, filum terminale or nerve roots, suggesting pial metastases,[51] various size nodules in the thecal sac, or filling of the entire subarachnoid space. Enhancement may be intense or subtle, underlying the need to acquire sagittal and axial oblique views. Contrast take-up is not specific for tumor; benign arachnoiditis may also show mild enhancement with gadolinium.[52] Visualization of the entire spinal canal and brain is also mandatory because tumor spread may be asymptomatic. Thus, MR, a non-invasive technique allowing entire neuraxis to be checked, should be preferred to myelography as first-step examination.

References

1. Russell DS, Rubinstein LJ, *Pathology of tumours of the nervous system*, 5th edn. (Edward Arnold: London 1989) 83–219.
2. Sloof JL, Kernohan JW, MacCarthy CS, *Primary intramedullary tumors of the spinal cord and filum terminale* (WB Saunders Co: Philadelphia 1964).
3. Epstein F, Epstein N, Surgical treatment of spinal cord astrocytomas of childhood. A series of 19 patients, *J Neurosurg* (1982) **57**:685–9.
4. Reimer R, Onofrio BM, Astrocytomas of the spinal cord in children and adolescents, *J Neurosurg* (1985) **63**:669–75.
5. Sonneland PRL, Scheithauer BW, Onofrio BM, Myxopapillary ependymoma: a clinicopathologic and immunocytochemical study of 77 cases, *Cancer* (1985) **56**:883–93.
6. Giudetti B, Mercuri S, Vagnozzi R, Long-term results of the surgical treatment of 129 intramedullary spinal gliomas, *J Neurosurg* (1981) **54**:323–30.

7. Cohen AR, Wisoff JH, Allen JC et al, Malignant astrocytomas of the spinal cord, *J Neurosurg* (1989) **70**:50–4.
8. Sze G, Twohig M, Neoplastic disease of the spine and spinal cord. In: Atlas SW, ed, *MRI of the brain and spine* (Raven Press: New York 1991) 921–65.
9. Kopelson G, Linggood RM, Intramedullary spinal cord astrocytoma versus glioblastoma, the prognostic importance of histologic grade, *Cancer* (1982) **50**:732–5.
10. Epstein F, Epstein N, Surgical management of holocord intramedullary spinal cord astrocytomas in children. Report of three cases, *J Neurosurg* (1981) **54**:829–32.
11. Goy AMC, Pinto RS, Raghavendra BN et al, Intramedullary spinal cord tumors: MR imaging, with emphasis on associated cysts, *Radiology* (1986) **161**:381–6.
12. William AL, Haughton VM, Pojunas KW et al, Differentiation of intramedullary neoplasms and cysts by MR, *AJNR* (1987) **8**:527–32.
13. Wagle WA, Jaufman B, Mincy JE, Intradural extramedullary ependymoma: MR pathologic correlation. *J Comput Assist Tomogr* (1988) **12**:705.
14. Halimi Ph, Sigal R, Doyon D, David Ph, Diagnostic des affections de la mœlle et du rachis, *Revue du Practicien* (1989) **39**:751–7.
15. Aboulker J. La syringomyélie et les liquides intrarachidiens, *Neurochirurgie* (1979) **25**(suppl 1):1–144.
16. Sigal R, Grenier N, Tumeurs. In: Sigal R, Grenier N, Doyon D et al, eds, *IRM de la moelle et du rachis* (Masson: Paris 1991) 107–46.
17. Kochan JP, Quencer RM, Imaging of cystic and cavitary lesions of the spinal cord and canal: the value of MR and intraoperative sonography. *Radiol Clin North Am* (1991) **29**:867–911.
18. Cooper PR, Epstein F, Radical resection of intramedullary spinal cord tumors in adults: recent experience in 29 patients, *J Neurosurg* (1985) **63**:492–9.
19. Bydder GM, Brown J, Niendorf HP et al, Enhancement of cervical intraspinal tumors in MR imaging with intravenous gadolinium-DTPA, *J Comput Assist Tomogr* (1985) **9**:847–51.
20. Enzmann DR, De La Paz RL, Tumor. In: Enzmann DR, De La Paz RL, Rubin JB, eds, *Magnetic resonance imaging of the spine* (CV Mosby: St Louis, 1990) 301–422.
21. Norman D, The spine. In: Brant-Zawadski M, Norman D, eds, *MRI of the central nervous system* (Raven Press: New York 1987) 289–328.
22. Rubin JM, Aisen AM, DiPietro MA, Ambiguities in MR imaging of tumoral cysts in the spinal cord, *J Comput Assist Tomogr* (1986) **10**:295–8.
23. Thulborn KR, Atlas SW, Intracranial hemorrhage. In: Atlas SW, ed, *MRI of the brain and spine* (Raven Press: New York 1991) 175–222.
24. Slasky BS, Bydder GM, Niendorf HP et al, MR imaging with gadolinium-DTPA in the differentiation of tumor, syrinx and cyst of the spinal cord, *J Comput Assist Tomogr* (1987) **11**:845–50.
25. Parizel PM, Balériaux D, Rodesch G et al, Gd DTPA enhanced MR imaging of spinal tumors, *AJNR* (1989) **10**:249–58.
26. Sze G, Krol G, Zimmerman RD et al, Intramedullary disease of the spine: diagnosis using gadolinium DTPA-enhanced MR imaging, *AJNR* (1988) **9**:847–58.
27. Breger RK, Williams AL, Daniels DL et al, Contrast enhancement in spinal MR imaging, *AJNR* (1989) **10**:633–7.
28. Aubin ML, Jardin C, Bar D et al, CT in 32 cases of intraspinal tumor, *J Neuroradiol* (1979) **6**:81–92.
29. Balériaux D, Parizel P, Segebarth C, Pathologie intrarachidienne et médullaire. In: Manelfe C, ed, *Imagerie du rachis et de la moelle*, (Vigot: Paris 1989) 499–545.
30. Gonzalez MG, Allut AG, Alonso CC et al, Intramedullary spinal neurofibroma diagnosed with computed tomography: report of a case, *Neurosurgery* (1985) **16**:543–5.
31. Wald U, Levy PJ, Rappaport ZH et al, Conus gangioglioma in a 2½-year-old boy, *J Neurosurg* (1985) **62**:142–4.
32. Larson TC, Houser OW, Onofrio BM et al, Primary spinal melanoma, *J Neurosurg* (1987) **66**:47–9.
33. Kendall B, Russel J, Hemangioblastomas of the spinal cord, *Br J Radiol* (1966) **9**:817–23.
34. Palmer JJ, Hemangioblastomas of the spinal cord. A review of 81 cases, *Acta Neurochir* (1972) **27**: 125–48.
35. Böker DK, Wassmann H, Solymosi L, Multiple spinal hemangioblastomas in a case of Lindau's disease, *Surg Neurol* (1984) **22**:439–43.
36. Enomoto H, Shibata T, Ito A et al, Multiple hemangioblastomas accompanied by syringomyelia in the cerebellum and the spinal cord, *Surg Neurol* (1984) **22**:197–203.
37. Sato Y, Waziri M, Smith W et al, Hippel–Lindau disease: MR imaging, *Radiology* (1988) **166**:241–6.
38. Seeger JF, Burke DP, Knake JF et al, Computed tomographic and angiographic evaluation of hemangioblastomas, *Radiology* (1981) **138**:65–73.
39. Costigan DA, Winkelman MD, Intramedullary spinal cord metastasis. A clinicopathological study of 13 cases, *J Neurosurg* (1985) **62**:227–33.
40. Grem JL, Burgess J, Trump DL, Clinical features and natural history of intramedullary spinal cord metastasis, *Cancer* (1985) **56**:2305–14.
41. Post MJ, Quencer RM, Green BA et al, Intramedullary spinal cord metastases, mainly of nonneurogenic origin, *AJR* (1987) **148**:1015–22.
42. Sze G, Abramson A, Krol G et al, Gadolinium DTPA in the evaluation of intradural extramedullary spinal disease, *AJNR* (1988) **9**:153–63.
43. Krol G, Sze G, Malkin M et al, MR of cranial and spinal meningeal carcinomatosis: comparison with CT and myelography, *AJNR* (1988) **9**:709–14.
44. Barloon TJ, Yuh WTC, Yang CJC et al, Spinal subarachnoid tumor seeding from intracranial metastasis: MR findings, *J Comput Assist Tomogr* (1987) **11**:242–4.

45. Bryan P, CSF seeding of intracranial tumors: a study of 96 cases, *Clin Radiol* (1974) **25**:355–60.
46. Berns DH, Blaser S, Ross JS et al, MR Imaging with Gd-DTPA in leptomeningeal spread of lymphoma, *J Comput Assist Tomogr* (1988) **12**:499–500.
47. Dorwart RH, Wara WM, Norman D et al, Complete myelographic evaluation of spinal metastases from medulloblastoma, *Radiology* (1981) **139**:403–8.
48. Sze G, Krol G, Zimmermann RD et al, Malignant extradural spinal tumors: MR imaging with Gd-DTPA, *Radiology* (1988) **167**:217–23.
49. Davis PC, Griedman NC, Fry SM et al, Leptomeningeal metastasis: MR imaging, *Radiology* (1987) **163**:449–54.
50. Yousem DM, Patrone PM, Grossman RI, Leptomeningeal metastases: MR evaluation, *J Comput Assist Tomogr* (1990) **14**:246.
51. Lim V, Sobel DF, Zyroff J, Spinal cord metastases. MR imaging with gadopentetate dimeglumine, *AJNR* (1990) **11**:977–82.
52. Johnson C, Sze G, Benign lumbar arachnoiditis: MR imaging with gadopentetate dimeglumine, *AJNR* (1990) **11**:763–70.

3

The pediatric central nervous system

Debra A. Gusnard

Introduction

In the pediatric population the central nervous system (CNS) is the most common site for the development of solid neoplasms.[1] Of all primary brain tumors, 15–20% arise in childhood.[2] The incidence and variety of histological tumor types in the pediatric CNS differ significantly from those in adults. For example, tumors of a primitive stem cell origin (e.g. primitive neuroectodermal tumors), tumors arising from abnormal cell rests (e.g. ependymoma, germinoma) and tumors arising from inclusions (e.g. teratoma, dermoid) are relatively common in children but rare in adults. Also, a child is more likely to suffer dissemination of his tumor through the subarachnoid space than is an adult. For these reasons, as well as the fact that the CNS is still immature, the child presents unique challenges for those attempting to treat him with surgery, radiation and/or chemotherapy. As a result, algorithms for appropriate imaging strategies of CNS tumors in children frequently differ from those used in adults.

This chapter addresses the general approach to the radiologic evaluation of pediatric CNS tumors as well as discussing in detail three key infratentorial tumors that illustrate differential points in imaging strategies. Also addressed are key issues regarding the imaging of several other CNS neoplasms.

The goals of radiologic assessment in the management of pediatric CNS tumors are:

- To identify the neoplasm at as early a stage as possible after the onset of symptoms, realizing that accurate pre-operative histopathologic identification, though desirable, is less important than accurate distinction of neoplasm from other non-neoplastic mass lesions (e.g. aneurysm, abscess) that necessitate markedly different management strategies.
- To accurately localize and define the extent, and the stage, of the neoplasm in order to aid the neurosurgeon in planning his operative approach and in his decision-making regarding biopsy vs. attempted total resection, as well as to help the radiation therapist avoid geometric misses with his radiation portal.
- To assess the impact of treatment modalities with regard to tumor response as well as possible complications.

Techniques and imaging strategies

The clinical presentation of a child with a tumor in the CNS will frequently determine the initial imaging evaluation (Diagram 3.1). For example, a child in extremis, with signs of increased intracranial pressure, will undergo CT scanning with and without contrast enhancement. The age and size of the child will help determine the thicknesses of the CT slices employed. For children less than a year old, 3–5 mm sections through the posterior fossa and 5 mm sections through the remainder of the brain are appropriate. For older children, 5 mm sections through the posterior fossa and 8–10 mm sections through the remainder of the brain suffice. This permits rapid assessment and generally provides information (e.g. detection of hydrocephalus) necessary for emergency intervention. With an unstable patient, MR is frequently not employed because of logistical difficulties and the need for speed.

CT is more than simply expeditious, however, since it occasionally provides information that MR does not. Neither CT nor MR has definite advantages with respect to tissue characterization, but CT more accurately screens for the presence of calcification within a mass[3] (common, for example, in ependymomas) as well as demonstrating some relatively characteristic contrast differences (e.g. the hyperdensity of the primitive neuroectodermal tumor before contrast administration).[4] Nevertheless, the multiplaner capability and greater contrast resolution of MR provide more sensitivity in tumor detection and better definition of tumor extent.[5–8] This makes MR the procedure of choice for imaging brain tumors in the stable patient.

The patient's presentation is often not acute. Patients may manifest subacute signs of increased intracranial pressure, such as the classical morning headache associated with vomiting. Seizures, another common presenting sign, are related to the cortical irritative effects from the tumor, but most patients with seizures, like those with headaches, will not have a brain tumor. However, nowadays most patients with focal seizures and even some with generalized seizures will at some point undergo an imaging study. For screening purposes, it is not debatable whether CT or MR should be employed.[9,10] MR is the more sensitive study. Having said this, logistics related to limited resources will often dictate the use of CT. In the majority of cases of brain tumors, the CT scan will provide the correct diagnosis. Nevertheless, small infiltrating neoplasms can go undetected on the initial CT scan (Figure 3.1). Consequently, if the CT scan is negative but clinical suspicion persists, a follow-up MR scan should be obtained.

When it is logistically feasible and clinical suspicion of a mass lesion (neoplasm) is high, an MR scan should be performed at the outset. At a minimum, 3–5 mm sagittal T1-weighted and axial proton density and T2-weighted images of the entire brain should be acquired. Coronal images are useful adjuncts when evaluating the inferior and medial aspects of the temporal lobes and the sella/parasellar region. At our institute, sagittal T2-weighted images are regarded as the most useful images for the design of the radiation portals. If an abnormality potentially indicative of neoplasm is discerned on such images, then gadolinium-DTPA (0.1 mmol/kg) is injected and axial or coronal T1-weighted images obtained. Like the iodinated contrast agents used in CT, gadolinium-DTPA crosses the abnormal blood–brain barrier and permits improved detection, and often characterization of the lesion by its pattern of enhancement or by a lack of enhancement.[11–16] Lesions that are enhanced are distinguished more clearly from surrounding edema (though it is recognized that infiltrating margins of tumor may extend beyond the region of abnormal signal intensity perceived on MR images, particularly in the case of glial neoplasms, whether enhancing or not enhancing.)[17,18] Tumor enhancement is more sensitive with gadolinium-DTPA and MR than it is with iodinated contrast and CT.[14] Enhancement of subarachnoid dissemination is much greater with enhanced MR than with enhanced CT.[19,20]

Once surgical intervention has taken place, we repeat CT or MR, with and without contrast, within the first 48 h after surgery. This is done in order to determine whether there is residual tumor and, in cases of subtotal resection, to assess its extent. Evidence of residual cerebellar astrocytoma prompts an additional surgical procedure (during the same hospitalization) with the goal of complete resection and cure; demonstration of residual neoplastic tissue yields useful information for other tumors as well, such as medulloblastoma and ependymoma, since the amount of residual tissue correlates inversely with prognosis. Post-operatively, the first 48 h are thought to be a window during which post-operative reactive changes and granulation tissue have not yet developed an altered blood–brain barrier, so that enhancing tissue is generally presumed to represent residual tumor. Non-enhancing tissue with mass effect could represent acute post-operative change as well as residual tumor. Obviously, comparison with the pre-operative, pre- and post-contrast CT or MR is important in aiding detection of residual tumor.

Beyond the early post-operative period, criteria other than simple contrast enhancement within the region of the surgical bed are utilized. This is because reactive gliosis ('scarring') can enhance as readily as residual or recurrent tumor, persisting in its enhancement for months to years, though ultimately fading with time. Scar appears as a linear focus of enhancement without mass effect (Figure 3.2A), while recurrent tumor manifests nodularity, which may enhance (Figure 3.2B) and which grows over time. It should be noted that, if the patient is receiving large doses of steroids, contrast enhancement of abnormal tissue (on CT or MR) can be suppressed.

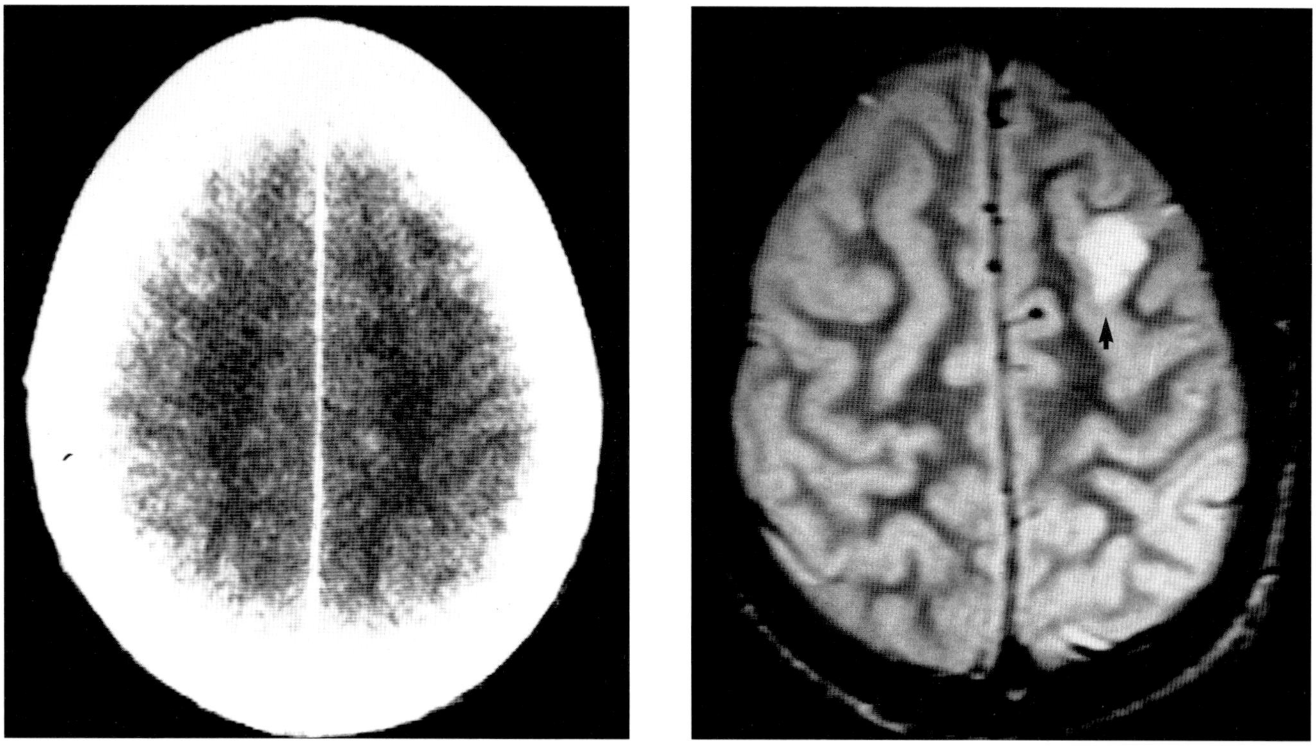

A

B

Figure 3.1

14-year-old male presenting with seizures.

A Contrast-enhanced axial CT image is negative.

B Axial T2-weighted MR image reveals a small, superficial high signal intensity mass lesion (arrow) in the posterior aspect of the left frontal lobe. This was surgically proven to be a ganglioglioma.

For patients with brain tumors that have a high likelihood of disseminating into the subarachnoid space (e.g. the primitive neuroectodermal tumor, pineoblastoma, ependymoma, malignant glioma, germinoma, choroid plexus carcinoma), complete radiologic staging also requires evaluation of the spinal canal. Myelography (± post-myelogram CT) has been the traditional method for evaluating for 'drop' metastases of the spinal canal (Figure 3.3A).[21,22] Myelography is generally performed at between 10 days and 2 weeks post-operatively. This is in order to minimize the risk of confusing post-operative blood clots in the spinal subarachnoid space with metastatic disease. However, contrast-enhanced MR is acquiring the role of a non-invasive alternative to myelography. After administration of gadolinium-DTPA, T1-weighted images can reveal 'drop' metastases as nodular deposits or as a coating of the nerve roots and spinal cord (Figure 3.3B).[12,23,16] Though MR appears to more sensitive than CT in the detection of metastatic deposits on the cord, it can be, for technical reasons, falsely negative for metastatic lesions along the nerve roots. Also, in our experience, metastatic (ependymoma) lesions may not always enhance when they are small. This compromises their visualization. Thus, while either a positive myelogram or contrast-enhanced MR is sufficient for confirming metastatic spread, neither a negative myelogram nor a negative MR is sufficient for excluding it. Consequently, the optimum strategy appears to be to employ MR, the non-invasive modality, first; and if the study is negative,

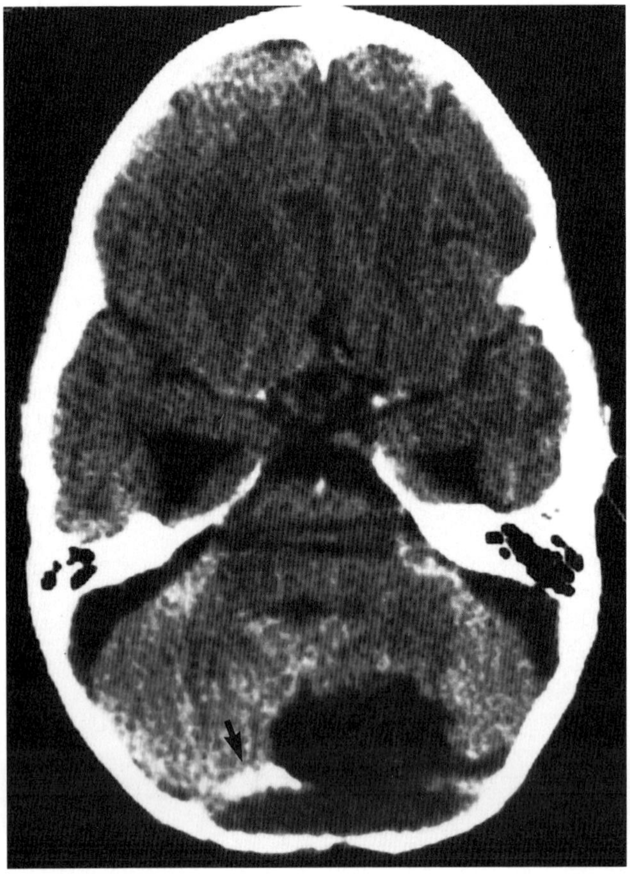

A

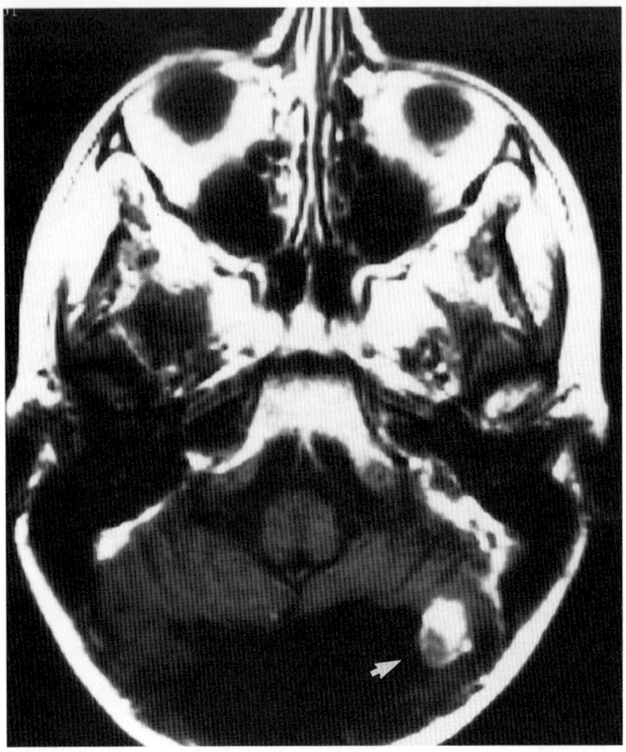

B

Figure 3.2

Scar vs. recurrent tumor.

A Contrast-enhanced CT demonstrates a linear enhancing focus (arrow) along the margin of the surgical bed of a previously resected low-grade astrocytoma without mass effect, compatible with scar.

B T1-weighted image after gadolinium demonstrates a focus of nodular enhancement (arrow) along the margin of the surgical bed of a previously resected anaplastic glioma, compatible with recurrent tumor.

proceed to myelography. It is worth noting that it has been shown that cerebrospinal-fluid (CSF) cytology may be negative in up to 50% of cases documented by imaging studies to be positive for metastatic disease.[22]

Finally, in the follow up of patients after various forms of treatment, complications need to be identified and distinguished from recurrent tumor.[24] Acute parenchymal injury in the radiation portal (occurring from several weeks to months after treatment) can be manifest as transient edema or gadolinium-DTPA enhancement within the white matter.[25–27] Radiation vasculitis and coagulative necrosis can occur months to years later. The former can result in focal brain infarcts, while the latter, though fortunately a rare occurrence, can appear mass-like and be radiologically indistinguishable from recurrent tumor, thus necessitating biopsy in some instances.[25–28] 'Functional' brain-imaging techniques such as positron emission tomography (PET) and single photon emission computed tomography (SPECT) may soon prove to be useful methods for making these distinctions noninvasively.[29]

Primitive neuroectodermal tumor – medulloblastoma

The primitive neuroectodermal tumor of the posterior fossa, also known as medulloblastoma (PNET-MB),[30] is the most common primary malignant

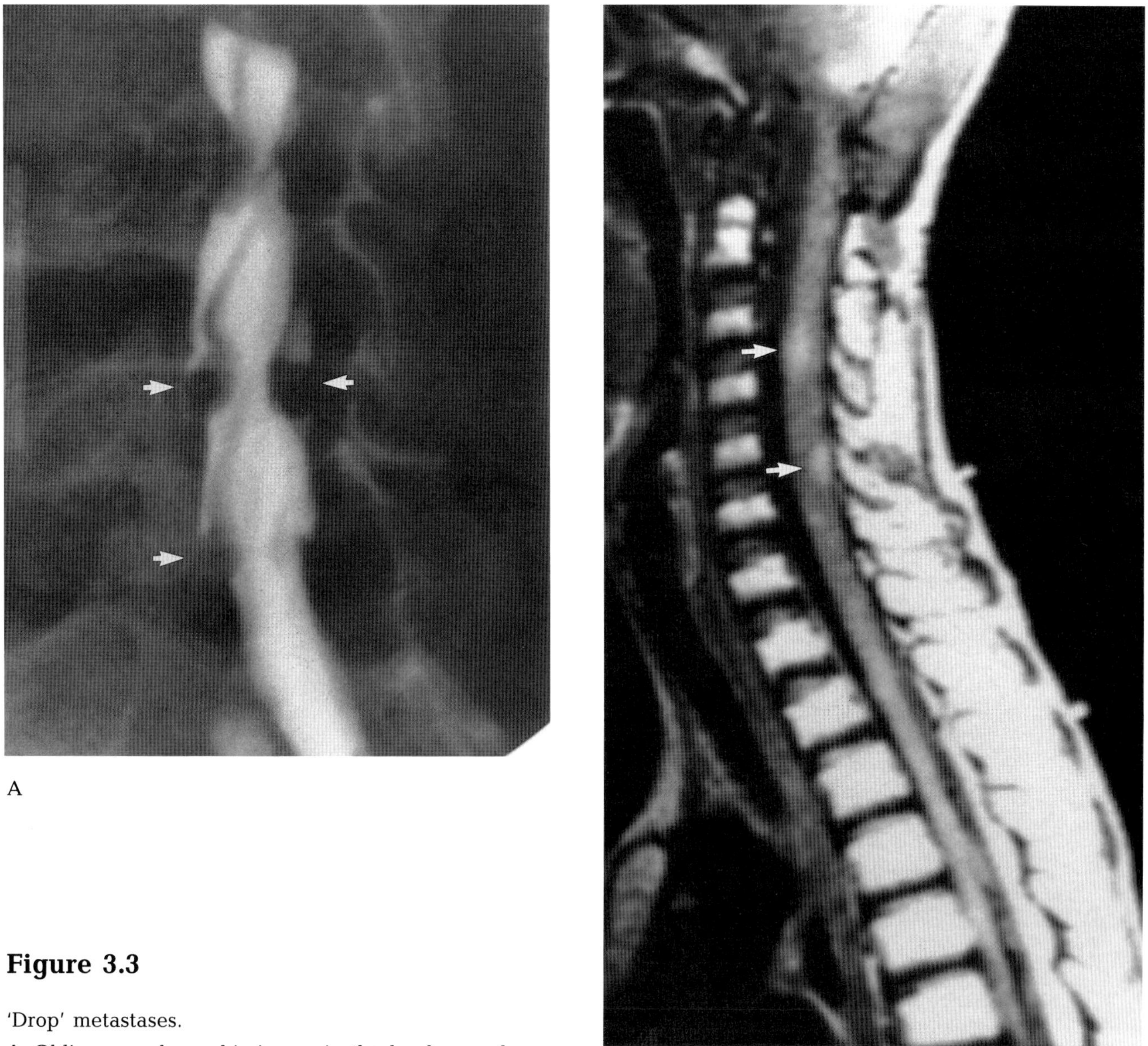

A

B

Figure 3.3

'Drop' metastases.

A Oblique myelographic image in the lumbosacral region demonstrates nodular filling defects along the exiting portion of multiple nerve roots (arrows).

B On this sagittal T1-weighted post-gadolinium image, fine patches of abnormal enhancement are seen coating the surface of the cervical cord (arrows).

brain tumor occurring in the pediatric population. Approximately 75% of these neoplasms present within the first decade of life. They are rapidly growing and generally present with symptoms or signs of less than 1 month in duration, for example, rapidly increasing head size in the infant, 'classical' headache from hydrocephalus and occasionally the even more specific sign of truncal ataxia in the older child. Frequently, its radiographic manifestations on CT are diagnostic,[31–33] the tumor typically appearing as a hyperdense midline vermian mass that enhances homogeneously with contrast; less commonly, it is isodense pre-contrast and/or enhances inhomogeneously. Cystic or necrotic areas are occasionally seen; calcification is visible in approximately 15% of cases.

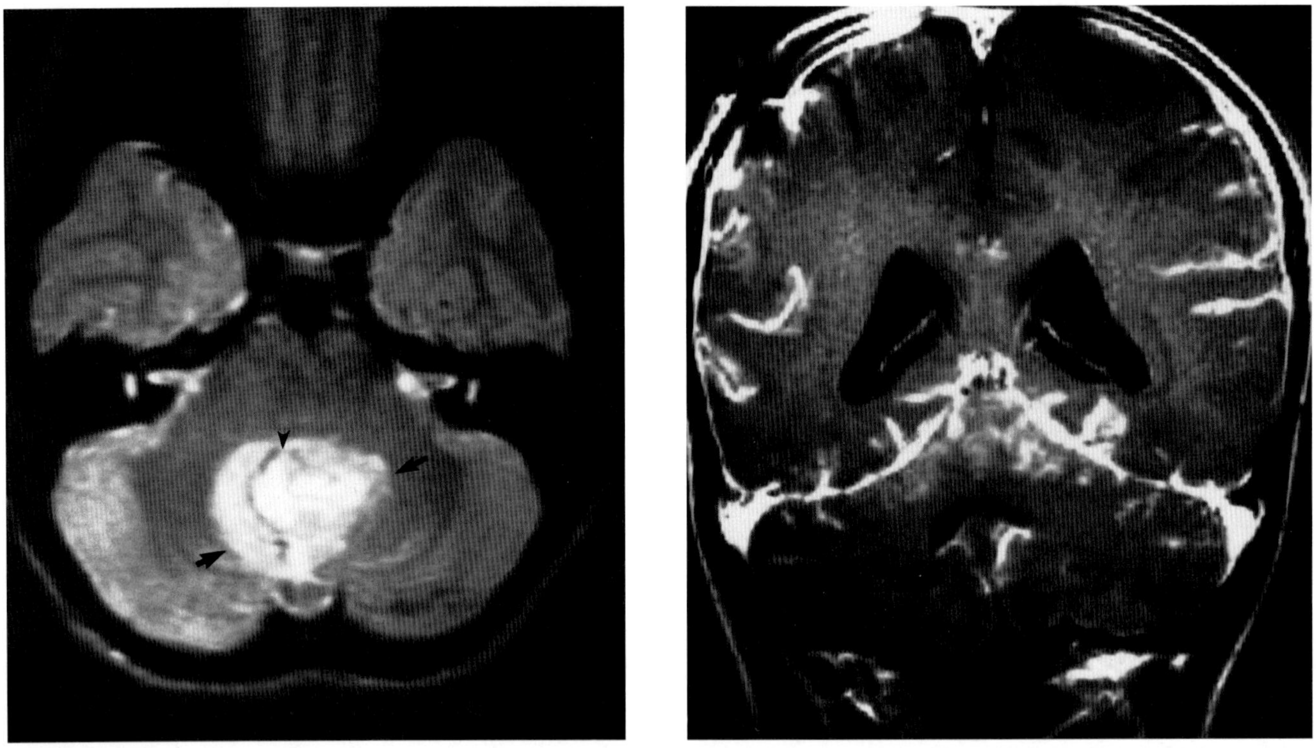

A B

Figure 3.4

Primitive neuroectodermal tumor – medulloblastoma.

A T2-weighted image in an 8-year-old female reveals a midline mass of inhomogeneous signal intensity in the posterior fossa. The outer rim of abnormal signal intensity corresponding to tumor tissue (arrows) is isointense to just slightly hyperintense to cortex. The central region of high signal intensity partially edged in low signal intensity (arrowhead) corresponds to focus of intratumoral hemorrhage.

B Coronal T1-weighted image after gadolinium administration in a 14-year-old male 2 years after primary tumor resection and radiotherapy demonstrates diffuse meningeal enhancement around both cerebral hemispheres and the cerebellum and along the margin of the 4th ventricle, consistent with widespread subarachnoid tumor seeding.

On MR, this tumor's appearance is less specific.[31] It sometimes may be seen to arise from the inferior medullary velum and/or appear as a relatively hypo- to iso-intense mass on T2-weighted images (Figure 3.4A) due to its unusually dense cellularity and high nuclear to cytoplasmic ratio. These are diagnostically helpful signs. It can sometimes appear simply as an enhancing midline vermian mass, iso- or hyperintense on T2-weighted images, much like the solid cerebellar (vermian) astrocytoma. Given this tumor's relative predilection for subarachnoid dissemination, when there is evidence of such tumor spread, the diagnosis of PNET-MB can be made with more certainty. Likewise, when there is evidence of hemorrhage within the mass (Figure 3.4A), it is more likely to be a PNET-MB than an astrocytoma. Occasionally, PNET-MB arises off the midline, in the cerebellar hemisphere. In this location the tumor has often been described as being 'desmoplastic',[34] a variant seen in older children and young adults.

Post-operatively, patients routinely undergo staging evaluation of the spinal canal with enhanced MR and/or myelography. Extraneural metastases (e.g. to bone, or lymph nodes) can occur, but are rare.[35] Consequently, the routine use of bone scans and bone marrow as staging procedures is not recommended.

Prognostic criteria for stratifying patients into poor-risk and average-risk categories have been developed.[22] Poor-risk patients are those who at diagnosis:

- have signs of tumor dissemination,
- are less than 4 years of age,
- have a tumor greater than 3 cm in size,
- have a tumor with features of histologic differentiation.

The standard treatment for all patients greater than 3 years of age consists of surgery and craniospinal radiotherapy at the time of diagnosis. This results in 5-year disease-free survival rates of approximately 60% in children with PNET-MB considered as a single group, and even higher rates in patients who fit the criteria of being at average risk. Due to the potentially damaging effects (adverse neuropsychologic and endocrinologic sequelae) of high-dose radiotherapy on the developing CNS, reduced radiotherapy dose, delayed administration and/or employment of adjuvant chemotherapy are frequently employed treatment options in children of less than 3 years of age.

The PNET-MB may recur at the primary site and/or disseminated within the subarachnoid space (Figure 3.4B). In their series, Zimmerman et al[31] observed tumor recurrence in some of their patients relatively early in the risk period (this being, according to Collin's Rule of Recurrence for Embryonic Tumors, a period equal to the age of the patient at diagnosis plus 9 months for gestation). This indicates that follow-up imaging studies (MR) for assessment for possible recurrence should begin shortly after treatment and be continued during the period of risk. Re-examination is warranted every 4–8 months, the frequency determined by the stage of the patient's tumor.

Cerebellar astrocytoma

The incidence of the cerebellar astrocytoma is just slightly less than that of the PNET-MB in most series of pediatric posterior fossa neoplasms. The most commonly used classification method distinguishes between the juvenile pilocytic astrocytoma (JPA) and the diffuse fibrillary type, which is more commonly associated with anaplastic change.[36–38] The JPA constitutes the vast majority of pediatric cerebellar astrocytomas and generally runs a benign course, being associated with a 25-year survival rate of approximately 90%. The rarer and less easily resectable diffuse fibrillary type more commonly occurs in the adolescent and young adult population and frequently runs a more aggressive clinical course, being associated with a 25-year survival rate of approximately 40%.

The cerebellar astrocytoma may have an acute or, more commonly, a subacute clinical presentation related to obstructive hydrocephalus and increased intracranial pressure. Over half are grossly cystic, most commonly with a mural nodule. The remainder are solid, generally with a necrotic center; a minority are completely solid. Over 80% arise within the vermis, with variable extension into adjacent cerebellar hemisphere. When grossly cystic, the tumor generally has a characteristic appearance on CT and MR (Figure 3.5).[31,39] The solid astrocytoma is frequently less specific in its appearance on MR, but on CT it is generally distinguishable from the other midline vermian mass, PNET-MB, by its hypodensity before contrast administration. The solid component of the JPA invariably enhances, while that of the fibrillary type is more variable in its enhancement, depending upon the degree of malignancy and relative deficiency in the blood–brain barrier. It is useful to look for signs of brain-stem invasion since, if present, they forewarn the surgeon that complete excision is not possible.

Post-operatively, appropriate imaging strategies depend upon the histologic findings in the tumor. The usual patient is one with JPA, who, at our institute, undergoes an early post-operative CT or MR to assess for residual tumor so that, if necessary, re-operation with total gross resection can be performed.[40] No additional treatment measures are offered in these cases under present-day regimens. Those cases with the rarer, fibrillary type of neoplasm, depending upon the degree of anaplasia, may undergo staging evaluation of their spinal canals. Generally, these patients also receive additional treatment in the form of either radiotherapy or chemotherapy. The frequency of follow-up imaging studies to assess for possible recurrence will, likewise, depend upon the tumor histology; for JPA, for example, this is approximately every 6 months for the first 2 years and yearly thereafter for several years, while the frequency is appreciably greater for those patients with potentially more aggressive tumors.

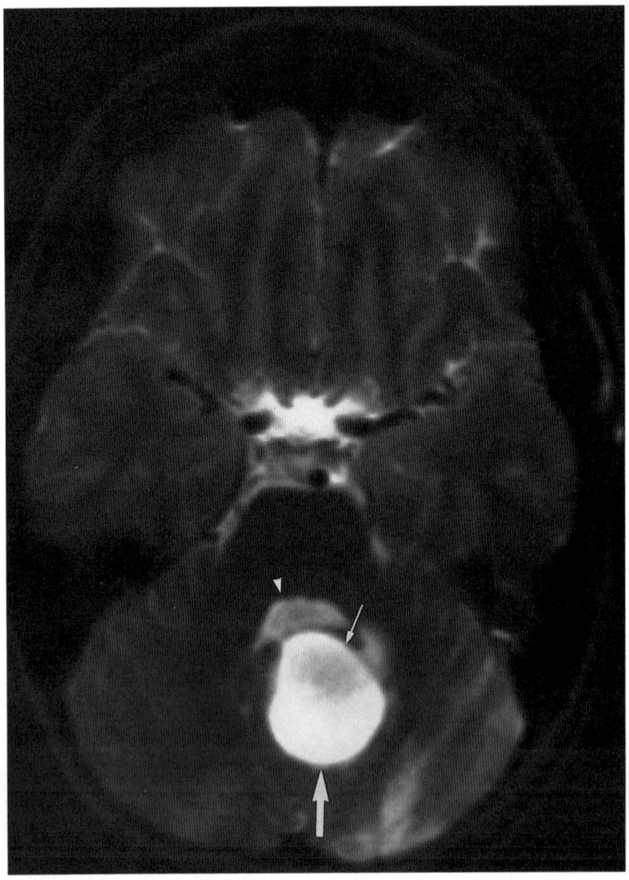

Figure 3.5

Cerebellar astrocytoma. This axial T2-weighted image reveals a vermian mass, with solid eccentric mural nodule (small arrow) and cystic component (large arrow), which is characteristically of even higher signal intensity than CSF; compare with CSF in the 4th ventricle (arrowhead).

Brain-stem glioma

The brain-stem glioma comprises 10–25% of pediatric CNS neoplasms.[41] As a group, prognosis is poor, there being at best a 5-year survival rate of only approximately 30%. However, differences with regard to histology, as well as with regard to location of the tumor and certain morphologic and radiographic characteristics, have recently been noted to be useful in distinguishing tumor subgroups in order to aid in refinement of prognosis as well as in tailoring treatment strategies; for example, tumors located in the midbrain are typically more benign histologically, enhance like other pilocytic variants and have a significantly better prognosis than the more common non-enhancing fibrillary type of pontine neoplasm.[42,43] Current imaging techniques generally permit diagnosis and treatment based on radiologic findings alone. Surgery is reserved for those tumors with atypical radiographic features[41] or with a large exophytic component amenable to debulking.

Brain-stem gliomas generally present with multiple cranial nerve palsies and long-tract signs; about a third of cases present with signs of increased intracranial pressure from associated hydrocephalus. A screening examination using CT may reveal either a hypodense or isodense mass enlarging the brain-stem; frequently the mass demonstrates no contrast enhancement.[44] Its mass effect upon the 4th ventricle and basilar cisterns may be helpful signs in its identification.[44] However, given the potential subtleties of its appearance on CT as well as the beam-hardening artifacts in the posterior fossa, MR is the modality of choice for defining these neoplasms (Figure 3.6). MR more accurately determines tumor location – critical for distinguishing tectal gliomas from pineal tumors, for example – and extent.[7,45] Histologically, the tumor may be the diffuse fibrillary type (80% of cases), which is highly susceptible to anaplastic change, or the pilocytic type (20% of cases); neither is generally associated with much edema. At the Children's Hospital of Philadelphia, the radiation portal is defined by a 2 cm margin around the tumor margins, calculated from sagittal T2-weighted images. Radiotherapy is the only proven effective treatment in these patients, though tumor response is only temporary in the majority of cases (the potential benefits of employing hyperfractionated radiotherapy and using adjuvant chemotherapy are presently under investigation).[7]

Follow-up MR examinations are performed 6–8 weeks after completion of radiotherapy, unless the clinical course is complicated in the interval. Brain-stem gliomas vary in their response: some may transiently disappear, while others progress. Most commonly, a partial response is seen, evidenced by a decrease in the area of abnormal signal intensity and associated mass effect. Post-treatment complications such as hemorrhage and cyst formation may be seen. Serial follow-up examinations are performed every 4–10 months.

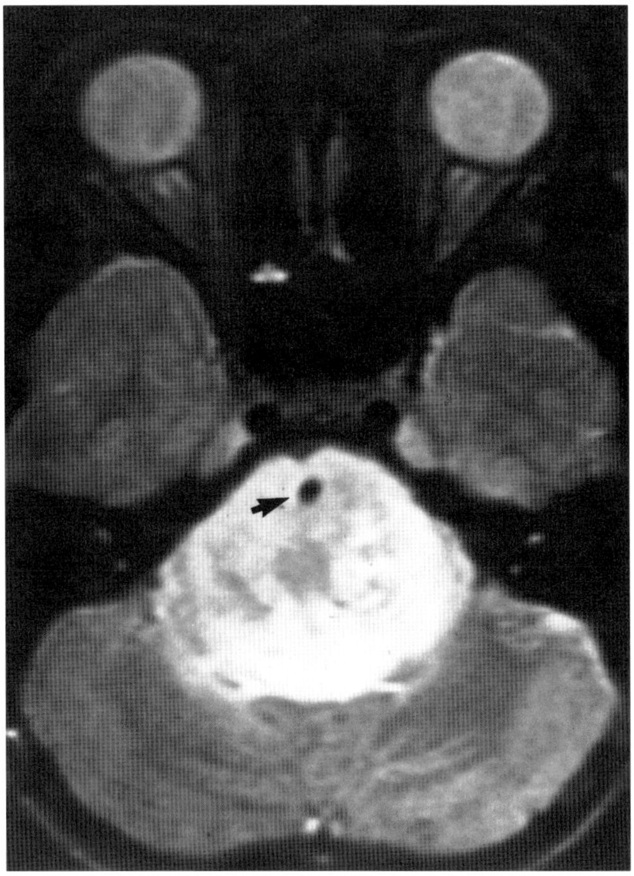

Figure 3.6

Brain-stem glioma. This axial T2-weighted image demonstrates large pontine mass slightly inhomogeneous in signal intensity; note encasement of the basilar artery (arrow) by the tumor mass.

Smith et al[7] have recently noted that the findings on these later examinations typically correlate well with clinical evaluation, though occasionally tumor progression on MR may precede clinical deterioration. Documenting tumor progression, for example, as increasing tumor bulk or new enhancement in a previously non-enhancing tumor, suggesting anaplastic degeneration, may permit more timely institution of adjuvant chemotherapy.

Other neoplasms

Limited space does not permit detailed discussion here of the remainder of the neoplasms arising within the pediatric CNS. However, important issues relating to imaging strategies in the management of several of them will be briefly described.

First of all, aside from differences in clinical presentation and surgical resectability related to differences in location, the imaging algorithms for astrocytomas of the cerebral hemispheres (the most common supratentorial tumors in children) are similar to those used for cerebellar tumors. Related tumors are the gangliogliomas, which are benign, slow-growing neoplasms that occur relatively frequently in the second decade of life, presenting most commonly with seizures.[46,47] Though they may be located anywhere within the brain parenchyma, typically they are manifest as small well-circumscribed lesions with minimal mass effect and no edema, located peripherally in a cerebral hemisphere (temporal and occipital lobes, most commonly), sometimes associated with overlying bony erosion.[48] They may be isodense (Figure 3.1) or hypodense on CT,[48] and of low to mixed signal intensity on T1-weighted and high signal intensity (Figure 3.1) on proton-density and T2-weighted MR images. Calcification and small cysts are frequently associated. Treatment is exclusively surgical. Given that many of the tumors fail to enhance, yearly post-operative imaging evaluation is best effected with MR, its greater contrast resolution being more sensitive in depicting the mass effect that distinguishes recurrence from scar.

Ependymomas are another relatively common neoplasm which may develop in the pediatric CNS, arising from ependymal rests in either the posterior fossa (60–80% of cases) or in the cerebral hemispheres.[49–52] Within the former, the masses typically 'insinuate' along CSF pathways, while supratentorially they typically develop in a completely intraparenchymal location. They vary widely in their radiologic features. On CT, they may be isodense or hypodense, and variably enhancing, with or without associated cysts and calcification.[53] On MR, they are characterized by their heterogeneity.[31] There is some predilection for dissemination,[50,54] thus warranting radiologic staging. In addition, these tumors are typically hypervascular.[52] Occasionally, such hypervascular tumors present acutely with intracranial hemorrhage. The parenchymal hematoma may be all that is visible radiographically. Consequently, in

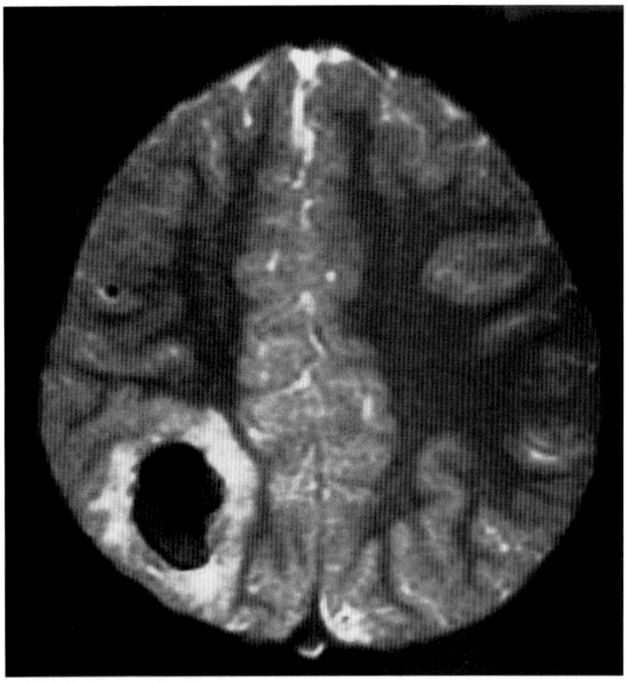

A

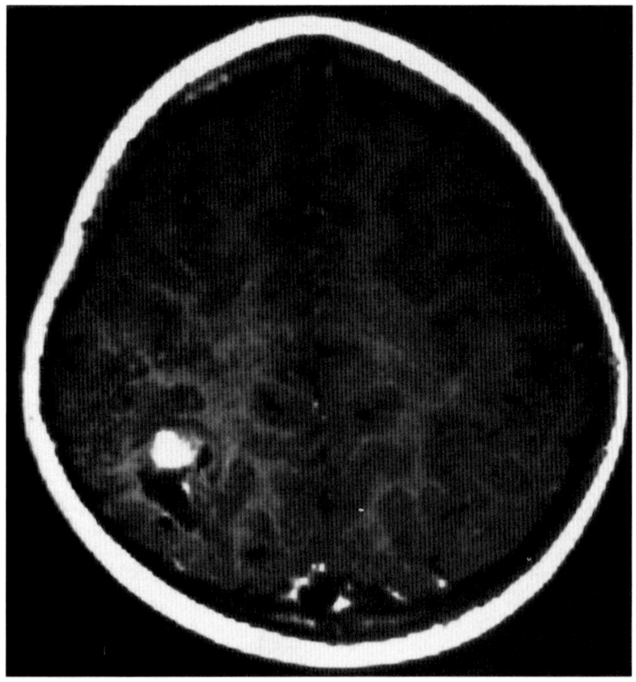

C

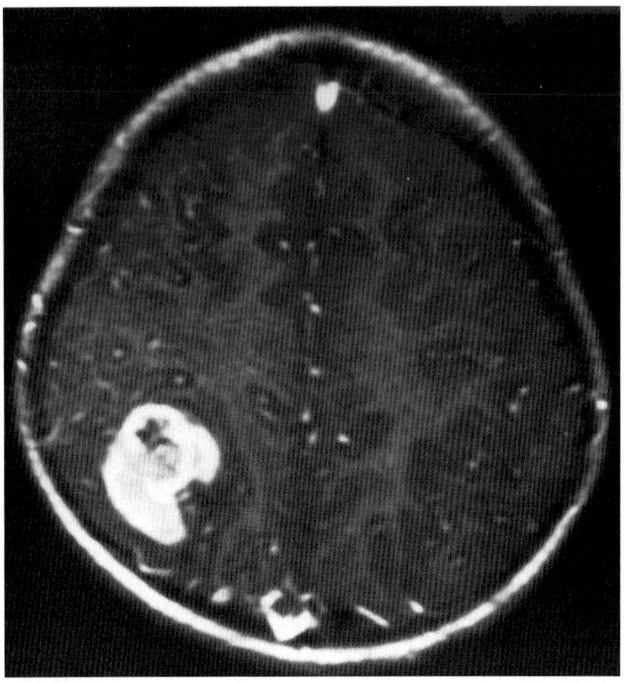

B

Figure 3.7

Parenchymal hemorrhage as a presenting sign of neoplasm (ependymoma).

A Axial T2-weighted MR image reveals lobulated focus of low signal intensity, corresponding to acute blood products (deoxyhemoglobin and intracellular methemoglobin) surrounded by high signal intensity of edema.

B The post-gadolinium T1-weighted image failed to demonstrate region of enhancement separable from high signal intensity hematoma (methemoglobin).

C On a follow-up examination 2 months after clot had evolved, a nodule of enhancement is visible along the anterior margin of the site of previous bleed, consistent with neoplasm (surgically proven ependymoma).

Figure 3.8

Spinal cord astrocytoma. Pre- (**A**) and post-gadolinium (**B**) sagittal T1-weighted images through the thoracic spine demonstrate enhancing soft tissue (arrows) within the substance of the cord, associated with a cyst (arrowheads) extending cranially and caudally (the entire length of the cord, which is not shown).

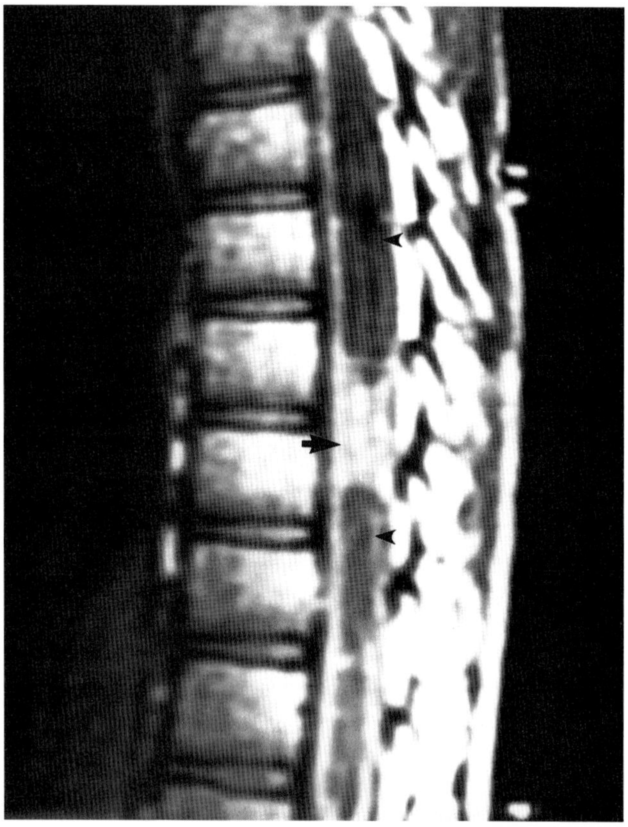

A

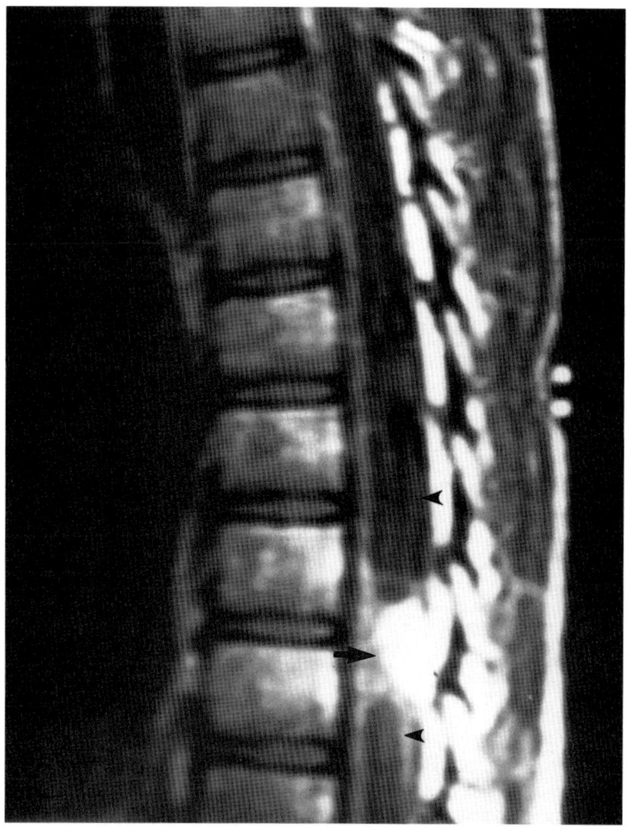

B

cases of unexplained hemorrhage, follow-up MR examination should be obtained 1–2 months later (sometimes serially) as the hematoma resolves in order to assess for a possible underlying lesion, for example, tumor (Figure 3.7) or vascular malformation.[55] Other tumors prone to hemorrhage are the oligodendroglioma, malignant glioma, choriocarcinoma and occasionally, the primitive neuroectodermal tumor.

The suprasellar/parasellar region is a common location for mass lesions in the pediatric population (for example, craniopharyngioma, Rathke's cleft cyst, germinoma, epidermoid, arachnoid cyst, hypothalamic/chiasmatic glioma and hamartoma of the tuber cinereum).[56–65] Imaging findings are frequently, though not invariably, diagnostic. Treatment of many of these lesions is controversial due to the complexity of surgery in this location as well as the potentially negative side-effects of radiotherapy. For screening, diagnostic evaluation and follow up of these tumors, MR is the method of choice. A caveat, however, is that CT may be a useful complement in the follow up of craniopharyngiomas, since it is more sensitive in the detection of calcification, which may be the first sign of this tumor's recurrence.

Metastases to the brain parenchyma from extracranial primaries are uncommon in the pediatric population. When they occur, they arise most frequently from a sarcoma or hepatoma and have a typical radiographic appearance. More commonly observed, however, is involvement of the skull and meningeal coverings by metastatic disease – neuroblastoma[66] and occasionally Ewing's sarcoma.

Finally, neoplastic involvement of the spinal canal and cord is usually a secondary phenomenon due to either the 'drop' metastases already mentioned or to the extradural extension of neuroblastomas, ganglioneuromas or sarcomas arising in the paravertebral area.[67] Intradural extramedullary neoplasms (e.g. neurofibroma, meningioma) are extremely rare except in patients with neurofibromatosis types 1 and 2.[56] Intramedullary neoplasms comprise less than 10% of the primary neoplasms arising in the pediatric CNS. Approximately two-thirds of spinal cord tumors are low-grade astrocytomas, the remainder being ependymomas, malignant gliomas and, occasionally, ganglioneuromas and oligodendrogliomas. MR is the pre- and post-operative imaging modality of choice (3–4 mm sagittal proton-density and T2-weighted images, as well as sagittal 3 mm and axial 3–5 mm T1-weighted images before and after gadolinium administration). The tumors may have a cystic component that is small or very extensive. Gadolinium-enhanced images are best for delineating the solid component of the tumor, which may or may not be subtle (Figure 3.8).[67,68] For this reason, these images are likewise critical for the complete evaluation of any unexplained cystic cavity within the cord, since they may reveal it to be due to an underlying neoplasm.

In conclusion, it is apparent that imaging strategies for pediatric CNS tumors vary significantly depending upon tumor type, location, idiosyncracies of tumor behavior and the treatment complications that they may develop. Given the diversity of such factors, only the general principles of such strategies have been offered here.

References

1. Farwell JR, Dohrmann GH, Flannary JT, Central nervous system tumors in children, *Cancer* (1977) **40:**3123–32.
2. Naidich TP, Zimmerman RA, Primary brain tumors in children, *Semin Roentgenol* (1984) **19:**100–14.
3. Atlas SW, Grossman RI, Hackney DB et al, Calcified intracranial lesions: detection with gradient-echo acquisition rapid MR imaging, *AJNR* (1988) **9:**253–9.
4. Segall HD, Batnitzky S, Zee C et al, Computed tomography in the diagnosis of intracranial neoplasms in children, *Cancer* (1985) **56:**1748–55.
5. Kucharczyk W, Brant-Zawadski M, Sobel D et al, Central nervous system tumors in children: detection by magnetic resonance imaging, *Radiology* (1985) **155:**131–6.
6. Lee BP, Kneeland JB, Cahill PT et al, MR recognition of supratentorial tumors, *AJNR* (1985) **6:**871–8.
7. Smith RR, Zimmerman RA, Packer RJ et al, Pediatric brainstem glioma: post-radiation clinical and MR follow-up, *Neuroradiology* (1990) **32:**265–71.
8. Zimmerman RA, Bilaniuk LT, Schut L et al, Medical imaging of pediatric brain tumors, *Prog Exp Tumor Res* (1987) **30:**61–80.
9. Sperling MR, Wilson G, Engel J et al, Magnetic resonance imaging in intractable partial epilepsy: correlative studies, *Ann Neurol* (1986) **20:**57–62.
10. Theodore WH, Dorwart R, Holmes M et al, Neuroimaging in refractory partial seizures: comparison of PET, CT and MRI, *Neurology* (1986) **36:**750–9.
11. Bird CR, Drayer BP, Medina M et al, Gd-DTPA-enhanced MR imaging in pediatric patients after brain tumor resection, *Radiology* (1988) **169:**123–6.
12. Cohen BH, Bury E, Packer RJ et al, Gadolinium-DTPA enhanced magnetic resonance imaging in childhood brain tumors, *Neurology* (1989) **39:**1178–83.
13. Felix R, Schorner W, Laniado M et al, Brain tumors: MR imaging with gadolinium-DTPA, *Radiology* (1985) **156:**681–8.
14. Graif M, Bydder GM, Steiner RE et al, Contrast-enhanced MR imaging of malignant brain tumors, *AJNR* (1985) **6:**855–62.
15. Powers TA, Partain CL, Kessler RM et al, Central nervous system lesions in pediatric patients: Gd-DTPA-enhanced MR imaging, *Radiology* (1988) **169:**723–6.
16. Zimmerman RA, Gusnard DA, Bilaniuk LT, Gadolinium-DTPA enhanced MR evaluation of pediatric brain tumors. In: Bleyer A, Packer RJ, Pochedly C eds, *New trends in pediatric neuro-oncology* (Raven Press: New York, 1990).
17. Earnest F IV, Kelly PJ, Scheithauer BW et al, Cerebral astrocytomas: histopathologic correlation of MR and CT contrast enhancement with stereotactic biopsy, *Radiology* (1988) **166:**823.
18. Johnson PC, Hunt SJ, Drayer BP, Human cerebral gliomas: correlation of postmortem MR imaging and neuropatholigic findings, *Radiology* (1989) **170:**211–17.
19. Enzmann DR, Tokye KC, Hayward R, CT in leptomeningeal spread of tumor, *J Comput Assist Tomogr* (1978) **2:**448–55.
20. Sze G, Soletsky S, Bronen R et al, MR imaging of the cranial meninges with emphasis on contrast enhancement and meningeal carcinomatosis, *AJNR* (1989) **10:**965–75.
21. George RE, Laurent JP, McCluggage CW et al, Spinal metastases in primative neuroectodermal tumors (medulloblastoma) of the posterior fossa: evaluation with CT myelograpgy and correlation with patient age and tumor differentiation, *Pediatr Neurosci* (1985–86) **12:**157–60.

22. Packer RJ, Sutton LN, D'Angio G et al, Management of children with primitive neuroectodermal tumors of the posterior fossa/medulloblastoma, *Pediatr Neurosci* (1985–86) **12:**272–82.
23. Sze G, Abramson A, Krol G et al, Gadolinium-DTPA in the evaluation of intradural extramedullary spinal disease, *AJNR* (1988) **9:**153–63.
24. Zeltzer PM, Friedman HS, Norris DG et al, Criteria and definition for response and relapse in children with brain tumors, *Cancer* (1985) **56:**1824–6.
25. Curness JT, Laster DW, Ball MR et al, Magnetic resonance imaging of radiation injury to the brain, *AJNR* (1986) **7:**389–94.
26. Dooms GC, Hecht S, Brant-Zawadski M et al, Brain radiation lesions: MR imaging, *Radiology* (1986) **158:**149–55.
27. Tsuruda JS, Kortman KE, Bradley WG et al, Radiation effects on cerebral white matter: MR evaluation, *AJNR* (1987) **8:**431–7.
28. Ball WS, Prenger EC, Ballard ET, Neurotoxicity of radio/chemotherapy in children: pathologic and MR correlation, *AJNR* (1992) **13**:761–76.
29. Schwartz RB, Carvalho PA, Alexander E III et al, Radiation necrosis vs. high-grade recurrent glioma: differentiation by using dual-isotope SPECT with ^{201}TI and ^{99m}Tc-HMPAO, *AJNR* (1991) **12**:1187–92.
30. Rorke LB, The cerebellar medulloblastoma and its relationship to primitive neuroectodermal tumors, *J Neuropath Exp Neurol* (1983) **42:**1–15.
31. Gusnard DA, Cerebellar neoplasms in children, *Semin Roentgenol* (1990) **25:**263–78.
32. Sandhu A, Kendall B, Computed tomography in management of medulloblastomas, *Neurorad* (1987) **29:**444–52.
33. Zimmerman RA, Bilaniuk LT, Pahlajani H, Spectrum of medulloblastomas demonstrated by computed tomography, *Radiology* (1978) **126:**137–41.
34. Russell DS, Rubenstein LJ, *Pathology of tumors of the nervous system*, 5th edn (Williams & Wilkins: Baltimore 1989) 251–79.
35. Arseni C, Ciurza AV, Statistical survey of 276 cases of medulloblastomas (1935–1978), *Acta Neurochir* (1982) **57:**159–62.
36. Lee Y, Van Tassel P, Bruner JM et al, Juvenile pilocytic astrocytomas: CT and MR characteristics, *AJNR* (1989) **10:**363–70.
37. Russell DS, Rubenstein LJ, *Pathology of tumors of the nervous system*, 5th edn (Williams & Wilkins: Baltimore 1989) 95–111.
38. Steinberg GK, Shuer LM, Conley FK et al, Evolution and outcome in malignant astroglial neoplasms of the cerebellum, *J Neurosurg* (1985) **62:**9–17.
39. Zimmerman RA, Bilaniuk LT, Bruno L et al, Computed tomography of cerebellar astrocytoma, *AJR* (1978) **130:**929–33.
40. Sutton LN, Current management of low-grade astrocytomas of childhood, *Pediatr Neurosci* (1987) **13:**98–107.
41. Reigel DH, Scarff TB, Woodford JE, Biopsy of pediatric brain stem tumors, *Child's Brain* (1979) **5:**329–40.
42. Albright AL, Guthkelch AN, Packer RJ et al, Prognostic factors in pediatric brainstem gliomas, *J Neurosurg* (1986) **65:**751–5.
43. Kun LE, Barkovich AJ, Krischer J et al, Correlation of MR imaging and outcome following hyperfractionated irradiation in brainstem gliomas: a three-center study. Presented at International Symposium Pediatric Neuro-oncology, Philadelphia, 1990.
44. Bilaniuk LT, Zimmerman RA, Littman P et al, CT of brainstem gliomas, *Radiology* (1980) **14:**89–95.
45. Packer RJ, Zimmerman RA, Luerssen TG, Brainstem gliomas of childhood: magnetic resonance imaging, *Neurology* (1985) **35:**397–401.
46. Demierre B, Stichnoth FA, Hori A et al, Intracerebral ganglioglioma, *J Neurosurg* (1986) **65:**177–82.
47. Sutton LN, Packer RS, Rorke LB et al, Cerebral gangliogliomas during childhood, *Neurosurgery* (1983) **13:**124–8.
48. Zimmerman RA, Bilaniuk LT, Computed tomography of intracerebral gangliogliomas, *CT: J Comput Tomogr* (1979) **3:**24–30.
49. Centeno RS, Lee AA, Winter J et al, Supratentorial ependymomas: neuroimaging and clinicopathological correlation, *J Neurosurg* (1986) **64:**209–15.
50. Kun LE, Kovner EH, Sanford RA, Ependymomas in children, *Pediatr Neurosci* (1988) **14:**57–63.
51. Liu HM, Boggs J, Kidd J, Ependymomas of childhood. I. Histological survey and clinicopathological correlation, *Child's Brain* (1976) **2:**92–110.
52. Russell DS, Rubenstein LJ, *Pathology of tumors of the nervous system*, 5th edn (Williams & Wilkins: Baltimore 1989) 192–219.
53. Swartz JD, Zimmerman RA, Bilaniuk LT, Computed tomography of intracranial ependymomas, *Radiology* (1982) **143:**97–102.
54. Salazar OM, Castro-Vita H, VanHoutte P et al, Improved survival in cases of intracranial ependymoma after radiation therapy. Late report and recommendations, *J Neurosurg* (1983) **59:**652–9.
55. Atlas SW, Grossman RI, Gomori JM et al, Hemorrhagic intracranial malignant neoplasms: Spin-echo MR imaging, *Radiology* (1987) **164:**71–7.
56. Braffman BH, Bilaniuk LT, Zimmerman RA, MR of central nervous system neoplasia of the phakomatoses, *Semin Roentgenol* (1990) **25:**198–217.
57. Fletcher WA, Imes RK, Hoyt WF, Chiasmal gliomas: appearance and long-term changes demonstrated by computed tomography, *J Neurosurg* (1986) **65:**154–9.
58. Hahn FJ, Leibrock LG, Huseman CA et al, The MR appearance of hypothalamic hamartoma, *Neuroradiology* (1988) **30:**65–8.
59. Jenkin RDT, Simpson WJK, Keen CW, Pineal and suprasellar germinomas, *J Neurosurg* (1978) **48:**99–107.
60. Kucharczyk W, Peck WW, Kelly WM et al, Rathke cleft cysts: CT, MR imaging, and pathologic features, *Radiology* (1987) **165:**491–5.
61. Packer RJ, Bilaniuk LT, Cohen BH et al, Intracranial visual pathway gliomas in children with neurofibromatosis, *Neurofibromatosis* (1988) **1:**212–22.

62. Pusey E, Kortman KE, Flannigan BD et al, MR of craniopharyngiomas: tumor delineation and characterization, *AJNR* (1987) **8:**439–44.
63. Rao KCVG, Fitz CR, Harwood-Nash DC, Craniopharyngiomas in children: neuroradiological evalution, *Rev Inter-Am Radiol* (1977) **2:**149–57.
64. Young SC, Zimmerman RA, Nowell MA et al, Giant cystic craniopharyngiomas, *Neuroradiology* (1987) **29:**468–73.
65. Zimmerman RA, Bilaniuk LT, Dolinskas CA, Cranial CT of epidermoid and congenital fatty tumors of maldevelopmental origin, *CT: J Comput Tomogr* (1979) **3:**40–50.
66. Zimmerman RA, Bilaniuk LT, Computed tomography of primary and secondary craniocerebral neuroblastoma, *AJNR* (1980) **1:**431–4.
67. Zimmerman RA, Bilaniuk LT, Imaging of tumors of the spinal canal and cord, *Radiol Clin N Am* (1988) **26:**965–1007.
68. Parizel PM, Balériaux D, Rodesch G et al, Gd-DTPA-enhanced MR imaging of spinal tumors, *AJNR* (1989) **10:**249–58.

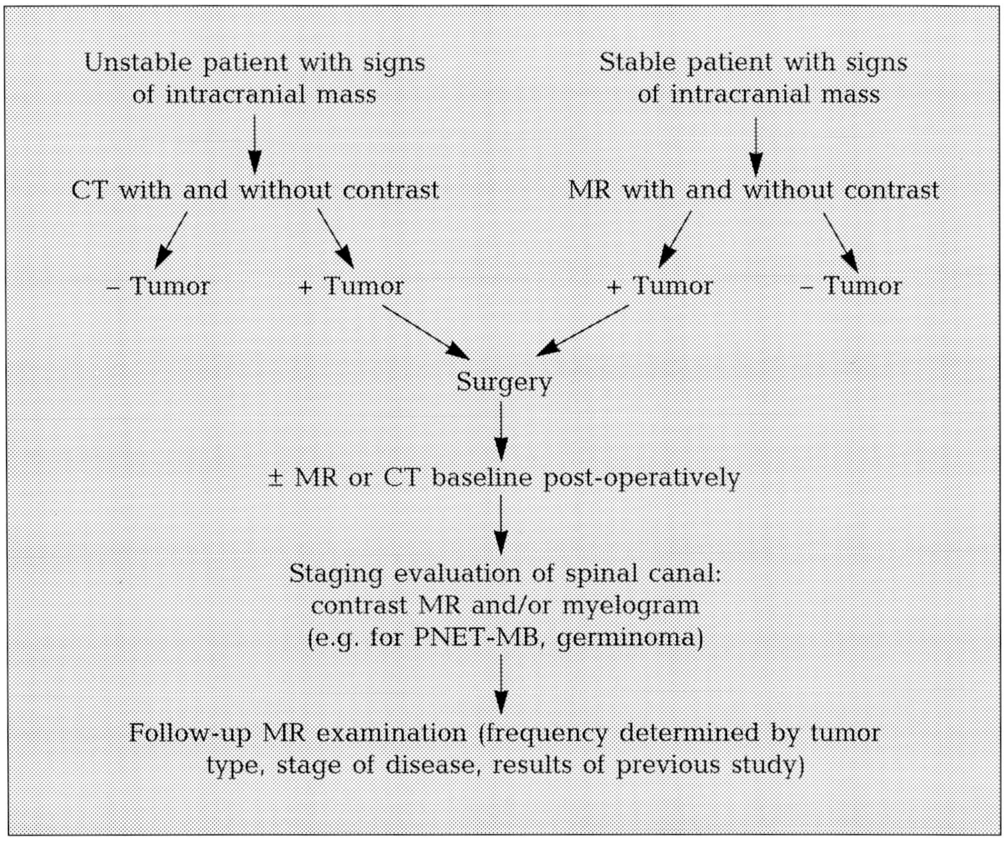

Diagram 3.1

Outline of imaging strategies of tumors of the pediatric central nervous system. PNET-MB, primitive neuroectodermal tumor–medulloblastoma.

4

The ear, nose and throat

Thomas Vogl and Stefan Dresel

Introduction

The diagnostic evaluation of the head and neck has undergone revolutionary changes in the past few years due to the introduction of CT scanning and MR imaging. The variety of methods available and their increased complexity necessitate new approaches to the imaging strategy and treatment planning for ear, nose and throat (ENT) tumors.

In imaging petrous bone and skull-base neoplasms, the use of high-resolution CT and MR has provided the radiologist with the unique opportunity to strengthen dialogue with otologic surgeons and neuro-otologists. The two new modalities have completely replaced polytomography. It has to be said, however, that CT scanning and MR imaging of the temporal bone, like so many types of radiologic imaging, involve careful physical monitoring if they are to be effective. Several further technical advances have been made, including direct sagittal CT and special MR techniques.

The complex pattern of spread of disease in the nasopharynx and paranasal sinuses, usually involving soft tissue and bony structures, requires an imaging method that reveals both tissue types well. New advances in MR have proved that its superior resolution in soft tissue depicts tumor margins in the nasopharynx and related spaces more accurately than does CT. Thus MR has remarkably improved our ability to diagnose lesions in this area, and with the introduction of paramagnetic contrast medium, the advantages of MR imaging might increase even further.

The radiologist plays an important role in choosing the best diagnostic and therapeutic approach for masses of the salivary glands. With the help of CT, ultrasonography or MR, decisions can be made by analyzing location, size and character of masses in both submandibular and parotid glands. Recently published data show that plain MR is superior to CT in the diagnosis of lesions in the parotid gland because MR provides better soft-tissue contrast and does not generate artifacts caused by metallic implants. Paramagnetic contrast is helpful in differentiating benign and malignant lesions.

The oropharynx, oral cavity and larynx are relatively accessible to the examining physician; the role of both CT and MR is to define the extent to which a disease has spread into the deep surrounding soft tissues.

Epidemiology and clinical science

Whereas there are no risk factors known for developing tumors of the petrous bone such as acoustic neuromas and glomus tumors, epidemiologic studies show squamous-cell carcinomas of the head and neck to be related to carcinogens, in particular human papillomaviruses (HPV) and tobacco use. The present evidence indicates that HPV has an etiologic role in at least an undefined subset of upper gastrorespiratory tract cancers. Although the accumulated data regarding the role of HPV in benign and malignant lesions is limited in terms of case numbers, the pattern of type specificity to particular lesion sites demands attention. It appears, nevertheless, that the presence of HPV is not limited to the lesion site: HPV is present in clinically and histologically normal epithelium in patients with recurrent respiratory papilloma, genital lesions and oral carcinoma.

The precise roles of cofactors such as tobacco, derivatives, irradiation, tissue trauma, coinfections and host immune factors invite investigation. The issue of spontaneous regression of benign and malignant lesions also requires clearer clinical documentation.

Many head and neck cancers may be regarded as the diseases associated with exposure to tobacco. If the latency period of carcinogenesis is allowed, the patterns of pharyngeal and laryngeal cancer incidence seem to be closely associated with lifelong consumption of cigarettes and reflects the dominant influence of tobacco in the etiology of the disease. The risk of cancer in long-term smokers of filter cigarettes is considered to be less than that for smokers of non-filter cigarettes. It has to be said, however, that the trends for buccal cavity cancer in males do not correlate well with reported changes in smoking prevalence. Interpretation of trends is further complicated by the synergistic role of alcohol in the etiology of these cancers, as well as the etiologic importance of chewing tobacco and snuff.

Patients diagnosed with an initial head and neck cancer incur extremely high risks of developing subsequent secondaries, particulary in tobacco-exposed epithelial tissues and especially if they continue to smoke. This pattern reflects epithelial susceptibility to carcinogenic activity and is highly site-specific. The risk is constant over time. Data suggest lower risks of metachronous lesions in patients who cease smoking.

Tumors of the face and nasopharynx are different. The male/female sex ratio is 2 : 1 instead of 10 : 1 for the other locations. Tobacco and alcohol play no role. Tumors do not occur in other locations during follow up. Adenocarcinomas of the face are frequent in workers on wood, a very long time after exposure (often more than 30 years). Undifferentiated carcinomas of the nasopharynx are very frequent in Southeast Asia (they are the most frequent cancers in Singapore) and North Africa; they occur at any age, even in young patients, and there is a history of infection by the Epstein–Barr virus.

The spectrum of head and neck pathology is wide and spans from the facial skull, rhinobasis (frontal portion of skull base) and otobasis (medial portion of skull base), to tumors of the esophagus and of the trachea. The clinically relevant basics are presented here in five topographically interesting regions.

Skull base and cerebellopontine angle

The diagnosis and differentation of neoplasms of the base of the skull and the posterior fossa has been improved significantly by the development of audiologic testing and new imaging techniques. The differential diagnosis includes several possibilities related to pathology in the region of the petrous bone. Pathology may arise from the temporal bone, the mastoid process and its communicating structures, such as the jugular vein, cranial nerves and meninges.

The acoustic neuroma is histologically a benign neoplasm, which arises from Schwann cells of the neurilemma of the main branches of the vestibular nerve. It has its origins at the junction of the peripheral ganglionic neurilemma and the brainstem neuroglia. Acoustic neuromas are divided according to site of origin into lateral, for example as tumors growing in the internal acoustic canal, mediolateral and medial tumors.[1]

The multitude of symptoms is produced by the pressure the tumor exerts on neighboring nerve structures.[2] The first functional deficits are to be expected in the vestibular and cochlear part of the 8th cranial nerve, because most tumors arise in the internal acoustic meatus.[3] Hence, early diagnosis of acoustic neuroma and other neoplasms in the cerebellopontine angle is an important interdisciplinary task for otoneurology and radiology.[2] Objective clinical symptoms of these tumors are general vestibular symptoms and a retrocochlear hearing loss. In advanced stages, symptoms due to compression of neighbouring structures, such as facial and abducens-nerve pareses, as well as symptoms of brainstem compression may also arise. The clinical diagnosis relies mainly on audiometry and vestibular tests. In spite of specific neuro-otologic and neuroradiologic examination methods, the diagnostic accuracy for small tumors was unsatisfactory before the introduction of MR.[3,5] Pre-operatively, however, accurate delineation of the neoplastic structure is indispensable.[2,6]

Tumors of the glomus jugulare are second most common in the region and originate from chemoreceptors (glomera) which can have numerous localizations throughout the human body.[7,8] Histologically, the tumors show precapillary arteriovenous shunts with a collection of non-chromaffin chemoreceptor cells. Most frequently, the glomera in the bulbus venae jugularis are affected, as well as the tympanic plexus and the bifurcation of the carotids.[9] The glomus tumors at the base of the skull are located in the region of the glossopharyngeal nerve extension (glomus tympanicum, jugulare and vagale). In pre-operative diagnosis of these tumors, determination of the exact topographical situation and the degree of vascularization is of importance. The clinical symptomatology of these tumors is diverse and depends on the localization of the neoplastic structure in the petrous part of the skull base.[10] Additionally, the existing of primary and secondary bone tumors, plasmocytomas and meningiomas must be taken into consideration when examining lesions in the petrous part. Infrequently, dermoid cysts, eosinophilic granulomas and other neoplastic structures may arise.

Nasopharynx and face

Of all malignant tumors of the head and neck region, 5% arise in the nasopharynx, of which 90% prove to be carcinomas on histological examination.[11] The most frequent type of malignant tumor in the nasopharynx is squamous-cell carcinoma. Lymphomas are more frequent in children. A characteristic of squamous-cell carcinomas is the early and extensive lymphatic metastasis.

Benign tumors in the nasopharynx are rare, the most numerous being the juvenile angiofibroma of the nasopharynx.[12] Although this fibroma is histiologically benign, clinically it behaves in a malignant manner due to its expansive growth.

Mesenchymal tumors are mostly represented in the group of the benign tumors of the nose and the nasal sinuses.[11] They are made up of papillomas, hemangiomas, fibromas and other rare tumors. The tumors originating in the intranasal mucosal membranes and the nasal sinuses make up less than 1% of all malignant neoplasms.

Histologically, the gross collective can be divided into squamous-cell carcinomas (60%), adenocarcinomas (20%), differentiated carcinomas (10%) and mesenchymal neoplasms (5%).[13]

Usually, the endoscopic findings are available when imaging is performed.

Salivary glands

The salivary glands may be divided into the parotid, submandibular and sublingual glands. Epithelial tumors represent 90% of all salivary gland neoplasms. The remaining 10% are composed of non-epithelial neoplasms, such as hemangiomas, lymphangiomas, periglandular tumors and malignant lymphomas.[14] Of the benign epithelial tumors, 85% are pleomorphic or monomorphic adenomas. Cystadenolymphomas (Warthin's tumor) and other tumors are less common. Malignant tumors develop in 25–30% of all tumors of the salivary glands and often show a typical symptomology with swelling, pain, firm infiltration and facial paresis. Of parotid lesions, 85% are benign, but 50% of the submaxillary lesions only. Histologically, acinus-cell tumors are found in 15% of all cases and mucoepidermoid tumors in 30%.[15] Carcinomas show a wide spectrum of histologies: adenoid cystic carcinomas (35%), adenocarcinomas (10%), squamous-cell carcinoma (10%) and other rare tumors.

Oropharynx and oral cavity

In spite of the fact that benign tumors occur rarely, all forms of neoplasms can occur in the region of the oropharynx and the oral cavity. Common epithelial benign neoplasms are papillomas, keratocarcinomas and adenomas. Congenital tumors are usually the hemangioma, lymphangioma and the goiters in the base of the tongue.[6,16] The vast majority of malignant tumors in the oral cavity and the oropharynx are squamous-cell carcinomas, rarely anaplastic carcinomas.[17] In the development of carcinomas in the oral cavity there are very few symptoms. Inspection, palpation and endoscopy are important in clinical diagnosis. Imaging methods are required to determine the exact extension in depth and infiltration into neighboring structures.

Hypopharynx, larynx and cervical soft tissue

Malignant tumors of the hypopharynx most frequently originate in the piriform sinus, less frequently on the posterior wall of the pharynx.[17] In over 40% of all cases the primary symptom of these tumors is a regional metastasis of laterocervical lymph nodes. Malignant tumors of the larynx show characteristic clinical findings, especially when they originate from the glottis level. Malignant carcinoma of the larynx is the most frequent among the head and neck tumors, representing 45%.[6,18] Laryngoscopy lays the base for decisions regarding operation, radio- or chemotherapy.

Table 4.1 **Tumor classification for squamous-cell carcinoma (ARA criteria)**

TX	The minimum requirements to assess primary tumor not met
TO	No evidence of primary tumor
T_{is}	Preinvasive carcinoma (carcinoma in situ)
T1	Tumour ≤2 cm in greatest dimension
T2	Tumor >2 cm, but not >4 cm in greatest dimension
T3	Tumor >4 cm in greatest dimension
T4	Tumor >4 cm in greatest dimension with extension to bone, muscle, skin, antrum or neck
NX	Regional lymph nodes cannot be assessed
NO	No regional lymph node metastasis
N1	Metastasis in a single ipsilateral lymph node, ≤3 cm in greatest dimension
N2a	Metastasis in a single ipsilateral lymph node, >3 cm, but not >6 cm in greatest dimension
N2b	Metastases in multiple ipsilateral lymph nodes, none >6 cm in greatest dimension
N2c	Metastases in bilateral or contralateral lymph nodes, none >6 cm in greatest dimension
N3	Metastases in a lymph node >6 cm in greatest dimension

Imaging techniques such as CT and MR have established themselves for the assessment of the primary tumors and the involvement of lymph nodes.

The classification of squamous-cell carcinomas related to the ARA criteria (TNM stages) is seen in Table 4.1.

Imaging modalities

Conventional radiography

Since the introduction of conventional radiography at the turn of the century a remarkable development in radiographic diagnosis of the skull and the pneumatic sinuses has taken place. The barium swallow is still the first diagnostic tool in patients with problems in swallowing. Conventional radiography has partly maintained its significance; conventional tomography has, however, disappeared from routine diagnosis. Dental films and orthopantography are still very useful for studying the maxilla and mandible. Anteroposterior (AP) and lateral views of the chest are mandatory in initial evaluation and follow up. CT of the chest may be useful if plain films are equivocal.

Angiography

The angiographic modalities are important non-invasive supplements to imaging classification of intensely vascularized processes and for vascular lesions in the head and neck region.[19,21] Conventional angiography has been replaced almost totally by digital subtraction angiography (DSA) in the last 5 years.[22] Intravenous DSA has not proved effective for the determination of vascular processes in the petrous part of the temporal bone and the facial skull. The reason for this lies in the simultaneous presentation of all craniocervical vessels and in the high susceptibility of this method to movement-induced artifacts. Arterial DSA has numerous advantages over conventional angiography: higher contrast resolution, higher picture frequency and the possibility of immediate reproduction of subtraction images through digital processing. Before a planned embolization, arterial DSA permits the precise analysis of the morphologic structure and the complex hemodynamic and angioarchitectural relations of vascular lesions and strongly vascularized tumors.[21] In spite of low complication rates in arterial DSA of the head and neck region, there still remain risks because of its invasiveness. Therefore, it should only be used when other interventional techniques are necessary, and not in routine diagnostic evaluation of neoplastic processes. With the establishment of arterial and venous MR angiography in the clinical routine, the numbers of angiographic examinations will continue to decrease.

Ultrasonography

The development of ultrasonography of the head and neck region took place in great leaps. Currently, ultrasound is used for different problems: in the craniocervical region as A-image sonography for the paransal sinuses, and as B-image sonography for the facial soft-tissue structures, salivary glands and cervical soft-tissue structures.[23] Sonographic examination of other regions, for example the larynx, the hypopharynx and the pharynx,[24] are in the experimental stage.

Radionuclide studies

Gallium scanning is useful in evaluating inflammatory conditions. Bone scan is applied in patients with a high risk of bone metastases (carcinomas of the nasopharynx, for instance).

Computed tomography

CT has allowed an obvious improvement of the local evaluation and follow up. The technical requirements are:

- small fields of view, less than 24 cm,
- 512 × 512 pixels matrix,
- reconstruction filter for soft tissues,
- double windows, for bone and soft tissues,
- slice thickness of 5 mm as routine, 1 mm for details.

Contrast-medium injection is almost always used, at high dose, to improve the contrast between the tumor, inflammatory reactions and normal tissues, to determine the vascularity of a lesion, to distinguish normal vessels from pathology (especially lymph nodes). When needed, two perpendicular planes (axial and coronal) are used (face, nasopharynx, oropharynx); three-dimensional reconstructions are available on recent equipment.

Magnetic resonance imaging

Technical requirements are:

- a small field of view, using a head coil or a surface coil,
- 256 × 256, or 192 × 256 pixels matrix
- a slice thickness of between 3 and 7 mm
- at least two perpendicular planes are acquired, sometimes three.

MR angiography, three-dimensional Fourier transformation and fat suppression techniques may be useful. There are usually T1, proton density and T2 acquisitions. Contrast medium is often used to increase the contrast between the tumor and inflammatory reactions, to decrease the acquisition time and to visualize perineural and meningeal extensions.

Comparison of computed tomography and magnetic resonance imaging

There is some competition between CT and MR. The choice depends on the location of the tumor and the state of the patient.

CT is more widely available, examination is faster and the patient experiences less claustrophobia than with MR. The acquisition time is much faster on CT, so motion artifact is rarely a real problem; this is especially true for the pharyngolarynx.

CT is simpler to perform and to interpret. Spatial resolution is usually better on CT, so bone and cartilage are usually better studied. CT shows calcifications better than MR. CT is especially efficient for detecting metastases in nodes, as hypodensity is well seen, and the whole neck is easily studied.

The main advantages of MR are the very high contrast, and the choice of the axis of the slices. The high contrast is especially helpful in differentiating tumor from inflammatory reactions (especially retention in a sinus) on T2-weighted sequences. Differentiating tumor from old fibrosis is also possible, but distinguishing between tumor and young inflammatory reaction is not usually possible. MR is very sensitive but not specific for the extension to the brain, the dura and along the nerves. MR is not as efficient as CT in detecting small bone lesions, although the changes of the fatty marrow are much easier to see on T1-weighted sequences. Again the distinction between tumor and inflammatory changes of the marrow is impossible to make. Nevertheless, MR has a number of advantages: it uses no ionizing radiation, imaging in any plane is possible and flow-sensitive procedures are available. There are some contraindications, however.

In summary, a choice between CT and MR must be made, the two techniques both being used only in rare selected cases. The technology of MR still is improving fast, and it is definitely better for the nasopharynx and face, and probably the salivary glands. CT probably remains the better technique for the pharyngolarynx and cervical nodes.

Imaging strategies and results

The main goal of imaging techniques is not usually lesion detection, which is conducted clinically and by endoscopy, nor is it diagnosis, which is made by biopsy, but it is instead mainly to define the extension of a lesion. Spread beneath intact mucosa is not visible to the endoscopist. Deep spread may be palpable but is difficult to evaluate precisely. For example, the extension of a tumor of oropharynx to the tongue-base muscles is often difficult to determine clinically, and easy to diagnose on CT or MR: it makes a probable T2 tumor a T4.

On CT the tumor is a mass which usually enhances after contrast medium is added. Some central hypodensities may represent necrosis. Inflammatory reactions around the lesion may enhance too, so the size of the tumor may be overestimated. On T2-weighted MR sequences, the signal of the tumor, although variable, is usually lower than that of inflammatory reactions. The tumor usually enhances on T1-weighted sequences after injection of contrast medium.

In the follow up, the detection of recurrences may be very difficult clinically as inflammatory reactions may hide the tumor and recurrences may be deep or under the mucosa. The main problem is to differentiate treatment-induced reactions from recurrences. This is usually impossible during the first 3 months after treatment, especially radiation therapy, because inflammatory reactions, as well as active tumor, may take up contrast medium. So the baseline examination should not be obtained sooner. Radio-induced changes give poorly limited, hypodense lesions on CT, heterogenous lesion on T2-weighted MR, or T1-weighted MR with contrast. After 6 months, if there is a mass taking contrast medium, it is usually a recurrence.

Temporal bone and skull base

Acoustic neuroma

In the primary diagnosis protocol, the clinical examination remains of paramount importance, as does the performance of neuro-otological examinations [audiology, evoked response audiometry (ERA), vestibular test].[25,26] Although conventional radiography (Schüller's and Stenvers's projection) provides the radiologist with low-specificity information, it can easily identify processes, especially in the area of the middle ear.[27]

So far, examination of the temporal bone has mostly been based on the use of CT, in some cases combined with air cisternography for intracanicular tumors. This technique, however, is limited in usefulness by a high ratio of false-positive findings, ranging between 5 and 12%.[28, 29] The high rate of false positives is often caused by structural anomalies, for example soft-tissue adhesions, arachnoidal cysts and abnormalities of the arachnoidal vessels, such as aneurysms or ectatic slings of the inferior cerebellar artery.[30]

The primary use of MR for tumorous masses within the internal auditory canal, the vessel nerve bundle and the cerebellopontine angle (Figure 4.1) is recommended because of the lack of invasiveness as well as the low costs in comparison to CT with air cisternography.[31,32] In MR, the demarcation of tumorous expansion is improved due to the superior soft-tissue contrast and the lack of signal by surrounding osseous structures. For optimal results, an appropriate head coil or a surface coil with a small diameter using a variable slice thickness have to be available. The results of several studies show that the sensitivity of MR, especially for intracanicular acoustic neuroma, can clearly be increased by the application of contrast medium.

Diagnostic results with the fast imaging technique and dynamic series over 7 minutes after application of contrast medium improve the diagnostic information concerning the differentiation of the lesions.

Classification

According to the clinical as well as the MR classification, three types of acoustic neuromas have to be differentiated. Type 1 represents the lateral, and intrameatally localized acoustic neuroma.[33] The area between gliacytes and Schwann cells of the superior vestibular nerve is the origin of this growth form. Type 2 represents the mediolateral, intra- and extrameatal tumor, the most frequent form in our own series (Figure 4.2). Type 3 represents the strictly medial type (extrameatal), which does not expand within the internal auditory canal and primarily originates from the nerve bundle in the cerebellopontine angle. The variable types of acoustic neuromas and their location with reference to the pyramid apex and the internal auditory canal allow an exact classification and differential diagnosis by the use of MR.

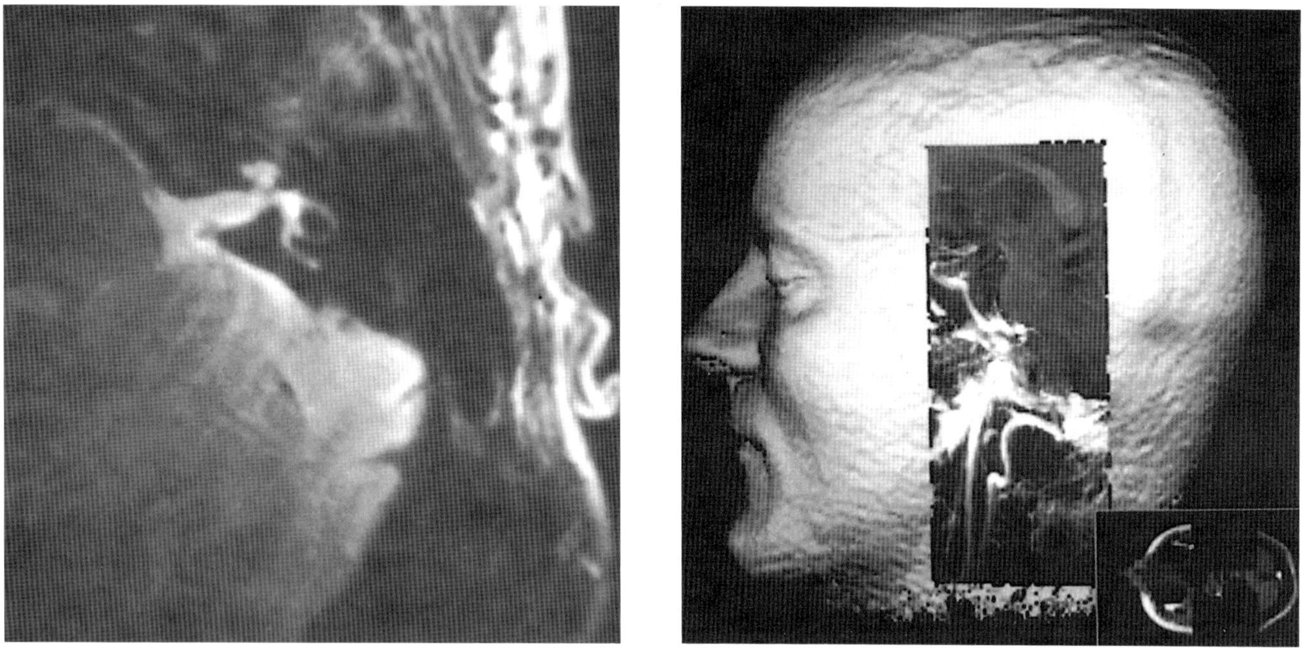

A B

Figure 4.1

Temporal bone.

A Axial MR (TR/TE = 2500/90). In the T2-weighted sequence the normal topographical relationship in the cerebellopontine angle and the middle skull base is illustrated. Note the high signal intensity of the cerebrospinal fluid.

B Three-dimensional MR, ray tracing reconstruction, magnetization-prepared rapid-acquisition gradient-echo (MPRAGE) sequence. In a sagittal reconstruction, the image demonstrates a normal topographic relationship of the intracranial and skull-base vessel structures. Due to the flow phenomenon the internal carotid artery and the vertebral artery are demonstrated via high signal intensity.

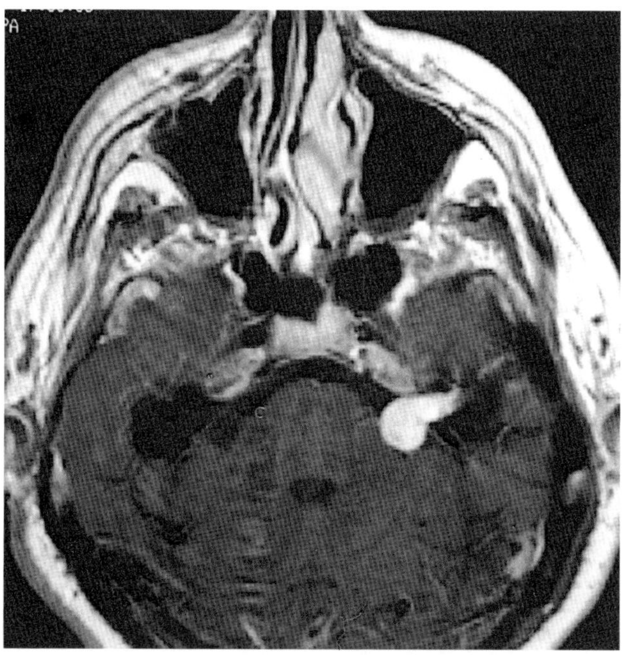

Figure 4.2

Acoustic neuroma. Transverse MR (TR/TE = 500/17) with contrast medium injection. Intra- and extracanalicular acoustic neuroma is demonstrated on the contrast-enhanced image. There is no evident compression of the brain stem.

Imaging appearance
Regularly the acoustic neuroma shows a comparable signal intensity to the brain parenchyma in T1-weighted sequences. Regressive changes of tumors, such as necrosis, show up as intratumoral areas of lower signal intensity. Recent or earlier hemorrhages are visualized as hyperintense areas. The demarcation of fluid, pons and the cerebellum is achieved via T2-weighted sequences. The comparative analysis of T2 relaxation times yields small variations between acoustic neuromas and other tumors of this area.

The highest overall accuracy is achieved for the diagnosis of the acoustic neuroma after application of contrast medium, which causes a signal increase in the tumorous area. With this technique, a neuroma as small as a few millimeters can be proved. Another important criterion, the percentage increase in signal intensity, is calculated in an analysis of enhanced and non-enhanced T1-weighted sequences.

Glomus tumors

Among glomus tumors of the middle skull base, tympanic and jugular glomus tumors have to be differentiated. The high resolution of CT can demonstrate their relationship with the cervical soft tissue as well as intratympanic and intracranial expansion. In the majority of the cases, glomus tumors can be differentiated from other skull-base diseases by dynamic CT and the time–density profile,[34,35] or, more easily, by angiography.

CT examination leads to a relatively high rate of false-negative and false-positive results, especially if the initial CT is carried out after intravenous infusion of contrast agent.[36] Small tumors, especially those originating from the tympanic glomus, render the diagnosis more difficult because they only show up as hypodense areas without osseous destruction. MR, with its superior soft-tissue contrast, proves to be superior for the evaluation of these tumors; the imaging of flowing blood due to the flow phenomenon constitutes its main advantages. Unenhanced CT is often also very accurate.

Jugular glomus tumors
The topographic relationship of the carotid syphon and the jugular bulb can reliably be diagnosed using plain MR.[37] One is able to discern between a glomus tumor and a jugular bulb located more cranially. These tumors, as well as their extension into the jugular vein, can be diagnosed on coronal sections.[38] The previously performed retrograde phlebography of the jugular vein has thus been completely replaced by MR.

Tumors of more than 1.5 mm in diameter can be precisely diagnosed as to localization and size. These tumors show a characteristically unclear outline and variable vascularization.

In some patients with small glomus tumors, plain MR yields limited diagnostic information. Angiography confirms the diagnosis in questionable cases. The use of the fast imaging technique and the application of contrast medium may be worth trying in difficult cases.

In the majority of cases, optimal imaging with exact demarcation of the vascularized parts of the tumor is achieved by application of contrast medium. In some patients with large tumors, no additional information is obtained with contrast enhancement. In the comparative analysis of MR and CT, the diagnostic accuracy, the topographic orientation, and the demarcation of jugular and tympanic glomus tumors have been evaluated. Especially in processes with infiltration of the middle skull fossa, coherent mastoiditis and small tympanic glomus tumors, enhanced MR shows its superior diagnostic potential. All patients with glomus tumors of the skull base or the temporal bone should undergo an additional angiographic study with DSA or perhaps MR angiography (MRA). The evaluation of the vascular supply provides important additional information on the exact vascularization of the tumor as well as the hemodynamic situation of the circulus willisii.

The MR characteristics of glomus tumors are:

- localization in the middle skull base and the cerebellopontine angle without involvement of the vestibulocochlear nerve,
- unclear outline,
- high grade of vascularization,
- prolonged T2 times in relation to the white matter,
- rapid increase in signal intensity after application of contrast agent and decrease in signal intensity after 300 s (wash out effect).

Tympanic glomus tumor
The most frequent benign tumors of the middle ear are the tympanic glomus tumors (Figure 4.3). Originating from the medial osseous border of the middle ear, tympanic glomus tumors are localized in the innervation area of the tympanic branch of the glossopharyngeal nerve (Jacobson's nerve) and the auricular branch of the vagal nerve (Amald's

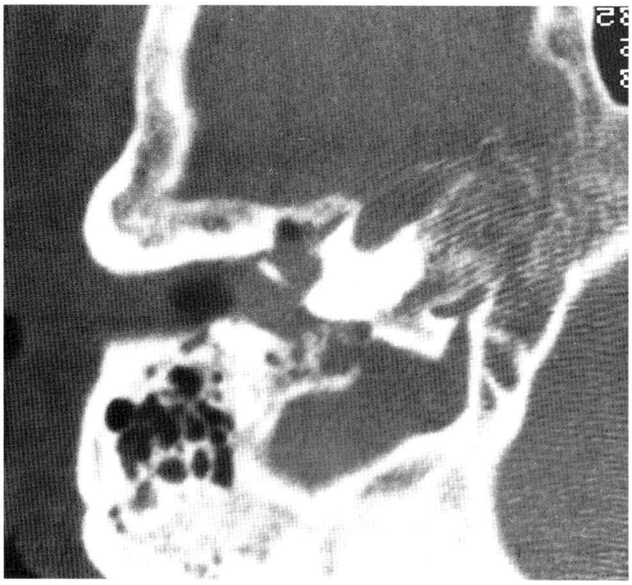

A

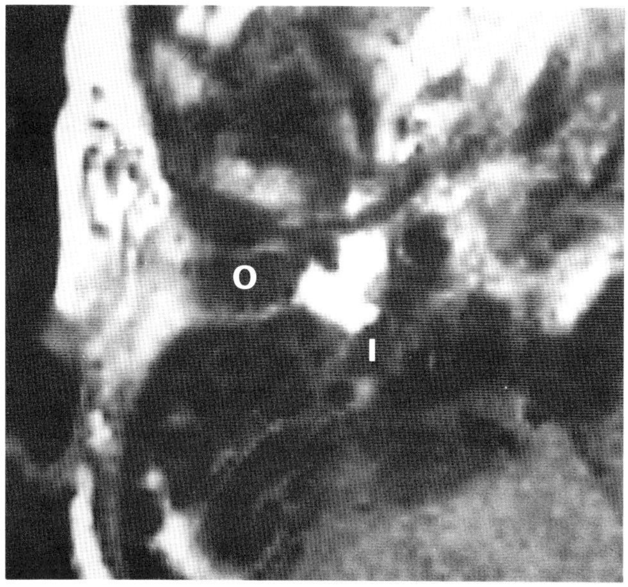

B

Figure 4.3

Tympanic glomus tumor: comparative evaluation of CT and MR with contrast medium injection.

A The contrast-enhanced CT scan in transverse orientation demonstrates a soft-tissue mass in the middle-ear cavity with some extension to the hypertympanic fossa. The mass is clearly located behind the tympanic membrane.

B On axial MR (TR/TE = 500/17) after contrast medium injection, the tumor demonstrates an enormous increase in signal intensity. Note the sharp border of the lesions and the exact demonstration of the extension within the middle ear and hypotympanic cavity. Note the neighboring structures, such as the outer ear canal (O) and the internal carotid artery (I).

nerve). These tumors are always clearly demarcated on MR and conform to the shape of the tympanic cavity by their rectilinear outline. Homogenous soft-tissue masses, they are located close to the cochlear promontorium as well as the carotid canal. The erosion of the cochlear promontorium, traceable on high-resolution CT, cannot be proved by MR.

The typical MR characteristics of tympanic glomus tumors are:

- localized in the tympanic cavity, adjacent to the cochlear promontorium or carotid canal,
- clear demarcation,
- homogenous signal intensity,
- high contrast agent uptake.

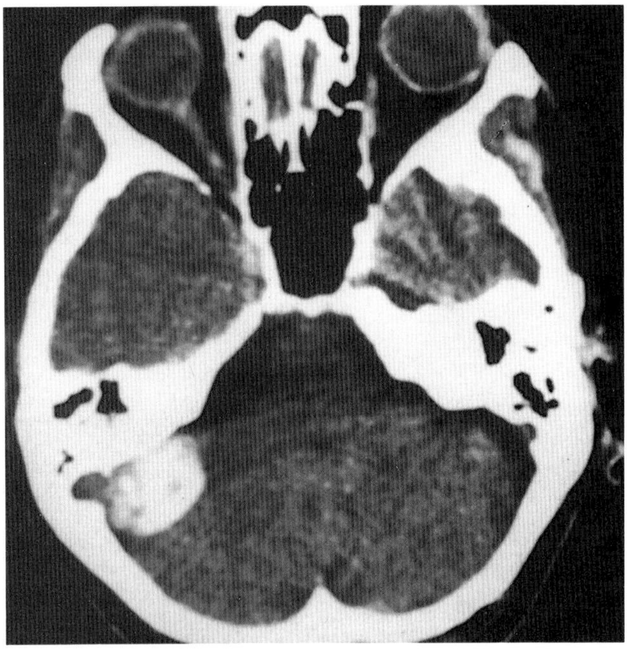

A

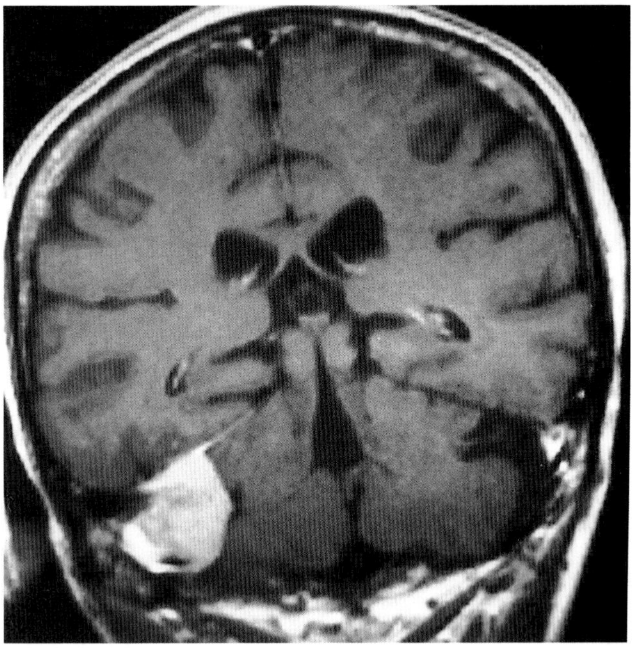

C

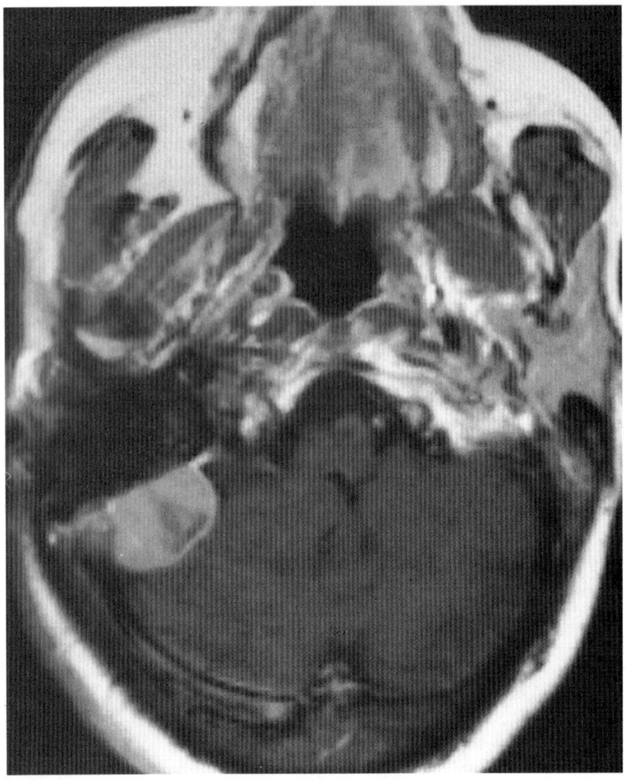

B

Figure 4.4

Meningeoma of the cerebellopontine angle: comparative analysis of CT and MR findings.

A The contrast-enhanced CT scan demonstrates a mass with high density growing along the posterior area of the pyramid apex.

B,C In gadolinium-enhanced MR (TR/TE = 500/17) in two slice orientations (axial and frontal) the exact topographic relationships of the meningeoma in the cerebellopontine angle are clearly demonstrated. Note the contrast enhancement of the adjacent dura. The structures of low intensity in the central part of the tumor are due to calcifications.

Other tumors of skull base

Primary tumors such as neuromas, meningeomas (Figure 4.4) and epidermoids originate from anatomic structures of the cerebellopontine angle and the internal auditory canal. In contrast to this, there are secondary tumors, extending from closely situated structures into the cerebellopontine angle and the internal auditory canal (jugular glomus tumors, chondromas, chordomas, cerebellar tumors, metastases and tumors of the hematopoietic system). The advantage of MR for evaluation of these tumorous lesions is its improved specificity and soft-tissue contrast as well as the facility to evaluate expansion of tumorous processes in all slice orientations. MR techniques yield useful information in the evaluation of these difficult tumorous lesions. As subtle lesions of bone are better seen on CT, a combination of CT and MR is often useful.

Diagnostic strategy

While in the primary stage of clinical testing, MR was rated as the only diagnostic instrument. Recently, specific use of this new imaging technique has been strongly recommended.[39–42] Because of the high diagnostic accuracy of this technique, a reliable evaluation of acoustic neuromas is achieved in an early stage.[43,44] This enables the surgeon to choose the transtemporal approach, which is less traumatic for the patient and improves the recurrence behavior of the tumor. In following primary and secondary tumors of the temporal bone, the cerebellopontine angle and the middle skull base, the following should be especially taken into consideration:

- *primary tumors:* neuroma, meningeoma, epidermoid;
- *secondary tumors:* glomus tumor, chondroma, chordoma, cerebellar tumors, metastases, plasmocytoma, osteoma.

Nasopharynx and paranasal sinuses

Malignant tumors of the nose and paranasal sinuses account for 0.2–0.8% of all malignancies; that is, there is one new case of maxillary sinus carcinoma diagnosed per 200 000 persons per annum. The majority (75%) of malignant tumors are squamous-cell carcinomas and adenocarcinomas. Malignant tumors of mesenchymal origin make up 15% of cases. In children, histiocytosis and rhabdomyosarcoma are observed quite frequently. Patients suffering from diseases of the nose, paranasal sinuses or nasopharynx can be examined by either indirect nasopharyngoscopy or direct flexible or rigid fiberoptic examination. The development of endoscopic devices has eased the early detection of small tumors of the nasopharynx. In case of impaired eustachian tube function or serious otitis media of unknown origin, a careful endoscopic evaluation of the nasopharynx is obligatory. Inflammatory diseases of the paranasal sinuses require ultrasonography or radiography.

In therapeutic planning for malignant tumors of the nose, paranasal sinuses and nasopharynx, it is essential to know about the extension of the lesion as well as the infiltration of the surrounding tissue. Due to the hidden localization of malignancies of the paranasal sinuses and nasopharyngeal space, tumors are often hard to detect by rhinoscopy or even endoscopy. Furthermore, it must be considered that a variety of tumors of the nasopharyngeal space occur in the submucosal tissue layer and will not be detected by rhinoscopic or endoscopic examination. MR has proved to be advantageous in documenting infiltrations. To improve the prognosis of these tumors, however, it is essential to establish a diagnosis as early as possible.

Squamous-cell carcinomas

Squamous-cell carcinomas of the nasopharynx originate at the lateral walls and particularly at the pharyngeal recess in 80% of cases. In almost all patients suffering from squamous-cell carcinomas, infiltration of the levator and tensor veli palatini muscles and destruction of the pharyngobasilar fascia are found (Figures 4.5 and 4.6). These tumors grow typically into the parapharyngeal space, the nasal cavity and the sinuses, and infiltrate the longus colli muscles dorsally.[45] Because of eustachian tube obstruction, 90% of these patients show fluid in the mastoid cells. Squamous-cell carcinomas can invade the sphenoid and cavernous sinuses and extend to the nasal cavity. Diffuse margins and necrotic areas are characteristic of these tumors. Low-intensity non-enhancing regions within the tumor mass often represent

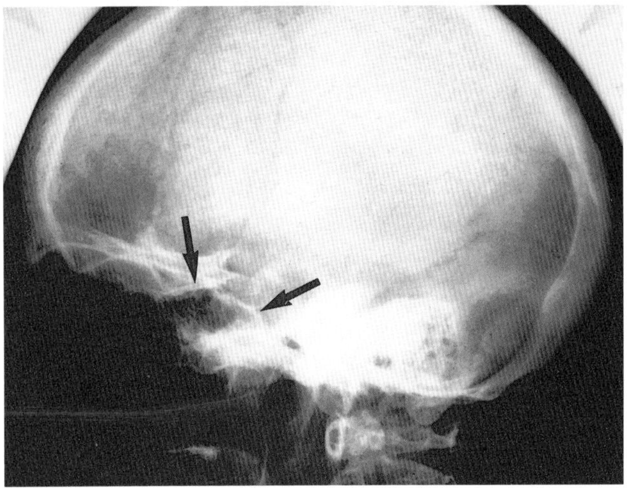

A

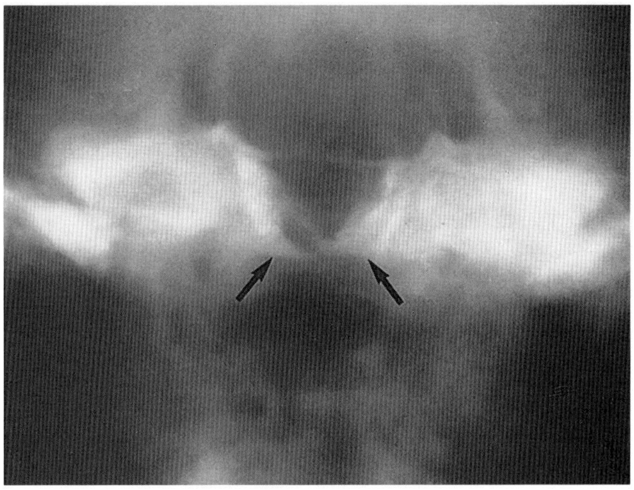

B

Figure 4.5

Squamous-cell carcinoma of the nasopharynx. Conventional radiography (**A**) and conventional tomography (**B**) show extended bony destruction on the bottom of the sphenoid sinus and the clivus. Soft-tissue lesion is demonstrated inside the sphenoid sinus (arrows).

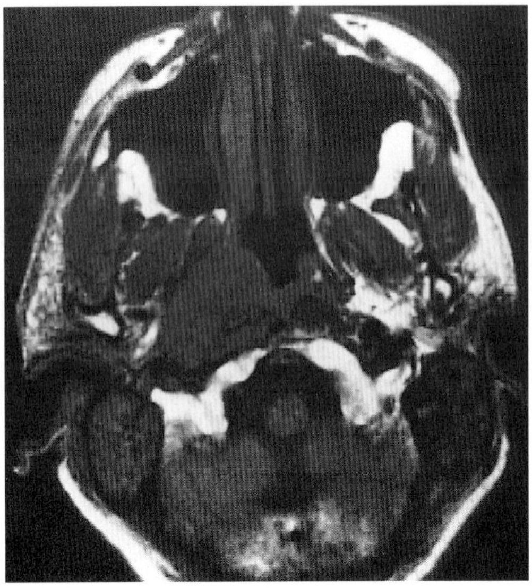

A

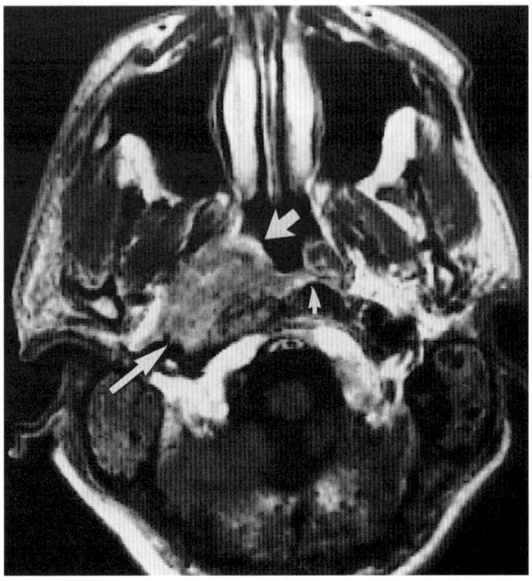

B

Figure 4.6

Squamous-cell carcinoma of the nasopharynx.

A Axial, plain MR (SE 500/25): right nasopharyngeal tumor of moderate signal intensity infiltrating the parapharyngeal space and the longus colli muscle. There is destruction of the antero-inferior portion of the right temporal bone and there is fluid in the mastoid cells. The tumor shows the same signal intensity as muscle. It can only be suspected that the tumor crosses the midline.

B Axial MR (SE 500/25) after contrast-medium injection: the tumor enhances inhomogeneously and less than the mucosa. There is infiltration and displacement of the sheath of the right carotid artery (long white arrow), of the longus colli muscle, torus tubarius, levator and tensor veli palatini muscle and of the pharyngobasilar fascia. There is also extension of the tumor to the right parapharyngeal space, with displacement of the pterygoid muscle. The midline has been crossed (small, white arrow), and there is infiltration of the left pharyngeal recess (thick, white arrow).

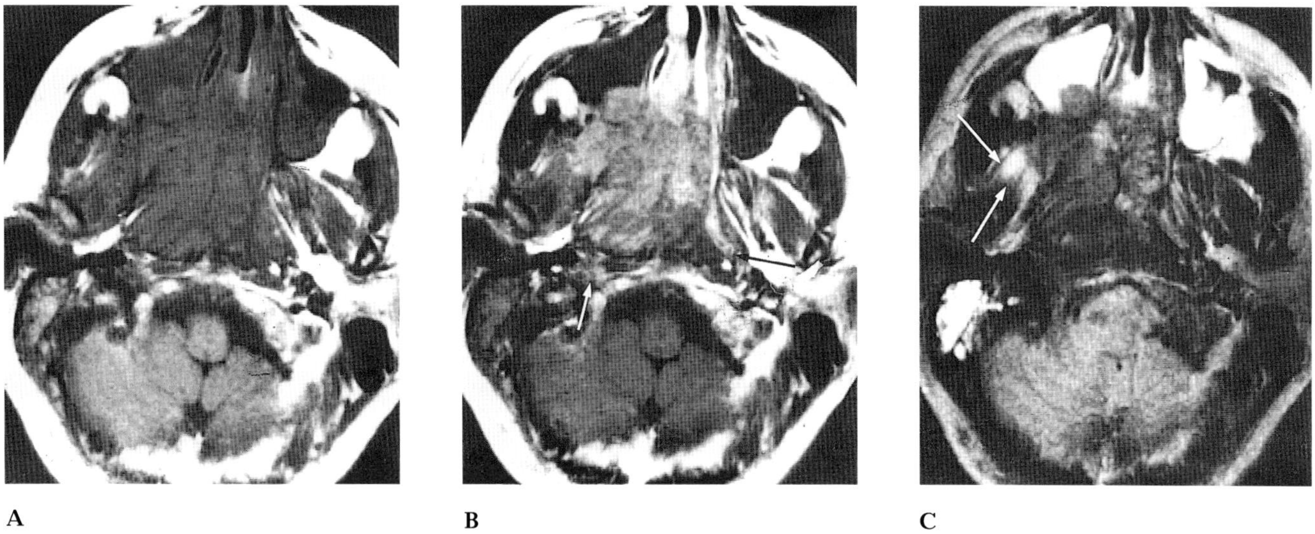

Figure 4.7

Squamous-cell carcinoma of the maxillary sinus.

A Axial, plain MR (SE 500/25): a large tumor has produced destruction of the posterior wall of the right maxillary sinus and has infiltrated the nasopharynx, parapharyngeal space and infratemporal fossa. The right pterygoid muscle appears infiltrated by tumor. Tumor shows low signal intensity and homogeneous pattern.

B Axial MR (SE 500/25) after contrast-medium injection: the tumor shows an increase in signal intensity in comparison to the fluid in the maxillary sinuses. In the anterior part of the nasal cavity, intact enhanced mucosa is identified. Tumor has destroyed the posterior part of the right maxillary sinus, the posterior part of the nasal cavity and the inferior aspect of the temporal bone (white arrow), and has infiltrated the prevertebral muscles. The middle third of the right lateral pterygoid muscle does not enhance as much as tumor (see **C**). The left parapharyngeal space and left pharyngeal recess appear uninvolved (black arrow).

C Axial, plain MR (SE 1600/90): the T2-weighted image allows good differentiation between tumor tissue and hyperintense fluid in the maxillary sinus. The middle third of the right pterygoid muscles shows high signal intensity (arrows), thought to represent edema at an edge of tumor. There is fluid in the mastoid sinus.

necrosis. A discrete crossing of the midline by the tumor can only be seen on the contrast-enhanced images, but might be suspected on the pre-enhanced images. In rare cases, tumor also invades the parotid space. Often the post-styloid compartment of the PPR is infiltrated, showing encasement and compression of the internal carotid artery. Additionally, involvement of cranial nerves 9–12 are seen, as well as extended lymph-node metastasis. Subtle extension of these tumors to the pterygoid muscles can be judged best in images with contrast-medium enhancement, because the signal intensity of squamous-cell carcinomas in the plain image is about the same as that of muscles. Calculation of the relaxation times gives moderate T1 and T2 values.[46] The exact delineation of the lesion is often only rendered possible by the application of contrast medium.[47]

The most frequent tumors of the nose and nasal sinuses are squamous-cell carcinomas of the maxillary sinuses (Figure 4.7). These lesions have a

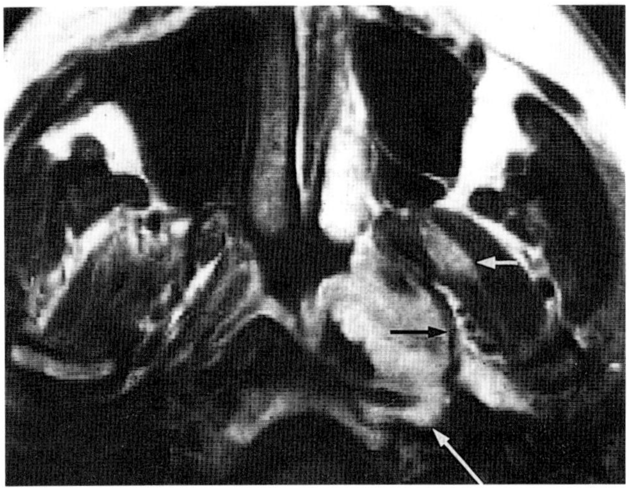

A

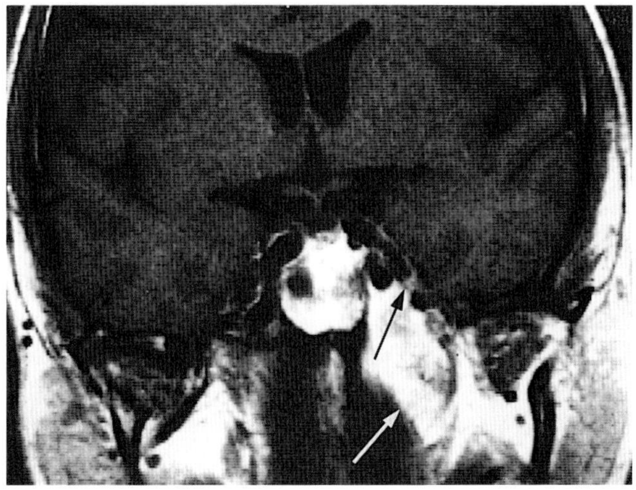

B

Figure 4.8

Adenoid cystic carcinoma of the nasopharynx.

A Axial MR (SE 500/25) after contrast-medium injection: there is marked enhancement of the tumor which destroys the skull base (white, long arrow), and infiltrates the levator veli palatini and the longus colli muscles on the left side. There is also infiltration of the left pterygoid muscles (white, short arrow). The differentiation of the tumor from the left turbinate, which is also enhanced is difficult. The left margin of the tumor is well demarcated by the muscles it has displaced, thus indicating expansion and not infiltration of the parapharyngeal space (black arrow).

B Coronal MR (SE 500/25) after contrast-medium injection: skull-base infiltration and involvement of cavernous sinus (black arrow) can be better demonstrated after enhancement of the tumor. Also after enhancement, there is a sharp interface between tumor and longus colli muscle (white arrow). However, the tumor and fat have similar intensity.

higher incidence in chronic inflammatory changes. For this reason, early symptoms of a neoplasms are often overlooked, thus the diagnosis is made in a late stage of the tumor, which already surrounds the bony walls. These tumors show similar characteristics to the primary nasopharyngeal carcinomas. In plain T1-weighted and in proton-density images, it is difficult if not impossible to differentiate tumor masses in the maxillary sinus from inflammatory changes and fluid. This differentiation can be made on enhanced MR and is also well-demonstrated on T2-weighted images, in which fluid appears bright and tumor is usually of lower intensity. If the posterior part of the tumor infiltrates the longus colli muscle, it can be judged best on enhanced MR images. Discrimination between inflammation and tumor in the anterior part is also possible in these images. Infiltration of the bony walls of the maxillary sinuses is better seen on CT, but the exact extension of the tumor can be judged better on MR.

A futher advantage of contrast-enhanced MR is the discrimination between solid tumor and fluid-containing cystic processes.

Adenoid cystic carcinomas

In comparison with squamous-cell carcinoma the rare adenoid cystic carcinomas show an aggresive growth pattern with early skull-base infiltration (Figure 4.8). This is typically found even in small lesions originating from the lateral or posterior walls of the nasopharynx. In contrast-enhanced image these tumors showed quite sharp margins with small necrotic areas. Adenoid cystic carcinomas have a variable signal on T2-weighted images, which seems correlated to the prognosis: the higher the signal and the better differentiated the lesion, the better the prognosis. Perineural extension is very frequent, explaining multiple recurrences.

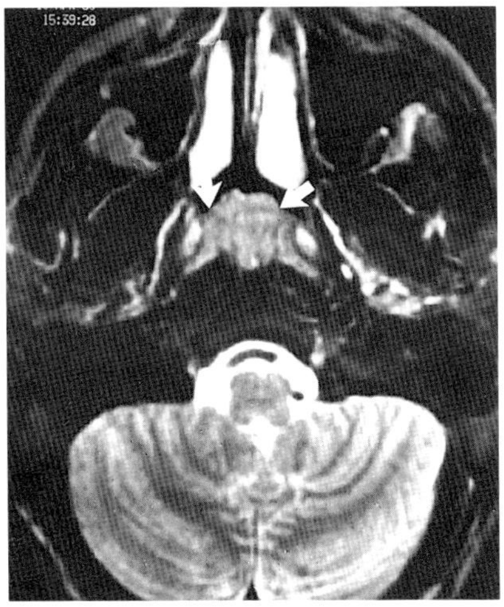

A

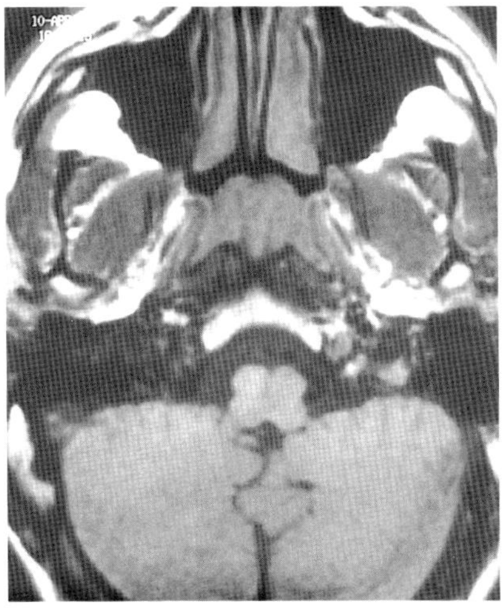

B

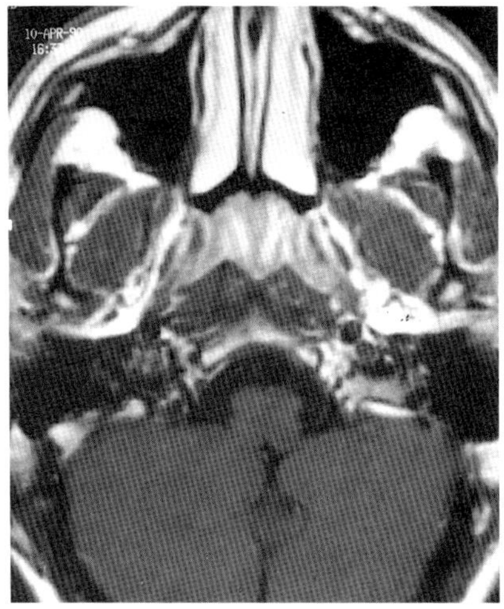

C

Figure 4.9

Lymphoid hyperplasia of the nasopharynx.

A Axial, plain MR (SE 1600/90): in the T2-weighted image the nasopharyngeal tissue is bright and shows slight inhomogeneity and scattered internal patterns. In distinction to the lymphoma, in the T2-weighted image the typical septae appear as areas of high signal intensity (arrows).

B Axial, plain MR (SE 500/25): the mass has a sharp margin, is symmetrical and is of homogeneous, low signal intensity. It has a similar appearance to that of the lymphoma shown in Figure 4.10.

C Axial MR (SE 500/25) after contrast-medium injection: the tumor shows moderate increase in signal intensity, with an inhomogeneous internal pattern mainly consisting of septae. As in lymphoma, there is compression of the veli palatini muscles on both sides.

Lymphomas and lymphoid hyperplasia

After the tonsil region, the nasopharynx is the second most frequent localization of lymphoid hyperplasia in the head and neck region. This disease is commonly seen in children causing airway obstruction. In adults, these hyperplasias are often found in patients suffering from chronic infections, such as HIV-positive patients.

On MR, lymphoid hyperplasia appears with high signal intensity in T1- as well as in T2-weighted images, with symmetric extension within the lumen of the nasopharynx (Figure 4.9). Characteristically, septae are found which are seen best in contrast-enhanced T1-weighted images.

The most important differential diagnosis is lymphoma of the nasopharynx (Figure 4.10). These lesions mostly belong to the group of non-Hodgkin's lymphomas. The growth pattern appears asymmetrical and usually there is no infiltration of surrounding tissues.[48,49]

Signal intensities on T1- and T2-weighted images are very similar to lymphoid hyperplasia. The contrast enhancement is medium and homogeneous, without the septa that are typical for the lymphoid hyperplasia.[46]

Rare lesions

A rare, but important neoplastic finding is the esthesioneurolastoma, originating from the neuroectoderm of the olfactory nerves (Figure 4.11). These lesions grow across the cribriform lamina and infiltrate the sphenoid sinus and maxillary sinuses, and extend intracranially to the anterior cranial fossa. On MR, these tumors reveal an inhomogeneous internal pattern, prolonged T1- and T2-relaxation times and an intense enhancement with contrast medium.

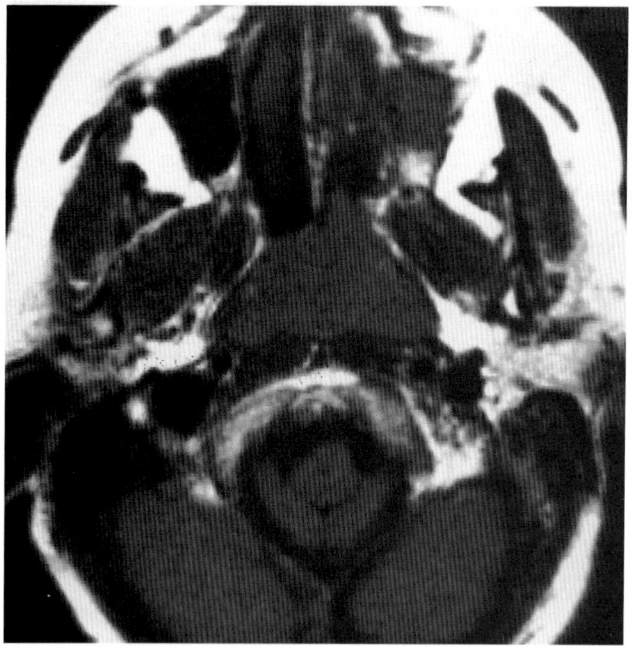

A

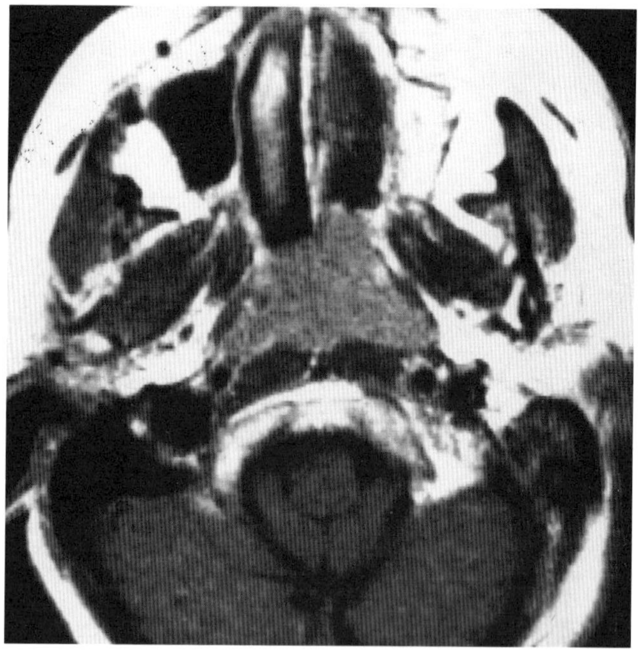

B

Figure 4.10

Lymphoma of the nasopharynx.

A Axial, plain MR (SE 1600/90): the nasopharynx is completely filled with quite homogeneous tissue. The proton density image (not shown) showed slightly higher signal intensity in the mass when compared to the signal intensity of muscles. There is fluid in the left maxillary sinus.

B Axial MR (SE 500/25) after contrast-medium injection: the tumor shows a homogeneous pattern of enhancement. There is no infiltration, but slight compression of the veli palatini muscles bilaterally.

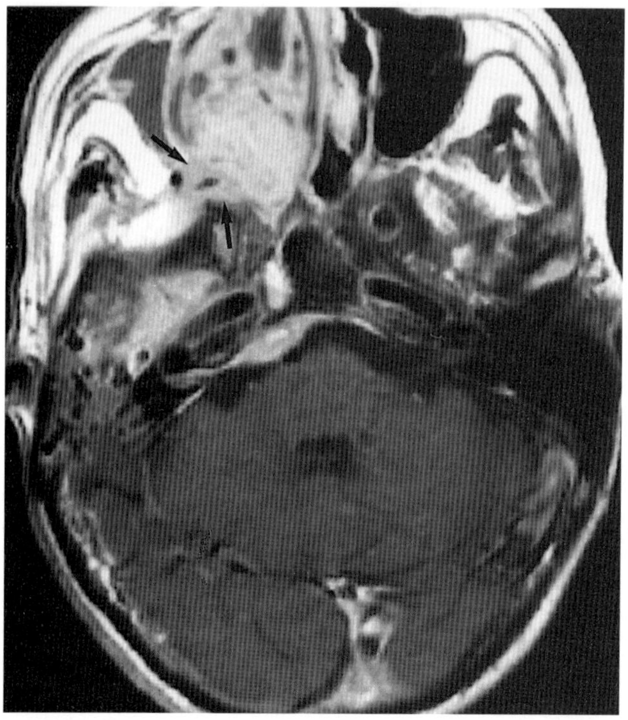

Figure 4.11

Esthesioneuroblastoma of the anterior skull base with infiltration of the paranasal sinus and nasal cavity. Axial, gadolinium-enhanced MR (TR/TE = 500/25): demonstrating a mass with high signal intensity, inhomogeneous inner structures and margins which infiltrate the nasal cavity and additionally show the tumor extension (arrows) to the retromaxillar space. Due to the obstruction of the eustachian tube, spaces within the mastoid are demonstrated to contain inflammatory fluid and findings offer a meningitis with increased signal intensity of the meninges.

In MR appearance, esthesioneuroblastomas are similar to meningiomas of the nasopharynx. The primary localization of meningiomas is commonly the brain or the skull base. However, meningiomas grow secondarily into the paranasal sinuses and the nasopharynx by eroding the bony skull base. Characteristically, they appear isointense to the grey matter of the brain. Meningiomas often show on MR images necrosis or calcifications, but appear without signs of an infiltrative growth pattern. Due to the disturbance of the blood–brain barrier, the administration of constrast medium leads to a high increase in signal intensities, providing the best diagnostic information in coronal and transverse images.

In the pre-operative diagnosis of meningiomas, CT and MR with contrast medium are equally effective; however, the topography is better demonstrated by MR.

Diagnostic strategy

In the differential diagnosis of tumors and inflammatory changes in the nasopharynx and paranasal sinuses, multisequence MR examination is superior to CT in most cases.[50,51] Therefore, MR examination must be carried out using T2-weighted sequences for demonstrating inflamed tissue and fluid-containing spaces. A further improvement has been achieved with the introduction of paramagnetic contrast medium: normal mucosa shows a middling to marked increase in signal intensity. Thus, better delineation of small anatomic details, such as the palatini muscles and the pharyngobasilar fascia, can be obtained. Whereas tumor and inflammatory tissues usually appear isointense on plain T1-weighted images, after contrast-medium administration the tumor shows in most cases a lower enhancement than do inflammatory changes. A cystic lesion with high signal intensity in the T2-weighted image reveals no enhancement in its central parts; however, the walls of cysts show a slight increase in signal intensity.

For tumors of the face, MR evaluates classical contraindications to radical surgery: osteolysis of a pterygoid process or body of the sphenoid and involvement of the middle part of the base of the skull, cavernous sinuses, pterygopalatine fossa, infratemporal space or brain, and optochiasmatic involvement. Involvement of the eye, cribriform plate, frontal sinus are relative contraindications; sagittal views acquired directly on MR, and reconstructed on CT, are especially helpful for detecting these.

In conclusion, the recommended diagnostic procedure is plain MR and MR with contrast medium for the primary diagnosis. CT may be performed additionally to demonstrate small bony details (Diagrams 4.1 and 4.2).

Salivary glands

The parotid gland is the most frequent site of salivary gland tumors, 80% of them occurring in the parotid gland, compared with 10% in the submandibular gland, 9% in the small salivary glands and 1% in the sublingual gland. On the other hand, only 30% of the parotid gland tumors are malignant, compared with 50% of submandibular gland tumors, 50% of small salivary gland tumors and 80% of sublingual gland tumors. The normal anatomy of this region is shown in Figure 4.12.

In total, salivary gland tumors make up 15% of head and neck tumors, but they represent the most complex and diverse group of tumors encountered by the head and neck oncologist. Pleomorphic adenoma (benign mixed tumor) is the most common of all salivary gland neoplasms, mainly located in the parotid gland. Warthin's tumor (papillary cystadenoma lymphomatosum) is another common tumorous lesion almost exclusively confined to the parotid gland. Cases of Warthin's tumor of the submandibular gland have, however, been reported.

Other benign tumors of the salivary glands are oncocytomas and monomorphic adenomas. The latter have to be distinguished from the pleomorphic adenomas, as they show a monomorphic feature.

Malignant salivary gland tumors are characterized by rapid growth, pain and—at an advanced stage—facial pareses and skin infiltration. Concomitant metastasis in cervical lymph nodes is also encountered in salivary gland malignancy.

Mucoepidermoid carcinoma is the most common malignancy of the parotid gland, while adenoid cystic carcinoma is most commonly found in the submandibular gland and in the minor salivary glands. Other, less common, malignant tumors of the salivary glands are acinus-cell carcinomas, adenocarcinomas, carcinoma in pleomorphic adenomas, squamous-cell carcinomas, undifferentiated carcinomas and salivary-duct carcinomas.

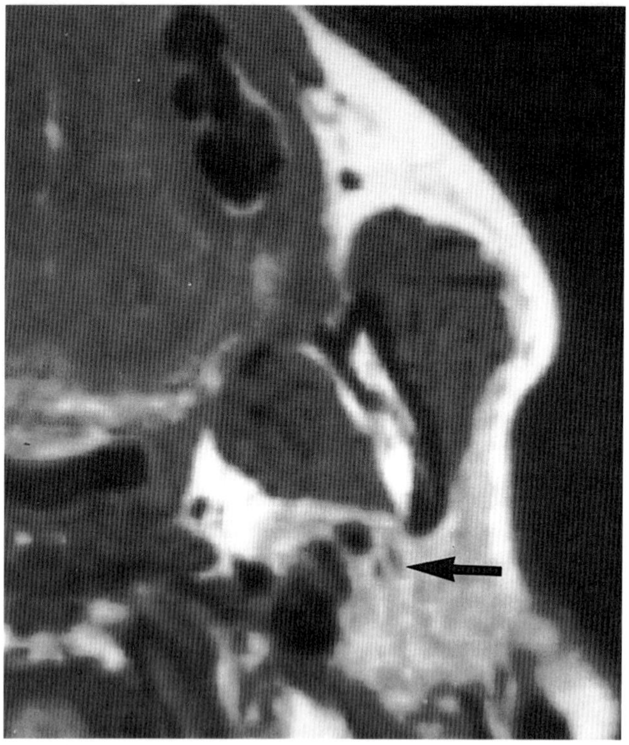

Figure 4.12

Normal anatomy of the parotid gland region. Transverse MR (SE, TR/TE = 500/25) after contrast-medium injection: the retromandibular vein appears as a structure of low signal intensity. The facial nerve is seen as a structure of lower signal intensity in the enhanced parotid gland lateral to the retromandibular vein (black arrow); the nerve appears already divided into its two major branches.

Clinical diagnosis

The diagnosis includes physical examination (inspection and bimanual palpation) as well as ultrasonography. The diagnostic value of needle biopsies of the parotid gland is controversial. Conventional radiography of the floor of the mouth, as well as sialography, might be indicated if sialolithiasis of the submandibular gland is suspected. However, sialography must not be performed in acute inflammation of the gland.[31]

Pleomorphic adenoma

Pleomorphic adenomas, the most commonly found benign tumors of salivary glands, usually grow slowly and without symptoms in middle-aged patients. In the parotid gland these lesion are found in the superficial lobe as well as in the deep lobe. On T1-weighted MR images adenomas appear as areas of low signal intensity within the parenchyma of the gland. The margins are distinct and without infiltration. On T2-weighted images the adenomatous tissue shows high signal intensity, representing fluid-containing spaces and showing a slightly inhomogeneous internal pattern. These lesions show the most increased T1 relaxation times and also prolonged T2 relaxation times. After contrast medium is introduced adenomas appear heterogeneous with areas of low signal intensity, representing necrosis (Figure 4.13).

Cystadenolymphoma (Warthin's tumor)

These benign tumors usually grow slowly and painlessly and appear in some cases in multiple areas. The lesions have sharp margins in all cases and, after infusion of contrast medium, high signal intensity in central areas, with less enhancement in the periphery. Plain images show decreased T1 and normal T2 relaxation times. No infiltrative growth is seen; the extension is usually limited to the parotid space. The retromandibular vein and the facial nerve are often medially displaced but are not compressed or infiltrated. T1-weighted images after administration of contrast medium are significantly better than plain T2-weighted images. The presumed benign character of Warthin's tumor can be confirmed using contrast medium, from the sharp margins, homogeneous appearance and the lack of malignant signs such as infiltrative growth.

Squamous-cell carcinoma

Squamous-cell carcinoma, more rare than pleomorphic adenoma or Warthin's tumor, has an unclear growth pattern and a quite inhomogeneous internal pattern (Figure 4.14). After contrast-medium administration, these tumors show areas of low signal intensity representing necrosis, which is overlooked in plain T2-weighted images. Small infiltrations of surrounding muscles and the exact

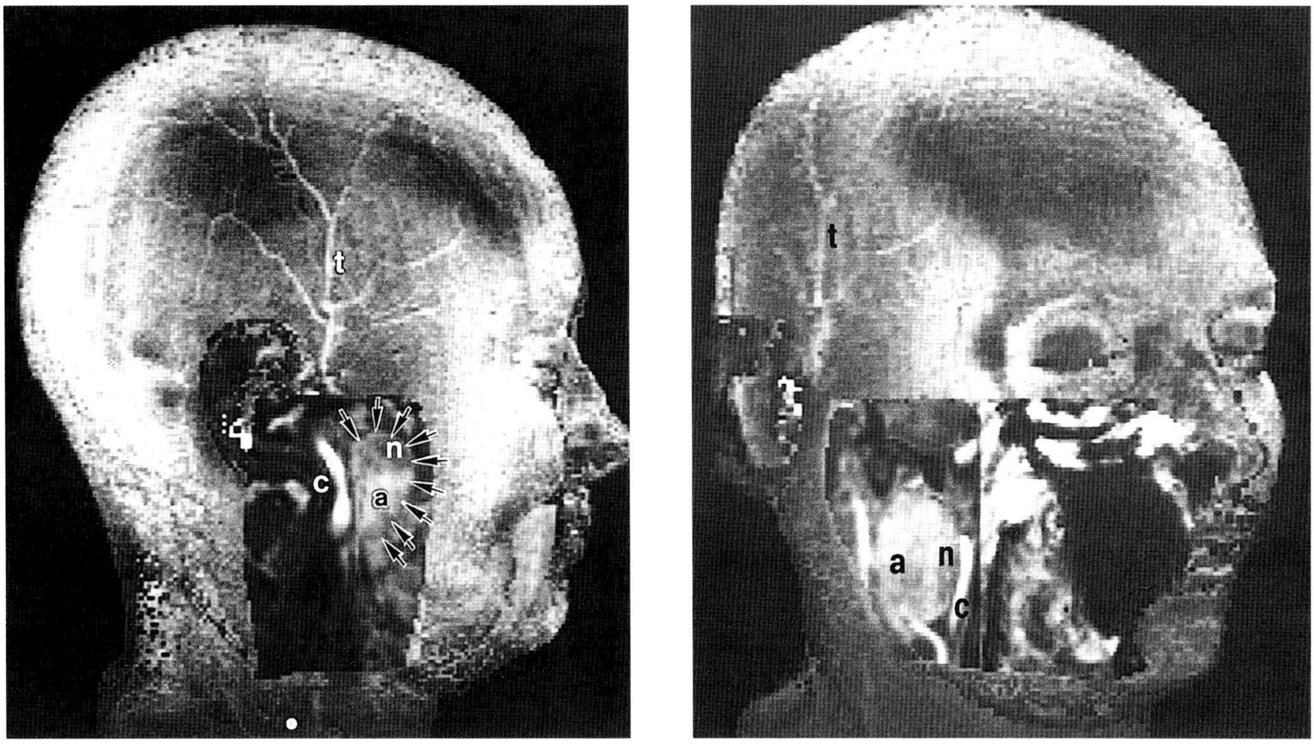

A B

Figure 4.13

Pre-operative MR-guided therapy planning of a pleomorphic adenoma of the parotid gland on the right side. The figures show MR reconstructions, using ray tracing technique, fast low-angle short imaging (FLASH) three-dimensional sequence, after contrast-medium injection. The reconstruction in the sagittal (**A**) and parasagittal (**B**) slice orientation demonstrates a 2 × 2 cm mass which lies anterior of the internal carotid artery (c); the mass is sharply delineated (arrows) and there are some inhomogeneous areas due to necrosis in the superior portion of the tumor (n). The MR findings and the topographic relationships are characteristic for pleomorphic adenoma (a). t, temporal veins.

margins are best recognized in contrast-enhanced T1-weighted images. Increased T1 and normal T2 relaxation times may be found.

Adenocarcinoma

One of the most common malignant tumors is adenocarcinoma. Pathologically, adenocarcinomas are classified as high-, intermediate- and low-grade lesions.[52,53] Low-grade adenocarcinomas appear similar to adenomas. In plain T1-weighted MR sequences, the margins of the more malignant adenocarcinomas cannot be clearly seen. After contrast-medium administration, a diffuse, infiltrative growth pattern can be recognized (Figure 4.15). Due to these infiltrations, the facial nerve can often be identified only by using contrast-enhanced T1-weighted sequences. Usually the nerve cannot be seen on T2-weighted plain images. In all cases, the retromandibular vein is either compressed or

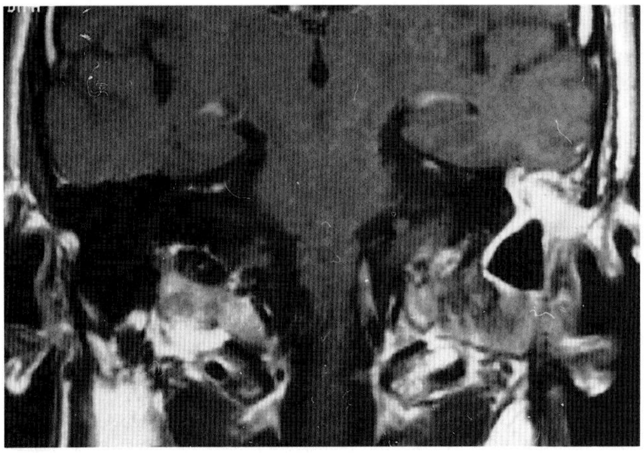

A

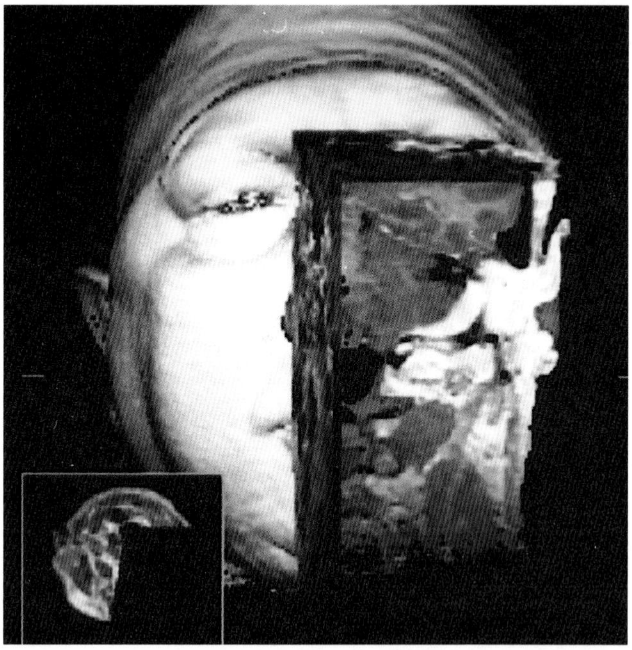

B

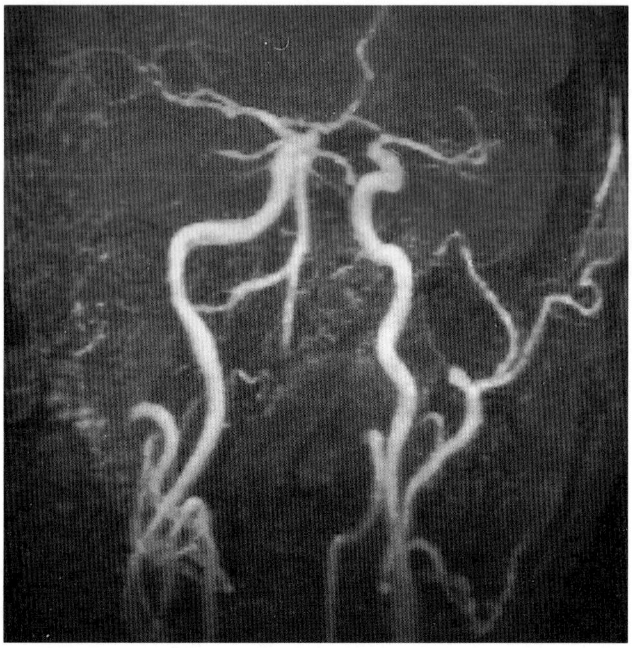

C

Figure 4.14

Recurrent tumor of a squamous-cell carcinoma of the parotid gland: comparative evaluation of spin-echo sequences, three-dimensional reconstruction and MRA.

A Coronal gadolinium-enhanced MR (TR/TE = 500/17): in the coronal slice orientation, an infiltrating mass is identified in the area of the middle-ear cavity and the mastoid. Centrally, an air-filled cavity is identified. The tumor is already infiltrating superior to the middle skull base.

B Three-dimensional, ray tracing, gadolinium-enhanced MR: the pre-operative image demonstrates a degree of infiltration of the temporal bone, the mastoid and the parotid space. Note the central portion of the tumor in the retromaxillary and infratemporal fossa. The sigmoid sinus also demonstrates a high signal intensity after contrast administration.

C MRA, using the fast imaging with steady procession (FISP) three-dimensional technique, head coil and parasagittal slice orientation: the arterial MRA after venous presaturation demonstrates the left external carotid artery as a complete structure after ligation. The course of the internal carotid artery on both sides appears normal, as does the course of the external carotid artery with the fascial branches.

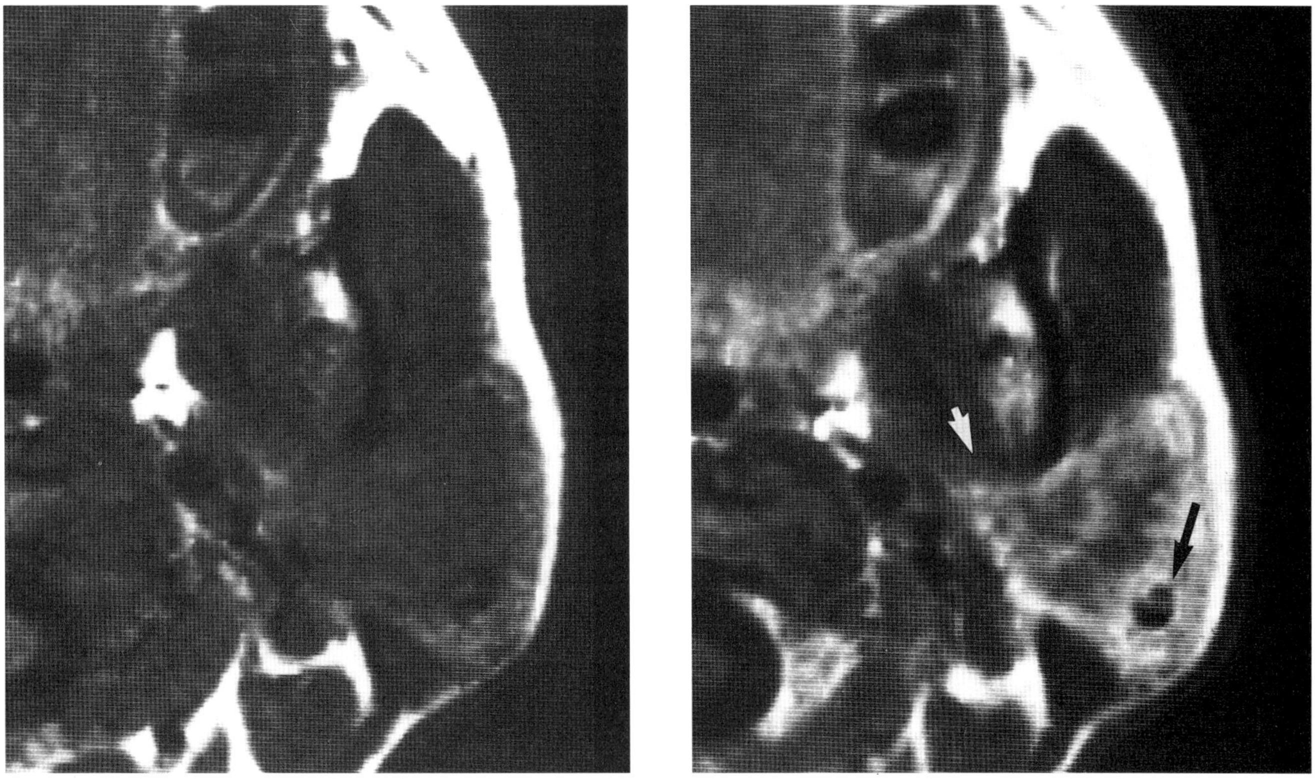

A B

Figure 4.15

Adenocarcinoma of the parotid gland.

A Transverse, plain MR (SE, TR/TE = 500/25): there is a lesion of the left parotid gland with unclear margins. It is not certain that the lesion is growing to the parapharyngeal space.

B Transverse MR (SE, TR/TE = 500/25) with gadolinium injection: inhomogeneous internal patterns become visible with displacement of the retromandibular vein (black arrow) and the masseter muscle. The tumor has already grown into the deep portion of the parotid gland (white arrow).

infiltrated. Adenocarcinomas can show extension to the mandible, with parapharyngeal growth and infiltration of the pterygoid muscles and the great vessels, best seen in contrast-enhanced T1-weighted sequences. Adenocarcinomas show increased T1 relaxation times and normal T2 relaxation times.

Adenoid cystic carcinoma

Adenoid cystic carcinoma is also found in the smaller submandibular and sublingual glands. Characteristically, they grow along the sheath of the 7th cranial nerve and show a high rate of recurrences. Adenoid cystic carcinomas present with a more aggresive growth pattern than that for squamous-cell carcinomas or adenocarcinomas. They grow diffusely into the parapharyngeal space as well as into the lateral facial skeleton and infiltrate the neck muscles, the masseter muscle and the mandible. In some cases, the disease is first seen at such an advanced stage that no remaining normal glandular tissue is identifiable. On plain T1- and T2-weighted MR sequences the muscles often appear not to be infiltrated. However, after contrast-medium administration, the infiltration of surrounding muscles can be easily diagnosed

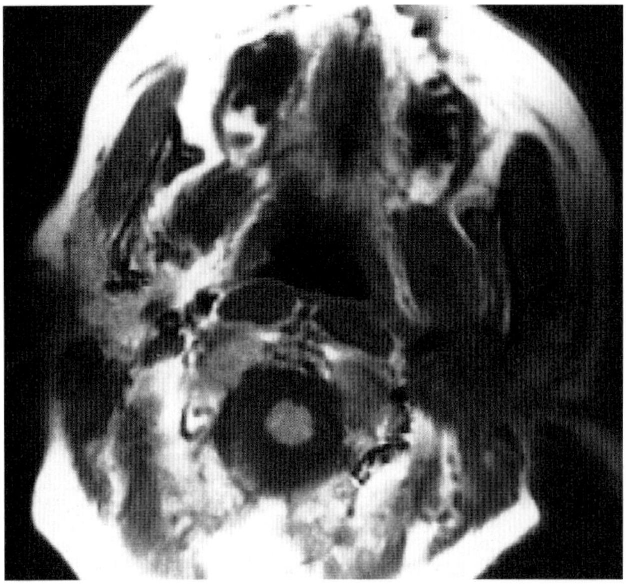

A

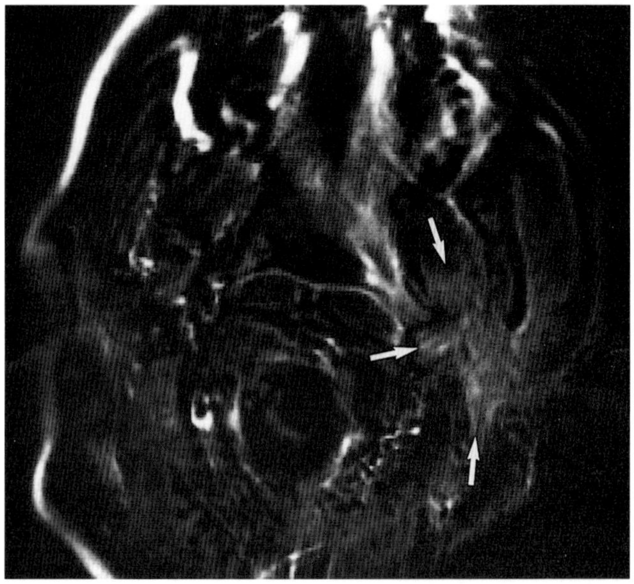

C

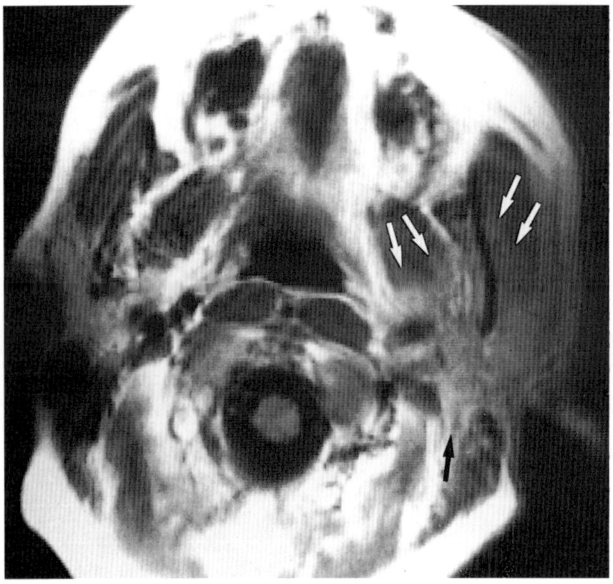

B

Figure 4.16

Recurring adenoid cystic carcinoma.

A Transverse, plain MR (SE, TR/TE = 500/25): there is a recurrent tumor in the operated-on left parotid space. The tumor tissue shows the same signal intensity as the surrounding muscle, presenting clear delineation.

B Transverse MR (SE, TR/TE = 500/25) after contrast-medium injection: the arrows show significant enhancement of the inhomogeneous lesion, with infiltration of the pterygoid muscles and the dura of the cerebellum. Early infiltration of the mandible is also shown.

C Transverse, plain MR (SE, TR/TE = 1600/90): this T2-weighted image does not allow clear delineation of the tumor margins (arrows)

(Figure 4.16). These infiltrations are often not seen on plain T2-weighted images. Usually the retromandibular vein is compressed and the facial nerve not detectable. T1 and T2 relaxation times are not helpful in differentiating adenoid cystic carcinoma from adenocarcinoma, due to similar increased T1 relaxation times and quite normal T2 relaxation times.

Lymphoma

Lymphomas belong to the rare space-occupying lesions of the salivary glands. An association is found between non-Hodgkin's lymphomas and a history of Sjögren's syndrome (Figure 4.17).

MR appearances of lymphomas can be divided in two different groups. The first group shows

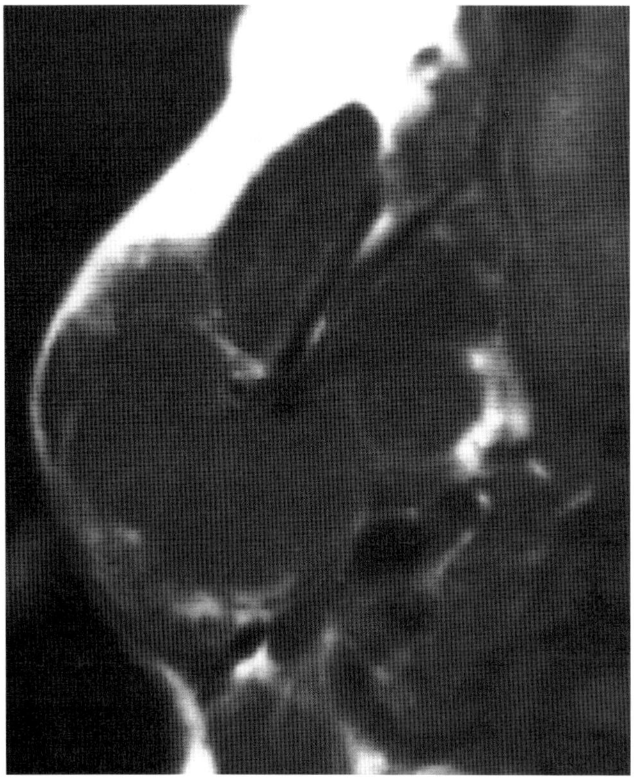

A

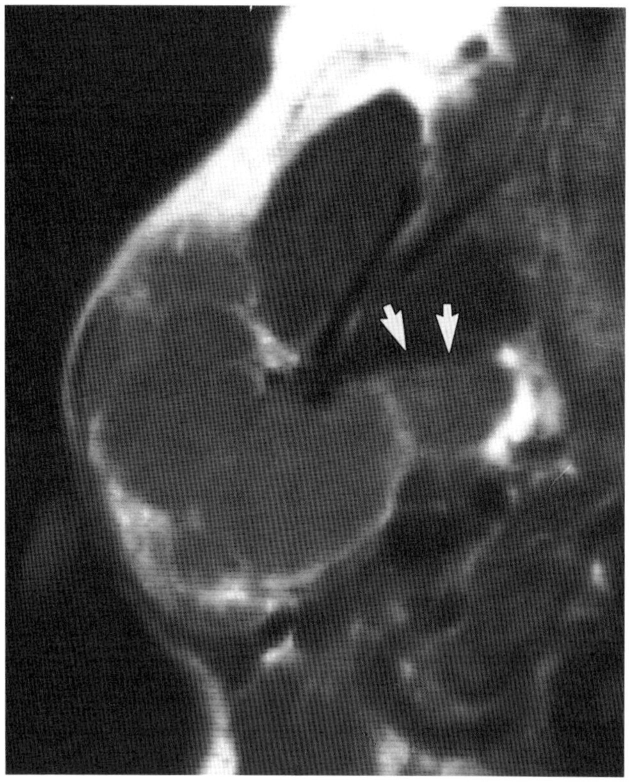

B

Figure 4.17

Lymphoma and Sjögren's syndrome of the parotid gland.

A Transverse MR (SE, TR/TE = 500/25) after contrast medium injection: a homogeneous space-occupying lesion of the right parotid gland with medium signal intensity is shown in this T1-weighted image.

B Transverse MR (SE, TR/TE = 500/25) after contrast-medium injection: only slight enhancement of the lesion is seen, due to the histology of a low-grade lymphoma. Tumor growth extends to the parapharyngeal space (arrows) with displacement of the pterygoid muscles and compression of the retromandibular vein.

small conglomerations of lymph nodes, visible at the medial margin of the parotid gland. On plain and contrast-enhanced images, the surrounding glandular tissue appears to lack signs of tumorous infiltration. The lymph nodes appear hypointense on T1- and hyperintense on T2-weighted plain images. In the second group, enlarged lymph nodes can be identified, completely displacing the normal tissue of the parotid gland. Lymphomas typically show small extensions to the parapharyngeal space, best seen in contrast-enhanced T1-weighted sequences. The contrast enhancement is comparable to that seen in squamous-cell carcinoma. The central part of the lymphomas show homogeneous medium contrast enhancement; the margins are significantly better enhanced. After adenomas, lymphomas show the most increased T1 relaxation times and unchanged T2 relaxation time. A differentiation of Hodgkin's and non-Hodgkin's lymphomas is commonly not possible by MR.

Diagnostic strategy and the value of magnetic resonance imaging

A differentiation of benign and malignant lesions is often suggested by using a combination of T2-weighted sequences and plain and enhanced T1-weighted images. A biopsy will always confirm the diagnosis. Unclear margins are a sure sign of malignancy.[54,55] Inhomogeneous internal pattern and necrosis can also be recognized in benign lesions; thus, these criteria cannot definitively identify malignancy.[56] Internal pattern and vascularization are better demonstrated after injection of contrast. Due to the high standard deviation of T1 and T2 values, an exact differentiation between types of malignant lesion is not possible.[54,57–59]

For diagnosing small lesions, plain MR often produces unsatisfactory results due to difficulties in delineation of the lesion from high-signal normal gland tissue.[59] After administration of contrast medium, the signal intensities change significantly. A marked contrast enhancement is suspicious of recurrence. In fibrous areas only a slight enhancement is found.

The diagnostic value of plain MR imaging of the parotid gland is superior to CT due to the lack of beam-hardening artifacts and the improved soft-tissue contrast.[60] Unlike other authors,[54,61] we find that administration of contrast medium proves to be advantageous in differential diagnosis of various neoplasms. Additionally, the delineation of lesions which are on plain images isointense to glandular tissue is improved.[58]

Oropharynx and oral cavity

Cancer of the oropharynx and oral cavity is a rather common disease. Alcohol and tobacco use are responsible and may account for the unequal male : female incidence of between 10 : 1 and 4 : 1.

The most common malignant tumor is squamous-cell carcinoma. The majority of these carcinomas arise in the tonsillar fossa. Deep extension can cause fixation to or erosion of the mandible, as well as infiltration of the pterygoid musculature. Infiltration of the parapharyngeal space can also cause functional loss of the caudal cranial nerves.

Other common sites of cancer growth within the oropharynx and oral cavity are the tongue, the base of the tongue, the vallecula epiglotta, the palatine arch, the pharyngeal wall, the anterior floor of the mouth and the gingiva.

Besides squamous-cell carcinomas, adenoid cystic carcinomas, mucoepidermoid carcinomas, adenocarcinomas and malignant pleomorphic adenomas have been described, as well as Hodgkin's and non-Hodgkin's lymphoma and, occasionally, sarcomas.

Clinical diagnosis

Patients with diseases of the oropharynx and oral cavity should be examined by either direct inspection or endoscopy. If there is suspicion of a malignant process, a biopsy should be taken; in addition, an inspection of the upper airway as well as the upper digestive tract (direct laryngoscopy, tracheoscopy, bronchoscopy and esophagoscopy) must be performed, to exclude multilocular growth of carcinomas. The risk of multiple primary cancer is generally increased in patients with malignant tumors of the upper gastrorespiratory tract. Additionally, as in the management of all malignant tumors of the head and neck, the patient has to be palpated for cervical lymph nodes. Sometimes ultrasound examination can also be helpful for the detection of hidden involvement of neck lymph nodes.

Squamous-cell carcinoma

Tonsils and oral cavity

In their early stages, carcinomas of the tonsils and oral cavity usually grow along nerve-vessel sheaths and muscle bundles. The most frequent localization is the anterior part of the tonsils, followed by the posterior part and the posterior wall of the pharynx (Figures 4.18 and 4.19). These tumors infiltrate cranially the soft palate (Figure 4.20), caudally the lateral wall of the pharynx and the tongue base, and laterally the parapharyngeal space and the mandible.

In small mucosal tumors (stage T2), infiltrations of the parapharyngeal space as well as infiltration of the tongue body are evident in more than 70% of cases. In more extended lesions, an infiltration of the longus colli muscles and a displacement of the pharynx are visible. Tumors of stage T1 and superficial growing lesions are hard to detect. Tumors of stages T2–T4 can be diagnosed positively in cases of good examination quality. Transverse as well as coronal slice orientation is diagnostically relevant in the exact documentation of craniocaudal and lateral extension of the lesion.

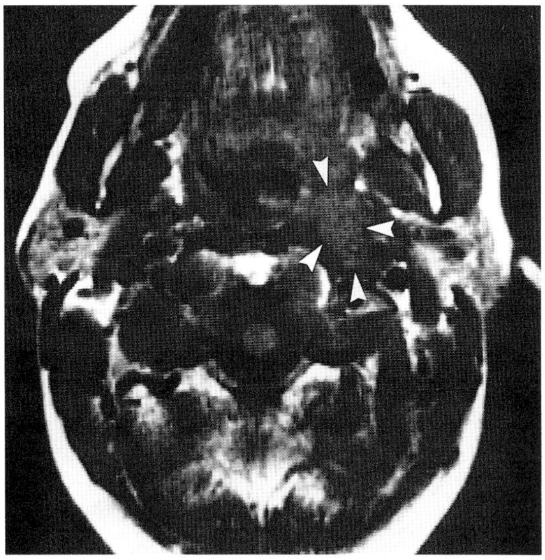

A

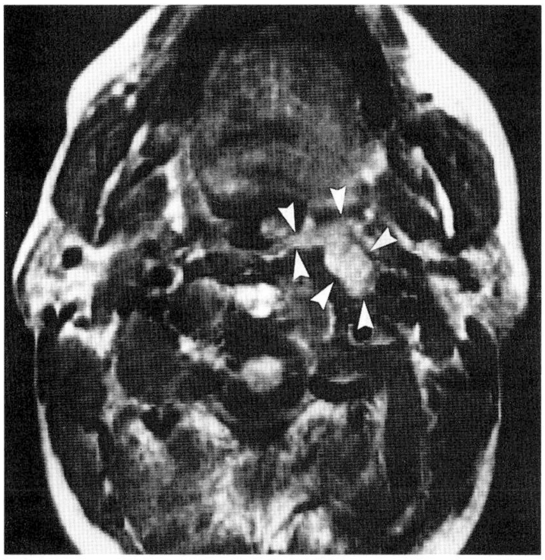

B

Figure 4.18

Squamous-cell carcinoma of the tonsil on the left side.

A Axial, plain MR (TR/TE = 500/17): a mass of low signal intensity (white arrowheads) is seen in the left tonsil and palatonsillar region. Note the lateral displacement of the internal carotid artery and jugular vein.

B Axial MR (TR/TE = 500/17) after contrast-medium injection: after contrast application, the tumor (arrowheads) and the posterior infiltrating mass show a significantly increased signal intensity. The parapharyngeal infiltration is better demonstrated after contrast application than by plain imaging.

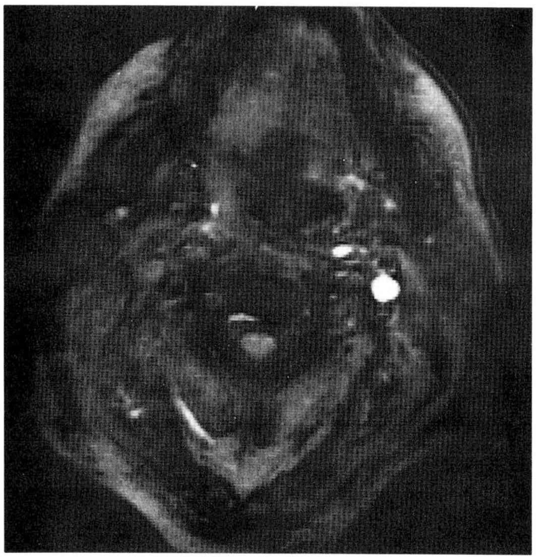

A

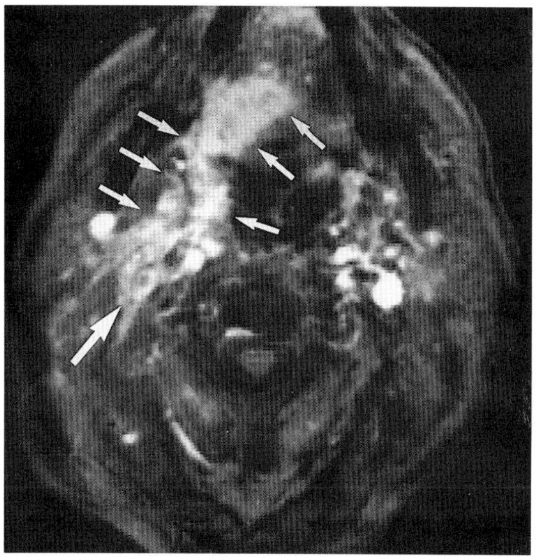

B

Figure 4.19

Recurrent tumor of a tonsillar squamous-cell carcinoma with infiltration of the oral cavity, oropharynx and parapharyngeal space: diagnostic value of fast sequence techniques. The MR images (TR/TE = 30/12, FLASH sequence) were taken before (**A**) and after (**B**) contrast medium injection. Using fast-sequence protocols and the paramagnetic contrast agent, there is delineation of a recurrent tumor on the right tonsillar fossa and oral cavity. Whilst it is difficult to delineate the tumor on plain MR, the infiltrated spaces are easy to recognize in the gadolinium-enhanced scan. Note the infiltration of the tongue, tonsillar fossa and parapharyngeal space (white arrows). The recurrent tumor was proved histologically.

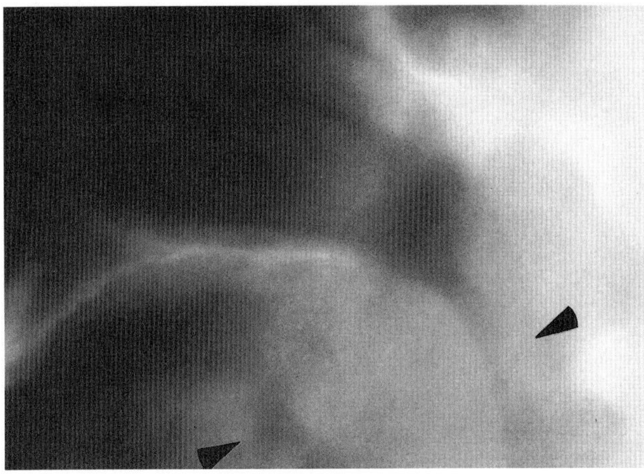

Figure 4.20

Squamous-cell carcinoma of the soft palate: conventional tomography in sagittal orientation. A huge mass, measuring 2 × 2 cm, is identified on conventional tomography in sagittal orientation. There is no infiltration of the bony palate, but it is difficult to exactly delineate the soft-tissue extension (black arrowheads) by using conventional radiography.

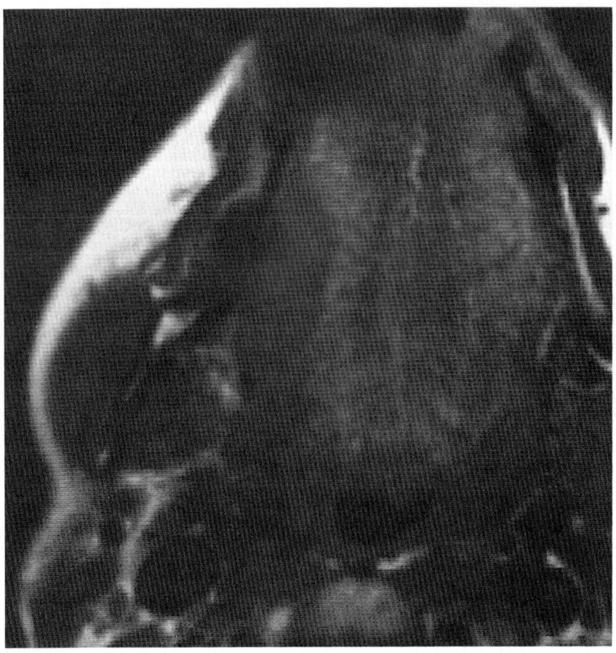

A

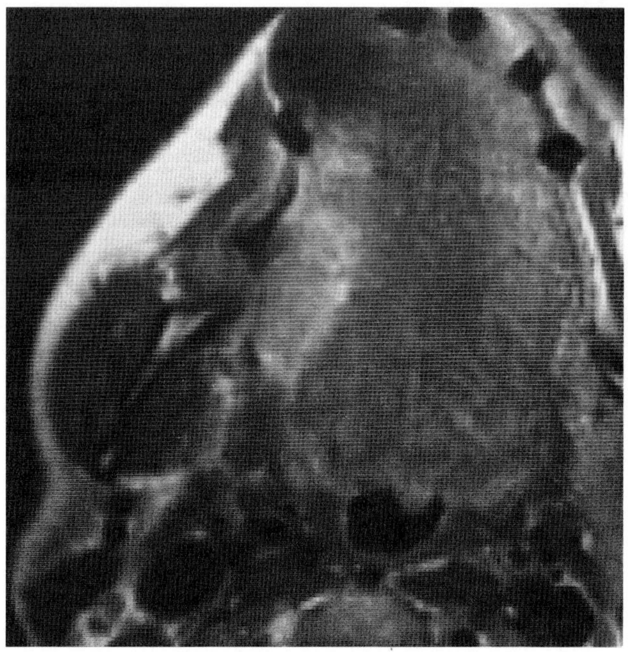

B

Figure 4.21

Carcinoma of the oral cavity with lateral tongue infiltration.

A Axial, plain MR (TR/TE = 500/25): the axial slice orientation demonstrates the normal tongue structures of the intrinsic and extrinsic muscles on the left side. On the right side a mass of low signal intensity 2 × 1 cm is identified.

B Axial MR (TR/TE = 500/25) after contrast-medium injection: there is a significant enhancement of the mucosal structures in the oral cavity and oropharynx. The tumor mass on the right tongue shows an inhomogeneous uptake. The exact delineation of the tumor border, the inner structures and the topographic relationships with the tonsillar fossa are well depicted.

Oral cavity and body of the tongue

Squamous-cell carcinomas of the tongue usually give rise to clinical symptoms in stage T2. Their growth is of a very destructive and infiltrative nature (Figure 4.21), therefore they tend to show a necrotic inner structure. An exact visualization of characteristic infiltrative direction is impossible using only plain T1- and T2-weighted sequences. But after application of contrast medium, the enhancement even of small infiltrative branches enables a clear delineation of infiltrated and normal muscles. Above all, the diagnostic value for tumors of a lower stage (T2) increases immensely. However, stage T1 tumors that do not bulk in the lumen cannot be diagnosed sufficiently by MR. Stage T3 and T4 tumors show only a slight displacement of normal anatomic structures due to the infiltrative character of the tumors. Nevertheless, osseous structures of the mandible and hyoid bone are eroded in the advanced stages.

The diagnostic results are obtained using axial and coronal slices in T1-weighted MR sequences. The use of contrast medium is indispensible for an exact tumor staging in the oral cavity and body of the tongue. Additional subtraction images pre- and post-contrast medium prove to be very helpful in doubtful cases. In T1- and T2-weighted sequences, the tumor has higher signal intensity compared with the muscles of the tongue. However, in only some cases of a questionably malignant cystic and inflammatory lesion do T2-weighted sequences add useful information; usually long sequences are not necessary. We have examined lesions of the tongue using the head coil, although other authors have achieved good results using a surface receiver coil.[16,27] In judging the posterior pharyngeal walls or an extension into the cranial nasopharynx, we feel that a head coil covering the complete region is of great advantage.

Vallecula and base of the tongue

Squamous-cell carcinomas of the vallecula show a primary infiltration of the floor of the mouth (Figures 4.22–4.24). Tumors of stages T3 and T4 enlarge their growth in the epiglottis, the supraglottic larynx and the intrinsic muscles of the tongue. A characteristic sign of low-stage tumors in this area is the displacement of normal anatomy, causing asymmetry evident on MR. The tumors are of relatively large size when infiltrating surrounding structures. An important differential diagnosis of lesions in the vallecula is the lymphatic hyperplasia.

Longer T2 relaxation times of lymphatic tissue and a similar signal intensity in T1-weighted images allow a certain differentiation of tumor and lymphatic tissue. Both structures assimilate contrast medium equally, but lymphatic tissue shows no inhomogeneous inner structure or signs of infiltration. The contrast-enhancement reaches 100%, causing intermediate T1 and increased T2 relaxation times. The combination of contrast-enhanced T1-weighted sequences and unenhanced T2-weighted sequences is required for the examination in the vallecula and base of the tongue. In this region, in addition to axial slices, a second sagittal slice orientation proves to be very helpful. In these images the extension to the epiglottis in its anterior/caudal to posterior/cranial plane is visualized best, and information concerning infiltration of the epiglottis is obtained.

Other manifestations

Kaposi's sarcoma

These semi-malignant tumors are associated with the acquired immune deficiency syndrome (AIDS).[61,62] They demonstrate only a low rate of infiltration; primarily they displace and narrow the pharyngeal cavity (Figure 4.25). They have characteristic morphology. Their T1 and T2 relaxation times are similar to squamous-cell carcinoma, therefore certain identification based only on the MR appearance is not possible. The diagnosis is revealed by biopsy in combination with the serological HIV antibody tests.

Glomus tumor

A characteristic sign of glomus tumor is an immensely high increase of signal intensity after application of contrast medium. This enhancement is caused by the enormous vascularization of these tumors. The tumors show a typical lobulated outline and a tendency to grow into the parapharyngeal space. The signal intensity in T1-weighted images shows an intermediate level equal to muscles; however, high T2 times due to the extreme vascularization allow a certain differentiation of glomus tumors from the other lesions arising in the oropharynx.

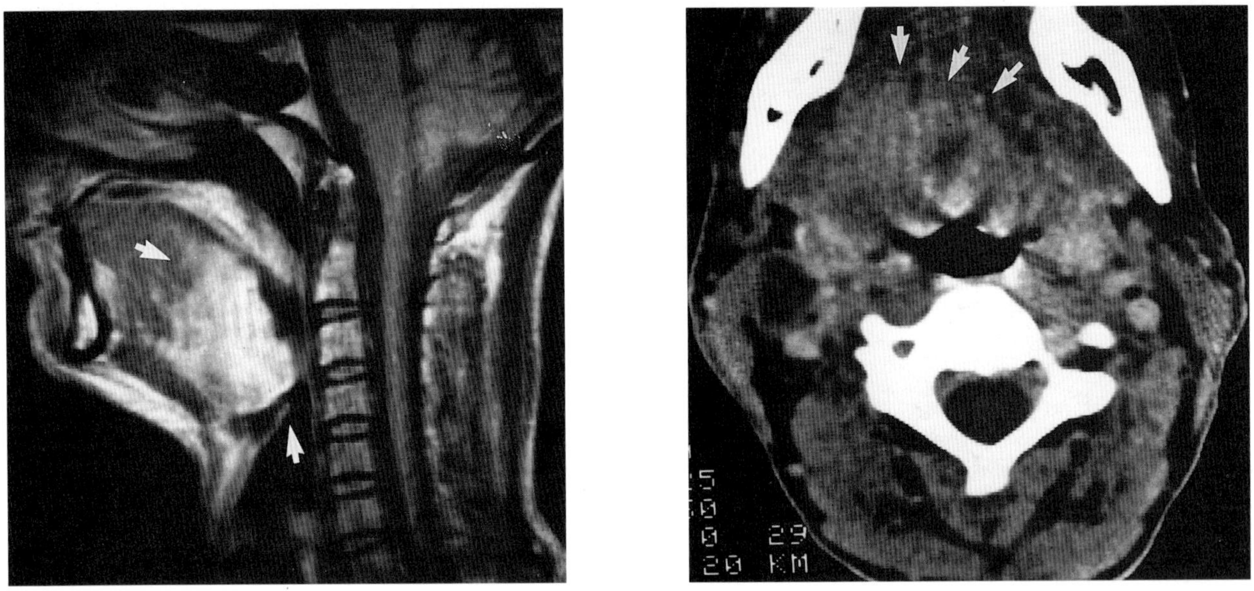

A B

Figure 4.22

Tongue-base squamous-cell carcinoma: comparative evaluation of CT and MR.

A Sagittal, plain MR (TR/TE = 1800/35): using a head coil, MR demonstrates mass of 4 × 3 cm in the tongue base, with anterior infiltration to the middle oral cavity. The pre-epiglottic space is free of tumor; the epiglottic cartilage (white arrow) is delineated precisely. The ventral border of the lower tumor is also seen (upper white arrow).

B Axial, contrast-enhanced CT scan: the tumor infiltration is difficult to interpret. The mass shows an inhomogeneous increase in density: additionally, huge lymph-node metastasis in the right cervical region is identified. (The tumor margins are marked by arrows.)

Lymph nodes

The differentiation of inflammatory and metastatic lymph nodes is still problematic. Lymph nodes can be regarded as pathologic, when they reach a size of 1 cm in smallest diameter, when more than three lymph nodes are bound together or if a necrotic inner structure is evident. On T2-weighted images, inflamed or metastatic lymph nodes exhibit high signal intensity comparable to the tonsils or other lymphatic tissue, and enhance after contrast medium administration.

Diagnostic strategy

MR is highly sensitive and specific for the diagnosis of disease of the oropharynx and the oral cavity because of its high soft-tissue contrast and the multiplanar views. CT is usually also very efficient, especially when coronal views are used in addition to axial views. CT is also accurate in studying bone erosion of the mandible, but MR depicts better the non-specific changes in bone marrow. The oropharynx is relatively accessible to the examining clinician, thus the role of imaging is to define the extent of a tumor into the deep, surrounding soft-tissue region. Several problems have to be solved: size and morphology of a tumor within the tongue, an estimate of encroachment upon the middle line, and the infiltration of tongue base or parapharyngeal space.[60,63–65] Paramagnetic contrast medium proves to be of high value in determining tumorous involvement. T2-weighted sequences often lead to a false tumor classification.

An exact delineation of tumors classified as stage T1 is extremely difficult, as the tumors do not

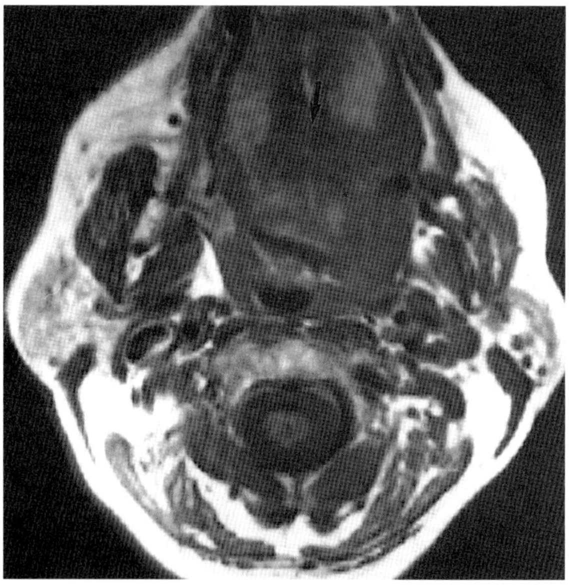

A

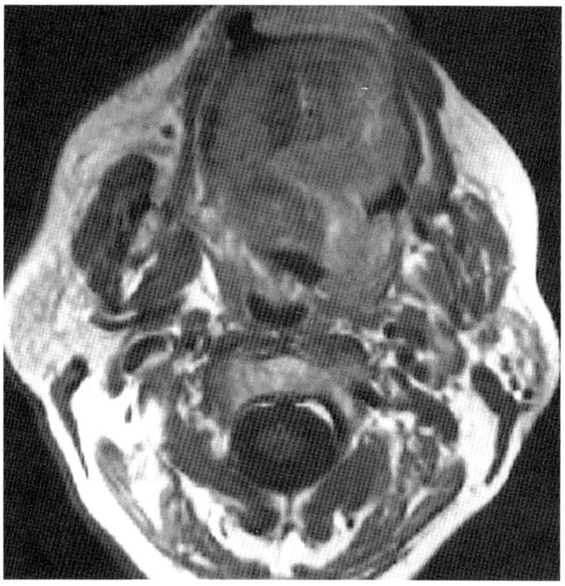

B

Figure 4.23

Squamous-cell carcinoma of the tongue with midline crossing and tumor ulceration.

A Axial, plain MR (TR/TE = 500/17): a linear lesion of low signal intensity is seen to be growing along the lateral side of the tongue muscle; within the intrinsic tongue muscle structure an area of low signal intensity is identified. Note the loss of signal of the lingual septum (arrow).

B Plain MR (TR/TE = 500/17) after contrast-medium injection: the gadolinium-enhanced scan allows the exact identification of the tumor infiltration. Note the anterior tongue infiltration, the crossing of the midline and the tumor ulceration on the lateral left side.

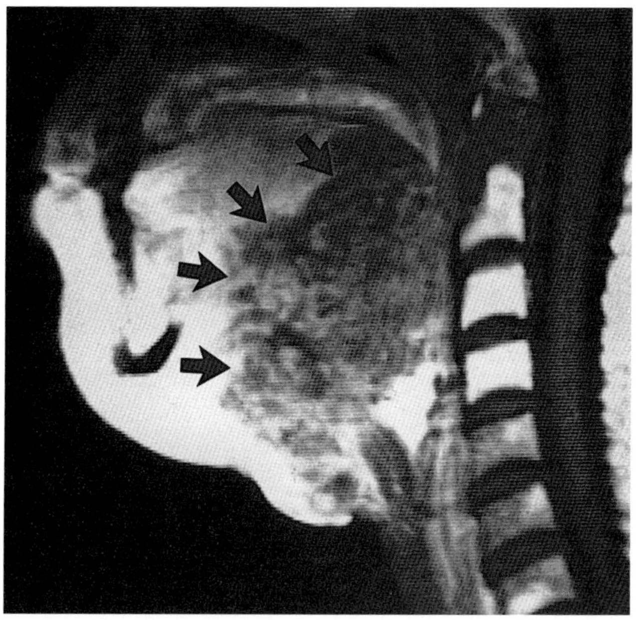

Figure 4.24

Recurrent squamous-cell carcinoma of the tongue and tongue base in a 42-year-old patient. Sagittal MR (TR/TE = 500/17) after contrast-medium injection demonstrates a huge mass with an inhomogeneous inner structure in the body of the tongue, tongue base and pre-epiglottic space. The anterior portion of the tongue is not infiltrated. (The margins of the necrotizing tumor are marked by arrows.)

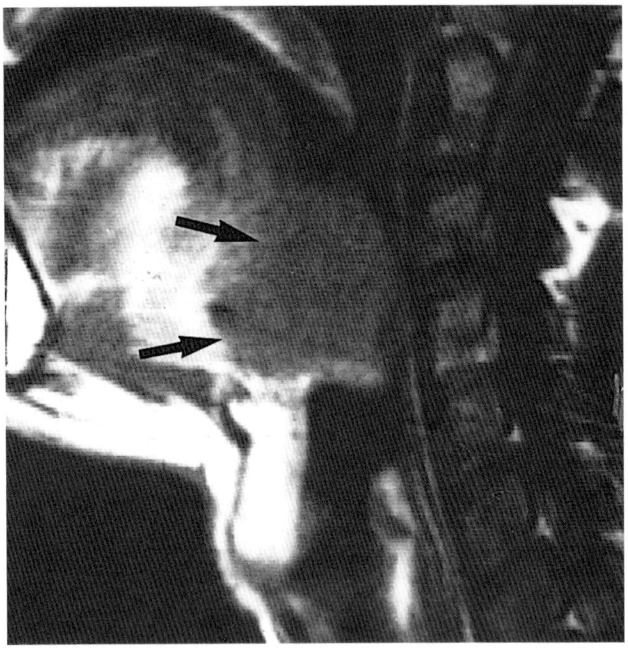

Figure 4.25

Kaposi's sarcoma of the tongue base. Sagittal, plain MR (TR/TE = 500/17) identifies a mass of low signal intensity, with diffuse borders, in the tongue base and pre-epiglottic space. The epiglottic cartilage is posterior; there is no clear infiltration (arrows).

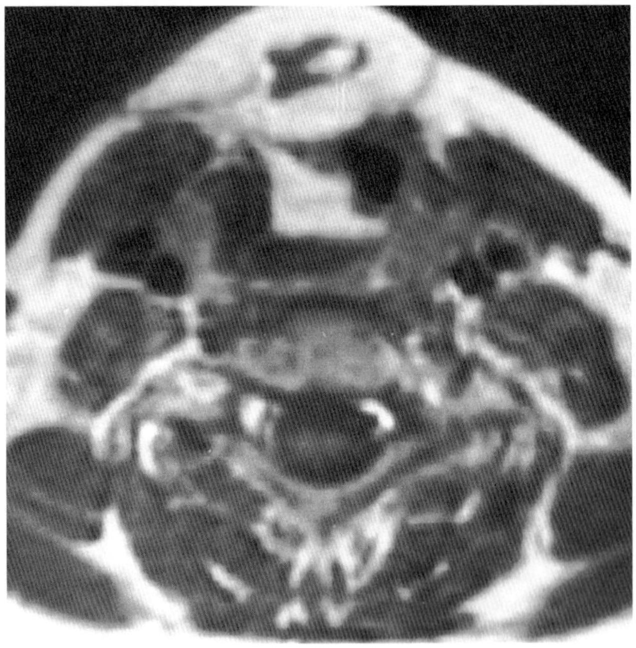

Figure 4.26

MR evaluation of a post-operative neck; the patient had undergone a total laryngectomy with soft-tissue transplantation. Axial, contrast-enhanced MR (TR/TE = 500/17) identifies a recurrent tumor mass. Structures of high signal intensity are due to fatty tissue layers. Note the adjacent signal intensity of the thyroid gland and the muscle structures on both sides. No recurrent tumor could be identified.

bulk into the lumen. In general, tumors of a higher stage can be visualized by the different MR techniques. Optimal results concerning the size and the character of the different lesions can be obtained using the combination of contrast medium T2-weighted enhancement sequences and at least two slice orientations.

In the primary diagnosis of oropharyngeal lesions, clinical and endoscopic examinations are still obligatory, because small and superficial stage T1 tumors cannot be diagnosed by imaging techniques. For pre-operative staging, T1-weighted sequences with contrast medium are of high value. Additional T2-weighted sequences are helpful to differentiate inflammatory and edematous reactions. Therefore MR is the method of choice for the diagnosis of high stage tumors in the oropharynx and complements the primary clinical examinations.

Larynx and hypopharynx

Layngeal disorders can cause a variety of different symptoms, depending on the site of origin as well as the disease.

The most common malignant neoplasm of the larynx is squamous-cell carcinoma. According to the National Cancer Institute of the United States, cancer of the larynx accounts for almost 1.3% of all new cancer diagnoses as well as 0.83% of all cancer deaths in the US. Several risk factors for the development of laryngeal cancer have been pointed out, including tobacco, alcohol and industrial or radiation exposition. Carcinomas of the larynx may also develop in patients with a history of laryngeal papilloma. In many cases, laryngeal carcinoma can be detected at an early stage, because, at least in tumors originating from the glottic level, a voice change will be the first symptom. Other symptoms may be difficult swallowing, throat pain, referred ear pain or hemoptysis. Depending on the tumor stage, the prognosis of endolaryngeal cancer is usually better than cancer of other regions of the upper gastrorespiratory tract.

The treatment of laryngeal cancer depends on the site and the extension of the tumor. Different surgical procedures including chordectomy, partial or hemilaryngectomy, or even total laryngectomy, may be necessary (Figure 4.26). Treatment can also be by radiotherapy. The hypopharynx has a close relationship to the larynx and is divided into the postcricoid area, the piriform sinus and the posterior pharyngeal wall.

Tumors of the hypopharynx occur less frequently compared to those of the larynx; the incidence rate is less than 1/100 000 of all newly diagnosed cancers.[66] Most of the malignant neoplasms are squamous-cell carcinomas. Swallowing disorders, throat pain, referred ear pain and hemoptysis may occur in patients suffering from a hypopharyngeal carcinoma; as these symptoms are not specific, they might be overlooked, and sometimes the appearance of a cervical lymph-node metastasis leads to the diagnosis. In many cases, parts of the larynx are already infiltrated at the time of diagnosis.

Depending on the site and extension of the tumor, it can be removed by either partial pharyngectomy or laryngectomy and partial pharyngectomy. In advanced stages combined radio- and chemotherapy can be performed. The long-term prognosis of carcinoma of the hypopharynx remains poor, however.

Clinical diagnosis

Disease of the larynx and hypopharynx require a thorough physical examination. Mirror and fiberoptic laryngoscopy of these structures is mandatory.

If a tumorous lesion of the endolarynx is suspected, the patient has to be examined under general anesthesia and a biopsy has to be taken endoscopically. During this procedure, the extension of the tumor has to be checked carefully to determine the adequate therapeutic approach. Sometimes the use of a binocular microscope can be helpful to determine the exact superficial borderlines of the lesion.[64,65]

Thorough palpation of the neck is obligatory for the detection of cervical lymph-node metastases, which can be an early symptom of hypopharyngeal cancer and can also appear in advanced laryngeal cancer.

Tumor classification

In giving a clear description of a certain tumor infiltration, a uniform classification of laryngeal and hypopharyngeal tumors is needed. Based on such information, appropriate therapy can be chosen. The most common classification of tumors is the TNM system, proposed by the International Union Against Cancer (UICC).

The TNM system defines stage T1 as tumor extension limited to a subsite of the tumor's topographic region, not transgressing supraglottic, glottic, subglottic or hypopharyngeal structures. Glottic tumors are subdivided into T1a (tumor confined to one vocal cord) and T1b (tumor affects both vocal cords).

T2 tumors extend to adjoining subsites of the laryngeal or hypopharyngeal region. Vocal cords show either normal or impaired mobility; the hypopharynx is not fixed on the larynx.

T3 tumors progress with an invasion, for example into the piriform sinus and pre-epiglottic space from supraglottic tumors, and into fixed vocal cords from glottic tumors.

T4 tumors invade structures beyond the larynx, such as the oropharynx or soft tissue of the neck and infrahyoid muscles. Glottic and supraglottic tumors invade through thyroid and/or cricoid cartilage, hypopharyngeal tumors through the epiglottis.

The definitions of the N categories follow the same scheme. N1 signifies metastasis in a single ipsilateral lymph node, 3 cm or less in greatest dimension, N2a 3–6 cm. Several homolateral lymph nodes, none more than 6 cm in greatest dimension, indicate N2b. In stage N2c there are bilateral or contralateral lymph nodes smaller than 6 cm in diameter. At least one lymph node more than 6 cm in greatest dimension is to be classified as stage N3.

The initial diagnostic tool for the pre-operative evaluation of location and extent of laryngeal and hypopharyngeal tumors is clinical laryngoscopy. The therapeutic procedure, such as operation, radiation or chemotherapy, is based on its results. In the last decade, additional imaging techniques, such as CT, sonography or MR have been established in the diagnosis of primary tumors and lymph node involvement.[60,63] CT is usually very efficient for studying the tumor and cervical nodes. Dynamic studies (apnea, inspiration, phonation, Valsalva's maneuver) are also easy using CT. MR is also efficient, but motion artifacts may be a real problem in 10–20% of patients. Coronal views are especially helpful for tumors near the ventricule (Diagram 4.3).

Squamous-cell carcinoma

Imaging provides vital information about laryngeal and hypopharyngeal anatomy in the following specific areas, which should be identified and evaluated for tumor extension:

- anterior and posterior commissures,
- supraglottic extension (pre-epiglottic space, paralaryngeal space, piriform sinuses, valleculae),
- infraglottic extension,
- vocal cord fixation,
- extralaryngeal spread (soft tissue of the neck and tongue base),
- cartilage invasion,
- carotid artery involvement,
- cervical adenopathy.

Laryngeal cancer can be divided into three groups based on location: supraglottic, glottic (true vocal cord) and infraglottic. Each group has a characteristic pattern spread. For instance, metastatic disease to lymph nodes is more common in supraglottic and infraglottic tumor than in glottic lesions. This reflects relatively poor lymphatic drainage of the vocal cords. Tumors of the piriform sinus, while actually of hypophryngeal origin, will be included in this discussion because of their close relationship to supraglottic lesions.

In the various types of laryngeal cancers, the laryngeal cartilages may be involved by tumor. Cartilage ossifies progressively with age: normal non-ossified cartilage should not be mistaken for involvement. Ossified cartilage may be involved by the tumor, non-ossified cartilage is usually not. Different patterns may be seen: osteosclerosis, which is non-specific and may be tumor or inflammatory reaction, erosion of the cortex and osteolysis. Expansion is rare and indicates tumor inside the cartilage.

Supraglottic carcinoma

CT scanning identifies the pre-epiglottic space as a low density area because of its high fat content. T1-weighted MR will show the tumor-to-fat contrast in the pre-epiglottic space to best advantage. Sagittal MR images will best show spread to the tongue base. Supraglottic tumors, arising anywhere from the false vocal cords to the epiglottis, comprise 20–35% of laryngeal cancers (Figure 4.27). Supraglottic tumors tend to spread to lymph nodes high in the neck, involving the internal jugular chain and often the jugular digastric nodes because of the abundant lymphatics in this region. Consequently, supraglottic cancers often present as more advanced tumors than glottic lesions.

- *Stage T1:* a supraglottic stage T1 tumor is hard to see on CT or MR. T1 tumors are limited to mucosal structures of the supraglottic region, for example the arytenoepiglottic fold or one false cord, either on the left or on the right side. The motion of the hemilarynx is not yet impaired.
- *Stage T2:* T2 tumors of the supraglottic larynx are the smallest tumors that can be diagnosed routinely, presuming excellent image quality is possible. The tumor tends to spread either cranially, infiltrating the hypopharyngeal region with epiglottis or the pharyngoepiglottic folds, or caudally into the glottic region and the lateral pharyngeal walls. The false cords may be fixed partially; the vocal cord is not impaired in its mobility.
- *Stage T3:* T3 tumors are a clear indication for imaging to determine the exact deep infiltration; imaging gives important information for determining therapy. Tumors of stage T3 often erode the thyroid cartilage or even the arytenoid cartilages. An overlapping of the tumor into pre-epiglottic space, valleculae or vocal cords, even with fixation of the cords, is quite common.
- *Stage T4:* T4 tumors are, according to the TNM classification, tumors infiltrating beyond laryngeal and hypopharyngeal structures. Starting from the supraglottic larynx, the base of the tongue together with tongue-base and geniohyoid muscles are frequently involved; in the dorsal direction, the piriform sinus and esophagus may be infiltrated. Because patients with a high-stage tumor often complain about dyspnea, shortness of breath and sore throat the MR images tend to be of a low quality due to motion artifacts: T2 and proton density images often do not contribute to the diagnostic findings because of severe motion artifacts. On the other hand, tumors of this size can be visualized by a CT scan in most cases. Therefore, CT may compensate for a MR examination; it is also of lower radiation load for the patient.

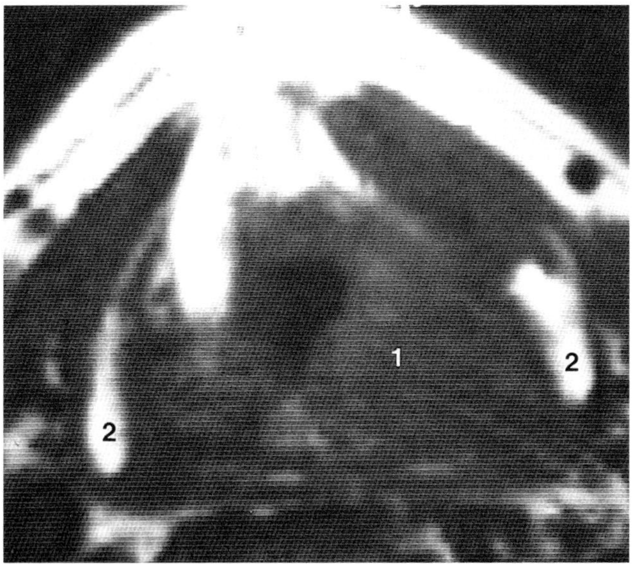

A

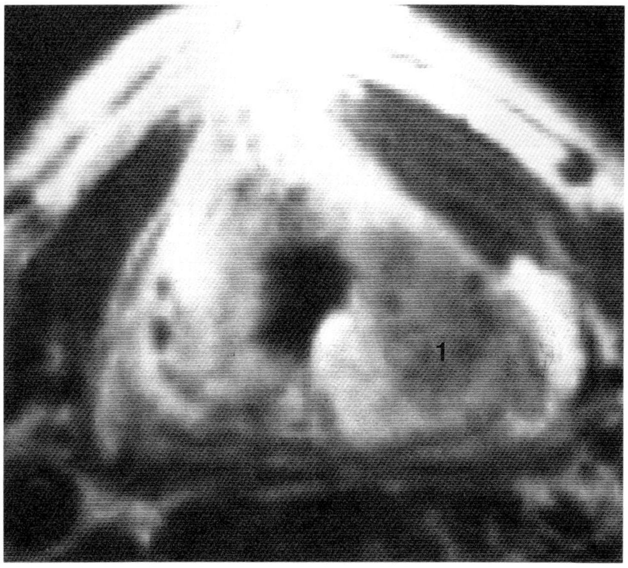

B

Figure 4.27

Supraglottic carcinoma on the left side, stage T3.

A Axial, plain MR (TR/TE = 500/17): there is a mass in the supraglottic portion of the larynx (1). The normal thyroid cartilage, with high signal intensity, is clearly demonstrated (2). The tumor does not cross the anterior commissura.

B Axial MR (TR/TE = 500/17) after contrast-enhanced injection: the inhomogeneous tumorous mass in the supraglottic portion of the larynx is identified on the left side. Note the high contrast enhancement of the surrounding mucosal structures. On the right side, some lymphoid hypoplasia is identified. There are no certain signs of infiltration.

Glottic carcinomas

Glottic tumors, arising from the true cords, are the most common laryngeal cancers. They comprise 50–70% of laryngeal malignancies and are usually well-differentiated, slow-growing lesions; 75% arise from the anterior half of the true vocal cord. Because of their early presentation and the ease of clinical examination, most glottic carcinomas do not require imaging studies. Nodal spread is uncommon because there is an absence of lymphatics along the free margin of the vocal cords. However, advanced lesions associated with cord fixation have a higher incidence of lymphatic involvement.

CT scans of small lesions may look normal or may show true cord thickening. CT density differences between non-enhancing tumor and muscle are not large enough in most instances to allow one to predict invasion of the true cord musculature. MR signals from tumor and muscle differ so much that the distinction between an exophytic and deeply infiltrating lesion is easier. Impaired mobility may be inferred from CT scans by diminished motion artifacts on the involved side as well as the typical paramedian position of the cord and more medially situated arytenoid. Both CT and MR provide an exquisite view of the anterior commissure and its relationship to the supraglottic and subglottic compartments. MR and CT may show invasion of the thyroid cartilage, which is a contraindication for partial laryngectomy and a relative contraindication for radiotherapy. More advanced glottic lesions will spread to the false cord, epiglottis, interarytenoid region; all of these are contraindications to vertical hemilaryngectomy. Coronal MR may prove superior to CT in showing this spread, because bulky lesions sometimes bulge upward and distort the false cord rather than invade it.

- *Stage T1:* normally, tumors of this low stage cannot be depicted with CT or MR imaging. The vocal cords are visualized as normal or cannot be differentiated from inflammatory or edematous lesions prospectively. Clinical symptoms such as hoarseness give support to a verdict of a tumor of the glottis and must be verified by clinical laryngoscopy. T1 is subdivided by definition into stage T1a, when the tumor infiltrates only one cord, and T1b, if both cords are infiltrated. The vocal cords are not impaired in their motion.
- *Stage T2:* glottic stage T2 tumors can be seen by CT or MR, provided that excellent image quality is available. Glottic tumors can spread in every direction; mostly the thyroid and arytenoid cartilages are involved. But infiltration of the false cords and the arytenoepiglottic folds are also very common. Another typical infiltration is dorsal, involving the cricoid cartilage and the dorsal parts of the piriform sinus. Even a caudal growth into the subglottic area is possible. The vocal cords are still free of motion restrictions, or at least the mobility is only slightly impaired.
- *Stage T3:* there is more advanced growth in stage T3 than in stage T2, but the tumors are still restricted to the topographic region of the larynx. The combination of the different MR techniques is very helpful to give a detailed description of the tumor with respect to the therapy that follows. The difference between stage T2 and stage T3 in tumor classification is based on the fixation of the vocal cords, which gives a classification of T3. Thus, dynamic CT examination can be helpful. Knowledge of the clinical symptoms and the progress of the patient's complaints is of great importance to the exact tumor classification.
- *Stage T4:* tumors staged T4 have already infiltrated anatomic structures beyond the larynx. The most common types of infiltration are dorsal, involving the esophagus, and ventral, reaching hyoid bone and the base of the tongue. Due to severe motion artifacts because of the long scan time, a CT examination may be considered instead of MR for patients with advanced clinical symptoms such as dyspnea.

Subglottic carcinomas

Infraglottic tumors arising between the true vocal cords and the inferior border of the cricoid cartilage (Figure 4.28) comprise 2–6% of laryngeal cancers. True infraglottic primary malignancies are

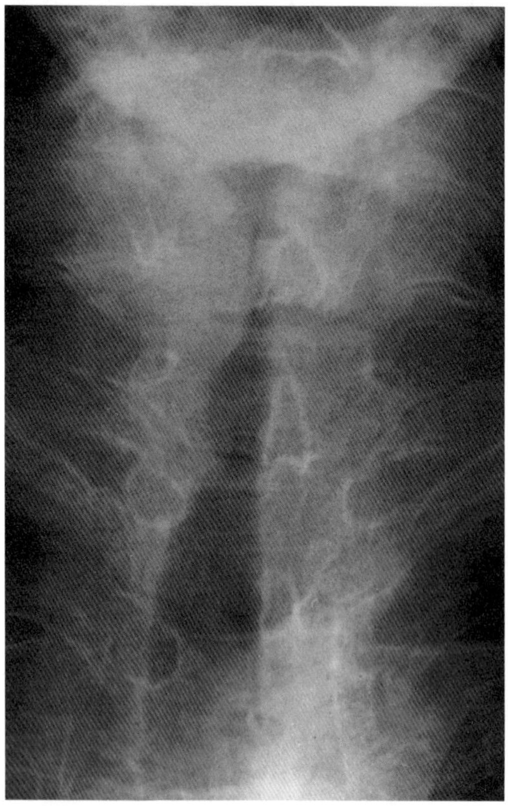

A

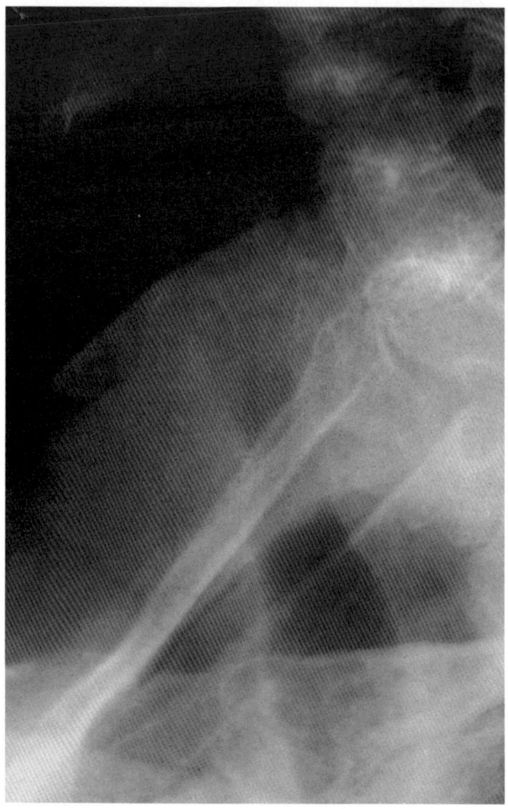

B

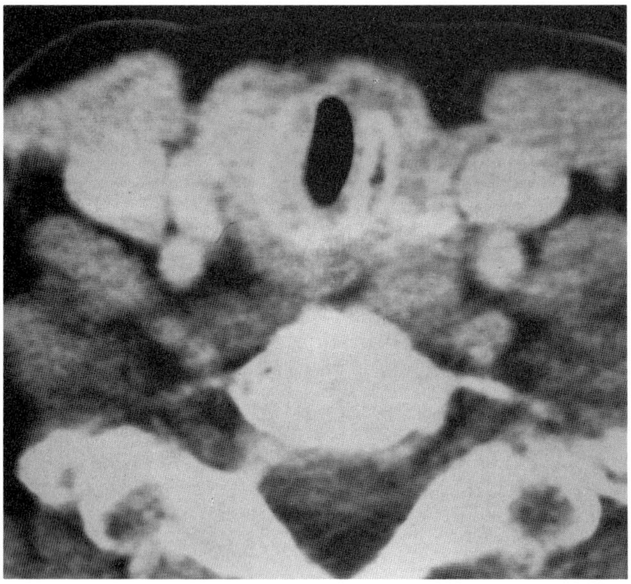

C

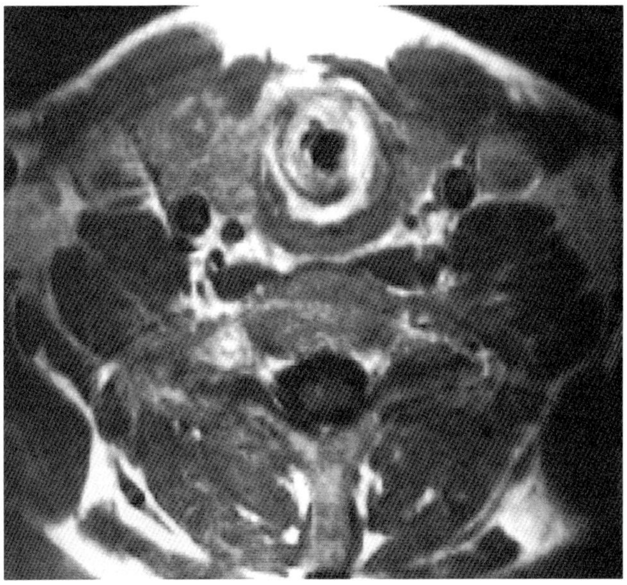

E

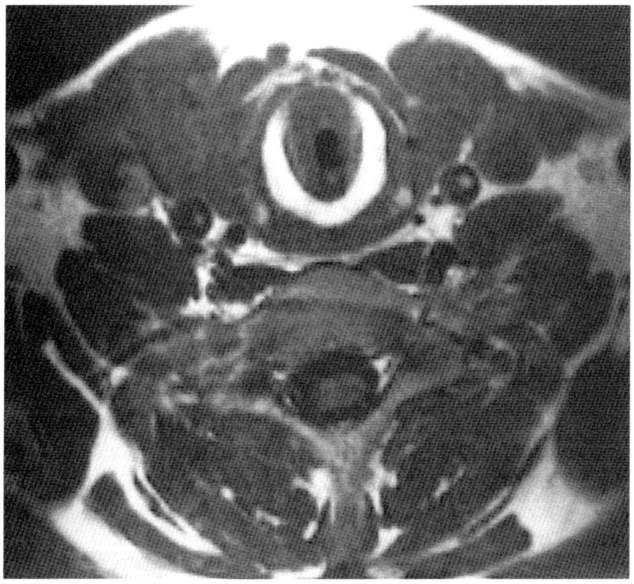

D

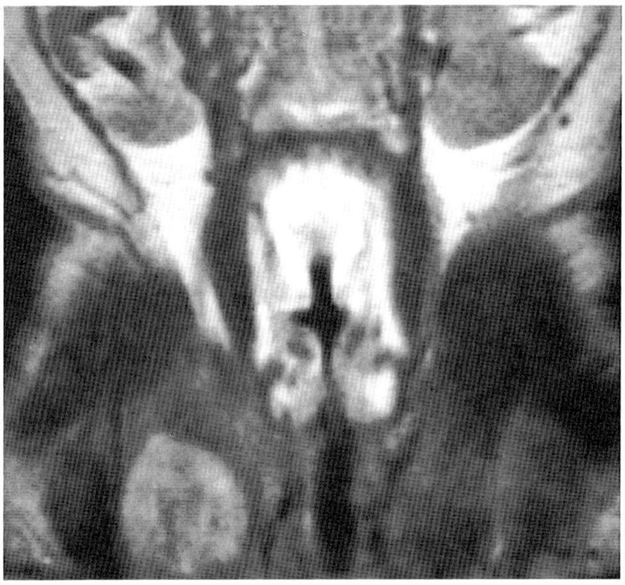

F

Figure 4.28

Subglottic laryngeal carcinoma: comparative evaluation of conventional radiography, CT and MR findings.

A,B Radiography (anterior, posterior and lateral) demonstrates some changes in the air-containing spaces of the subglottic larynx and upper portion of the trachea. A mass cannot be clearly delineated.

C CT scan after contrast application shows a widening of the subglottic mucosal structures mainly on the right side. The cricoid cartilage is not infiltrated.

D–F MR (TR/TE = 500/17)—axial, plain (**D**), axial, enhanced (**E**), coronal, enhanced (**F**). Plain MR (**D**) demonstrates a narrowing of the subglottic level of the larynx. Adjacent cricoid cartilage shows normal signal intensity structures. After contrast-medium injection (**E**), the soft-tissue mass of the mucosal structures shows an inhomogeneous and diffuse contrast enhancement. The coronal section (**F**) additionally shows the normal false vocal cords, the normal sinus of Morgagni and the contrast-enhancing tumorous mass in the subglottic level of the larynx. Note additionally a thyroid adenoma with high signal intensity in the right thyroid lobe.

rare, and tumors arising from this area spread easily to the trachea, thyroid, hypopharynx and lateral-compartment lymph nodes. Infraglottic tumors are most often due to inferior extension of glottic and occasionally supraglottic cancers. On scans below the true vocal cords, any soft tissue between the cricoid cartilage and the airway is abnormal and may represent subglottic extension. The conus elasticus is an anatomic barrier that separates deep tumors from mucosal lesions. Tumors infiltrating deep to the conus elasticus (for example, transglottic tumors) tend to remain on its deep surface (paralaryngeal surface), while those beginning on its mucosal side tend to remain mucosal.

Generally, if an infraglottic tumor extends more than 1 cm caudal to the true cords, a total laryngectomy is indicated because it is necessary to remove the cricoid cartilage to obtain a clear margin of excision. With more aggressive voice conservation techniques, parts of the superior rim of the cricoid lamina may be excised, leaving the cricoid ring intact to preserve laryngeal function. In advanced lesions the cricoid cartilage may be eroded, and total laryngectomy is then necessary.

Transglottic tumors are defined as those involving the true cords and subglottic space, or those that cross the laryngeal ventricles. Involvement of the true and false vocal cords may cause vocal cord fixation. A few transglottic tumors begin in the laryngeal ventricle; many more originate from the true vocal cord with laryngeal spread. Transglottic tumors have an increased incidence of thyroid cartilage invasion and extension through the cricothyroid membrane. Treatment is usually total laryngectomy with or without radiation therapy.

The use of thin-section CT, overlapped if necessary, makes the depiction of tumor margins relative to the cricoid cartilage extremely accurate.

Hypopharyngeal carcinomas

Piriform-sinus tumors (Figure 4.29) behave more aggressively than endolaryngeal lesions and comprise 10–20% of laryngeal cancers. They are usually squamous-cell cancers of inferior hypopharyngeal origin. Early nodal disease occurs because of the rich lymphatics anterior to the piriform sinuses. Piriform-sinus tumors grow in two major patterns. Lateral-wall lesions invade the thyroid cartilage and soft tissues of the neck, forming bulky masses about the piriform sinus. Medial-wall lesions extend into the paralaryngeal space and vocal muscle, resembling marginal supraglottic lesions. Less commonly, piriform-sinus cancers invade the pre-epiglottic space and extend across the midline. Tumors of either piriform sinus wall may spread supramedially to the arytenoepiglottic fold, again simulating marginal supraglottic lesions.

There is no clear evident definition, differentiating supraglottic laryngeal carcinomas from hypopharyngeal ones. Usually it is difficult or even impossible to identify the original anatomic site of the tumor growth.

- *Stage T1:* hypopharyngeal tumors of stage T1 are often clinically undetectable. On CT and MR, the tumors are too small to be diagnosed with sufficient assurance, because they are hidden in the mucosal layer coating the complete hypopharynx. Even clinical laryngoscopy does not give 100% detection of T1 tumors: the complex anatomy often obstructs the laryngoscopical view into the complete hypopharynx.
- *Stage T2:* T2 tumors of the hypopharynx can be evaluated exactly with CT or MR. The most common locations of tumor growth are the piriform sinus on both sides, the pharyngoepiglottic fold and the posterior wall of the hypopharynx. In stage T2, the tumor infiltrates one or several of these structures, often eroding the epiglottis, but is not yet fixed at the hemilarynx.
- *Stage T3:* the T3 tumor is characterized by increased size and infiltration. Posteriorly developed tumors have infiltrated the piriform sinus and the posterior pharyngeal wall; cranially spreading tumors can be found in epiglottis, the pharyngoepiglottic folds and the valleculae epiglotticae. If the tumor reaches the laryngeal area, it tends to infiltrate the post-cricoid area, the false cords and the arytenoid cartilage, and is fixed at the hemilarynx.
- *Stage T4:* a stage T4 tumor is defined by infiltration of anatomic structures beyond the hypopharynx. Usually the base of the tongue and tongue-base and geniohyoid muscles are reached first by the tumor. The hyoid bone is often affected, and erosions of the thyroid area can be found. Infiltrations of the cricoid cartilage or soft tissues of the neck are further criteria for stage T4 hypopharyngeal tumors. In MR, particularly large tumors of the hypopharynx show a characteristic necrotic inner structure. The necrotic tissue is visualized best using contrast medium. The diagnosis can be made on CT with the same accuracy in stage T4.

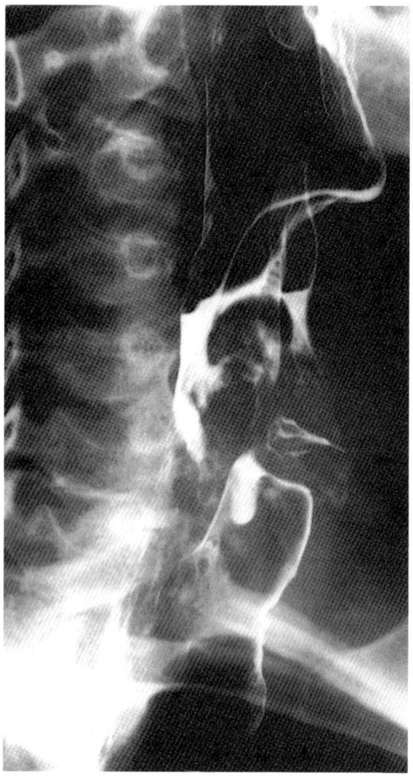

A

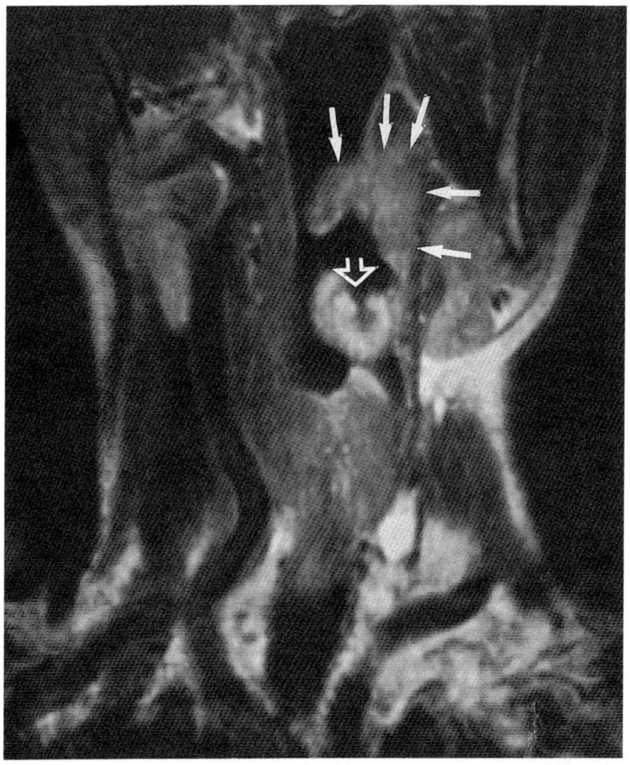

B

Figure 4.29

Hypopharyngeal carcinoma.

A Barium swallow examination: after contrast application, the pre-epiglottic space and the hypopharyngeal structures are identified. Note a huge mass with displacement of the vallecula and the hypopharyngeal folds. Using conventional radiography, the exact topographic relationship of the tumorous mass cannot be clearly evaluated.

B Coronal MR (TR/TE = 500/17) after contrast-medium injection: the use of coronal MR helps to delineate soft-tissue extension in hypopharyngeal carcinomas. MR allows the delineation of two polypoid tumor masses, one is identified at the hypopharyngeal entrance (white arrows), the other is lying in the hypopharyngeal space (open arrow).

Lymph-node disease of the neck

Lymph-node metastases of head and neck tumors (Figure 4.30), as well as lymph nodes in Hodgkin's and non-Hodgkin's lymphomas may present as cervical swellings. Particularly in patients with risk factors such as chronic alcohol and nicotine abuse, metastatic lymph nodes in the neck may present as an early manifestation of a cancerous lesion in the nasopharynx, the oral cavity, the oropharynx, the hypopharynx or the larynx. At least 10% of pathologic nodes are missed clinically, thus CT or MR from the skull base to the upper inlet of the thorax should be performed in patients suffering from malignancies of the head and neck. CT is usually easier to perform, as the coil used on MR to study the primary tumor may be inappropriate to study the whole neck simultaneously.

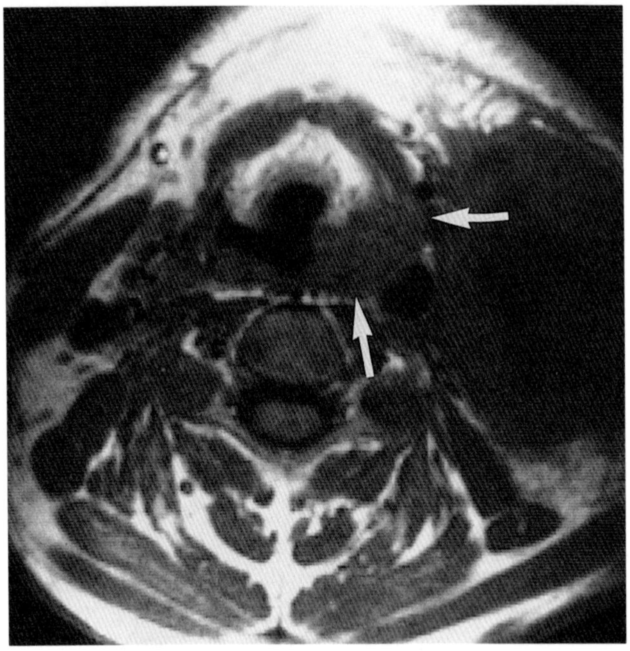

A

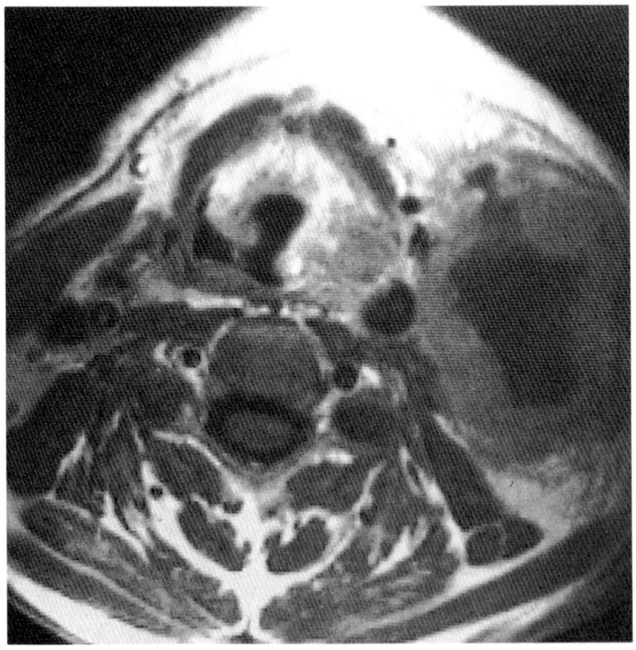

B

Figure 4.30

Hypopharyngeal carcinoma (stage T2) with huge lymph-node metastasis (stage N3).

A Axial, plain MR (TR/TE = 500/17): there is a soft-tissue mass in the left vallecula and the hypopharyngeal entrance is identified (arrows). In the left lateral neck, a huge mass with diffuse margins and inhomogeneities is clearly depicted.

B Axial MR (TR/TE = 500/17) after contrast-medium injection: the exact depth of infiltration of the vallecula and hypopharynx is demonstrated. The huge lymph-node metastasis is clearly diagnosed by inhomogeneous necrosis.

Clinical diagnosis

In the diagnostic evaluation of cervical swellings, a thorough physical examination, including inspection and palpation, is absolutely mandatory. In many cases, physical examination and the patient's history will enable the physician to establish the diagnosis. Ultrasonography can be useful as a screening method in cervical tumors, and especially to guide needle biopsies.

If a patient with a cervical mass has a history of alcohol and nicotine use, a biopsy of the lesion must be made. In addition, the upper gastrorespiratory tract has to be checked carefully. Even if the patient does not complain of any symptoms, an endoscopic evaluation of the nose, the nasopharynx, the oropharynx and oral cavity, as well as the hypopharynx and larynx, the trachea and the esophagus, must be undertaken to exclude cancerous growth in one of these regions that might be responsible for the metastatic lymph node.

Disease of the lymphatic system in the neck region can be subdivided into primary (Hodgkin's and non-Hodgkin's lymphoma) and secondary tumors and inflammatory lesions. The grading of lymphomas follows the Ann Arbor classification. The lymph node groups of the neck have very complex discharge pathways, alongside the venous system. Hence the most important leading structure in the neck is the internal jugular vein.

Lymphadenopathy appears above all other symptoms, with lesions in the areas of oropharynx, hypopharynx and supraglottic larynx. In systemic diseases, an infiltration of the supraglottic lymph nodes, which are the connection between the jugular and cervicoposterior lymph nodes, is typical.

Malignant lymphomas

Lymphomas show a preference for the lymphatic tissue of the deep vessel-nerve layer of the neck, reaching a vast size on both sides (Figure 4.31). On CT, a thickening of the soft tissues of the neck can be detected. Sometimes there are conglomerates of lymph nodes visible. The density does not significantly differ from the surrounding tissues and the lesion enhances only slightly after administration of intravenous contrast medium. Peripheral rim enhancement may occur, but central necrosis is rare. At CT, they are indistinguishable from reactive nodes or non-necrotic nodes of other etiologies. On plain MR T1-weighted sequences, a low signal can be detected. Plain T1-weighted images allow a distinction of tumorous parts from fatty tissue, while in T2-weighted images a differentiation of tumor from muscle is possible, due to increased T2 relaxation times. After therapy a low signal intensity on T1- and T2-weighted sequences is to be viewed as an expression of response to therapy. Signal intensity reaction after contrast medium application reveals a homogeneous enhancement of the altered tissue.

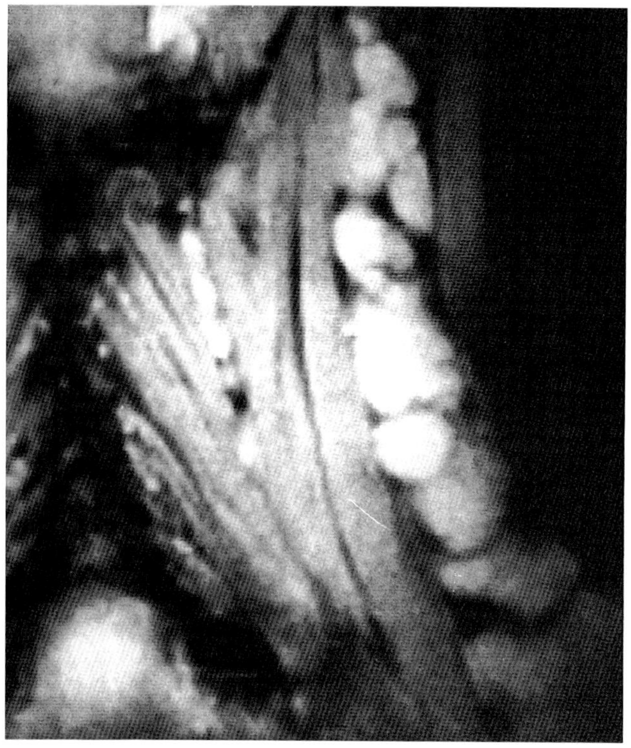

Figure 4.31

Hodgkin's lymphoma of the right lateral side of the neck. Coronal plain MR (FLASH sequence, TR/TE = 30/12): the fast imaging protocol demonstrates a chain of lymph nodes of increased diameter and increased signal intensity. All show homogeneous inner structures, sharp margins and low infiltration of the neighboring structures.

Metastatic cancer

Areas predisposed to metastasis are the lymph nodes of the cervicojugular and cervicoposterior group. Clinical assessment of the cervical lymph nodes in patients with squamous-cell carcinoma in the head and neck region is difficult. The overall error rate for detection by palpation is more than 20%. Thus the clinical N0 stage is controversial. If there is a high risk of occult cervical lymph-node metastases, surgical treatment of the neck is often done, but around 75% of the dissections are free of disease. On the other hand, if cervical nodes are not treated, up to 32% of patients with clinically negative nodes will develop lymph-node metastasis. So the imaging evaluation is especially helpful.

Size is a very useful criterion. The minimum diameter in the axial plane is the most accurate size criterion for predicting lymph-node metastasis. A minimum diameter of 10 mm is the best criterion for differentiating normal and metastatic nodes. Groups of three or more borderline nodes increase the sensitivity.[63,65]

On CT, nodes are homogeneous in 25% of the patients only. On MR T1 and T2 relaxation times resemble those of normal lymph nodes, with a long T1 and an average T2 relaxation time. T2-weighted sequences improve the signal : noise ratio. An extension of echo and repetition time produce a decrease in contrast with a masking of the tumor,

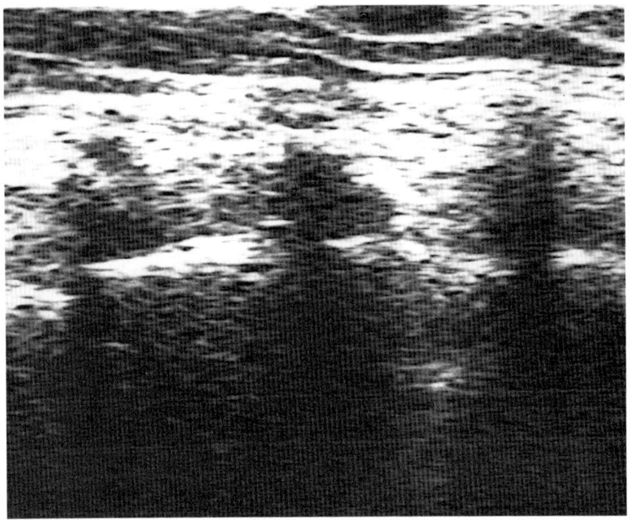

A

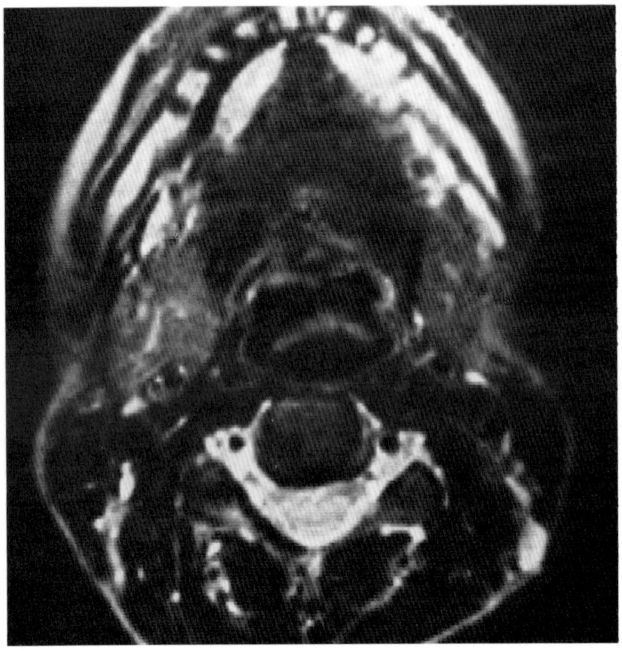

B

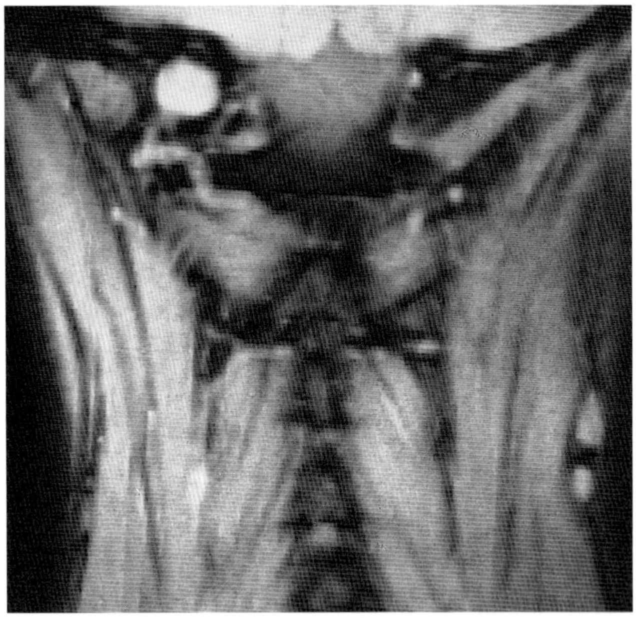

C

Figure 4.32

Lateral neck cyst on the left side: comparative evaluation of ultrasound and MR findings.

A Coronal ultrasound (5 MHz): the elliptical mass with low echogenicity is identified in the lateral portion of the neck. An increased echogenicity is seen in the posterior portion of the neck structures.

B Axial, plain MR (TR/TE = 3000/90): the T2-weighted image demonstrates a cystic structure in the left lateral neck area. Note that the signal intensity is nearly equivalent to that of the cerebrospinal fluid.

C Fast sequence coronal MR technique (FLASH, TR/TE = 30/12): due to its excellent soft tissue contrast, the FLASH sequence allows the exact differential diagnosis of a neck cyst with internal fluid, which is located on the left side of the neck.

due to the signal reduction by fatty tissue and a simultaneous signal increase by the metastasis. Metastases, which are surronded by little or no fatty tissue (for example retrolaryngeal lymph nodes), are distinguished best with a T2 sequence or a T1/T2 mixed sequence. Differential diagnostic considerations should include lateral neck cysts, which do not show contrast enhancement (Figure 4.32). After contrast medium administration, metastatic lymph nodes show enhancement and increase signal intensity in T1- and T2-weighted images, in the course of which even heterogeneous structures can be discerned (Figure 4.33).

A central hypodensity on CT is seen in 75% of patients with metastasis, and almost only in tumorous nodes. So it is possible to diagnose a normal-

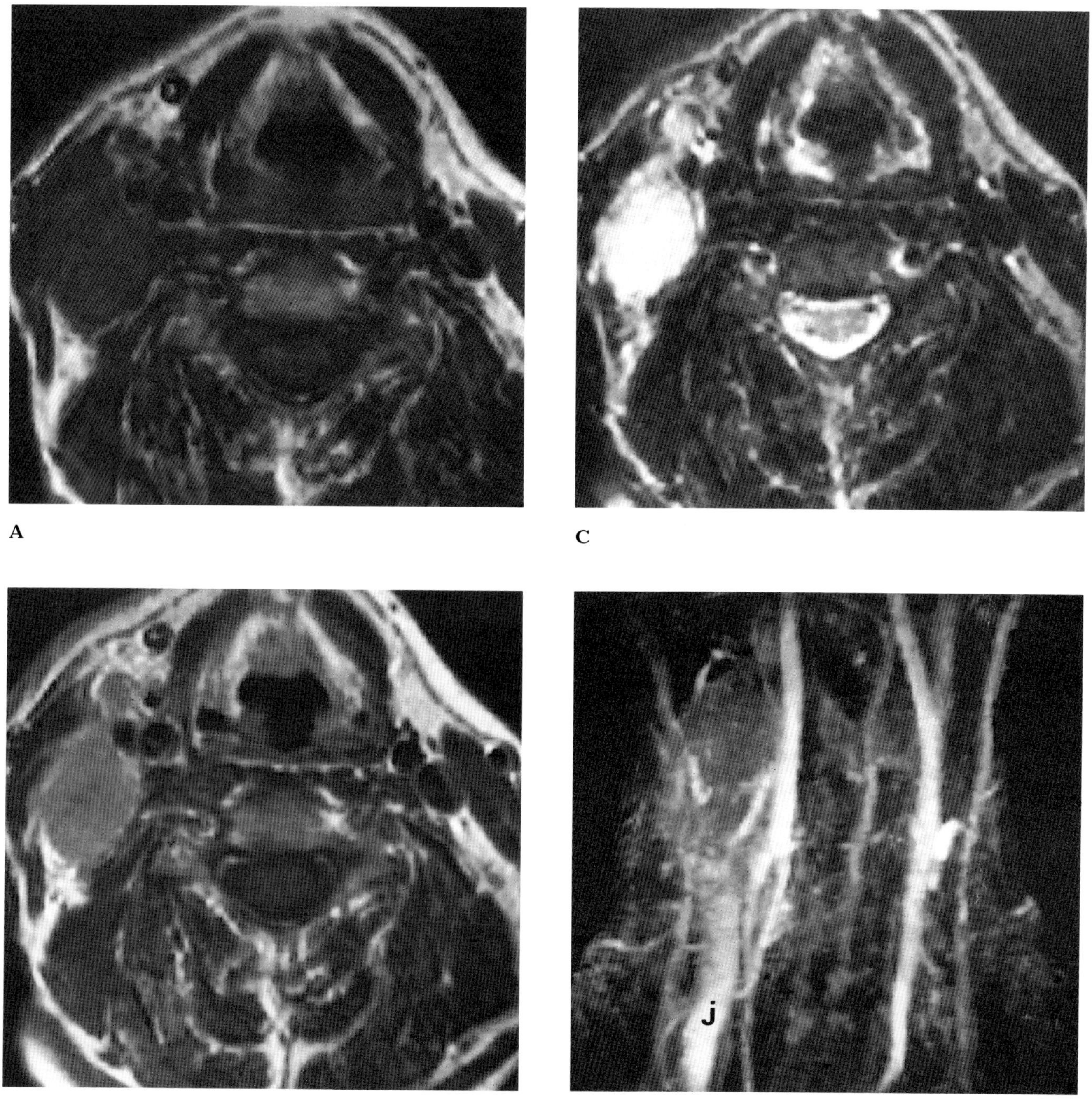

A C B D

Figure 4.33

Lymph-node metastasis from unknown primary tumor.

A Axial, plain MR (TR/TE = 500/17): plain MR is characterized by low tissue contrast; the tumorous mass is identified by the deep cervical structures on the right side.

B Axial MR (TR/TE = 500/17) after contrast-medium injection: the tumorous mass shows a medium increase in signal intensity. Note that anterior of the internal carotid artery another lymph-node metastasis is clearly detected.

C Axial, plain MR (TR/TE = 2000/90): in the T2-weighted image, the lymph-node metastasis on the right lateral neck is identified via masses of high signal intensity. Note the tumor in the hypopharynx or larynx.

D Venous MRA, arterial presaturation (FLASH two-dimensional technique, TR/TE = 25/6, FLIP angle 20°): lymph-node metastasis is identified via low signal intensity structures. The right jugular vein (j) is obstructed, and collateral vessels are visualized over the external jugular vein and paravertebral venous structures.

sized metastatic node. The hypodensity may indicate necrosis, poorly vascularized tumor stroma, or even keratin after treatment. Whatever the cause, hypodensity is correlated with a worse survival rate. Hypodensity is also seen on MR after contrast enhancement. A poor limitation of the borders of the nodes is also very useful, indicating a probable capsular rupture.

Conclusion

The unique topography of the head-and-neck region is the reason for the outstanding possibilities of use of imaging examination methods. In a small space there are located a multitude of different tissue structures and sense organs which have to simultaneously control physiologic processes and movements. The task of imaging methods of this complex region is especially to identify tumorous masses and their expansion.[67]

The main use of imaging techniques is local evaluation, since the deep aspects of the tumor may not be visible or palpable. However, when the surgeon's clinical and endoscopic assessment of the mucosal extent of the tumor is combined with CT or MR assessment of the deep tissue extent, an accurate pre-treatment staging can be achieved.

Both CT and MR can be applied to primary tumor and nodal evaluation. The choice of which technique to use is based on the clinical questions, availability of equipment, the patient's ability to cooperate, and relative costs. In addition, imaging techniques can help in diagnosing recurrences, and in searching for an unknown primary. The best use of the new imaging modalities is obtained through close cooperation with the clinical disciplines.

Acknowledgments

We wish to thank W Steger, J Balzer, M Juergens and M Vorbuchner.

References

1. Fisch U, Die Mikrochirurgie des Felsenbeins, *HNO* (1977) **25**: 193–7.
2. Plester D, Wende S, Nakayma N, *Kleinhirnbrückenwinkeltumoren – Diagnostik und Therapie* (Springer-Verlag: Berlin, 1978).
3. Fisch U, Transtemporal surgery of the internal auditory canal, *Adv Otorhinolaryngol* (1970) **17**: 203–40.
4. Kurze T, Doyle JB, Extradural intracranial approach to the internal auditory canal, *J Neurosurg* (1962) **19**: 1033–77.
5. Young IR, Hall AS, Pallis CA et al, Nuclear magnetic resonance imaging of the brain in multiple sclerosis, *Lancet* (1981) **ii**: 1063–6.
6. Silverberg E, Luvera J, Cancer statistics, *CA* (1987) **37**: 2–19.
7. Hildmann H, Tiedjen KV, Zur Differentialdiagnose des Glomustumors, *Laryng Rhinol Otol* (1983) **62**: 502–4.
8. Gastpar H, Die Tumoren des Glomus caroticum, Glomus jugulare tympanicum und Glomus vagale, *Acta Otolaryngol* (1961) **167** (suppl) 1–23.
9. Tidwell H, Montague ED, Chemodectomas involving the temporal bone, *Radiology* (1975) **116**: 147.
10. Valavanis A, Schubinger O, Naidid TP, *Clinical imaging of the cerebello pontine angle* (Springer-Verlag: Berlin, 1987).
11. Lovrencic M, Kalousek M, Marotti M et al, Tumors of nasopharynx: a CT evaluation of 52 patients. In: *Digital radiology* (Springer-Verlag: Berlin, 1987) 265–9.
12. Bloch F, Hansen WW, Packard M, Nuclear magnetic resonance, *Phys Rev* (1946) **69**: 127–38.
13. Lloyd G, Land V, Phelps P et al, MRI in evaluation of nose and paranasal sinus disease. *Br J Radiol* (1987) **60**: 957–68.
14. Mandelblatt S, Bron IF, Davis PC et al, Parotid masses: MR imaging, *Radiology* (1987) **163**:411–14.
15. Casselman JW, Mancuso AA, Major salivary gland masses: comparison of MR imaging and CT, *Radiology* (1987) **165**: 183–9.
16. Lufkin RB, Wortham DG, Dietrich RB et al, Tongue and oropharynx: findings on MR imaging, *Radiology* (1986) **161**: 69–75.
17. Spiessl B, Hermanek P, Scheibe O et al, *TNM-Atlas, UICC* (Springer-Verlag: Berlin, 1982).
18. Kleinsasser O, *Tumoren des Larynx- und Hypopharynx* (Thieme: Stuttgart, 1987).
19. Lajaunias P, Moret J, Normal and nonpathological variables in angiographic aspects of the arteries of the middle ear, *Neuroradiology* (1978) **15**: 213–19.
20. Lloyd TM, Van Aman V, Johnson JC, Aberrant jugular bulb presenting as middle ear mass, *Radiology* (1979) **131**: 139–41.
21. Valavanis A, Praeoperative embolization of the head and neck, indication, patient selection, goals and precautions, *Am J Neuroradiol* (1986) **7**: 943–52.
22. Valavanis A, Intraarterielle DSA in der interventionellen Neuroradiology. In: Nadjimi M ed, *Digitale*

Subtraaktionsangiographie in der Neuroradiologie (Thieme: Stuttgart, 1986) 239–46.
23. Hajek PC, Salomonowitz E, Türk R et al, Lymph nodes of the neck, evaluation with US, *Radiology* (1986) **158**: 739–42.
24. Frühwald F, Salomonowitz E, Neuhoff A et al, Tongue cancer: sonographic assessment of the tumor stage, *J Ultrasound Med* (1985) **6**: 121–37.
25. Bender A, Bradac GB, Erfahrungen in der radiologischen Diagnostik kleiner Akustikusneurinome, *Röntgenblätter* (1986) **39**: 36–9.
26. Daniels DL, Schende JF, Forster Th et al, Surface-coil magnetic resonance imaging of the internal auditory canal, *Am J Roentgenol* (1985) **145**: 469–72.
27. Castelijns JA, Doornbos J, Verbeeten B et al, Magnetic resonance imaging of the normal larynx, *Comput Assist Tomogr* (1985) **9**: 919–25.
28. Brash RC, Methods of contrast enhancement for NMR imaging and potential applications: a subject review, *Radiology* (1983) **147**: 781–3.
29. Bydder GM, Steiner RE, Young IR et al, Clinical NMR imaging of the brain: 140 cases, *AJR* (1982) **139**: 215–36.
30. Felix R, Schoerner We, Laniado M et al, Brain tumors: MR imaging with gadolinium-DTPA, *Radiology* (1985) **156**: 681–8.
31. Hansson LG, Johansen CC, Biörklund A, CT sialography and conventional sialography in the evaluation of parotid gland neoplasm, *J Laryngol Otol* (1983) **102**: 163–8.
32. Kazner E, Wende S, Grumme T et al, *Computed tomography in intracranial tumors* (Springer-Verlag: Berlin, 1982).
33. Young JR, Bydder GM, Hall AS et al, The role of NMR imaging in the diagnosis and management of acoustic neuroma, *ANJR* (1983) **4**: 223–4.
34. Bentson J, Combined gascisternography and edge enhanced computed tomography of the internal auditory canal, *Radiology* (1980) **136**: 777–9.
35. Mathew GD, Faser GW, Symptoms, findings and method: a diagnosis in patients with acoustic neuroma, *Laryngoscope* (1987) **88**: 1893–1903.
36. Mafee MF, Valvassai GE, High resolution and dynamic sequential computed tomography, *Arch Otolaryngol* (1983) **109**: 691–6.
37. Bauer WM, Baierl P, Vogl Th et al, Contrast-enhancement in intercranial tumors—a comparison of CT and MR, *Radiology* (1985) **157**: 126–30.
38. Weber AL, Davis KR, Nadol JB, Chemodectomas of the glomus jugulare, glomus vagale and carotid body, *Ann Otol Rhinol Laryngol* (1982) **91**: 666–9.
39. Beimert U, Grever G, Vogl Th, Zum Stellenwert der digitalen Subtrakionsangiographie bei der Diagnostik von Glomustumoren, *Arch Otorhinolaryngol* (1988) suppl II: 100–1.
40. Carr DH, Brown J, Lenng WL et al, Iron and gadolinium chelates as contrast agents in NMR imaging: preliminary studies, *Comput Assist Tomogr* (1984) **8**: 385–9.
41. Felix R, Schoerner W, Laniado M et al, Kontrastmittel in der magnetischen Resonanztomographie, *RÖFO* (1985) **143**: 9–14.
42. Lenz M, König H, Sauter R et al, Kernspintomographie des Felsenbeins und des Kleinhirnbrückenwinkels, *RÖFO* (1985) **143**: 1–8.
43. Runge VM, Clanton JA, Price AC et al, The use of GD-DTPA as a perfusion agent and marker of blood–brain barrier disruption, *Magn Reson Imaging* (1985) **3**: 43–55.
44. New PF, Badow TB, Wismer GL et al, MR imaging of the acoustic nerves and small acoustic neuromas at 0.6 Tesla, *Am J Roentgenol* (1985) **144**: 1021–6.
45. Mancuso AA, Bohmann L, Hanafee WN et al Computed tomography of the nasopharynx: normal and variants of normal, *Radiology* (1980) **137**: 113–21.
46. Vogl Th, Dresel S, Kang K et al, Nasopharyngeal and adjacent tumors, MRI with Gd-DTPA, *Am J Neuroradiol* (1990) **11**: 187–94.
47. Vogl Th, Mees K, Grevers G, Die diagnostische Wertigkeit der Kernspintomographie bei Raumforderungen des Pharynx, *Laryng Rhinol Otol* (1987) **66**: 543–6.
48. Silver JA, Mawad ME, Hilal SK et al, Computed tomography of the nasopharynx and related spaces. I. Anatomy, *Radiology* (1983) **147**: 725–31.
49. Silver JA, Mawad ME, Hilal SK et al, Computed tomography of the nasopharynx and related spaces. II. Pathology, *Radiology* (1983) **147**: 733–8.
50. Teresi LM, Lufkin RB, Hanafee WN et al, MRI imaging of the nasopharynx and floor of the middle cranial fossa. I. Normal anatomy, *Radiology* (1987) **164**: 811–16.
51. Teresi LM, Lufkin RB, Hanafee WN et al, MRI imaging of the nasopharynx and floor of the middle cranial fossa. II. Malignant tumors, *Radiology* (1987) **164**: 817–21.
52. Bryan RN, Miller RM, Ferreyro RJ et al, Computed tomography of the major salivary glands, *AJR* (1982) **139**: 547–54.
53. Dillon WP, Applications of magnetic reasonance imaging to the head and neck, *Semin US CT MR* (1986) **7**: 202–9.
54. Gademann G, Semmler G, Bachert-Baumann P et al, ^{31}P-Spectroscopy follow up studies of human tumor after chemotherapy. In: *Works in progress (*Society of Magnetic Resonance in Medicine. Sixth annual meeting and exhibition. Book of abstracts: Berkeley, California, 1987) 506.
55. Mancuso AA, Bohmann L, Hanafee WN et al Computed tomography of the nasopharynx: normal and variants of normal, *Radiology* (1980) **137**: 113–21.
56. Tereis LM, Lufkin RB, Warthan DG et al, Parotid masses: MR imaging, *Radiology* (1987) **163**: 405–9.
57. Som PM, Braun JF, Shapiro MD et al, Tumors of the parapharyngeal space and upper neck, *Radiology* (1987) **164**: 823–30.
58. Vogl Th, Dresel S, Kang K et al, Kernspintomographie der Glandula parotis: Nativdiagnostik und Gd-DTPA, *Digitale Bilddiagn* (1989) **5** (suppl): 59–68.

59. Riederer A, Müller-Höcker J, Wilmes E et al, Die aggressive Fibromatose im Kopf-Hals-Bereich, *Arch Otorhinolaryngol* (1988) **321** (suppl).

60. Lufkin RB, Hanafee WN, MRI of the head and neck, *Magn Reson Imaging* (1988) **6**: 69–88.

61. Gademann H, Haels J, Semmler W et al, KST bei Erkrankungen er Parotis, *Laryng Rhinol Otol* (1988) **67**: 211–16.

62. Riderer A, Vogl Th, Wilmes E et al, Wertigkeit der KST bei Symptomen der HIV 1-Infektion im Kopf-Hals-Bereich, *HNO* (1989) **1**: 100.

63. Lufkin RB, Larsson SG, Hanafee WN, Work in progress: NMR anatomy of the larynx and tongue base, *Radiology* (1983) **148**: 173–5.

64. Lufkin RB, Hanafee WN, MR reveals subtleties of head and neck pathology, *Diagn Imaging* (1986) **8**: 98–104.

65. Van Der Brekel NWM, Stel HV, Castelijins JA et al, Cervical lymph node metastasis: assessment of radiologic criteria, *Radiology* (1990) **177**: 379–84.

66. In: Wilson JD, Braumwald E, Isselbacher KJ, eds, *Harrison's principles of internal medicine*, 12th edn (McGraw-Hill: New York, 1991).

67. Vogl T, Steger W, Grevers G et al, MRI with Gd-DPTA in tumors of larynx and hypopharynx, *Eur Radiol* (1991) **1**: 58–84.

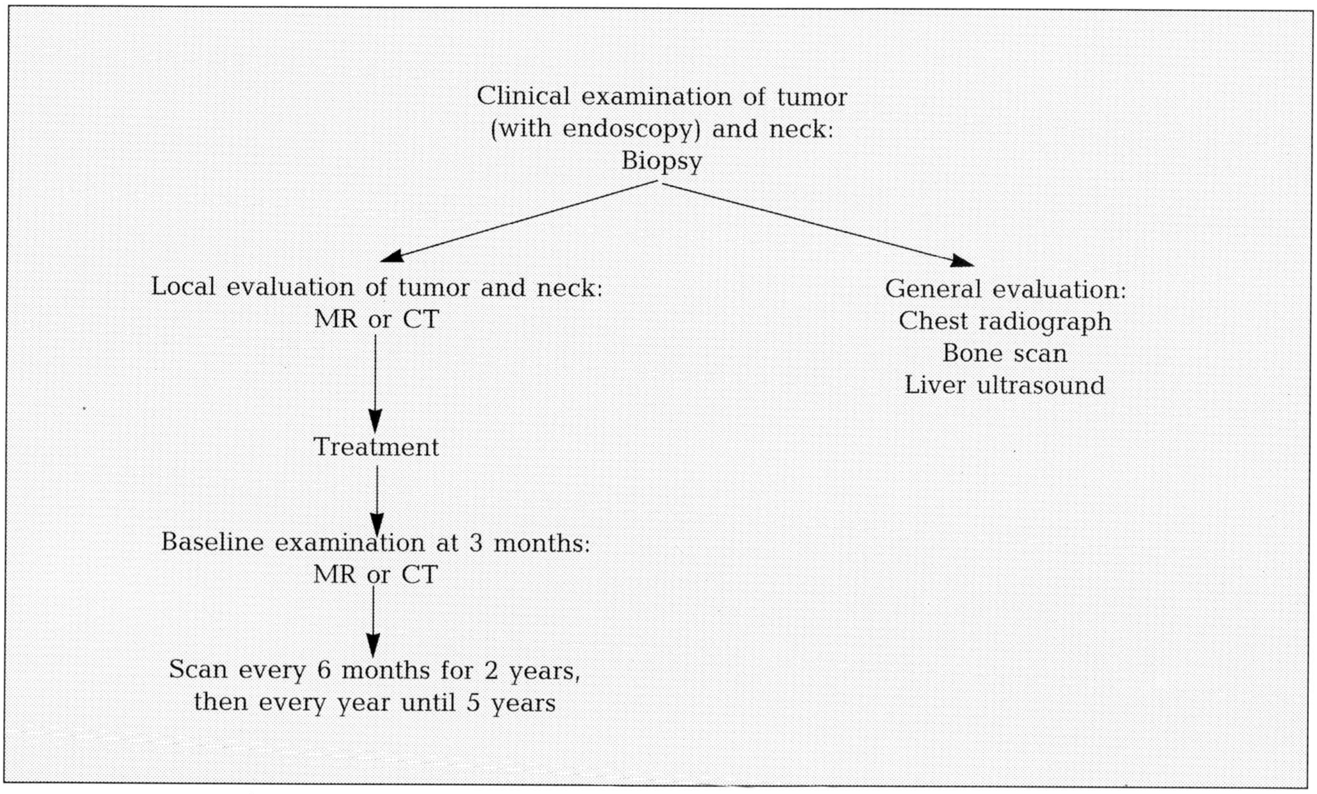

Diagram 4.1

Imaging strategy for carcinoma of the nasopharynx.

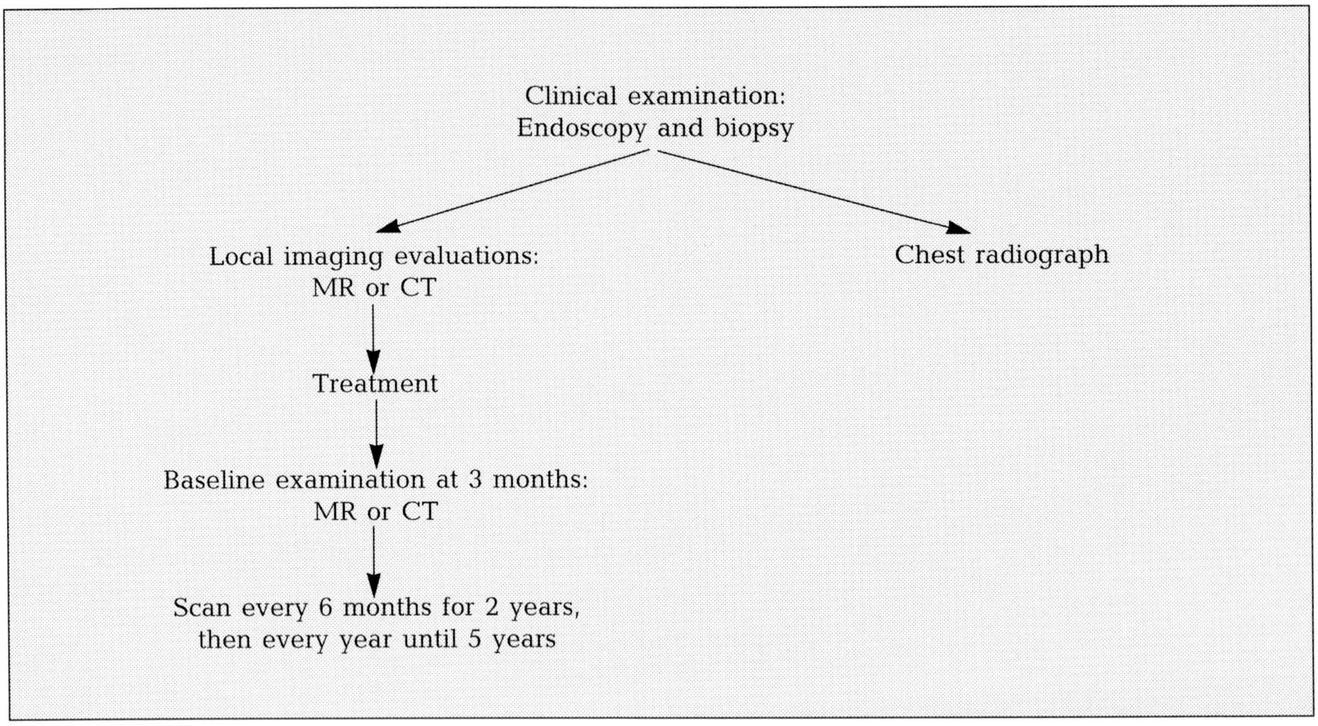

Diagram 4.2

Imaging strategy for tumors of the face.

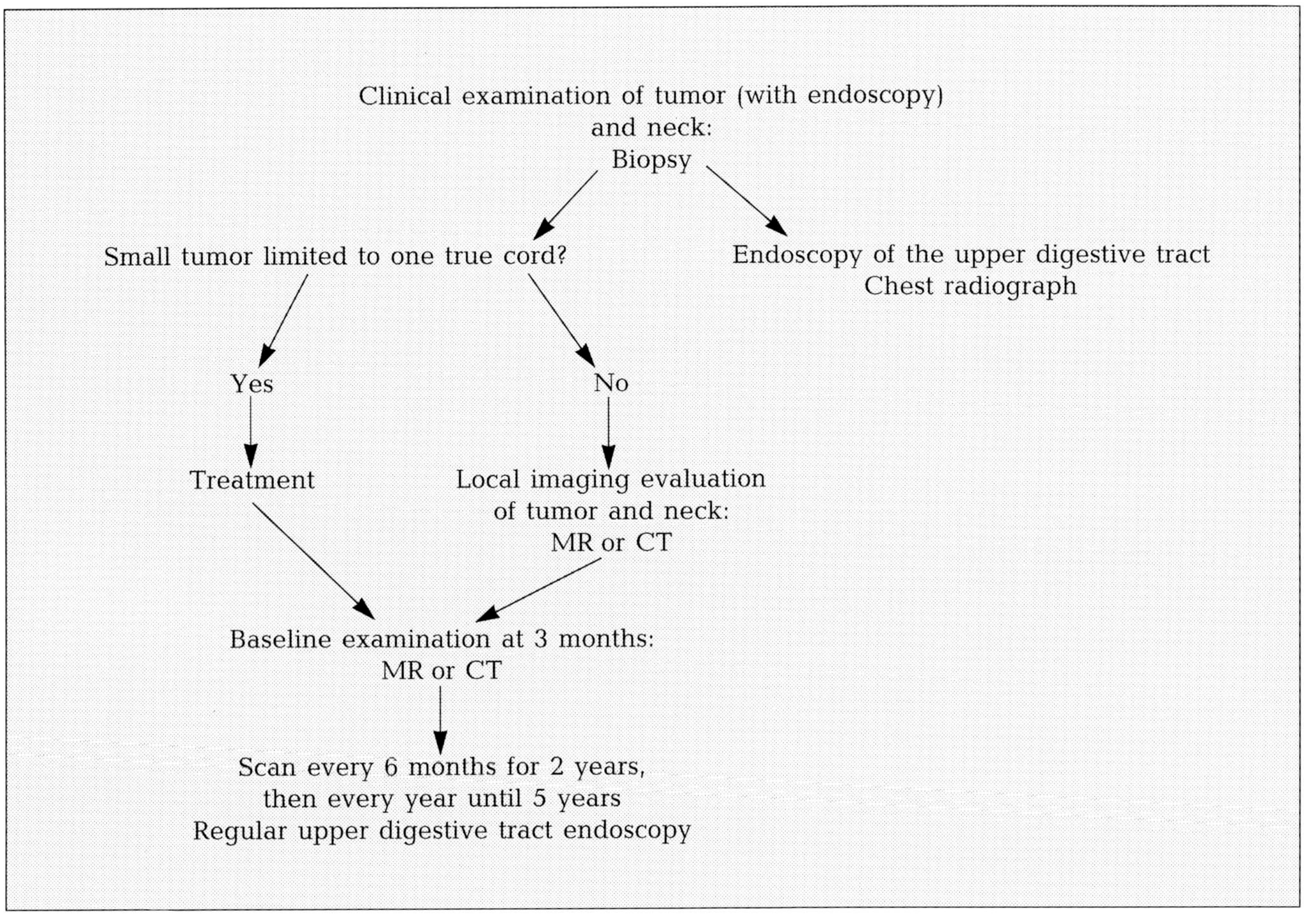

Diagram 4.3

Imaging strategy for tumors of the pharynx and larynx.

5

The thyroid

Cecilia Francese and Martin Schlumberger

Introduction

Two main problems pertaining to imaging in thyroid carcinoma will be discussed. First, at presentation in a patient with a thyroid nodule, is surgery warranted and what is the usefulness of pre-operative diagnostic tests? Second, after initial treatment, what is the optimal protocol for follow up of thyroid carcinoma patients that permits the early discovery of relapses?

Diagnosis

Thyroid nodule[1–3]

Palpable thyroid nodules are present in 4–7% of the adult population in areas in which goiter is non-endemic. Most surgical series report a cancer incidence of 5–20% in patients with no history of radiation exposure, for whom surgery was selected on clinical grounds. Furthermore, 40–50% of adults reaching the age of 50 years will have some thyroid abnormalities as shown by high resolution ultrasonography. Therefore, it is neither practical nor necessary to remove every nodule in order to exclude malignancy, and investigations are directed to select for surgery those with an increased risk of malignancy (Diagram 5.1).

Most thyroid carcinomas present as an asymptomatic, slow-growing nodule. Several clinical arguments may give rise to the clinical suspicion of malignancy in patients with a solitary thyroid nodule: a history of external irradiation to the neck, young age, progressive though not sudden growth, hoarseness due to an ipsilateral vocal cord paralysis, adherence of the nodule to surrounding tissues, presence of palpable neck lymph nodes, etc. These patients should be operated upon, as well as those with large nodules (>3 cm), irrespective of the results of diagnostic tests. In contrast, a long-standing familial goiter without a dominant mass is likely to be benign.

Thyroid scans are currently performed with ^{99m}Tc or ^{123}I and are able to demonstrate the lack of uptake in palpable (cold) nodules (Figure 5.1). The prevalence of carcinoma in these cold nodules is 5–10%, but less than 1% in hot nodules. In case of uptake with ^{99m}Tc (warm nodules), these should also be explored with ^{123}I or ^{131}I since some of these nodules are unable to retain radioiodine at 6 or 24 h and should therefore be considered as cold nodules.

Other tools, such as thyroglobulin measurement, iodine content measured by X-ray fluorescence, thallium scintigraphy, CT scan and MRI are not useful for distinguishing malignant from benign lesions.

When a cold nodule is solitary, needle aspiration or ultrasonography should be used to search for the existence of a cyst. (The risk of cysts being malignant becomes practically negligible when the nodule shrinks completely after aspiration and does not reappear.) All cystic fluids, either bloody or clear yellow, should be sent for cytologic review as either can be found in papillary carcinoma. However, this fluid is frequently insufficient for diagnosis, and so surgery should be performed if the cyst recurs, if it fails to resolve completely or if there is clear-cut ultrasound evidence of local invasion.

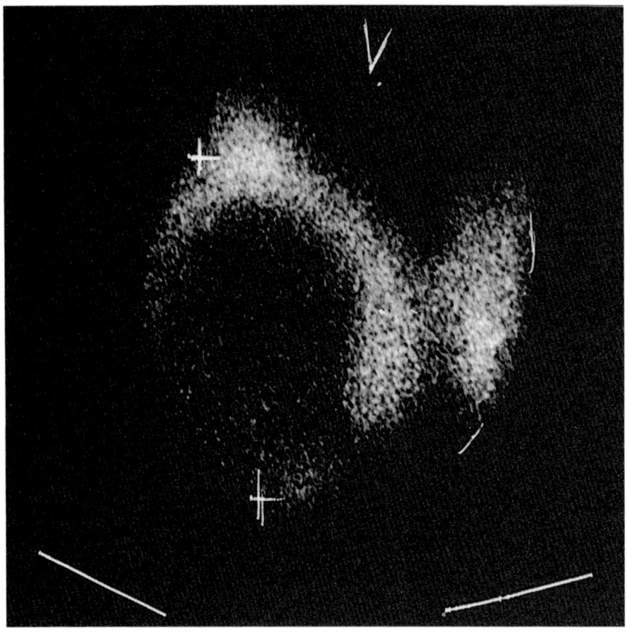

A

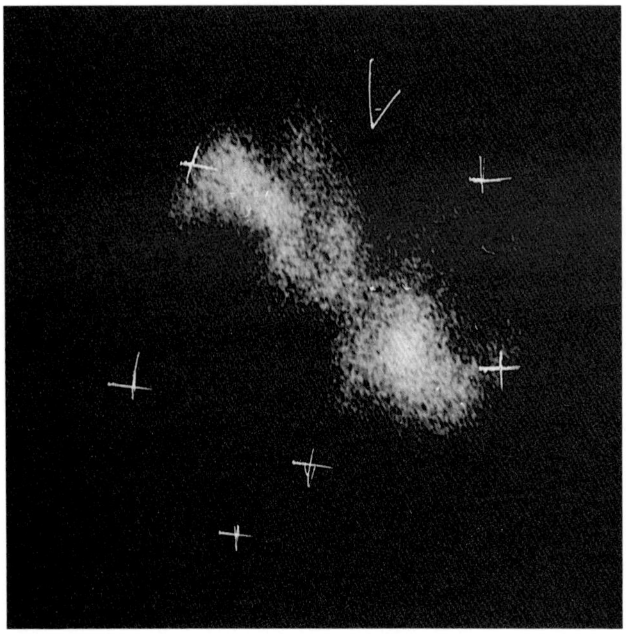

B

Figure 5.1

Thyroid scan.

A Cold nodule in the right lobe as shown by ^{99m}Tc scan.

B Multinodular goiter with a cold nodule in the right and in the left lobes.

When a cold nodule is at least in part solid, the most useful method is aspiration cytology by fine-needle biopsy. This shows a good correlation with the histology of tissue removed at operation. The technique requires practice in obtaining samples and making the smear preparations and the skills of an expert cytologist. Technical failures due to insufficient material do occur in 5–10% of patients, who should then be considered candidates for surgery. On adequate smears, cytologic results can be scored as benign, indeterminate or malignant; these account for 60, 35 and 5% of cases, respectively. A false-positive report of malignancy is rare but the rate of false negatives, that is tissue thought to be benign but found to show malignant changes at surgery, is 5–10%. This is largely because of the difficulty in distinguishing cells from benign adenoma, atypical adenoma and follicular carcinoma. Thus, a safe policy is to regard all such lesions as indeterminate and to advise surgical exploration.

Such a selective approach, operating only patients with indeterminate or malignant nodules on the basis of clinical grounds and cytology, reduces the number of patients requiring surgery by a factor of three. However, the risk of neglecting a cancer, although small, is not totally avoided. In the absence of surgery, the patient is usually followed up at 6-month intervals, with or without suppressive therapy. Whether repeated cytology is warranted in benign nodule, is still a matter of debate. An increase in nodule mass should, however, be regarded as an indication for surgery.

Particular conditions

The discovery of a thyroid nodule in a patient with distant metastases from an unknown primary warrants a complete work up, despite the fact that benign thyroid nodules are frequent and metastases from thyroid carcinoma are rare. A biopsy of a metastasis, with histological and immunohistological examination, is often the only means to discover the primary. The presence of lymph-node metastases in which fine-needle aspiration or biopsy has shown the presence of thyroid cells or papillae should dictate the search for the thyroid nodule, which may be found only at surgery.

Ultrasonography is the most sensitive tool in detection of non-palpable thyroid abnormalities. This method has proved to be useful for the follow up of subjects who have had previous external radiation of the neck, in those with lymph node metastases in the neck from a papillary carcinoma and in the familial screening of relatives of patients with medullary thyroid carcinoma. However, ultrasonography is currently used with a great frequency in subjects complaining only of non-specific symptoms. If a non-palpable thyroid nodule (<1 cm in size) is discovered, a follow up is advisable with neck palpation and ultrasonography 1 year later.

Follow up of patients with differentiated thyroid carcinoma

Differentiated thyroid carcinomas represent 90% of all malignant thyroid tumors. Long-term results in patients with metastatic thyroid carcinoma have shown that prognosis is strongly related to the tumor burden at discovery of the metastases. Thus detection at an early stage of distant metastases[4] and relapses in the neck, when radiographic findings are still normal, is to be encouraged. This became possible with the advent of the combined use of serum thyroglobulin (Tg) measurement and total body ^{131}I scan.[5–7]

Relapses are discovered with a maximal frequency during the first years of follow up, but they may also emerge clinically after decades of apparent complete remission. Therefore follow up should intensive during the first 2–3 years and should also be pursued throughout the patient's life.

Clinical evaluation

Neck recurrences are often discovered by palpation or ultrasonography, but prior external irradiation of the neck may hamper clinical examination. Thus, CT scan or scintigraphy of the neck may be required, and fine-needle aspiration is helpful to determine the nature of any abnormal mass.

The lungs and bones are the most frequent locations of distant metastases. Metastases in the brain, liver or skin tend to appear late in patients who already have multiple bone or lung metastases. Clinical symptoms usually indicate large metastases, that is, macronodular lung metastases, pleural effusion or bone abnormalities on X-ray.[4]

Radiological findings

In nearly all patients with lung metastases, the serum Tg level has increased before metastases are visible on chest radiographs. Therefore, the routine use of chest radiographs appears to be unnecessary. In patients with normal chest radiographs and diffuse ^{131}I uptake in lungs, lung computed tomography detects a few peripheral micronodules in only half of the patients (Figure 5.2).

Most bone metastases are osteolytic and therefore difficult to find on skeletal survey radiographs. More sensitive is a ^{99m}Tc diphosphonate bone scan, but this also may be falsely negative. This should not be performed systematically but only in case of suspicion of bone involvement (pain, iodine uptake, etc.).

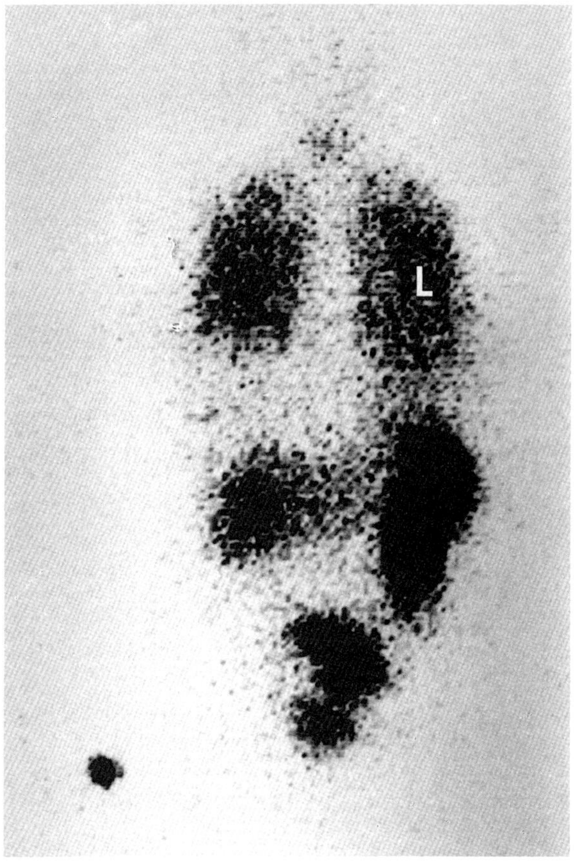

Figure 5.2

^{131}I Total body scan performed 5 days after the administration of 100 mCi in a patient with a normal chest radiograph. Uptake of ^{131}I in lungs is clear (L). There is also some accumulation of ^{131}I in the stomach and in the colon.

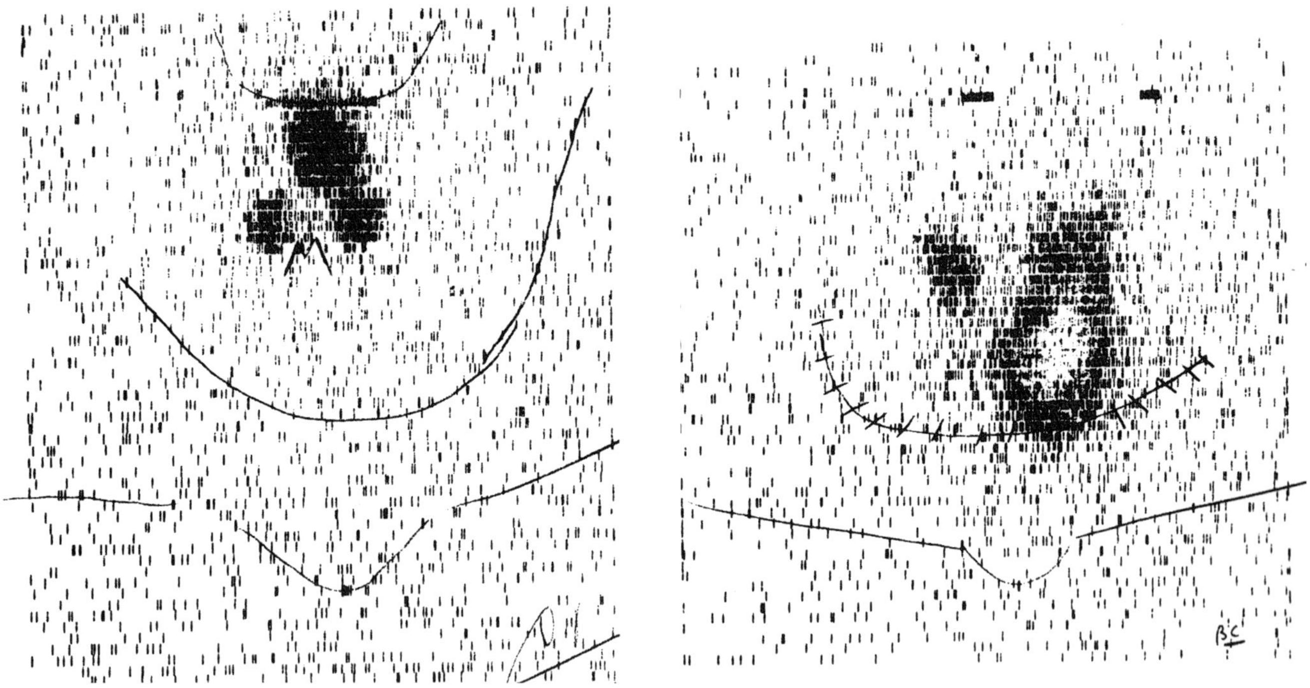

A B

Figure 5.3

^{131}I Thyroid scan using 2 mCi.

A Thyroid remnants after total thyroidectomy.

B Left lobe and upper pole of the right lobe after loboisthmectomy.

Serum Tg measurement

Serum Tg is a reliable marker of differentiated thyroid carcinoma during follow up;[5, 6] divergent results reported in some series appear to have been due to insufficient sensitivity or accuracy. Endogenous anti-Tg antibodies are found in about 15% of cancer patients. They may interfere in the assay and so prevent the determination of the actual Tg level. However, with immunoradiometric assay (IRMA) methods using monoclonal antibodies, interference is found in only 5% of the sera tested. Anti-Tg antibodies should be systematically sought, and only results from sera without interference should be used clinically.

The serum Tg level is detectable in nearly 100% of patients with large metastases during T4 treatment. However, it is undetectable in 10–20% of patients, or detectable but at a relatively low level, in patients with metastases that are not visible on radiographs and in those with involvement of neck lymph nodes only. Measurement must therefore be adequately sensitive to reliably detect these low Tg levels. This underlines the need for systematic lymph node dissection at initial treatment, and thereafter for a systematic post-operative ^{131}I total body scan to search for foci of ectopic uptake (Figure 5.3).

The serum Tg level increases following thyroid-stimulating hormone (TSH) stimulation even in patients whose metastases do not take up ^{131}I. False-negative Tg measurements are very rare in this situation, and some may be due to technical problems in Tg assays. In some series, false-positive Tg measurements appeared to be more frequent in patients without thyroid remnants during T4 treatment, and even more frequent following thyroid hormone withdrawal. However, the Tg level remains relatively low in most patients with no other evidence of disease, whereas it increases to significantly higher levels in patients with metastatic disease. Furthermore, when interpreting these results, it should be remembered that thyroid cancer has a slow growth rate. Therefore, an increased Tg level may be detected long before metastases become detectable, in particular when they do not take up ^{131}I.

During the follow up of patients who have undergone a lobectomy only, serum Tg measurement during T4 treatment is less specific. However, no relapse has been observed among patients without a detectable serum Tg level and the probability of relapse has been found to be significantly correlated with Tg level. Therefore, Tg measurement during T4 treatment is useful for detecting relapse and for avoiding total body ^{131}I scan in the 60% of patients with low or undetectable Tg levels. In the case of a detectable Tg level, ultrasonography should be performed since it frequently detects non-palpable nodules in the remaining lobe. The interpretation of an increased Tg level following TSH stimulation is more difficult in these patients, as Tg can be released either by normal thyroid remnants or by neoplastic foci.

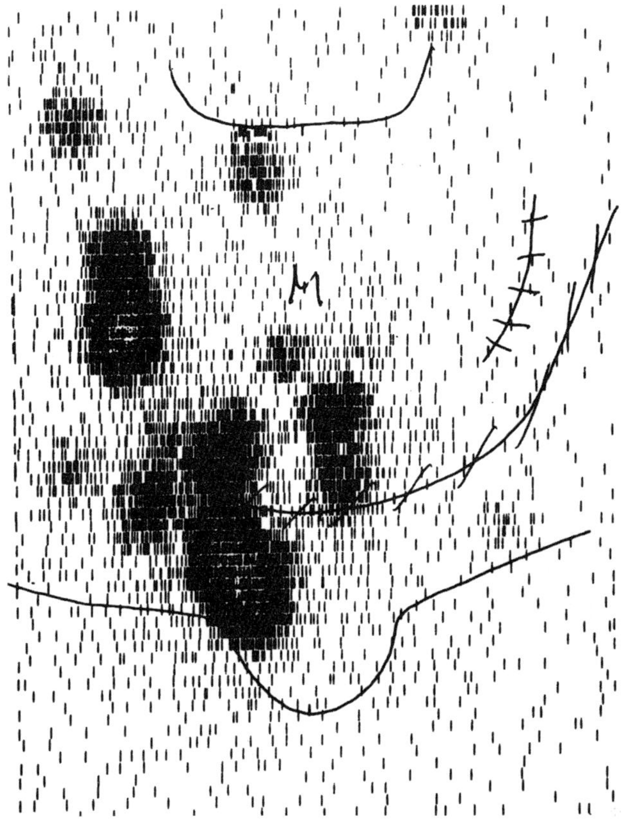

Figure 5.4

Neck scintigraphy performed 5 days after the administration of 100 mCi. There is a clear uptake of ^{131}I in lymph node metastases and in normal thyroid remnants.

^{131}I Total body scan

As the efficacy of total body scan depends upon the ability of malignant tissue to take up ^{131}I, iodine overload should be avoided and stimulation by TSH is of critical importance.[5] In practice, patients are taken off T4 treatment and receive T3 for 3 weeks. Thereafter, T3 is withdrawn for 14 days; T3 withdrawal for more than 2 weeks is unnecessary and may be harmful. The serum TSH level should be measured before the scan is performed because, in some patients, TSH fails to reach an adequate level. In these particular patients, the best technique is the use of exogenous TSH. The ^{131}I dose generally used in testing is 2–5 mCi. Usually the optimal scanning time is 72 h later, when the background activity is lower and the uptake or secretion in organs such as the nasopharynx, salivary glands, stomach, breast and bladder have diminished. A diffuse liver uptake at this time results from the concentration of labeled iodoproteins. False-positive images are very rare, but only two-thirds of patients with distant metastases are able to take up ^{131}I. The scintigram may be performed with either a rectilinear scanner or a gamma camera, but quantitation of uptake is mandatory. A post-therapeutic total body ^{131}I scan is warranted in all patients treated with high activities of ^{131}I, as it may detect occult neoplastic uptake not shown by conventional scintigrams with 2–5 mCi (Figure 5.4).

Follow-up strategy

A strategy has been developed for the follow up of patients without interferences in Tg assay (Diagram 5.2).[7] A total thyroidectomy increases the sensitivity of both Tg measurement and ^{131}I total body scan, and is advocated in patients at high risk of developing relapses. An ^{131}I total body scan is performed each year for 2 years after initial therapy. Thereafter, in patients with undetectable or low Tg levels after thyroid hormone withdrawal, follow up is resumed with clinical evaluation, TSH and Tg measurements, once a year, while on T4 therapy. The principal aim of the post-operative administration of an ablative dose of ^{131}I in such patients is to allow for a post-therapy total body scan, 5 days after the ^{131}I dose. This may detect occult neoplastic foci for which further treatments may be warranted.

After a total thyroidectomy, when a Tg level is detectable during T4 treatment, neck ultrasonography, ^{131}I total body scan (with 2 or 5 mCi) and chest X-ray are performed, and Tg is measured again after thyroid hormone withdrawal. Patients with positive total body scan are treated with 100 mCi ^{131}I. In those patients with a negative ^{131}I total body scan, where Tg levels increased significantly after thyroid hormone withdrawal, additional attempts to localize thyroid tissue are made (bone scintigraphy, neck and thorax CT scan). Administration of 100 mCi of ^{131}I with a total body scan 5 days later is particularly useful in these patients and permits the detection of unknown normal or neoplastic thyroid tissue which could be subsequently cured in most of them.

In patients with thyroid remnants, whose Tg levels are elevated during T4 treatment, a complete work up should be performed, starting with ultrasonography of the residual lobe and of the cervical lymph node areas.

Thallium-201 total body scan appears to be less reliable than ^{131}I total body scan for the routine follow up. Venous sampling catheterization does not reveal any Tg concentration gradient in these patients, and scanning with the ^{131}I-labeled anti-Tg monoclonal antibody has not proved to be useful.

Since the advent of routine use of the serum Tg assay, systematic chest X-ray appears not to be useful and the number of ^{131}I total body scans performed has been reduced. ^{131}I total body scans are more effective because their indications are better defined, allowing an earlier discovery of relapse; this should improve the long-term results of treatment.[4,7]

References

1. Molitch ME, Beck JR, Dreisman M et al, The cold thyroid nodule: an analysis of diagnostic and therapeutic option, *Endocrinol Rev* (1984) **5:**185–99.
2. Rojeski MT, Gharib H, Nodular thyroid disease: evaluation and management, *N Engl J Med* (1985) **313:**428–36.
3. Van Herle AJ, Rich P, Ljung BM et al, The thyroid nodule, *Ann Intern Med* (1982) **96:**221–32.
4. Schlumberger M, Tubiana M, De Vathaire F et al, Long-term results of treatment of 283 patients with lung and bone metastases from differentiated thyroid carcinoma, *J Clin Endocrinol Metab* (1986) **63:**960–7.
5. Ashcraft MW, Van Herle AJ, The comparative value of serum thyroglobulin measurement and iodine-131 total body scan in the follow up study of patients with treated differentiated thyroid cancer, *Am J Med* (1981) **71:**806–14.
6. Schlumberger M, Tubiana M, Serum Tg measurements and total body ^{131}I scans in the follow-up of thyroid cancer patients. In: Hamburger JL, ed., *Diagnostic methods in clinical thyroidology* (Springer-Verlag: New York 1989) 147–57.
7. Schlumberger M, Parmentier C, De Vathaire et al, ^{131}I and external radiation in the treatment of local and metastatic thyroid cancer. In: Falk SH, ed., *Thyroid disease: endocrinology, surgery, nuclear medicine, and radiotherapy* (Raven Press: New York 1990) 537–52.

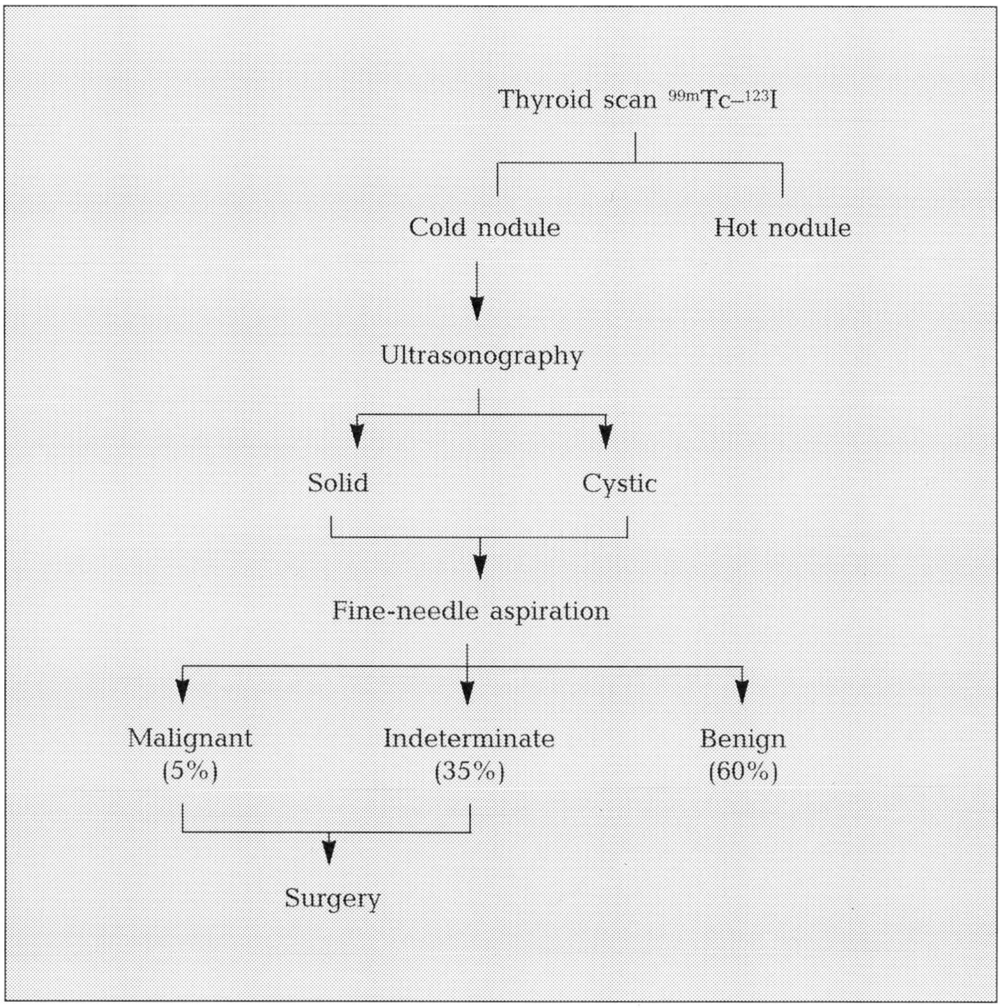

Diagram 5.1

Diagnostic strategy in patients with thyroid nodule.

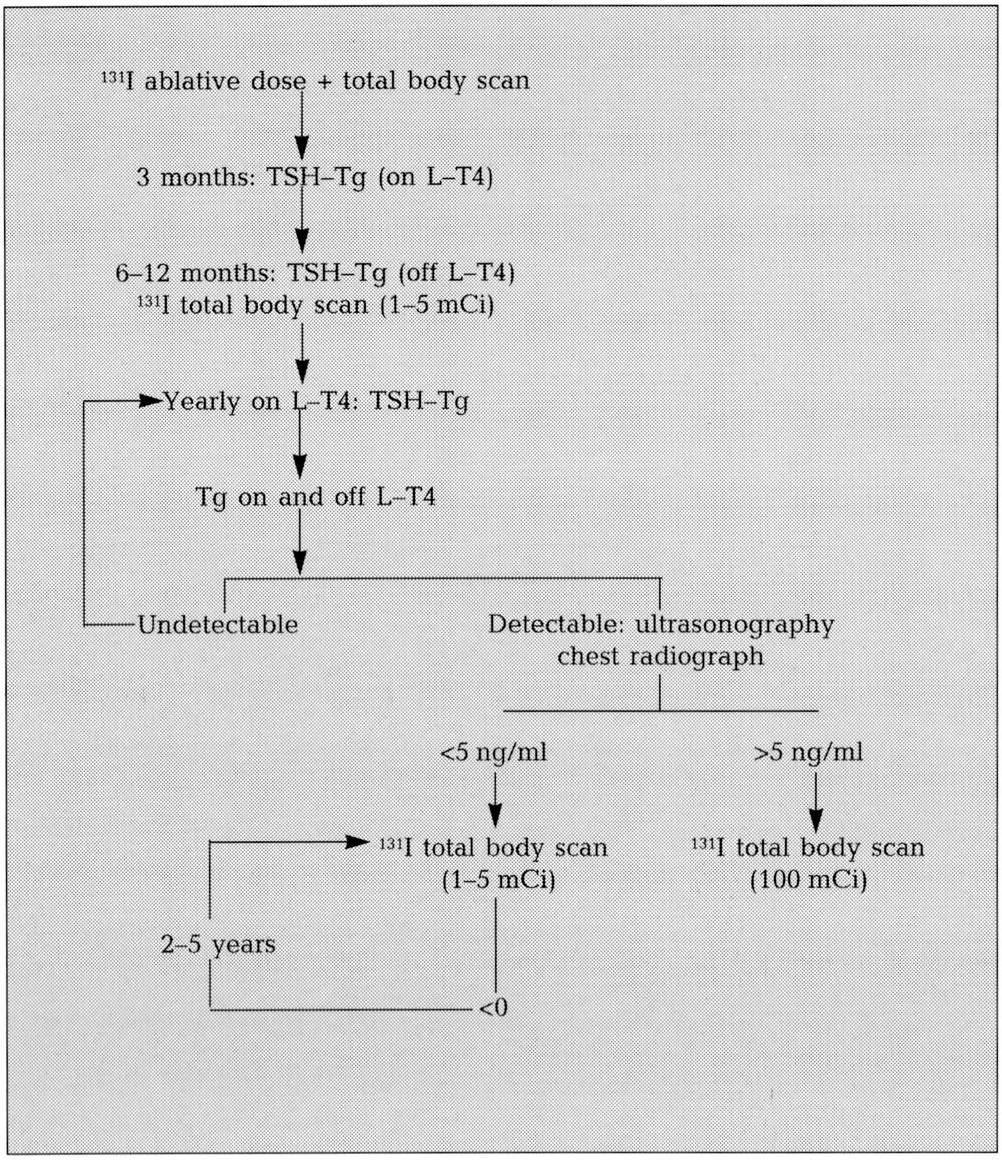

Diagram 5.2

Strategy of follow up in thyroid cancer patients without thyroid remnants. The same strategy is used in patients who have undergone a total thyroidectomy without ^{131}I-ablation of thyroid remnants. TSH, thyroid-stimulating hormone; Tg, thyroglobulin.

6

The lung, pleura and chest wall

David G. Bragg

Introduction

The routine chest radiograph forms the window through which almost all neoplasms involving the thorax are initially detected. This chapter will focus on the fundamental techniques and will review the applications of imaging in the initial detection and post-treatment follow up of the benign neoplasms and malignant primary and major metastatic tumors of the lung and pleura, as well as those of the chest wall, focusing on adult thoracic neoplasms.

Techniques

The routine posterior/anterior (PA) and lateral chest radiographs are usually the initial examination that detects the solitary nodule or the multiple bilateral nodules that suggest metastatic disease. In the patient with a solitary pulmonary nodule (coin lesion), the elliptical radiographic density is conventionally described as being less than 5 cm in diameter. In a patient with solitary or even multiple non-calcified pulmonary nodules, no radiographic features allow one to suggest a specific histologic diagnosis. Histologic verification is essential prior to assuming the lesion to be of neoplastic origin.

In the patient with a solitary pulmonary nodule, age is an important discriminator in structuring a differential diagnosis. In the patient of less than 10–12 years of age, a congenital origin for the neoplasm or a pyogenic inflammatory lesion almost invariably explains the radiographic abnormality. In the patient with a similar radiographic abnormality but of an older age group (20–30 years), however, a granulomatous inflammatory process is statistically a more likely explanation. In contrast, a solitary pulmonary nodule in a patient over the age of 50, particularly if there is a smoking history, should be assumed to be a primary lung cancer until proven otherwise[1] (see Diagram 6.1).

Routine chest radiographs

Routine chest radiographs should be obtained with a high kilovoltage technique [120–140 kilovolts peak (kVp)], using either a grid or air-gap separation to avoid scatter radiation. The high kVp technique reduces anatomic noise from normal structures and enables the viewer to detect nodular lesions with greater accuracy than the older, low kVp techniques. A variety of scatter-reduction techniques have been applied, with the aim of further improving nodule detection, some of which are now commercially available.[2]

Only two plain film radiographic characteristics allow characterization of a solitary pulmonary nodule as benign or malignant. These are the presence of dense, central calcifications and the absence, over a period of observation exceeding 2 years,[3] of interval enlargement of the nodule.

Calcifications are difficult to detect in high kVp radiographs, so it is necessary to use either low kVp fluoroscopic spot radiographs or CT evaluation. Benign types of calcifications are those which are dense and central or laminated. Occasionally, certain cancers which are metastatic to the lung may develop calcification or ossification as matrix within the tumor. Calcifications also have been described in association with bronchioloalveolar cell carcinomas (described later).

The growth characteristics of radiographic masses can prove valuable as benign–malignant discriminators, as initially described by Nathan.[4] In general, nodular lesions that exhibit rapid growth (doubling in less than 30 days) or extremely slow growth (unchanged in 24 months) are almost invariably benign in nature. One strategy, then, is that the individual suspected of having a benign pulmonary nodule may occasionally be followed to determine doubling time and growth characteristics.

One should always make certain that the nodule apparent on a chest radiograph is not superimposed from the skin surface, such as a nipple shadow, skin nodule or artifact. The easiest way to confirm the intrathoracic location of the nodule is to obtain shallow PA oblique radiographs, with nipple markers in place. In addition, every effort should be made to obtain previous chest radiographs to make certain the detected abnormality was or was not present on earlier films and also determine the growth characteristics of the mass.

Computed tomography

In 1980, Siegelman et al described the application of CT in the evaluation of the solitary pulmonary nodule.[5] They suggested that the density of the nodule might allow characterization of the lesion histologically, into either a probably malignant or benign category. Differences in CT equipment and lack of standardization frustrated the effort of others to verify the initial observations of Siegelman et al and led to the cooperative study that standardized the approach, despite differing CT equipment, based on a phantom used as a reference standard.[5,6] The techniques may have some limited application in the individual with a small nodule (less than 2 cm in size) with relatively well-defined margins, or in the patient with some medical contraindications to operative intervention and aggressive therapy. The criteria for assuming benignancy based on CT densitometry incorporate the size of the mass, its marginal characteristics and its density. In most institutions, however, this technique is seldom utilized.

The primary role of CT scanning in the evaluation of the patient with primary lung cancer is one of staging and post-treatment follow up.

Magnetic resonance imaging

To date, the application of MR in the assessment of thoracic neoplasms has been limited, there being few advantages over CT. MR has no use in the evaluation of the nodule that is found centrally in the lung. Nevertheless, some reports have suggested a slight advantage of MR over CT in the assessment of chest wall invasion as well as mediastinal penetration, particularly if involvement of the central major vascular structures of the mediastinum is suspected. In addition, MR has a theoretical advantage over CT in the assessment of pericardial penetration. In the post-treatment follow up of thoracic neoplasms, particularly those treated with radiation therapy, MR may have some advantage over CT in following the signal characteristics of the neoplasm and comparing post-treatment to pre-treatment echo characteristics.[7,8] In the evaluation of the pulmonary hilum, MR would seem to be the modality for separating vascular structures from enlarged, abnormal lymph nodes. Although this is true in theory, generally the experienced observer can make this assessment almost as well using CT. In addition, the staging yielded by the assessment of the hilum is generally of less consequence than the similar evaluation of the mediastinum.[9]

In general, MR has no practical advantage over CT in the assessment of the patient with primary lung cancer.

Lung biopsy

Percutaneous transthoracic needle biopsy can be used to verify the histology of a pulmonary nodule in lesions as small as 5 mm in size. The approach to percutaneous transthoracic needle biopsy (PTNB) will vary with the operator, both with regard to the preferred type of needle and the use of CT as opposed to fluoroscopy for guidance. In most instances, where the lesion is clearly visible on plain films, fluoroscopy is recommended. In contrast to CT, fluoroscopy is more readily available, simpler, less expensive and allows the procedure to be performed more rapidly in most instances.

As a general rule, PTNB should be utilized in those individuals who are not candidates for primary resection or who are suspected of having metastatic disease to the lung. With primary lung cancers, when sputum cytology is negative, histologic verification should be reserved for the individual with a more peripheral location of the nodule. Bronchoscopy is usually a more effective diagnostic tool when the primary lung cancer is located in the first- to third-order divisions of the bronchial tree. In the patient suspected of having a nodular presentation of an infectious process, percutaneous biopsy is less accurate and useful than bronchoscopy.[10]

The major contraindication to PTNB is the uncooperative patient. Other relative contraindications are patients with pulmonary arterial hypertension or chronic obstructive pulmonary disease. The incidence of pneumothorax will vary, depending upon the location of the biopsied lesion within the thorax (a somewhat higher incidence of pneumothorax with apical lesions), the number of needle passes through the pleura and the needle calibre. In most instances, reported pneumothoraces occur in approximately 15–25% of PTNB procedures.[11,12] Tube thoracostomy is probably necessary in fewer than 5% of these cases.

Needles for PTNB range in size from 20 to 23 gauge. Generally, small needle sizes are safer. Following local anesthesia, the needle is directed, under fluoroscopic or CT guidance, over the upper (cranial) margin of the rib closest to the nodule. During suspended respiration, the needle tip is placed at the edge of the lesion or within its outer margin. Samples of tissue are obtained during aggressive rotation, combined with in-and-out motion of the needle during suspended respiration and suction. The suction is released as the needle is withdrawn, while the patient again suspends respiration. The material is then expressed into the appropriate medium, depending upon whether one is interested in bacteriologic analysis or merely in cytologic/histologic diagnosis. If possible, the pathologist/cytopathologist should be available in the procedure room at the time of the PTNB, to determine whether the specimen is adequate for diagnosis. After the procedure is complete, the patient should then be placed in a recumbent position, with the needle entry side down, for at least 4 h following the procedure. Verification radiographs should be obtained immediately post-biopsy and in 4 h to check for complications such as pneumothorax and hemorrhage: approximately 98% of the post-procedure pneumothoraces are visible by the time of the 4 h film. Patients whose lung biopsy is performed on an outpatient basis, without evidence of a pneumothorax 4 h after the procedure, can be safely discharged home with appropriate instructions and precautions.[13]

The accuracy of PTNB varies with the institution reporting, the diagnostic composition of the patients population and the approach utilized. With primary lung cancers, the diagnostic accuracy should approach 90%. Specific histologic stratification of the cell type of the primary lung cancer may not be possible, particularly between the non-oat cell types; however, from the standpoint of planning treatment, this may not be a critical limitation. The lymphomas are not as easy as primary lung cancer to characterize with tissue obtained through PTNB. Generally, the more differentiated the cell type of lymphoma, the more difficult it is to histologically characterize the tumor by needle biopsy.

Close teamwork and cooperation are required for PTNB. A decision to attempt the needle biopsy of a lung nodule should be made in cooperation with the clinician and surgeon, and the patient should understand clearly the implications and limitations of the technique.

Benign neoplasms of the lung

The most common benign neoplasms of the lung are summarized in Table 6.1. More than half of these benign lesions will be found to be bronchial

Table 6.1 Benign neoplasms of the lung.

Type	*Characteristics*
Bronchial adenoma (carcinoid/ cyllindroma)	Most common: carcinoid type (85%) Locally aggressive (10–25%)
Hamartoma	3rd to 6th decade, 25% calcify
Papilloma	Pre-pubertal child: tracheo-bronchial tree, atelectasis and bronchiectasis
Lieomyoma	? Smooth muscle origin or metastatic. Slow growing, well marginated
Fibroma	No distinctive features
Lipoma	Bronchial, parenchymal or intrapleural
Hemangioma	Solitary (usually). Multiple. Peripheral

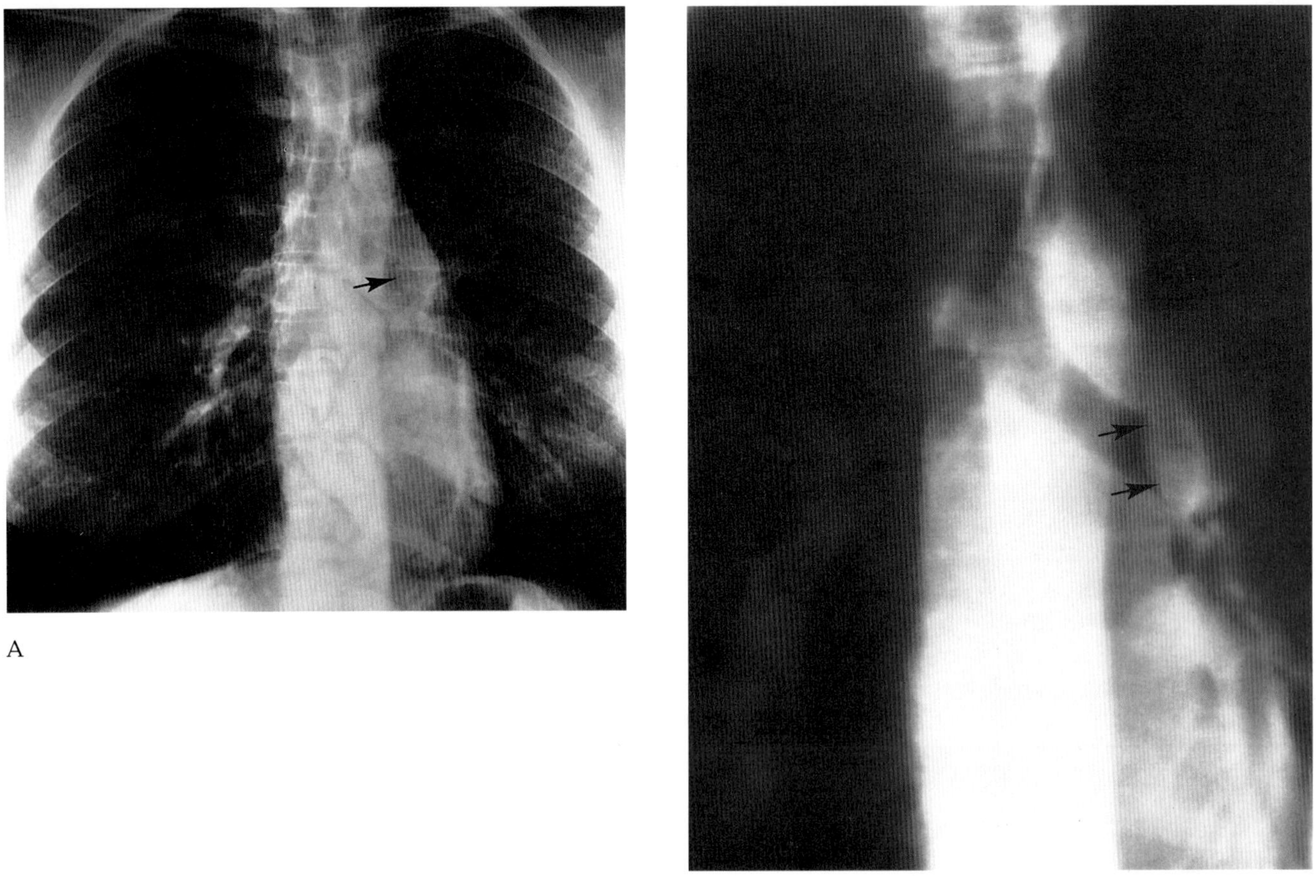

A

B

Figure 6.1

Bronchial adenoma. This 27-year-old initially was seen for unilateral wheezing, treated as asthma.

A The initial chest radiograph showed mediastinal shift from right to left with, in retrospect, a mass lesion visible in the left mainstem bronchus (arrow).

B The tomogram better shows the 'iceberg' tumor mass nearly completely occluding the left mainstem bronchus (arrows). This lesion is a typical appearance for a bronchial adenoma, found at surgery to be a carcinoid tumor.

adenomas. Few have characteristic radigraphic features that suggest a specific diagnosis. Most benign tumors are randomly found in patients in the cancer-prone age group (late teens to late 70s). A few of the more common benign neoplasms will be reviewed.

Bronchial adenoma

Bronchial adenomas are said to comprise nearly 50% of all benign neoplasms of the lung.[14] These bronchial adenomas represent between 5 and 10% of all thoracic neoplasms. They have some fascinating characteristics, both clinically and pathologically, with few distinguishing radiologic features. A broad age range has been reported in patients with bronchial adenomas, ranging from late teens to patients in their late 70s. Most

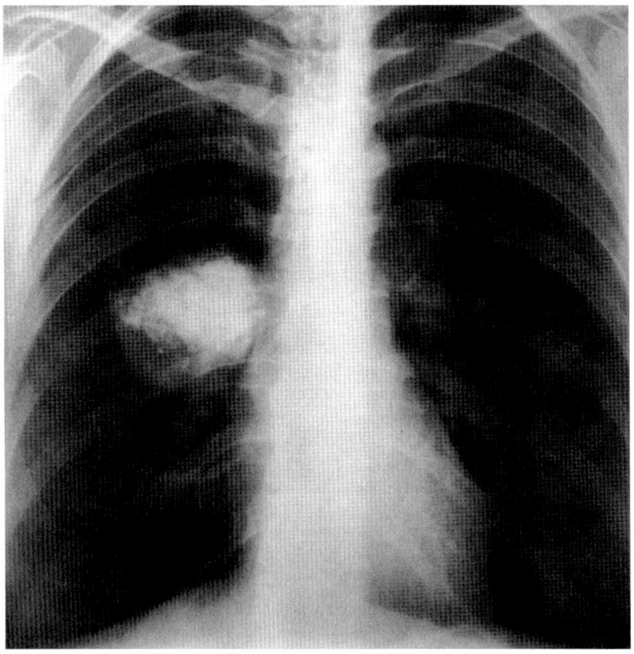

Figure 6.2

Hamartoma. Radiograph of a 42-year-old female found on routine chest radiography to have a 6 cm right mid-lung mass with typical dense calcifications radiologically characteristic of a hamartoma.

bronchial adenomas are found to be within the central, larger calibre segments of the bronchial tree. Patients therefore tend to present radiologically and clinically with evidence of atelectasis and/or hemoptysis. The tumors are contained within the elements of the bronchial wall, described as 'iceberg' tumors, with only a fraction of the volume of the mass protruding into the bronchial lumen. These neoplasms are often highly vascular, so that bronchoscopic biopsy may be followed by brisk hemorrhage (Figure 6.1).

Nearly 85% of bronchial adenomas are of the carcinoid type, the remainder being cylindromas.[15] There is a variable incidence of reported metastases from these neoplasms, ranging from 10% to as high as 50%. There is also a curious relationship histologically with Kulchitsky's cells, which are found in the bronchial mucous glands, and the undifferentiated small cell anaplastic primary lung cancers.[16]

The carcinoid syndrome has been reported to occur with bronchial carcinoids in the absence of extrathoracic metastases.[17] Occasionally, adrenocorticotrphic hormone (ACTH) producing bronchial carcinoid tumors may occur. Computed tomography and MR may be used to detect small lesions when a clinical syndrome of ACTH production is present and the chest radiograph is normal.[18]

Hamartoma

The pulmonary hamartoma is not a true neoplasm, but rather a lesion thought to arise from an embryonic rest. A hamartoma will appear to enlarge in the second to fifth decades of life and therefore will often present in much the same way that a patient with a primary lung cancer might. This growth pattern is unusual and poorly understood, considering the embryologic origins of the hamartoma.

Hamartomas are said to appear more frequently in males. The mass is pathologically characterized by a disorganized collection of different types of tissue, including smooth muscle and cartilage. It is usually located in the periphery of the lung, and is rarely found in an endobronchial location. The characteristic 'popcorn' calcifications are radiologically apparent in a minority of the lesions, estimated to range from 25 to 30% of reported cases (Figure 6.2). Fat is very suggestive of the diagnosis and can be characterized on CT in 5% of reported cases.[19]

Papilloma

Tracheobronchial papillomatosis is a very uncommon condition that occurs in the pre-pubertal child. Benign growths stud the tracheobronchial mucosa, causing peripheral atelectasis, distal pneumonia and bronchiectasis. Occasionally, cavitation or pneumatoceles can also be seen. These lesions are difficult to manage. Often they spontaneously disappear following puberty.[14]

Leiomyoma

Leiomyomas are curious solitary or multiple, well-marginated nodules found in the lower half of the lungs, almost invariably in women. The tumors grow very slowly and seldom cavitate. It is debatable as to whether these lesions arise spontaneously in the lung from the smooth muscle surrounding the pulmonary blood vessels or whether they are metastatic foci from uterine leiomyosarcomas (occasionally found upon review to have been misdiagnosed as leiomyomas).

Malignant primary neoplasms of the lung and pleura

Primary lung cancer remains one of the largest unresolved problems in the entire field of medicine. The awesome proportions of this disease are best illustrated by its ever rising incidence, estimated to represent 161 000 new cases and 143 000 deaths in the USA in 1991.[20] The incidence in females continues to escalate, having surpassed the death rate for breast cancer in the USA in 1985. The age-adjusted cancer death-rate curve for males began to plateau in the same year. Unfortunately, there has not been shown to be any mortality advantage to justify the application of available screening techniques to the patient at risk of lung cancer. Our imaging procedures should therefore be focused on challenges of staging and post-treatment follow up in the patient with lung cancer.

Histology

The histologic classification of primary lung cancers is broadly subdivided into oat cell and non-oat cell cancers. This subdivision is primarily performed to separate the differing staging, prognostic and treatment challenges of these two groups of patients. The localized non-oat cell cancers are treated surgically yet virtually all of the oat cell cancers will be treated with non-surgical techniques. Exceptions to this include those very uncommon peripheral oat cell lesions without evidence of extra thoracic disease, which may be treated with aggressive surgical techniques.

The primary cell types characterizing the most common lung cancers are adenocarcinoma, squamous cell carcinoma, large cell anaplastic and small cell anaplastic cancer. Bronchioalveolar cell carcinomas are generally included as subtypes of adenocarcinomas. The prevalence of adenocarcinomas now exceeds that of squamous cell carcinomas in most reported series. This is believed to be a consequence of several factors, including the increased incidence of women with lung cancers, histologic classification differences, the possible impact of filter cigarettes eliminating larger carcinogenic particles, allowing the smaller particles to extend more peripherally in the lungs, as well as other unknown factors. Although the dominant cell type can be identified in the majority of patients with primary lung cancers, many of these neoplasms contain mixed histologic features which may not be evident with limited sampling techniques.

Generally, the squamous cell carcinomas and small cell anaplastic cancers tend to present in the central, larger divisions of the bronchial tree. In contrast, adenocarcinomas and large cell anaplastic cancers tend to present as peripheral mass lesions. Few if any distinguishing radiologic features allow accurate recognition of these cancers. The majority of patients with a small cell anaplastic cancer will have extrathoracic metastatic disease when the tumor is initially detected. It is for this reason that these cancers are generally regarded as non-surgical, with a different staging challenge from the non-oat cell cancers (Table 6.2).

Squamous cell carcinomas and small cell anaplastic cancers tend to arise centrally and may resemble each other radiologically. Thereafter, their behavior is quite different. The aggressive, small cell anaplastic carcinoma metastasizes early and, in over 75% of patients, extrathoracic metastatic disease will be detected at the time of initial presentation. A very small percentage of small cell anaplastic cancers are peripheral and localized on initial presentation and may be amenable to surgical resection and control.

The aggressive small cell anaplastic cancers arise within the bronchial wall, obstructing the

Table 6.2 Primary lung cancer.

Type	*Frequency (%)*	*Appearance and characteristics*
Squamous cell carcinoma	30–35	Central: obstructive atelectasis, most common cavitary tumor, central nodal spread
Adenocarcinoma	35–40	Peripheral, uncommonly cavitate, bronchioloalveolar cell subtype, early brain metastases, pathologically difficult to distinguish primary and metastatic cancers, more commonly seen in women
Small cell anaplastic carcinoma	25–30	Central, rarely cavitate, arise within bronchial wall and obstruct bronchi and lymphatics, 75–80% have extra-thoracic metastatic disease upon initial presentation
Large cell anaplastic carcinoma	10–15	Peripheral, large, uncommonly cavitate, may be a subtype of adenocarcinoma (clinically and radiologically similar)

bronchi and lymphatics, often leading to dramatic chest radiographic findings when the tumor is initially detected. The tumor site may be concealed by the peripheral obstructive manifestations evident on the initial radiograph. These cancers uncommonly cavitate, in contrast with the squamous cell cancer which is the most frequent cell type to undergo excavation. Squamous cell cancers tend to extend centrally to the hilar and mediastinal lymph node chains prior to extending the extrathoracic metastatic sites.

Adenocarcinomas and large cell anaplastic cancers appear similar radiologically and may behave in quite the same way clinically. Both types are usually peripheral and rarely excavate, with a reported tendency for adenocarcinomas to metastasize to the central nervous system early in the course of their disease.[21–23]

Detection

In most instances, lung cancer tends to be a slow-growing neoplasm, the notable exception being the small cell anaplastic lung cancer. It is believed that repetitive stimuli (smoking, environmental factors, genetic predisposition, chemicals, etc.) stimulate cells to transform into their neoplastic counterparts, leading to a series of cell doublings and an exponential growth of the cancer. It is estimated that some 30 doublings are necessary for the cancer to reach the threshold size visible radiologically, i.e. 1 cm. The margins of the primary lung cancer are usually ill defined and represent very difficult objects for the observer to recognize. It has been estimated in a variety of reported series that detection errors and the inconspicuous margins of primary lung cancers cause them to be overlooked in 30–70% of the cases. In the USA, the National Cancer Institute supported a major three-center trial program analyzing serial chest radiographs and pooled sputum cytology in patients at high risk of developing lung cancer. Control and study populations analyzed over 5 years showed no significant survival or mortality advantage between the study and control groups, leading to the abandonment of these trials. None the less, 85% of the primary lung cancers were detected by the screening chest radiograph, with only the centrally located 15% of the lung cancers detectable by sputum cytology. In retrospective analysis of the serial chest radiographs of the study population, the shadow of the primary lung cancer could be detected in nearly 90% of the cases once its location was known.[24,25]

There are no specific distinguishing radiographic features allowing a precise diagnosis of primary lung cancer. All of the characteristics seen on chest radiographs and defined as 'typical of primary lung cancer' have been described in non-neoplastic entities, most often inflammatory

Table 6.3 The TNM system of staging lung cancers (see Diagram 6.2).

Primary tumor (T)	
[ ] TX	Primary tumor cannot be assessed, or tumor proven by presence of malignant cells in sputum or bronchial washings but not visualized by imaging or bronchoscopy
[ ] T0	No evidence of primary tumor
[ ] Tis	Carcinoma in situ
[ ] T1	Tumor 3 cm or less in greatest dimension, surrounded by lung or visceral pleura, without bronchoscopic evidence of invasion more proximal than the lobar bronchus
[ ] T2	Tumor with any of the following features of size or extent: > 3 cm in greatest dimension Involves main bronchus, 2 cm or more distal to the carina Invades the visceral pleura Associated with atelectasis or obstructive pneumonitis which extends to the hilar region but does not involve the entire lung
[ ] T3	Tumor of any size that directly invades any of the following: chest wall (including superior sulcus tumors), diaphragm, mediastinal pleura, parietal pericardium; or tumor in the main bronchus less than 2 cm distal to the carina but without involvement of the carina; or associated atelectasis or obstructive pneumonitis of the entire lung
[ ] T4	Tumor of any size invading any of the following: mediastinum, heart, great vessels, trachea, esophagus, vertebral body, carina; or tumor with a malignant pleural effusion
Lymph node (N)	
[ ] NX	Regional lymph nodes cannot be assessed
[ ] N0	No regional lymph node metastasis
[ ] N1	Metastasis in ipsilateral peribronchial and/or ipsilateral hilar lymph nodes, including direct extension
[ ] N2	Metastasis in ipsilateral mediastinal and/or subcarinal lymph node(s)
[ ] N3	Metastasis in contralateral mediastinal, contralateral hilar, ipsilateral or contralateral scalene or supraclavicular lymph node(s)
Distant metastases (M)	
[ ] MX	Presence of distant metastases cannot be assessed
[ ] M0	No distant metastases
[ ] M1	Distant metastases

processes. One should never attempt to confidently and specifically diagnose a primary lung cancer based only on plain film criteria.

At the present time, routine screening of the patient at risk of primary lung cancer cannot be recommended. Imaging procedures should therefore be reserved for staging and post-treatment follow up.

Staging

The TNM system of staging cancers has now been adopted worldwide and forms the language universally accepted by oncologists. It was most recently modified in 1986 (Table 6.3).[26] The radiologist should be familiar with the TNM staging system and should include the criteria for the definition of each compartment as a part of the radiologic report.

The definition of the primary tumor (T) can be derived almost entirely from the PA and lateral chest radiograph. The elements characterizing the T compartment relate to the size of the tumor, its proximity to the carina, involvement of the chest wall (which is inaccurately defined by even the most sophisticated imaging techniques), the presence or absence of atelectasis, and the involvement or invasion of critical mediastinal structures and/or the presence of a malignant

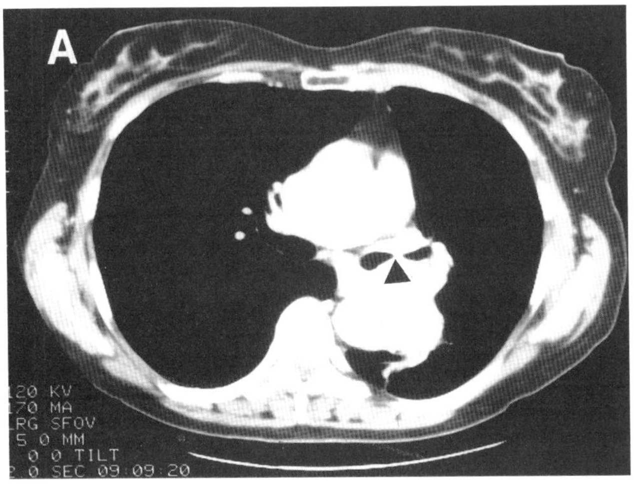

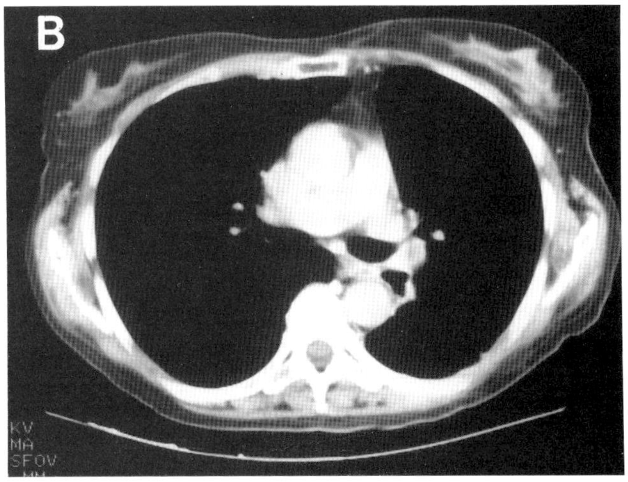

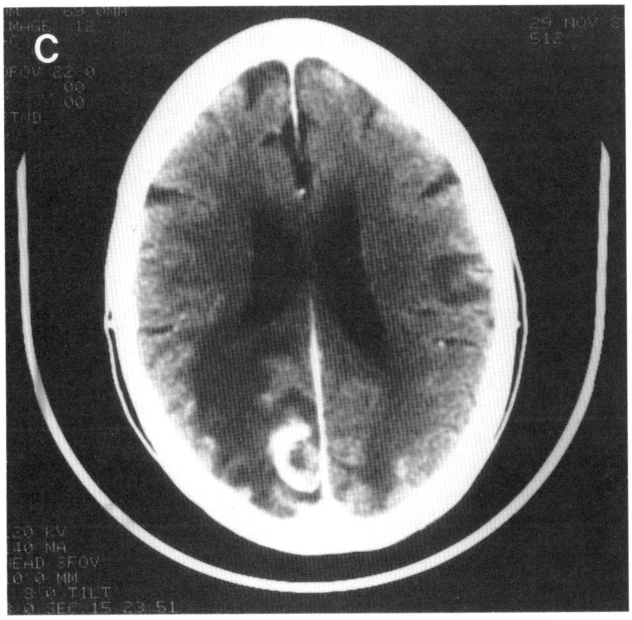

Figure 6.3

Adenocarcinoma, left lower lobe—brain metastases. This 45-year-old female was noted to have a mass surrounding the left hilum.

A Initial CT staging showed a mass surrounding the left main stem bronchus (arrowhead) almost completely obstructing the orifice. The mass extended centrally to involve the aorta and was found at surgery to be unresectable secondary to aortic wall attachment.

B The patient was placed on chemotherapy and restaged by CT 3 months later, when the mass had nearly completely regressed, allowing re-expansion of the left lower lobe. Upon surgical re-exploration the tumor was found to be resectable.

C Two months later, metastatic brain cancer was found.) This illustrates the propensity of adenocarcinomas to develop brain metastatic disease, suggesting evaluation of this site prior to aggressive treatment.

(Reproduced from Bragg,[22] courtesy of W.B. Saunders.)

pleural effusion. Invasion of the chest wall can be defined with confidence only when bone destruction is noted or frank penetration of the chest wall can be documented. Penetration of the mediastinum and invasion of critical mediastinal structures probably is best assessed with MR, this being one of the very few instances in which MR may have a slight advantage over CT in staging the patient with primary lung cancer. Pleural effusions are used as an element in defining T4 status only when malignant cells are identified.

The nodal (N) status of the patient is the critical staging element for the thoracic surgeon. Nonresectability can be established when contralateral lymph node involvement is verified histologically. Some thoracic surgeons feel that the low survival associated with even unilateral lymph node involvement does not warrant the morbidity associated with extensive mediastinal dissection. The radiologist should therefore carefully understand the implications of the N compartment staging process using cross-sectional imaging techniques. Magnetic resonance has no advantage over CT in staging the mediastinal compartment except in the definition of mediastinal vascular invasion.[27] Hilar lymph node involvement is a less critical determinant, changing only the choice of the surgical procedure to be utilized (local resection versus pneumonectomy).

The evaluation of extrathoracic disease extension (metastatic, M, category) should be reserved for the patient with an oat cell carcinoma or for the patient who has symptoms suggesting extrathoracic disease with a non-oat cell cancer. Random screening cannot be cost-justified in the asymptomatic patient. A possible exception might be patients with adenocarcinoma, since they have a somewhat greater incidence of brain metastatic disease within the first 3 months of initial presentation (Figure 6.3). The evaluation of a patient with a small cell anaplastic carcinoma is affected by the behavior of the neoplasm. In the majority of individuals, extrathoracic extension of the cancer has already occurred by the time of initial clinical presentation. Rare exceptions to this axiom relate to the occasional, peripheral T1 presentation of small cell anaplastic cancers which appear amenable to resection and have no evidence of extrathoracic disease. Extrathoracic staging in the patient with small cell anaplastic lung cancer should include MR scans or contrast-enhanced CT scans of the brain, bolus-dynamic contrast-enhanced CT scans of the liver and radionuclide bone scans. When cross-sectional imaging techniques (either MR or CT) are utilized, inclusion of the adrenal gland should be made a part of the staging process in view of the prevalence of asymptomatic adrenal metastases in patients with lung cancer on initial presentation. Unfortunately, CT cannot reliably separate benign from malignant causes of adrenal enlargement. Initial experience with MR suggests this distinction may be possible in certain instances, but histologic verification of adrenal abnormalities will be required, just as with abnormally enlarged mediastinal lymph nodes found during the staging process.

Recommendations for the application of cross-sectional imaging techniques in staging the patient with lung cancer have changed over the years and will vary with the individual institution and surgeon. The prevalence of involved mediastinal lymph nodes increases with the size of the primary cancer and its proximity to the central, hilar region of the lung. In most institutions, the patient suspected of having a primary lung cancer, presenting with a small (<2 cm) peripheral mass, who is medically operable, with a normal hilum and mediastinum on chest radiographs, generally will go straight to surgery rather than undergo routine CT scanning for staging. Cross-sectional imaging, using CT, is usually reserved for the patient with a large, central cancer, an abnormal mediastinum on plain films or in an individual who is at greater surgical risk or has a higher likelihood of having something other than a primary lung cancer (Figure 6.4).

The technique for CT scanning in staging the patient with lung cancer must be carefully established and monitored. Axial, 10 mm sections are obtained from the lung apex through the upper abdomen to include the adrenal glands (Figure 6.5). Intravenous contrast material is injected, with a bolus of 50 ml and dynamic, thin (5 mm) sections obtained through the pulmonary hilum. The criteria for determining enlarged, abnormal lymph nodes must be tailored to the location within the mediastinum where the lymph node is found. Normally, lymph nodes will be larger the closer they are to the hilum. A mediastinal lymph node found greater than 1.5 cm must be viewed as suspicious for metastatic disease, histologic verification prior to anticipated thoracotomy for resection of the cancer being recommended. The location within the mediastinum of the abnormal lymph node must be made known to the thoracic surgeon so that the appropriate mediastinal exploratory procedure is utilized. There are certain blind areas in the posterior mediastinum for specific surgical procedures, for example mediastinotomy cannot adequately visualize the posterior mediastinum, subcarinal or anteropos-

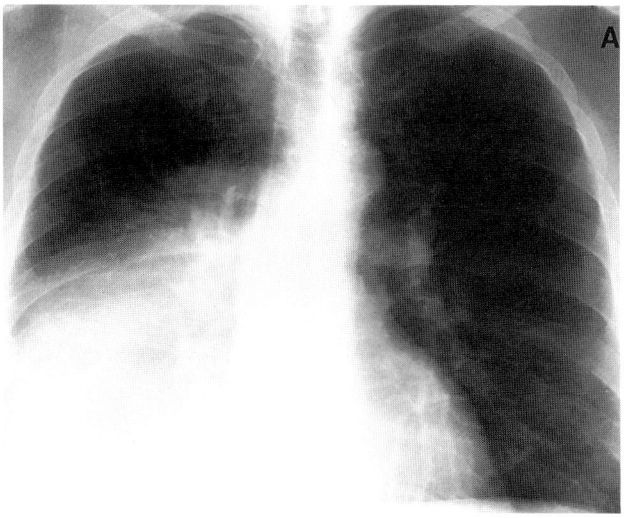

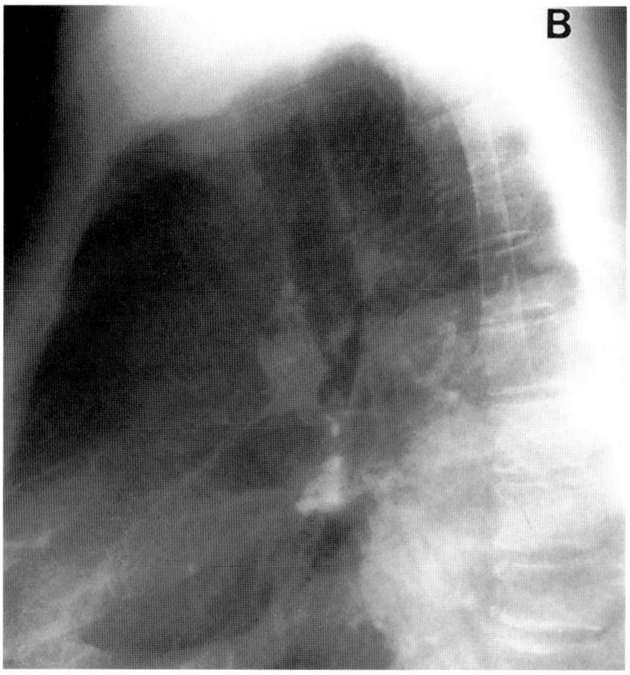

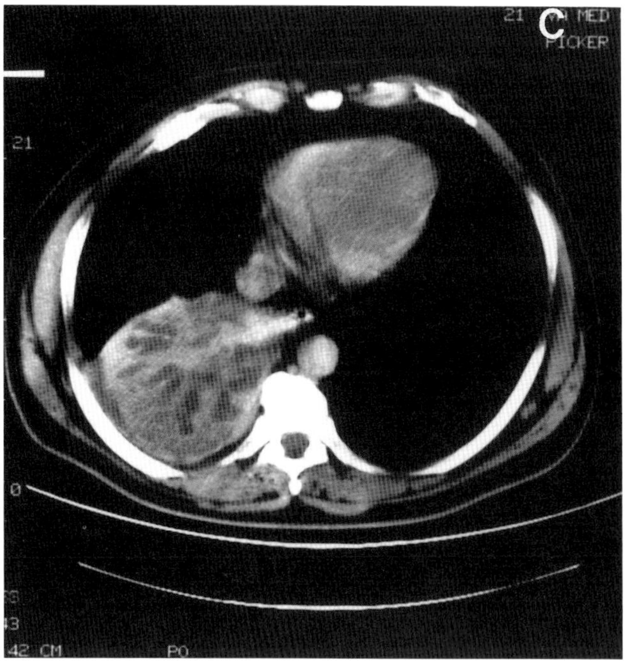

Figure 6.4

Squamous cell cancer—drowned lung.

A,B The plain film characteristics typical of a 'drowned lung' involving the right lower lobe on PA and lateral chest radiographs.

C The axial contrast-enhanced CT scan, showing the tubular dilated structures of the bronchial tree, filled with mucin, surrounded by the collapsed right lower lobe. This post-obstructive 'pneumonia' is not found to be secondarily infected on pathologic examination. The absence of an air-filled bronchial tree implies a central bronchial obstruction, in this case, secondary to a squamous cell carcinoma.

(Reproduced from Bragg,[22] courtesy of W.B. Saunders.)

terior window regions. It should be emphasized that there is no imaging procedure that can specifically define the presence or absence of metastatic cancer within a lymph node. All abnormally enlarged lymph nodes must therefore be histologically verified prior to assuming that they contain metastatic cancer.[28]

Follow up

As in the initial detection in the patient suspected of having a primary lung cancer, the plain film remains the dominant imaging technique in follow up. Abnormalities detected on serial, plain-film follow up should be further evaluated with cross-

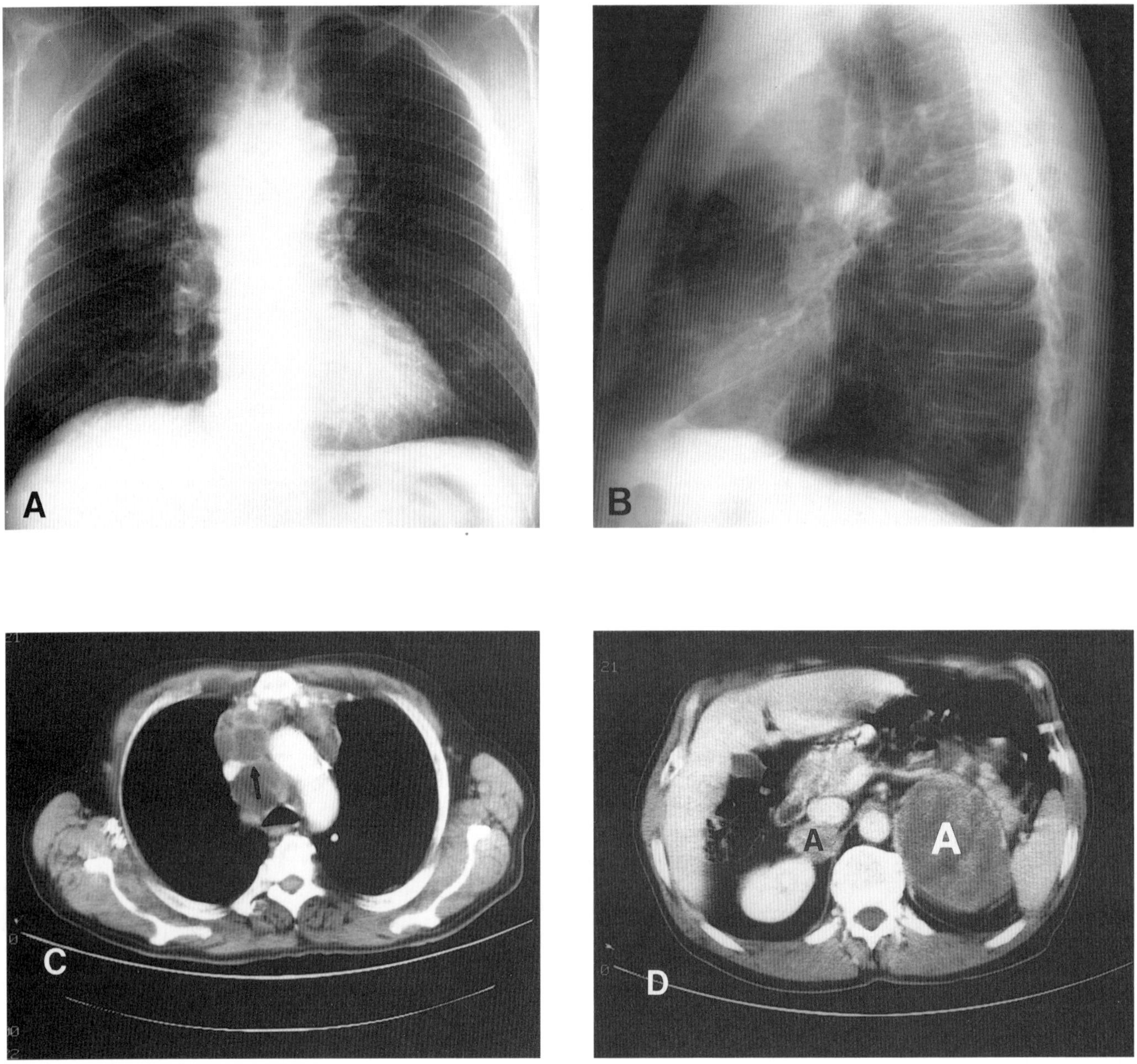

Figure 6.5

Staging process, primary lung tumor. This 67-year-old male was found by sputum cytology to have a squamous cell carcinoma of the lung, with an abnormal mediastinum on routine chest radiographs.

A,B The peripheral right mid-lung nodular density measured 3.2 cm. Lobular mediastinal abnormalities were present bilaterally. This individual therefore appears to have a T2, N3 (stage IIIb) primary lung cancer utilizing plain film alone.

C,D CT scans confirmed the presence of bilateral hilar adenopathy, distorting the superior vena cava (arrow on **C**). Surprisingly, bilateral adrenal metastatic lesions were proven by percutaneous biopsy ('A' on **D**). This confirms the need to routinely extend the axial CT sections, through the upper abdomen to include the liver and adrenal areas.

(Reproduced from Bragg,[22] courtesy of W.B. Saunders.)

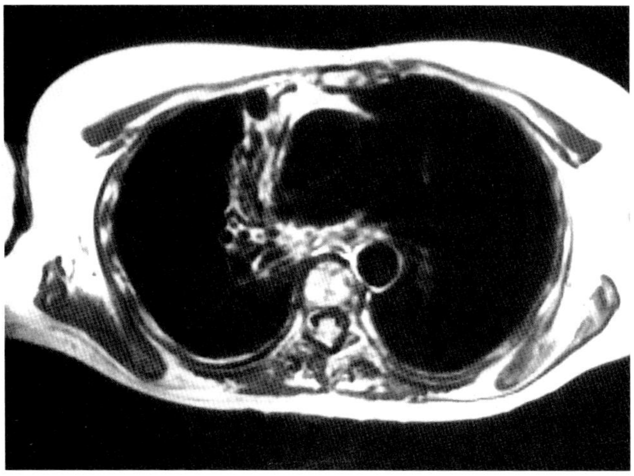

Figure 6.6

Radiation changes—MR T2-weighted image. This 61-year-old female was treated with radiation therapy for unresectable right upper lobe adenocarcinoma. Serial chest radiographs suggested abnormal widening in the right mediastinum. These T2-weighted images reveal the characteristic changes of radiation injury to the lung, sharply limited by the treatment port margins.

sectional imaging techniques. Again, CT will be adequate to explore most of the abnormalities found on plain films. In the patient who has had radiation therapy, mediastinal and contiguous lung changes resulting from radiation may create plain film changes that are difficult to discriminate from recurrent tumor. In these instances, MR scans may allow more easy distinction of the lower intensity signal of radiation fibrosis from that of recurrent tumor[29] (Figure 6.6).

Superior sulcus (Pancoast's) tumors

The superior sulcus or Pancoast's tumor is a neoplasm arising in the apex of the lung with specific clinical and radiographic characteristics. This lesion was originally described by the radiologist Henry Pancoast, who first theorized that its location was responsible for the unusual clinical attributes, including Horner's syndrome, brachial plexopathy, shoulder pain and an apical location of a mass lesion in the lung.[30,31]

The type of neoplasm responsible for the superior sulcus tumor or Pancoast's syndrome is varied, although usually is caused by primary lung cancer, most often of the squamous cell type. Uncommonly, metastatic tumors, inflammatory lesions and even lymphomas have been reported to cause a Pancoast's syndrome.

The presenting symptoms and apical location of a mass lesion should suggest the diagnosis. Staging is best performed with a combination of both CT and MR. Computed tomography will allow characterization of bone destruction (Figure 6.7), MR being better for assessing vascular invasion and nerve root/spinal cord extension.

Pleural neoplasms

Benign and malignant neoplasms of the pleura share many common imaging features. The discussion below will focus on the appearance and staging of primary malignant mesothelioma, an uncommon mesenchymal tumor involving the pleura.

The primary histologic types of malignant mesothelioma of the pleura are epithelial, mixed and sarcomatous in origin, generally decreasing in frequency in this order.[32] Mesotheliomas are usually considered as either diffuse (virtually always malignant, comprising 75% of the group) or simple (usually benign, not related to asbestos exposure, forming the remaining 25%).

Diffuse malignant mesothelioma is usually detected in the patient found to have a record of asbestos exposure. The tumor tends to encase the pleural surface, extending locally, rather than exhibiting distant metastatic disease outside of the

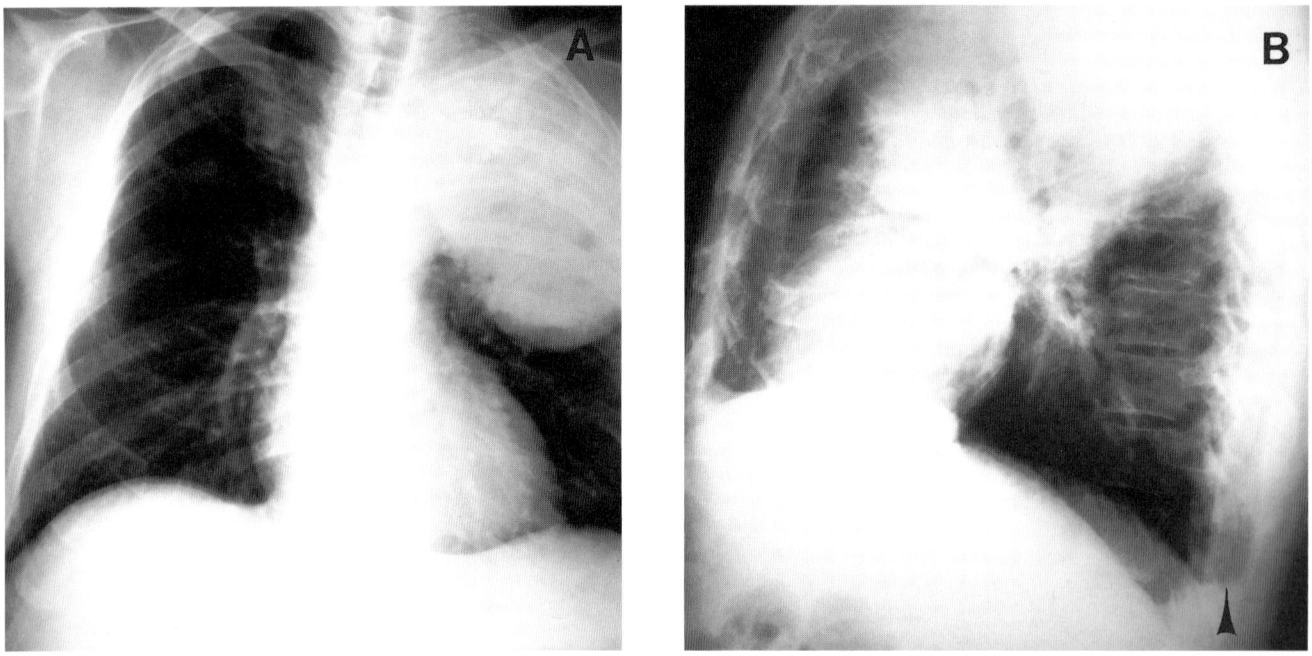

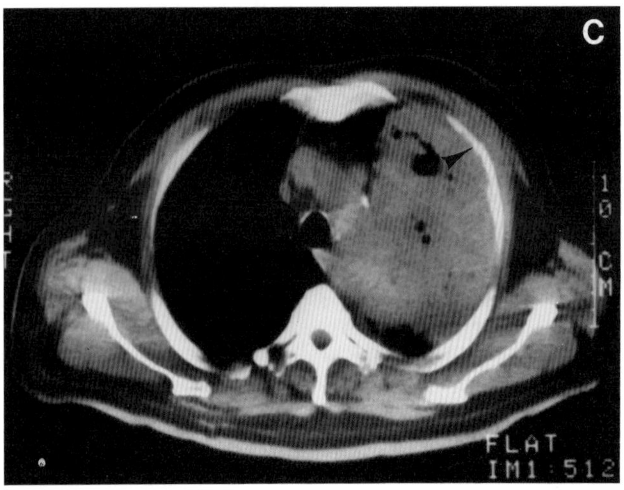

Figure 6.7

Superior sulcus (Pancoast's) tumor.

A,B A 57-year-old male initially presenting with complaints of shoulder and chest wall pain was found to have a large left apical mass lesion, posteriorly located on the lateral film (arrowhead on **B**).

C On CT scanning, rather extensive bone destruction, not evident on plain films, was found eroding the ribs (arrowhead) and extending to involve the brachial plexus. This was an unresectable squamous cell carcinoma of the lung.

(Reproduced from Bragg,[22] courtesy of W.B. Saunders.)

thorax. In spite of the proximity of the mesothelioma to the rib cage, osseous metastatic disease or bone destruction is not commonly seen until late in the course of the neoplasm. The plain-film radiographic and CT appearance of diffuse malignant mesothelioma is characterized by a lobular mass lesion, nodular pleural thickening and an associated pleural effusion. Histologic verification is usually difficult, as much of the mesothelioma is found to contain fibrous tissue with no distinguishing cellular features. It is for this reason that percutaneous needle biopsy is not recommended as an initial diagnostic approach to the patient suspected of having a malignant mesothelioma.

It is far more common to encounter metastatic pleural disease than diffuse malignant mesothelioma. With limited biopsy material, the pathologist may occasionally have difficulty separating metastatic adenocarcinoma from malignant mesothelioma.

The primary staging process for malignant pleural mesothelioma is dependent on CT evaluation of the thorax. Extension into critical mediastinal compartments, as well as the local extent of the neoplasm, is best seen by axial CT.[33] Separation of the tumor mass from critical mediastinal structures may be more accurately performed by MR.

Metastatic disease in the lung and pleura

The imaging challenges presented by suspected metastatic disease are centered in two primary clinical settings: surveillance of the patient with a primary tumor known to metastasize to the chest and the initial detection of metastatic disease. The lung is usually the first organ to be found to harbor metastatic disease; this is due, in large part, to its rich blood supply, the initial capillary bed being available to trap migrating cancer cells. In addition, there is a propensity of certain tumors such as melanomas and sarcomas to seek or prefer the 'soil' of the lung. The hematogenous route of spread of cancer to the lung is usually characterized by nodular disease, with lesions in the lung bases, where perfusion is the greatest, being of greater density and size.

Lymphangitic metastatic disease is a pathologic expression of metastatic tumor secondary to involvement of the lymphatic elements of the lung parenchyma. The primary cancer cell type responsible for a lymphangitic tumor is nearly always an adenocarcinoma: it is believed that the metastatic adenocarcinoma reaches the lung through the vascular compartment and subsequently overwhelms the lymphatic system leading to obstruction. The routine chest radiographic features are non-specific and may be indistinguishable from interstitial pulmonary edema of heart failure. High resolution CT scans may allow one to be more specific about the diagnosis of a pattern suggesting lymphangitic tumor spread. Their features have been described as a peripheral interstitial pattern with an abnormal infiltration of the bronchovascular bundles, leading to a 'spoked wheel' appearance. Septal lines may be visible with ill-defined nodularity in the lung parenchyma and, often, pleural effusions.[34]

The imaging features of nodular metastatic disease are quite non-specific, seldom allowing metastatic disease to be identified by imaging criteria alone. Histologic proof is necessary to confirm the diagnosis as a number of benign neoplastic and inflammatory lesions may exactly mimic the imaging features, for example lesions of viral infections, lymphoid granulomatosis or histoplasmosis.

The predominant blood supply to metastatic pulmonary lesions is derived from the pulmonary circulation, with only infrequent bronchial arterial supply.[35] This feature is occasionally helpful during the CT evaluation of a patient with metastatic nodular disease. The branches of the pulmonary arterial tree may be seen to enlarge and extend directly to the location of the peripheral, nodular metastatic lesions.

Occasionally, metastatic nodular lesions to the lung will undergo excavation. In most instances, the histology of these metastatic cancers will prove to be squamous cell in type, most frequently from primary tumors in the head and neck or the uterine cervix. Other nodular neoplastic lesions that undergo excavation may occur in patients with sarcomas and, occasionally, lymphomas.

Computed tomography is the most sensitive, accurate means for detecting metastatic pulmonary disease. A strategy has to be developed to apply the appropriate imaging techniques to the patient suspected of pulmonary metastatic disease; it should be based on the primary tumor, the anticipated therapeutic options for the patient, the age and status of the patient and the stage of the cancer. As an example, in the individual with an osteosarcoma, who is a candidate for extensive reconstructive surgery, initial CT evaluation of the chest should be obtained in a definitive search for metastatic disease, prior to definitive treatment. In other individuals whose primary cancer therapy would not be affected by the detection of metastatic pulmonary disease, routine chest radiographs will suffice for screening purposes. Follow-up imaging strategies should take advantage of similar clinical, pathologic considerations.

The appearance of specific metastatic lesions is governed by the histology of the cancer and, occasionally, therapeutic interventions. Sarcomatous metastatic lesions have sharp borders and often can easily be surgically extracted from the lung parenchyma. Adenocarcinomas tend to have ill-defined margins that make them more difficult to detect on plain films. The margins of metastatic lesions can also be made indistinct by surrounding hemorrhage or edema, such as in patients with choriocarcinomas metastatic to the lung.

Unusual features of metastatic tumors can occasionally be found in imaging studies. Young patients with primary sarcomas may experience a spontaneous pneumothorax as the initial, clinical and radiologic presentation of their metastatic disease. This results from the subpleural location

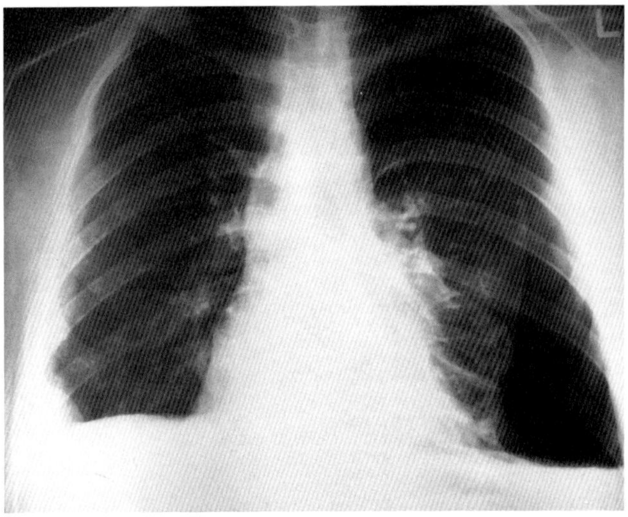

Figure 6.8

Metastatic malignant fibrous histiocytoma. This 17-year-old male had undergone limb salvage surgery with resection of the proximal humerus and distal clavicle (note the clips and absence of the right calvicle). Follow up chest radiographs showed no evidence for disease extension. The patient was re-evaluated in the emergency room after the development of acute shortness of breath and left chest pain. The radiograph shows a hydropneumothorax. The nodular metastatic lesions can be seen in the immediate subpleural regions.

of these metastatic deposits which may develop a bronchopleural fistula and result in a pneumothorax. Calcification or ossification may be seen on CT evaluation of certain metastatic lesions; this matrix formation is associated with metastatic deposits from bone- and calcium-producing tumors such as osteosarcomas and chondrosarcomas. Occasionally, mucin-producing adenocarcinomas of the colon may be noted on CT evaluation to have faint calcific densities within them.

Metastatic disease to the pleura is usually expressed clinically and radiologically by pleural effusions, which are found on analysis to contain recognizable neoplastic cells. The most common tumor associated with a malignant pleural effusion is metastatic breast cancer. Seldom are the pleural nodules of metastatic disease visible in any imaging study. Occasionally, in the patient with a spontaneous pneumothorax secondary to metastatic disease, one will be able to identify the subpleural nodules with the lung separated from the chest wall (Figure 6.8). In most instances, the metastatic pleural involvement is microscopic, not macroscopic.

Pleural effusions may occur as a result of tumor seeding from extensive deposits of the cancer involving the peritoneal surfaces of the abdomen. The existing anatomic apertures in the diaphragm may allow the passage of tumor cells into the pleural space by direct extension. This is seen in patients with advanced cancers of both the ovary and colon, in whom tumor deposits seem to initially attach to the diaphragmatic pleural surface and then extend along the chest wall, mimicking the appearance of a mesothelioma (described above). Occasionally, the pathologist may have difficulty separating metastatic adenocarcinoma and mesothelioma in both the lung and pleura.

Sometimes metastatic disease to the thorax will be visible on the chest radiograph as an extrapleural mass of considerable size. These masses are almost always secondary to a destructive metastatic focus within a contiguous rib. The site of bone destruction may not initially be obvious. When a large, extraosseous soft tissue mass and a metastatic rib lesion are found, the possibility of either an unusual metastatic cancer or, more likely, multiple myeloma should be considered.

Occasionally, a very frustrating clinical problem presents, the patient with a metastasis to the lung from an unknown primary site. In this instance, the goal of the clinician and radiologist is to determine the histology of the metastasis (lung biopsy) and direct a limited search for the occult primary tumor. For example, if the nodular metastatic pulmonary lesion proves to be an adenocarcinoma, the likely site in a female is the breast, uterus or colon. In the male, the lesion is more likely to be secondary to an occult primary in the pancreas, colon or kidney. The search for the primary site should be limited as, even at post-mortem examination, these clinically occult primaries may prove difficult to detect.[36]

Chest wall neoplasms

Chest wall neoplasms are uncommon clinical, pathologic and radiologic problems which are dominated by the common benign lesions, traumatic rib fractures and metastatic disease or myeloma. Within this broad spectrum of lesions lie a number of uncommon entities that share some common imaging features and occasionally have unique imaging features. Table 6.4 summarizes the more common benign, malignant and chest wall neoplasms, the term 'neoplasm' being used with editorial license. Some of these benign lesions are obviously congenital, traumatic or infectious in origin, merely mimicking a true neoplasm clinically or radiologically.

These chest wall neoplasms may present as either a palpable mass clinically or an incidentally detected abnormality on a routine chest radiograph. Since the high kVp chest radiographs limit bone detail, once an abnormality is detected, low kVp radiographs of rib detail should be obtained. If the diagnosis is not obvious from these initial films, more sophisticated axial imaging techniques should be utilized; however, bone detail is difficult to access due to the oblique course of the ribs and resulting challenge in imaging these structures by CT and MR. If a metastatic lesion is suspected, the obvious imaging study to obtain next is confirmatory clinical history and a radionuclide bone scan.

Benign neoplasms

The more common benign abnormalities involving ribs are summarized in Table 6.4. By far the most common are unusual manifestations of rib fractures that may not have been adequately immobilized or may have been subjected to multiple episodes of trauma and incomplete healing. In these instances, abundant callus may form, distorting the fracture site and rib ends or may even be palpable. In the child, the possibility of abuse should be suspected and other manifestations of skeletal injury sought.

It is said that the two most common benign rib neoplasms are enchondromas and fibrous dysplasia. Enchondromas are extremely uncommon and are characterized by a faintly calcified matrix as is encountered in their more common locations in the short tubular bones of the hands and feet. Deposits of fibrous dysplasia are represented by an expanded rib with a very thin cortex and a 'ground glass' texture to the involved rib.

In my experience, congenital exostosis are typical on plain films but often mistakenly diagnosed. The exostosis develops in childhood; as the thorax expands, the cartilaginous cap is drawn toward the lung parenchyma, appearing in adult life as a densely calcified 'granuloma'. If one looks closely, the donor site of the exostosis in the rib, usually anteriorly, can be detected.

Paget's disease may occasionally involve the thorax and is characterized by enlargement of the entire circumference of the affected bone, with disorganized bone architecture that is usually much denser than the surrounding skeleton bones. In the chest wall, the shoulder girdle is most commonly affected, usually the clavicle.

Osteomyelitis of the thorax is the most troublesome entity to detect and confirm radiologically. The imaging features of osteomyelitis closely resemble those of primary bone tumors. Osteomyelitis involving the thorax is usually bacterial in origin and most often caused by a staphylococcal organism. Occasionally, secondary chest wall involvement may occur secondary to blastomycosis, actinomycosis, cryptococcosis or tuberculosis.

Radiation bone injury is less often seen nowadays than in earlier years when the radiation therapy equipment available was less sophisticated, with lower energy sources that damaged bone more frequently than the newer, supervoltage sources. Osteoblasts are destroyed by radiation doses in excess of 4000 rads (40 Gy). In the adult, the osseous skeleton contained within radiation ports treated to doses above this level gradually demineralize within the treatment field, developing a Paget-like texture. These radiation-injured bones are less able to defend against both trauma and infection. Fractures that develop within radiation-damaged bone may heal but, if the bone is not immobilized, often progress to non-union. If skin breakdown occurs over the radiation-injured skeletal parts, an aggressive osteomyelitis and bone destruction may result, often with dystrophic calcification. These destructive bone lesions may be confused with radiation-induced sarcomas of bone.[37]

The immature skeleton subjected to radiation expresses different changes to the adult. The cartilaginous elements of the growing skeleton and, specifically, chondroblasts are more sensitive to radiation than the osteoblasts. It is therefore the growth centers which are affected in the child, deforming the growing bone exposed to the radiation beam. When possible, growth centers should not be exposed to radiation doses in excess of 2000 rads (20 Gy), to avoid subsequent growth distur-

Table 6.4 Chest wall neoplasms.

Neoplasm	*Feature*
BENIGN	
Rib fracture	
Enchondroma	Calcified matrix
Fibrous dysplasia	Expanded rib, thin cortex, 'ground glass' texture
Exostosis	Cartilaginous cap extends into lung
Paget's disease	Enlargement of bone, disorganized trabeculae
Brown's tumor	
Hemangioma	
Eosinophilic granuloma	
Osteomyelitis	May resemble a destructive sarcoma
Congenital (bifid rib)	
Aneurysmal bone cyst	Expansile, intact cortex
Radiation bone injury	Confined to treatment port, demineralized with Paget-like texture, exostoses
MALIGNANT	
Malignant round cell tumors	
Ewing's sarcoma	Most common malignant childhood rib tumor
Askin's tumor	Similar to Ewing's, neuroepithelial tumor, spreads along sympathetic chain
Chondrosarcoma	Adult tumor, tendency to involve contiguous ribs
Non-Hodgkin's lymphoma	Extranodal site, young females, resembles Ewing's sarcoma
Malignant fibrous histiocytoma	Low-grade sarcoma, older patient
Myeloma	Destructive lesion, large soft tissue mass, older patient
Desmoid tumor	Low-grade sarcoma, calcifies, extends over chest wall in women
Osteosarcoma/fibrosarcoma	
Metastatic cancer	

bances. The expression of growth disturbances will vary depending upon whether the axial or appendicular skeleton is included in the treatment port. Occasionally, osteocartilaginous exostoses may develop within the radiation field.[38]

Malignant neoplasms

The most common destructive rib lesions in adults are caused by metastatic cancer. These lesions are usually not associated with a significant or prominent soft-tissue mass visible on routine chest radiographs. If a destructive rib lesion with a large surrounding soft tissue mass visible on plain films is found in an older patient, multiple myeloma should be suspected.

The most common primary malignant chest wall neoplasms are the primary malignant round cell tumors, including Ewing's sarcoma and Askin's tumors. These cancers behave in a similar manner and may be variations of the same neoplasm. In the case of Ewing's sarcoma, a destructive rib lesion is usually found to be associated with a very large surrounding soft tissue mass. Occasionally, a soft-tissue Ewing's sarcoma may appear in the absence of a visible destructive rib lesion. Askin's tumor is a neuroepithelial neoplasm and the initial

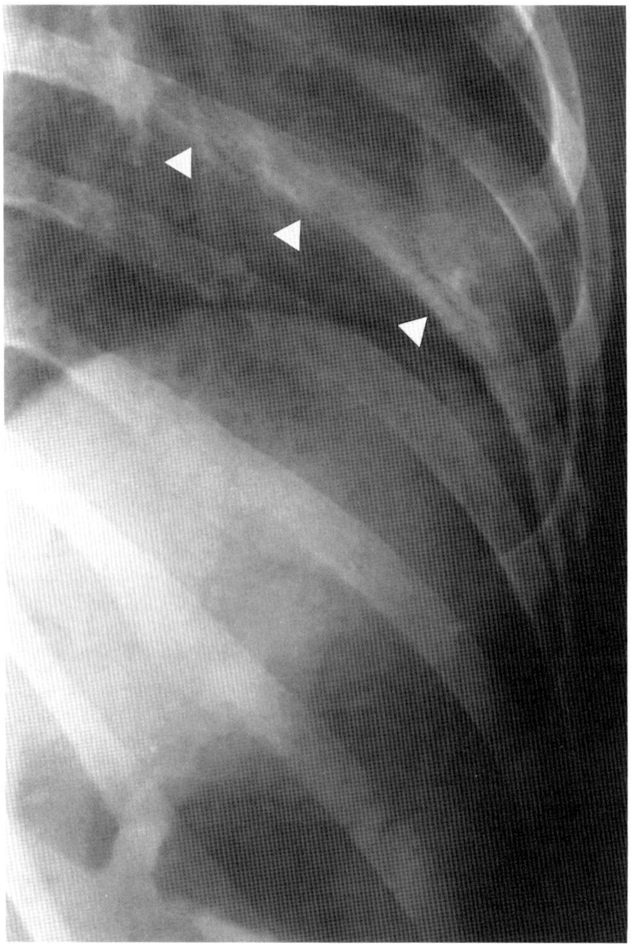

A

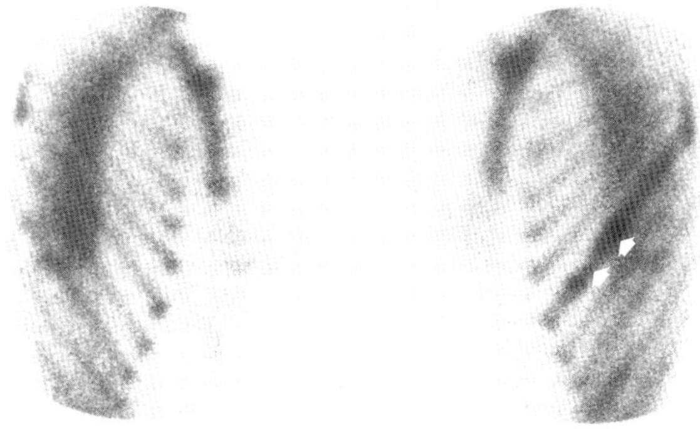

B

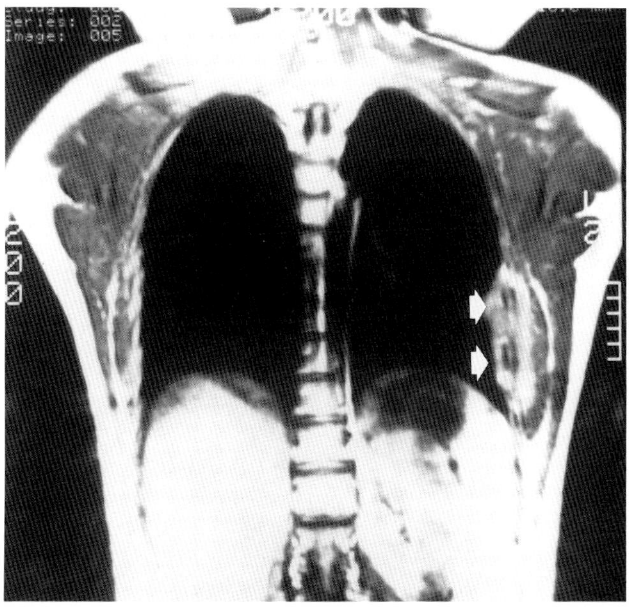

C

Figure 6.9

Non-Hodgkin's lymphoma—chest wall. This 18-year-old female complained of chest wall pain for nearly a year prior to the films.

A There was an abnormal texture to the rib with areas of both destruction and apparent new bone formation (arrowheads).

B The radionuclide bone scan showed a single area of increased activity (arrows).

C The MR scan showed the soft-tissue mass of high signal intensity (arrows) surrounding this mass. The radiographic features were consistent either with a malignant round cell tumor or a non-Hodgkin's lymphoma; at surgery it was found to be the latter.

(Reproduced from Devita VT, Jr, Hellman S, Rosenberg SA, eds, *Cancer, Principles and Practice of Oncology*, 3rd edn, courtesy of J.B. Lippincott.)

destructive lesion is similar in appearance to Ewing's sarcoma. The metastatic extension of the Askin's tumor tends to follow the course of the sympathetic chain.

A very similar appearing chest wall neoplasm to the small malignant round cell tumor is the extranodal chest wall expression of a non-Hodgkin's lymphoma.[39] These tumors also tend to occur in young women and cause destructive rib lesions with a surrounding soft-tissue mass (Figure 6.9). In all of these malignant chest wall tumors, it should be recalled that osteomyelitis has a similar appearance radiologically. Osteomyelitis and most destructive chest wall tumors may closely resemble each other both clinically and radiologically.

The other malignant chest wall tumors are infrequently seen; they are summarized in Table 6.4. In an older individual, malignant fibrous histiocytoma may involve the chest wall, giving a radiologic appearance similar to the malignant round cell tumors.[40,41] A curious, rare tumor, the desmoid tumor, is a low-grade sarcoma, which has a tendency to involve the chest wall in women. It spreads over the chest wall, occasionally exhibiting rather profound calcifications and deformity of the ribs where the tumor intersects the bony thorax.

References

1 Trunk G, Gracey DR, Byrd RB, The management and evaluation of the solitary pulmonary nodule, *Chest* (1974) **66**:236–9.

2 Sorenson JA, Mitchell CR, Armstrong JD, et al, Effects of improved contrast on lung-nodule detection: a clinical ROC study, *Invest Radiol* (1987) **22**:772–80.

3 Webb WR, Radiologic evaluation of the solitary pulmonary nodule, *AJR* (1990) **154**:701–8.

4 Nathan MH, Management of solitary pulmonary nodules, an organized approach based on growth rate and statistics, *JAMA* (1974) **227**:1141–4.

5 Siegelman SS, Khouri NF, Leo FP, et al, Solitary pulmonary nodules: CT assessment, *Radiology* (1986) **160**:307–12.

6 Zerhouni EA, Stitik FP, Siegalman SS, et al, CT of the pulmonary nodule: a cooperative study, *Radiology* (1986) **160**:319–27.

7 Webb WR, The role of magnetic resonance imaging in the assessment of patients with lung cancer: a comparison with computed tomography, *J Thorac Imag* (1989) **4**:65–75.

8 Spritzer C, Gamsu G, Sostman HD, Magnetic resonance imaging of the thorax: techniques, current applications and future directions, *J Thorac Imag* (1989) **4**:1–18.

9 Webb WR, Radiologic imaging of the pulmonary hila, *Postgrad Radiol* (1986) **6**:145–68.

10 Webb WR, Radiologic evaluation of the solitary pulmonary nodule, *AJR* (1990) **154**:701–8.

11 Westcott JL, Percutaneous transthoracic needle biopsy, *Radiology* (1988) **169**:593–601.

12 Perlmutt LM, Johnston WW, Dunnick NR, Percutaneous transthoracic needle aspiration, a review, *AJR* (1989) **152**:451–455.

13 Perlmutt LM, Braun SD, Newman GE, et al, Timing of chest film follow-up after transthoracic needle aspiration, *AJR* (1986) **146**:1049–50.

14 Fraser RG, Paré JAP, *Diagnosis of disease of the chest*, 3rd edn (Saunders: Philadelphia 1991).

15 Giustra PE, Stassa G, The multiple presentations of bronchial adenomas, *Radiology* (1969) **93**:1013–19.

16 Forster BB, Muller NL, Miller RR, et al, Neuroendocrine carcinomas of the lung: clinical radiologic and pathologic correlation, *Radiology* (1989) **170**:441–5.

17 Oates JA, Carcinoid syndrome, *N Engl J Med* (1986) **315**:702–4.

18 Doppman JL, Pass HI, Nieman LK, et al, Pulmonary hamartoma: CT findings, *Radiology* (1986) **160**:313–18.

19 Siegelman SS, Khouri NF, Scott WW, et al, Detection of ACTH-producing bronchial carcinoid tumors: MR imaging vs. CT, *AJR* (1991) **159**:39–43.

20 Boring CC, Squires TS, Tong T, Cancer statistics, *CA, Cancer J. Clinicians* (1991) **41**:19–36.

21 Bragg DG, Rubin P, Youker JE, *Oncologic imaging* (Pergamon Press: New York 1987).

22 Bragg DG, Imaging and primary lung cancer, the roles of detection, staging and follow-up, *Semin Ultrasound, CT MR* (1989) **10**:453–66.

23 Bragg DG, Applications of imaging in lung cancer, *Cancer* (1991) **67**:1165–8.

24 Muhm JR, Miller WE, Fontana RS, et al, Lung cancer detected during a screening program using four month chest radiographs, *Radiology* (1983) **148**:609–15.

25 Fontana RS, Sanderson DR, Woolner LD, et al, Screening for lung cancer: a critique of the male lung project, *Cancer* (1991) **67**:1155–64.

26 Beahrs OH, Henson DE, Hutter RVP, Myers MH, *Manual for staging of cancer*, 3rd edn (J.B. Lippincott: Philadelphia 1988).

27 Webb WR, Gatsonis C, Zerhouni EA, et al, CT and MR imaging in staging non-small cell bronchogenic carcinoma: report of the Radiologic Diagnostic Oncology Group, *Radiology* (1991) **178**:705–13.

28 Poon PY, Bronskill MJ, Henkelman RM, et al, Mediastinal lymph node metastases from bronchiogenic carcinoma: detection with MR imaging and CT, *Radiology* (1987) **162**:651–6.

29 Gamsu G, Sostman D, Magnetic resonance imaging of the thorax, *Am R Resp Dis* (1989) **139**:254–75.

30 Pancoast HK, Importance of careful roentgen-ray investigation of apical chest tumors, *JAMA* (1924) **83**:1407–11.

31 Pugatch RD, Shaffer K, Primary pulmonary neoplasms. In: Freundlich J, Bragg DG, eds, *A radiologic approach to diseases of the chest* (Williams & Wilkins: Baltimore 1992).

32 Adams VI, Krishnan KU, Muhm JR, et al, Diffuse and malignant mesothelioma of pleura, diagnosis and survival in 92 cases, *Cancer* (1986) **58**:1540–51.

33 Mirvis S, Dutcher JP, Haney PJ, et al, CT of malignant pleural mesothelioma, *AJR* (1983) **140**:665–70.

34 Munk PL, Muller NL, Miller RR, Ostrow DN, Pulmonary lymphangitic carcinomatosis: CT and pathologic findings, *Radiology* (1988) **166**:705–9.

35 Milne ENC, Zerhouni EA, Blood supply of pulmonary metastases, *J Thorac Imag* (1987) **2**:15–23.

36 Kagan AR, Steckel RJ, Diagnostic imaging in clinical cancer management: metastases from unknown primary tumors, *Invest Radiol* (1988) **23**:545–7.

37 Bragg DG, Shidnia HH, Chu FCH, et al, Clinical and radiographic aspects of radiation osteitis, *Radiology* (1970) **97**:103–11.

38 Libshitz HI, Cohen MA, Radiation-induced osteochondromas, *Radiology* (1982) **142**:643–74.

39 Bragg DG, Colby T, Ward JH, New concepts in non-Hodgkin's lymphomas: radiologic implications, *Radiology* (1986) **159**:289–304.

40 Franken EA, Smith JA, Smith WL, Tumors of the chest wall in infants and children, *Pediatr Radiol* (1977) **6**:13–18.

41 Fink IJ, Kurtz DW, Cazenav EL, et al, Malignant thoraco-pulmonary small-cell (Askin) tumor, *AJR* (1985) **145**:517–20.

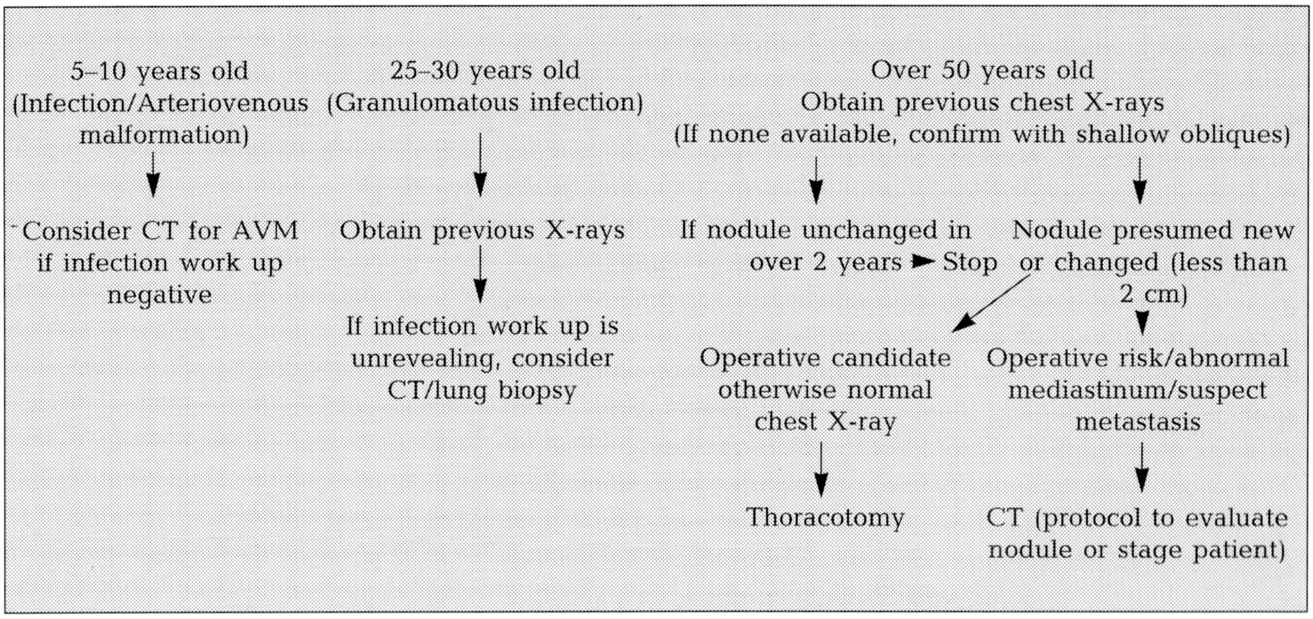

Diagram 6.1

Imaging strategy for a solitary pulmonary nodule: radiologic work up by age of patient. AVM, arteriovenous malformation.

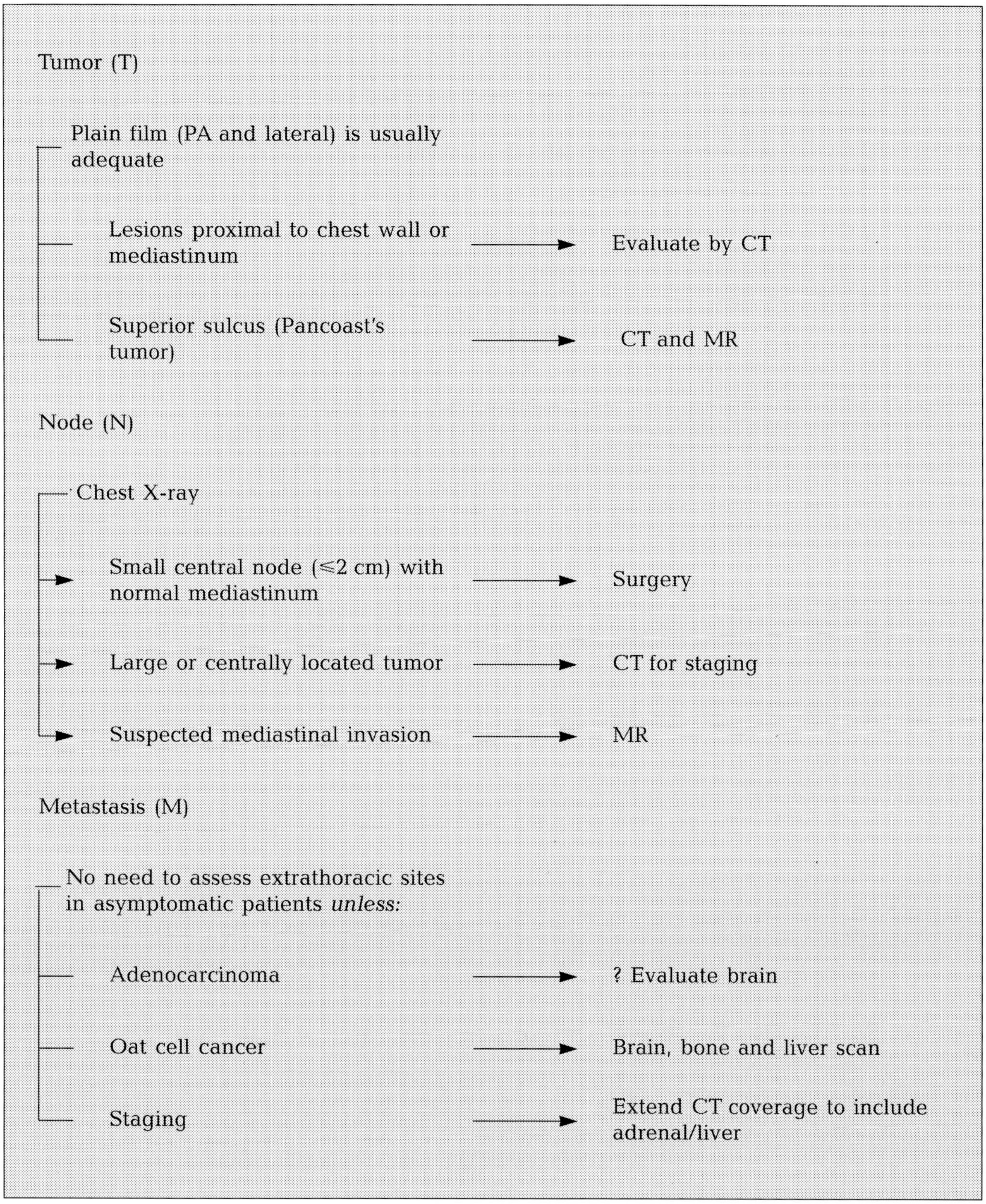

Diagram 6.2

Imaging strategy for staging lung cancer.

7

The breast

Marie Hélène Dilhuydy, Alain Le Treut, Jean Marie Dilhuydy, Michèle Kind

Introduction

Epidemiology and pathogenesis

Breast cancer is the most common form of cancer in women in the industrialized regions such as the USA and Western Europe, where it accounts for 27% of all cancers in women. In certain American states, its incidence is 80–90 per 100 000 per year.[1] In France, incidence is between 70 and 73 per 100 000, with higher rates in urban and industrial areas.[2] Incidence increases with age, with two peaks occurring at 55 and 70 years, and is increasing by 2% per year in the Western World. In Asia and Africa, the incidence, especially of postmenopausal forms, is much lower but is perhaps underestimated because of difficulty in compiling reliable data.[3] However, it is increasing rapidly in countries which are becoming industrialized.

Breast cancer is the main cause of female mortality due to cancer in industrialized nations—17% of deaths. It accounts for 35% of all deaths from cancer between 35 and 54 years of age, and is also the leading cause of overall female mortality.[2] The mortality rate is approximately 30 per 100 000 per year in the USA and France.

The pathogenesis of breast cancer depends on many factors—genetic, hormonal or environmental—affecting mammary tissues, which undergo periodic variations at different stages in the life cycle. A direct family history of breast cancer (mother, sister, daughter) multiplies the risk factor by 2 or 3 and two first-degree relatives by 12 or 15. The risk is even greater if family cancers are premenopausal and/or bilateral.[3] Benign mastopathies are frequent but are rarely investigated histologically and their prognostic significance is variable. A relationship between some of these lesions such as atypical hyperplasia or lobular carcinoma in situ and different types of cancer is probable but difficult to prove. The multiplicity of etiological factors and the complexity of mechanisms limit attempts at prevention. The identification of risk factors allows individual management but cannot define a high-risk population with a view to screening. Although certain women have a higher risk factor, there does not exist a low-risk population which can be omitted from screening.[4]

The role of imaging techniques

Imaging techniques play a vital role in early diagnosis, on which chances of breast conservation and cure depend. Diagnosis has been transformed during the past 20 years, due to progress in such techniques: less bulky tumors are identified—more minimal breast cancers which are infracentrimetrical or in situ. The existence of imaging techniques leads to the possibility of mass screening.

Progress in treatment is derived from locoregional, functional and esthetic results and from the integration of general treatment in curative procedures. The complexity of indications relying on the evaluation of prognostic factors increases the importance of pre-treatment assessment, in which imaging techniques play an essential role. The frequency of conservative treatment, the extension of survival, the possibility of treating relapses and a better understanding of the readaptation of patients emphasizes the importance of follow up, both during and after treatment, in which imaging is also a determining factor.

Classification of breast cancer

Cancer can be classified in a homogeneous prognostic group. The most widely used classification is the TNM clinical classification of the International Union Against Cancer (UICC), revised in 1988 (Table 7.1). This clinical classification, which is supplemented by the acquisition of other prognostic factors, especially histologic factors and receptors, allows the evaluation of individual prognosis and the deduction of therapeutic indications.

Prognosis and therapeutic assessment

In 98% of cases, histologically, breast cancer is more or less differentiated adenocarcinoma. Certain rare histologic forms have a favorable prognosis, such as mucinous, medullary, papillary or cylindromatous carcinoma or juvenile secreting carcinoma. Prognosis correlates closely with the histoprognostic grading. The most widely used grading is that of Scarff, Bloom and Richardson, which divides cancers into three grades:[5] I - favorable prognosis, II - intermediate and III - unfavorable, according to the amount of tubular structures, anisocaryosis and the number of mitoses. This grading does not apply to in situ and medullary forms.

Axillary lymph node invasion is the main prognostic factor. Survival is reduced in proportion to the number of lymph nodes involved, falling from 79% after 5 years for one to three nodes to 39% for 10 or more. Fifty to sixty per cent of carcinomas present axillary invasion, and involvement increases with the size of the tumor. Invasion can be minimal, partial or total, with or without capsular rupture. It progresses via adjoining lymph nodes from the lower groups to the top of the armpit.[6] No other criteria, such as size, the extent of invasion, capsular rupture or the reactional state of other lymph nodes, apart from the number of lymph nodes involved, have been shown to have any prognostic value. The estrogen and progesterone receptor rate is a contributive prognostic factor, a low rate being significantly correlated with poor prognosis. Other factors such as ploïdy, S-phase, cathepsin D, EGF receptors and *HER-2* oncogene, are still being evaluated.

Table 7.1 The TNM clinical classification of breast cancer.

T	**Primary tumor**	
Tis	In situ cancer or isolated Paget's disease of the nipple	
T0	No evidence of primary tumor	
T1	<2 cm	**a** <0.5 cm
		b >0.5–1.0 cm
		c >1–2 cm
T2	>2–5 cm	
T3	>5 cm	
T4	any size with	**a** = extension to the chest wall
		b = edema, ulceration of the skin or satellite skin nodules
		c = **a** + **b**
		d = inflammation
N	**Regional adenopathies**	
N0	No adenopathies	
N1	Mobile homolateral axillary adenopathies	
N2	Fixed homolateral axillary adenopathies	
N3	Internal homolateral mammary adenopathies	
M	**Distant metastases**	
M0	No known distant metastasis	
M1	Distant metastases present: supra- or infraclavicular adenopathies are included in this category, as are contralateral lymph nodes	

After assessment and before treatment, prognostic estimation can be resumed thus:

- Immediate surgery is possible and the tumor is less than 30 mm: conservative treatment can be used. The global metastatic risk is 30% after 5 years, but can be estimated more precisely from prognostic factors, to decide on indications for general treatment.
- Immediate surgery is possible and the tumor is more than 30 mm: the risk is approximately 50% after 5 years and should be estimated more precisely from prognostic factors to decide on general treatment. Locoregional control can be obtained with mastectomy, or general treatment can contribute to conservative treatment.

- The tumor is more than 60 mm and/or has invaded the skin and deep-seated tissues and/or is accompanied by fixed axillary adenopathies: the metastatic risk is 70–80% after 5 years. General treatment is essential and can help to obtain better local control.
- There are signs of inflammation and/or rapid growth: the metastatic risk is about 100% after 3 years. Local treatment is integrated into general treatment.
- There are distant metastases: general treatment is essential and local treatment incidental.

Imaging techniques

The breast being an exterior organ facilitates the use of imaging techniques, but in practice only mammography and ultrasound are used.

Mammography

This necessitates films of perfect quality, which depends on contrast, the sensitivity of the detector, spatial resolution and background noise. These have a direct influence on the diagnostic value of the examination. All the elements of the radiographic chain should be optimized; the variations in the size and structure of the breast exclude global optimization and necessitate individual adaptation for each case. The dose delivered to the breast should remain within acceptable limits.[7] Magnification, by moving the breast away from the film, thus interposing an air gap, is reliable. It allows a better analysis of calcifications and a better spreading of architectural structures.

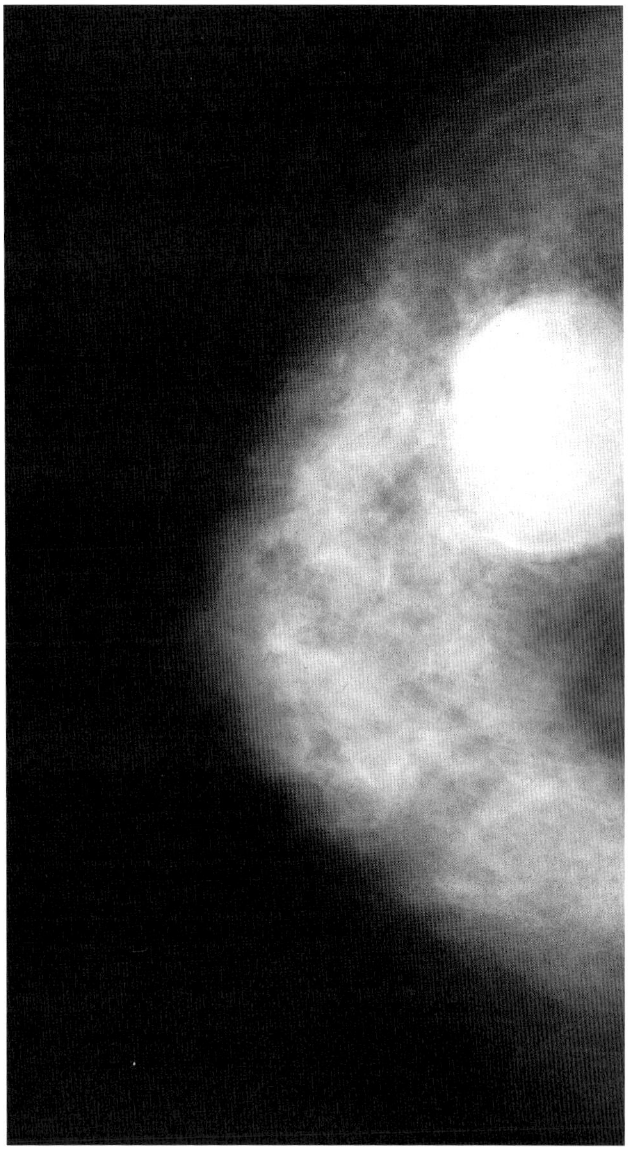

Figure 7.1

Recent discovery of a round, smooth and mobile mass in the medial quadrant of the left breast in a 39-year-old woman. Mammography (craniocaudal view) shows a smooth-bordered, rounded opacity. The histology was poorly differentiated, grade III, adenocarcinoma.

Round opacities

These are frequently discovered. Although suggestive of benign lesions, they prove malignant in 8% of cases.[8] In order to permit detection, they have to be silhouetted on a fatty density, but part of the outline can remain indistinct because of the dense structures. The visibility of the opacity depends on the density of the breast: an obvious lesion in a transparent breast can pass unnoticed in a dense or heterogeneous breast.

Round opacities can either be fluid lesions or solid tumors. Cystic lesions are regular, rounded, homogeneous and often multiple. The walls are invisible on mammography, and endoluminal tumors are missed.

Solid lesions are made up of epithelial and conjunctive tissue in variable proportions, the cells of which may either be normal or malignant

Table 7.2 Etiology of round masses.

Type of mass	*Etiology*
Anatomical structures	Nipple (incorrect incidence) Circumscribed conjunctive structure Intramammary lymph node
Cutaneous or subcutaneous tumors	Wart, naevus Neurofibroma Sebaceous cyst Angioma etc.
Benign lesions	Adenofibroma, adenofibromatosis Cysts, fibrocystic diseases Intraductal papilloma Phyllode low-grade tumor Hamartoma Galactoceles, lymphoceles Collected abscess—tuberculosis Hematomas, hemangiomas Real adenoma Leiomyoma
Malignant lesions	Adenocarcinoma Colloid carcinoma Medullar carcinoma Metastases Lymphomas Sarcomas

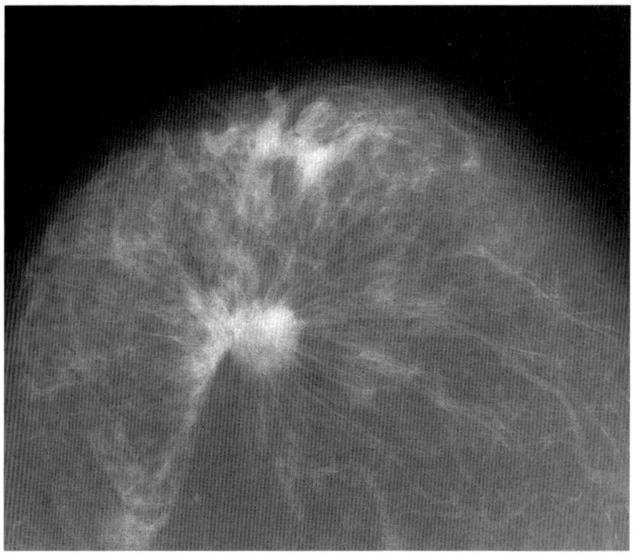

Figure 7.2

A bulky lesion (7 cm), clinically malignant in the upper quadrant of the left breast of a 62-year-old woman. Mammography (craniocaudal view) shows a spiculated opacity with microcalcifications. The histology was well-differentiated, grade II, adenocarcinoma.

(Figure 7.1). These lesions usually have centrifugal growth patterns and displace the parenchyma.

Diagnosis should include an analysis of density, shape, outline, size, evolution, localization and number of lesions. Associated signs, such as calcifications, cutaneous or areolar modifications, and edema, should be sought, and clinical indications, such as age, or the existence of a palpable mass especially taken into account. Ultrasonography is reliable. The main etiologies of round opacities are given in Table 7.2.

Spiculated opacities

A stellate appearance is one of the most reliable patterns on mammography. The lesion consists of a center and spiculae (Figure 7.2).

The center often has irregular borders because of implantation of the base of the spiculae, and can be rounded or crenellated. Its density depends on its size, on the type of lesion and on other factors: a carcinoma often has an opaque center, but the center of a radial scar is lighter and more heterogeneous. There may be no dense center if it is formed by converging spiculae, but this does not justify the elimination of cancer as a diagnosis.

The number of spiculae varies, as does their length, which can be several millimeters or a few centimeters, and they can either be thin or thick. Their distal extremity disappears into the glandular parenchyma, fastening onto the inner surface of superficial planes or curving without being attached. They are formed from a conjunctivoelastic framework which may be colonized by malignant cells.

The visibility of the spiculated pattern depends on the density and homogeneity of the breast and the quality of the image, but only part of its outline may be visible (Figure 7.3) and supplementary views are therefore necessary.

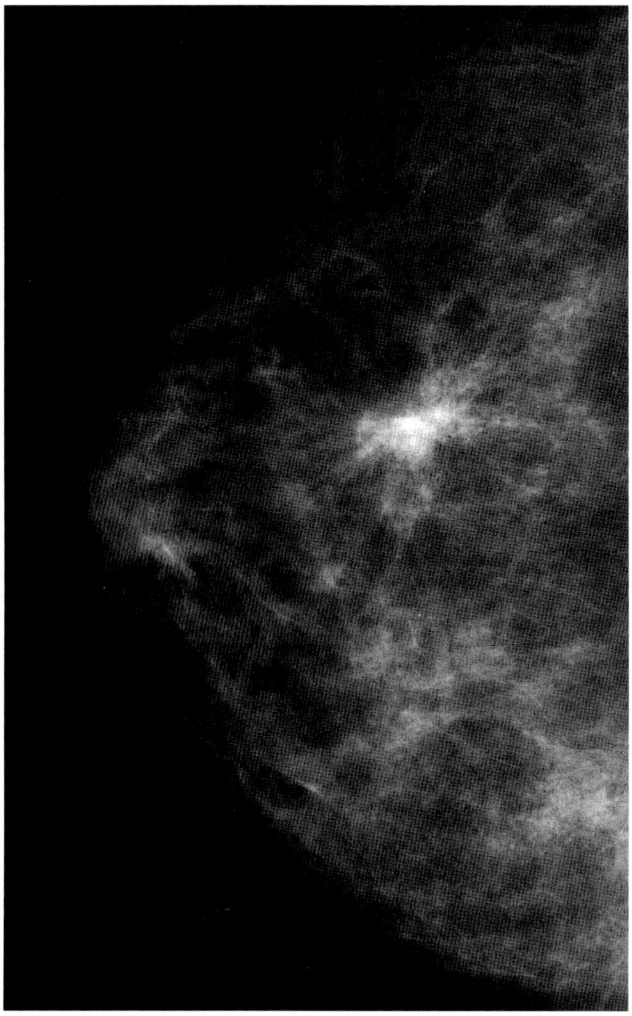

Figure 7.3

Clinically there was a slight asymmetry in the upper quadrant of the left breast of this 52-year-old woman. Mammography (craniocaudal view) shows a poorly limited opacity with short and thick spiculae. The histology was infiltrating intraductal carcinoma, grade III.

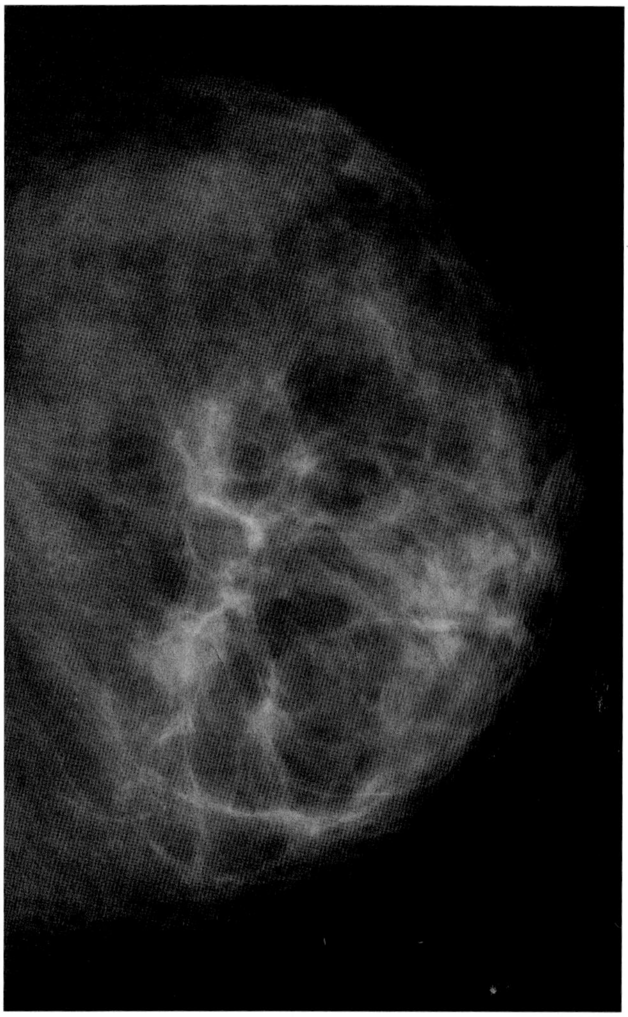

Figure 7.4

Soft mass in the lower quadrant of the left breast of a 49-year-old woman. Mammography (lateral view) shows distortion of breast architecture. The histology was infiltrative lobular carcinoma.

The diagnostic work up includes clinical examination and a search for associated signs such as microcalcifications, thickening and retraction of the skin or edema (ultrasonography is reliable). A spiculated opacity should be considered as carcinoma until it has been proved otherwise. The main differential diagnoses are a radial scar, a fibrous scar or sclerosing adenosis.

Architectural disruption

Various pathologic processes can modify the architecture of the breast to a greater or lesser degree (Figure 7.4). All constructed patterns based on a single film should first be eliminated, by repeating the basic film with spreading and different compression and with oblique views.

Architectural distortion is shown by opaque heterogeneous structures which are more or less convergent, and destroy conjunctive harmony. Their extension is variable, as they can be focalized, triangular at the summit of the nipple, reminiscent of galactophoric topography, extended, diffuse or multicentric. They should be analysed in relation to the contralateral breast.

Diagnosis necessitates careful consideration of clinical findings. These can correspond either to badly systematized carcinoma or to a benign mastopathy, as well as to inflammation such as secreting ductal ectasia or a scar. In 15% of cases, such findings are the only sign of a subclinical cancer.

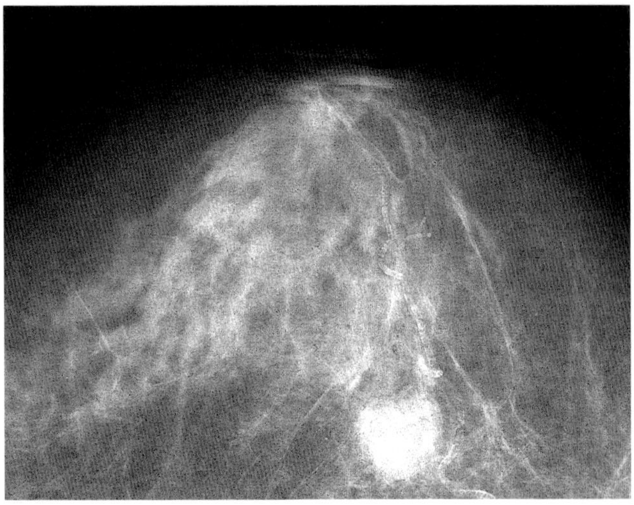

Figure 7.5

A palpable mass. Mammography shows an opacity with a poorly defined border. The histology was infiltrating intraductal carcinoma, grade III.

Poorly localized and asymmetrical opacities

The identification of poorly localized (Figure 7.5) and asymmetric opacities is difficult and depends on the global density of the conjunctivoglandular cone, as well as on the quality of the examination. Interpretation should take clinical and echographic data into account, as well as density and the asymmetry of the pattern, associated signs and whether the lesion is recent or fast growing. Interpretation should also be circumspect, especially in the case of isolated lesions with no clinical signs or asymmetrical size or density.[10]

Clear patterns

These are usually benign: lipomas or hamartomas. Butyric cysts and encysted fat necrosis are more interesting from the oncological point of view, since they are often observed during follow up after plastic surgery or conservative treatment: they show a clear round pattern with distinct borders which may be calcified, and they are seldom bulky.

A stellate tumoral pattern is sometimes surrounded by a clear halo which outlines its borders. According to certain authors, this results from peritumoral dehydrated fat, but others think it is simply an optical phenomenon.

Table 7.3 Mammary macrocalcifications (>1 mm).

Type of calcification	*Origin*
Linear calcifications	Vascular Ductal (secreting ductal ectasia) Parasitic (filariosis)
Gross or granulous calcifications	Adenofibroma Adenofibromatosis Cyst Papillomatosis Ductal carcinoma Epidermoid tumor Osteogenic tumor Hemangioma
Circular calcifications	Cyst Subcutaneous liponecrosis Fat necrosis

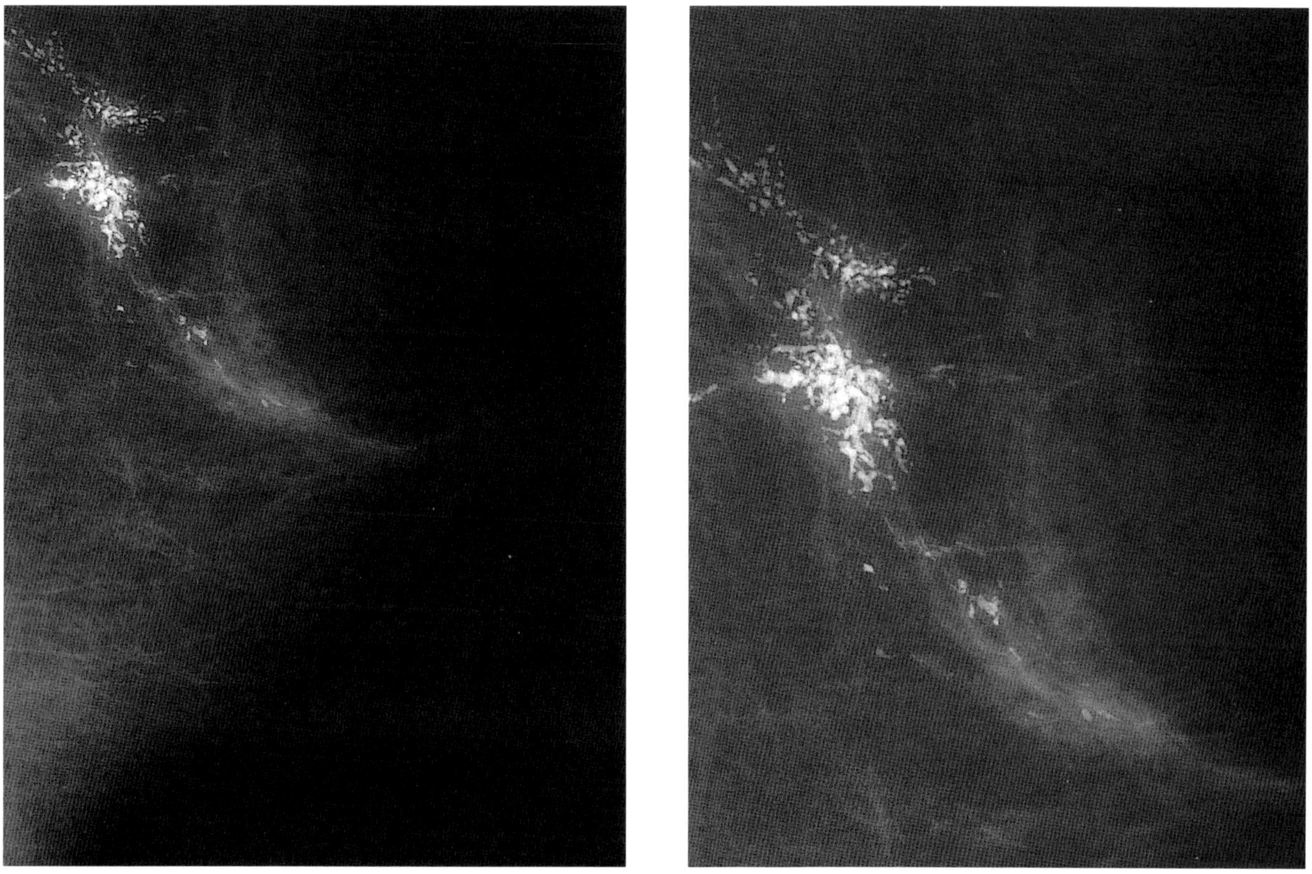

A B

Figure 7.6

Mammographic appearance of typical intraductal microcalcifications. Lateral view of the right breast (**A**) and magnification (**B**) show a triangle-shaped cluster. The histology was infiltrating intraductal carcinoma.

Calcifications

These deposits are easily distinguishable because of their high differential density. After having eliminated the possibility of foreign bodies, artifacts or skin blemishes, their size, shape, number, topography and grouping should be analysed. Their significance varies according to whether or not they are associated with a palpable tumor and a radiologically visible opacity. It is usual practice to distinguish between macrocalcifications of more than 1 mm and microcalcifications of less than 1 mm.

- Macrocalcifications can be linear, gross or granulous, or circular, like an egg-shell. They are usually benign and their origin is often evident (Table 7.3).
- Microcalcifications are the best markers of subclinical cancers, half of which are observed only because of these microcalcifications (Table 7.4, Figures 7.6–7.8).

Recent improvements in techniques allow excellent visualization of microcalcifications, and lead to the risk of biopsies being carried out unnecessarily. The discovery of isolated microcalcifications should

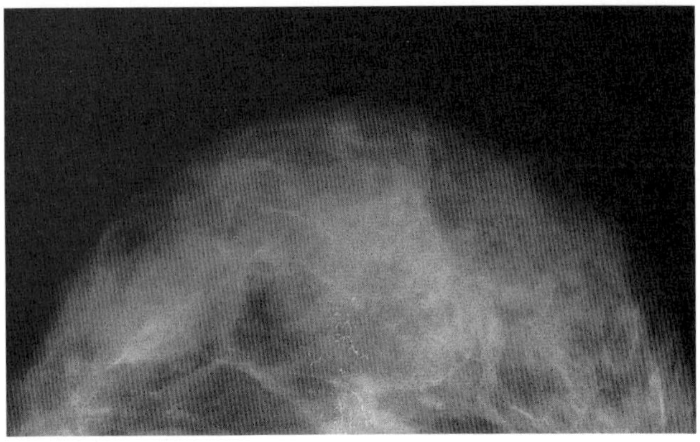

A

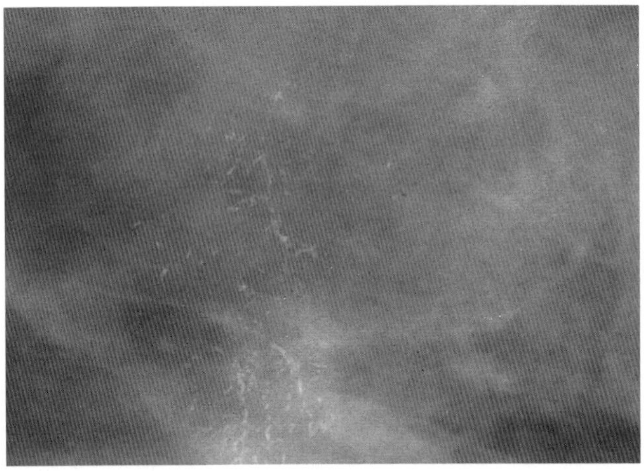

B

Figure 7.7

Mammography in an asymptomatic 42-year-old woman. Craniocaudal view (**A**) and magnification (**B**) show branched linear V-shaped microcalcifications. The histology was non-infiltrative intraductal carcinoma.

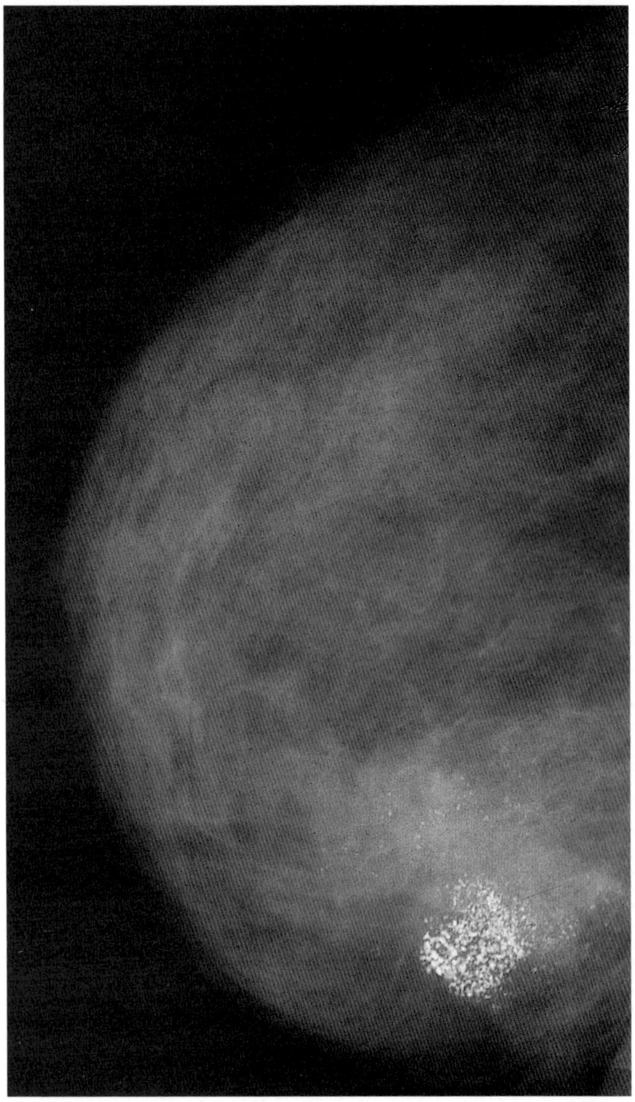

A

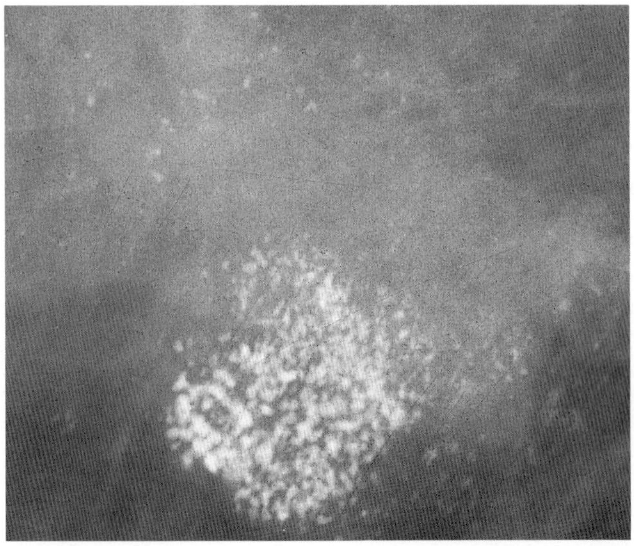

B

Figure 7.8

Mammography of a poorly delimited mass in the upper quadrant of the left breast. Lateral view (**A**) and magnification (**B**) show a poorly limited opacity with clustered microcalcifications. The histology was infiltrating ductal carcinoma.

Table 7.4 Mammary microcalcifications (<1 mm).

	Morphology	*Grouping and number*	*Topography*
Malignant	Branched calcifications	Several groups, >30 elements	Segmentary groups triangular at the summit nipple
↓	Gross polymorphous		
	Pulverulent		
	Regular punctiform	1 group, <20 elements	Round cluster
Benign	Annular, cup of tea	Multiple, dispersed	Diffuse, scattered bilateral

lead to a precise diagnostic work up to evaluate the probability of malignancy and to deduce the necessity of a biopsy. This includes the analysis of the number and grouping, topography and morphology of the microcalcifications[11,12] (Table 7.4).

The radiologist can now distinguish between calcifications which are probably benign or malignant. There nevertheless remains a certain number of patterns whose significance is more difficult to determine, for which biopsy or follow up are necessary.

Stereotaxic guided needle puncture

Stereotaxic devices allow us to perform fine-needle aspiration cytology of suspicious mammographically detected abnormalities. Even for experienced operators, the rate of unsatisfactory samples reaches 40%. Technical improvements now allow us to perform biopsies ('Tru-cut', biopty gun) for histologic samples.

Cystography

Cystography is radiography of a cystic cavity insufflated with contrast gas after evacuation of the liquid which it contained (see Figure 7.9). It comprises at least one anteroposterior (AP) and one lateral view to show the complete evacuation of the cyst.

This technique allows a precise analysis of the morphology of the cyst and its walls. It can show intracystic growths, which may be sessile or pedunculated, with or without local or diffuse thickening of the walls. Because of the radiotransparency obtained with this method, it facilitates a more accurate analysis of the adjoining gland and can show occult lesions not seen with mammography because of cystic opacity. Cystography should be avoided in an infectious or inflammatory context, as the risk of septic complications is far from negligible. It has become less useful because of the progress of ultrasonography.

Galactography

Galactography permits the observation of the galactophorous ducts after opacification with a water-soluble contrast medium. It is always used after initial mammography. It is indicated in case of serous or bloody secretion from a single duct (Figures 7.10 and 7.11), and should help determine the necessity for surgery and, before surgery, identify the pathological duct.

Galactography gives an opaque picture of a tubular cavity and patterns observed are those of ductal pathology:

- Dilatation extending throughout the whole galactophoric system or only localized, suggests secreting ductal ectasia.
- Stenosis, which may be complete or not, is often observed with inflammation or dystrophy, as well as with benign papillomas or malignant tumors.
- Lacunae, either a single one or several, are most often associated with benign papillomas but sometimes are observed with intraductal carcinomas.

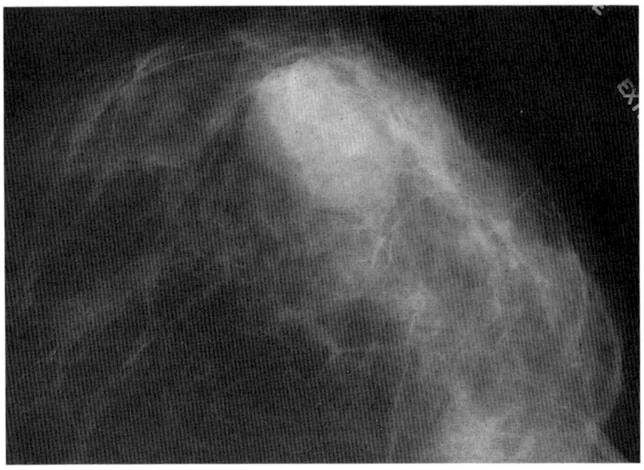

A

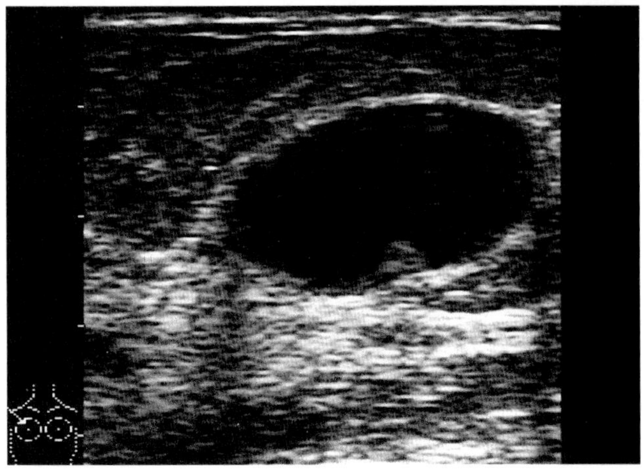

B

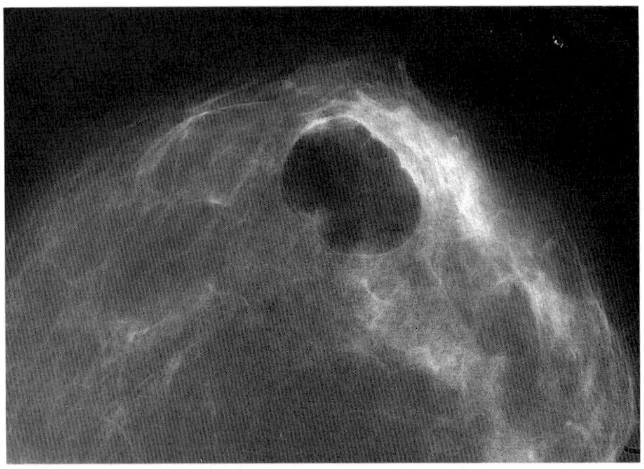

C

Figure 7.9

A round mobile mass in the upper quadrant of the right breast of a 48-year-old woman.

A Mammography shows a well-limited, lobulated opacity (40 mm).

B Ultrasonography (7.5 MHz) demonstrates a cystic oval, homogeneous, anechoic lesion with posterior reinforcement. There is an intracystic vegetation on the posterior wall.

C Pneumocystography after evacuation of 8 cm^3 of green fluid. The histology was benign papilloma.

- Additional patterns, either round and regular, may be seen, such as opacified microcysts, or extravasation of a duct which is already fragile because of inflammation, dystrophy or a tumor.
- Rigidity, compression or deviation may be present.

These elementary aspects are often associated with each other or with other mammographic abnormalities, such as microcalcifications or architectural alterations. The biopsy decision depends on the clinical finding, cytology and associated signs. Galactography is in fact only slightly specific and is mainly useful for locating lesions before surgery.

Ultrasonography

Real-time ultrasonography can often prove a useful supplementary examination to mammography and, in view of recent technological progress, is sometimes indispensable.

Technique

The patient is in a slightly oblique position so that the breast is lying flat. Linear high-resolution (7.5–10 MHz) probes have to be used. Scopic time

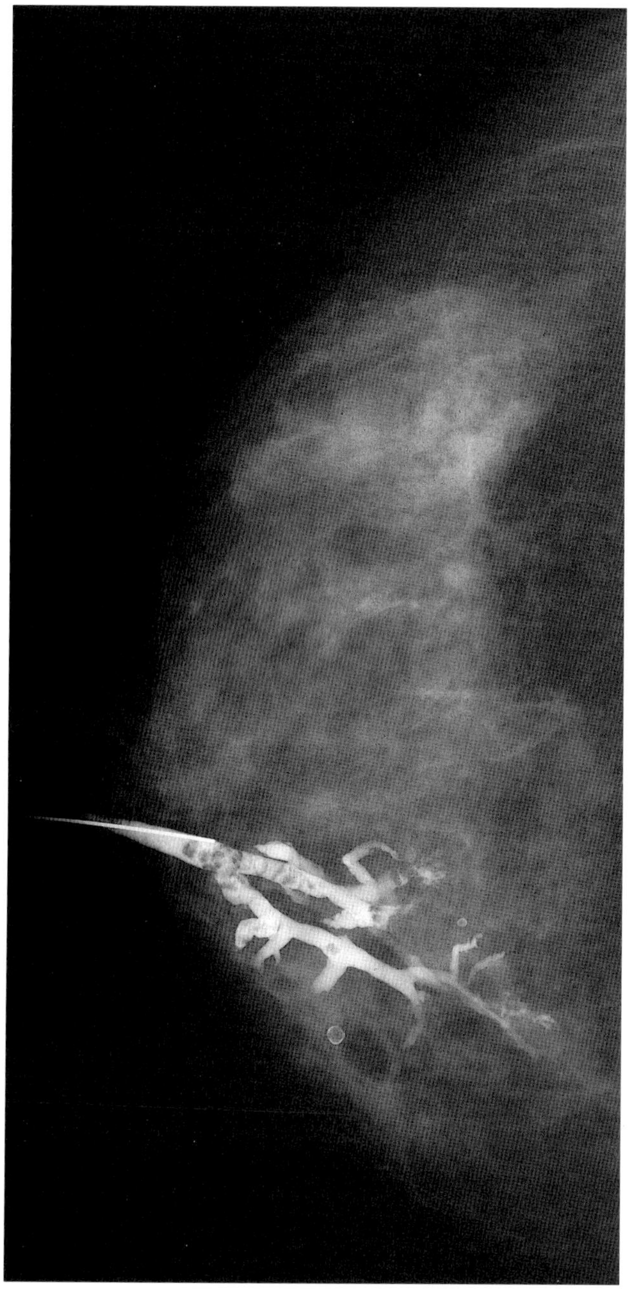

Figure 7.10

Bloody unicanalar nipple discharge of the right breast of a 53-year-old woman. Mammography was normal. Galactography (lateral view) shows multiple proximal and peripheral defects. The histology was multiple papilloma (benign).

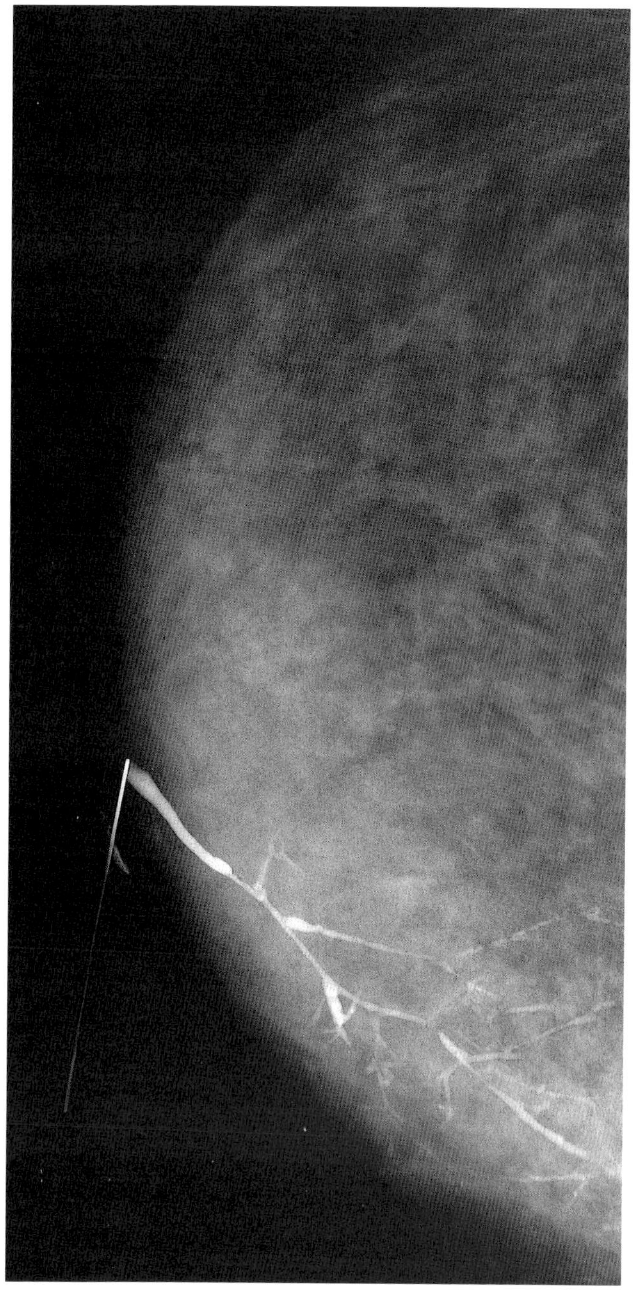

Figure 7.11

Serous unicanalar nipple discharge of the left breast of a 61-year-old woman. Mammography was normal. Galactography (lateral view) shows dilatation, irregularities and stenosis. The histology was intraductal carcinoma without invasion.

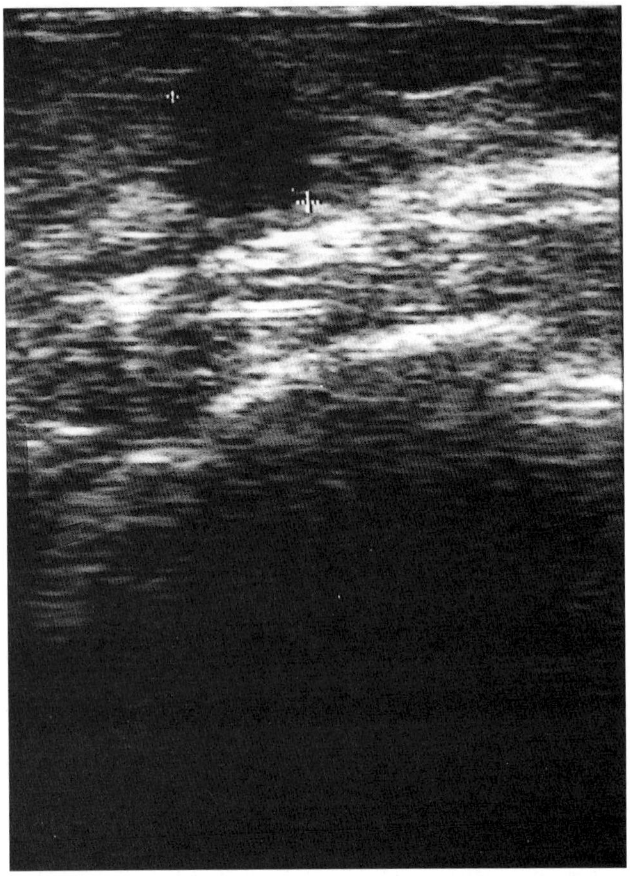

Figure 7.12

A barely palpable mass. Ultrasonography (7.5 MHz) shows a poorly limited, heterogeneous and hypoechoic mass (11 mm) without attenuation of the beam (cancer).

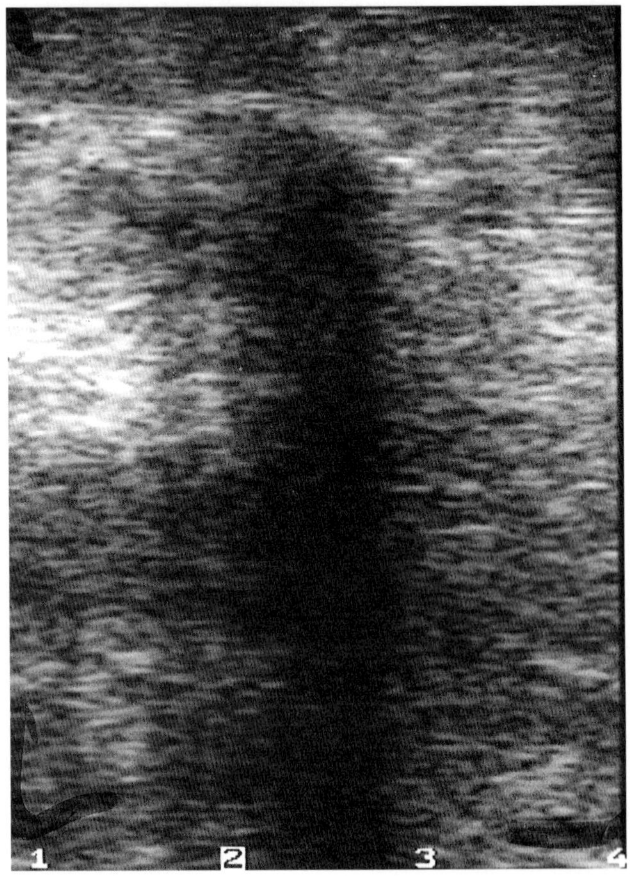

Figure 7.13

A 20 mm palpable mass in the outer quadrant of the left breast. Ultrasonography (7.5 MHz) shows a poorly limited, heterogeneous and hypoechoic mass with markedly reduced posterior transmission (cancer).

is an essential factor and should be reported exactly. Films should provide images of the lesion (or lesions), localize it and give an exact indication of its measurements. As opposed to mammography, images are difficult to reproduce during successive examinations. Control films should be carried out by the same operator, as far as possible, and with the same machine. One of the limitations of this method is the degree of operator dependence, since the value of the examination depends on the quality of the machine and the experience of the operator.

Findings

In 70–80% of cases, breast cancer is characterized by a heterogeneous hypoechoic image,[13] with an irregular shape and indistinct outlines (Figures 7.12 and 7.13). A peripheral hyperechoic halo may be observed, although the image is not always so typical: 13% of benign lesions have a heterogeneous infrastructure, 30% of cancers a homogeneous structure[13] and some have regular outlines, especially colloid and medullary forms. The ratio thickness:width is often equal to or more than 1, that is the lesion is rounded or else its largest axis is perpendicular to the skin; this is one of the most determining factors in favor of malignancy, especially for small cancers.

With ultrasonography, all the dimensions of a tumor can be measured accurately and reproduced and this can also be used as a basis for follow up during treatment. The size shown on ultrasonography is often smaller than that observed clinically or with mammography, and its use is therefore restricted in the diagnosis of extremely small cancers.

A posterior shadow, which was initially considered one of the best indications of malignancy, is only observed in 30% of cancers, since it depends on the absorption of the ultrasonic beams by the lesion and may be the only ultrasonic manifestation of small cancers.

Indirect signs have been observed, often difficult to distinguish, such as thickening of the cutaneous border, reduction of the anterior fatty layer, disruption or thickening of the Duret crests, small echoic spiculated chains, etc. The echoscopic impression of rigidity seems more valuable, since a malignant lesion is neither deformed nor displaced by the probe, unlike benign lesions.

Finally, in cases of intracystic cancer, ultrasonography gives a precise analysis of the fluid cavity, endocavitary growths and abnormalities of the wall.

Ultrasound as a supplementary examination to mammography

Ultrasonography, useless in fatty breasts, is an ideal supplement to mammography, as it compensates for the limitations and deficiencies of mammograms in dense breasts. Furthermore, the systematic study of dense breasts with echography is in question. It is used for:

- The study of the posterior part of the breast and relations with the chest wall.
- Determination of the type of tumor or infraclinical opacity, either solid or liquid, and the need for cystography.
- Examination of breasts containing prostheses, which are always difficult to examine with mammography.
- Study of inflammatory masses, where a collected abscess can be shown and aspirated.
- Examination of breasts after surgery and/or radiotherapy when problems arise in the interpretation of the mammograms.
- Guiding of cytological punctures and investigations before surgery.

Biopsy guided by ultrasonography

Ultrasonography allows three-dimensional localization and puncture with scopic observation of an infraclinical echovisible lesion.[14] For experienced operators, the rate of unsatisfactory samples varies between 10 and 20%.

Other techniques

Thermography

Infrared thermography was greeted with an initial wave of enthusiasm, but its lack of sensitivity in the identification of small cancers led to it being abandoned in routine diagnosis.[15] Short-wave thermography is probably more efficient but remains at the experimental stage.

The prognostic value of thermography, the existence of an intense thermic signal correlating with unfavorable prognosis, is not a determining factor, since it also correlates with other main prognostic factors such as the size of the tumor and lymph-node invasion.[16]

Transillumination

Direct viewing (diaphanoscopy) or recording of images (diaphanography) is less effective than mammography and contributes no supplementary data. Its sensitivity is insufficient for it to be used in diagnosis or screening.

Positron emission tomography

The positron-emitting machine opens up possibilities for research into tumoral metabolism, since there would appear to be a correlation between the rate of estrogen receptors and tumoral fixation.[17] This method is still at an experimental stage.

Computed tomography

Diagnostic mammary CT has been the object of several preliminary studies which do not appear to

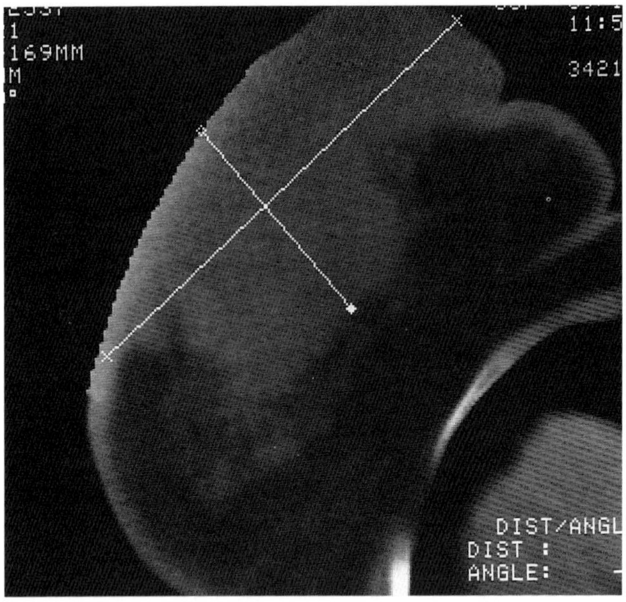

A

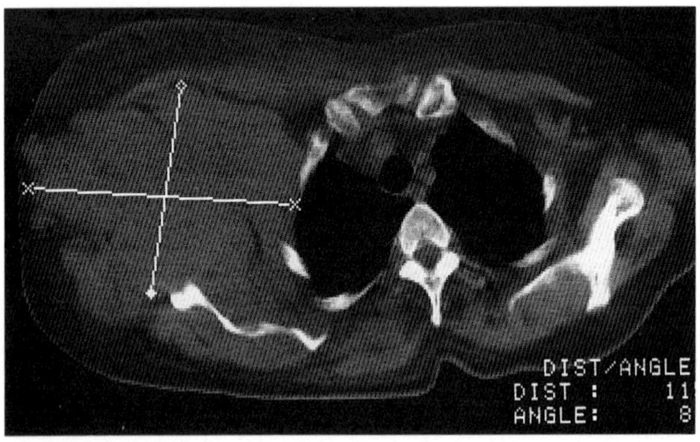

B

Figure 7.14

Huge ulcerated tumor of the right breast. Local evaluation can only be done on CT: the tumor can be measured (**A**) and the axillary extension visualized (**B**). The histology was lymphoma.

be decisive. The time taken over the examination, the lack of definition and irradiation mean that indications for the use of CT are rare and are more for pretherapeutic assessment than for diagnostic purposes: the study of the relation of a deep-seated mass with the chest wall, assessment of bulky lesions, especially with axillary extensions (Figure 7.14), investigation of internal mammary adenopathies, assistance with configuration and dosimetry for radiotherapy.

Magnetic resonance imaging

The results before introduction of the use of a contrast medium were very poor, as microcalcifications could not be seen, and specificity was very low. The use of a contrast medium allowed the differentiation of carcinomas and fibroadenomas with a considerable increase in signal intensity from scars. Since 1986, the use of fast sequences combined with a contrast medium in 'dynamic measurements' has improved specificity. A considerable increase in the signal within the first minute is suggestive of a cancer. This technique can probably be proposed whenever a biopsy is planned for a lesion which does not appear particularly suspect.[18,19]

Imaging strategy

Imaging techniques play an essential role throughout the various stages of the disease: diagnosis, screening, pretherapeutic assessment, and follow up during and after treatment.

Diagnosis in symptomatic patients

Presence of a palpable mass

Over 80% of breast cancers are revealed by the presence of a palpable mass. Physical examination is the essential element of diagnosis.

Mammography is the first additional examination used, and is systematically carried out in the presence of mammary tumefaction, except in very young women with a clinically benign mass, in which case ultrasonography can be used first. The diagnostic strategy based on physical examination and mammography, supplemented if necessary with ultrasonography and cytology, is summarized in Diagrams 7.1 and 7.2.

This diagnostic procedure is extremely efficient, if carried out under satisfactory conditions, and diagnoses approximately 97% of palpable cancers. It has, however, certain limitations.

First, in order that a cancer can be observed, it must have a differential density (i.e. there are calcifications), deform conjunctive tissue (i.e. there is distortion) or it must overlap it into the layer of fat (i.e. give opacity). Some 3% of cancers which are poorly localized and/or situated in dense heterogeneous conjunctive tissue (either in slim young women or in cases of mastopathy) are not shown radiologically, and may also show up poorly on ultrasonography. The essential rule resulting from this is that an assessment which does not show signs of malignancy does not necessarily prove a palpable mass to be benign. In the presence of a clinically suspicious lesion, signs which are normally considered to have little significance, such as density gradient, asymmetry or heterogeneous architecture, can be taken into consideration; this study necessitates a completely reliable technique, with perhaps additional tangential or oblique views and magnifications.

Second, imaging is not histology. A radiologic view that appears to indicate malignancy cannot be considered as a certainty, and there are exceptional differential diagnoses: a spiculated opacity can correspond to mammary tuberculosis, fibromatosis or an Abrikossoff's tumor. There therefore results a second essential rule: it is unthinkable to begin oncologic treatment such as radiotherapy or chemotherapy without histologic proof, even with positive cytology.

Paget's disease

Paget's disease of the nipple, with or without associated tumefaction, is a clinical diagnosis. Mammography should be used first, as it can show a single or several tumoral opacities and/or microcalcifications.

Images with a pyramidal topography, with the nipple as the summit, are typical, with a disorganized increased density and microcalcifications. But even if mammography is normal, this does not dispense with the need for a biopsy: if the diagnosis of Paget's disease is histologically confirmed, there is almost always an infiltrating or in-situ subjacent cancer which can be subclinical and subradiological. The main differential diagnosis is erosive adenomatosis of the nipple.

Discharge from the nipple

This is rarely an isolated sign of cancer (less than 1% of cases). However, 25% of intraductal cancers have some discharge.

Once galactorrheas and diffuse discharge resulting from mammary dysfunction, such as secreting ductal ectasia or sclerocystic disease, have been eliminated, discharge suggestive of ductal pathology coming from one orifice is often spontaneous and recurrent; its color can vary from whitish, greyish or clear, through yellow, pink and reddish-brown to black. In 90% of cases, it results from a benign lesion.

The appearance of the discharge and cytology are fundamental. The first additional examination to use is mammography. This may show one or several tumoral opacities, architectural disruption or microcalcifications; in this case, galactography is only used with a view to conservative treatment, in order to locate the duct in relation to radiological abnormalities.

Mammography often shows no focalized abnormality, which does not exclude the hypothesis of malignancy; galactography is thus carried out in second place. Pyramidectomy is indicated according to clinical and cytologic findings, especially in view of the fact that galactography is not particularly specific; an observation suggestive of ectasia without any other abnormality does not permit the elimination of intraductal carcinoma.

Inflammation of the breast

A clinically and radiologically obvious cancer can be accompanied by inflammation, but this can also be the only clinical sign of cancer whose differential diagnosis from that of inflammatory or infectious mastitis proves difficult. Physical examination and anamnesis differentiate between acute, subacute or chronic inflammation, or panmastitis, segmentary mastitis or focalized inflammatory reaction. Clinical signs are sometimes reminiscent of malignant lesions, such as tumors or adenopathies, but the pattern is often not especially specific.

Bilateral comparative mammography is the initial examination, as it shows signs of inflammation, such as edema or thickening of the skin, and sometimes a tumoral opacity or microcalcifications. The examination is difficult from a technical point of view (compression, choice of radiologic constants), because of edema and pain. However high quality is necessary, in order not to miss the slightest sign of malignancy.

Ultrasonography can determine whether a focalized abnormality exists: it can help differentiate between a malignant tumor and an abscess, it can show a lesion to be benign by showing ductal dilatation (inflammatory granuloma with ectasia), an infected cyst or galactocele. It also helps direct the cytologic puncture of a solid or cavitary mass (puncture in the center in order to evacuate a cavity or in the periphery for cytologic purposes).

Examinations based on the introduction of a contrast medium (cystography, galactography) are not indicated because of the risk of infectious complications.

The main differential diagnoses are bacterial mastitis, whether or not collected, and inflammatory granuloma: secreting ductal ectasia with complications (plasmocyte mastitis), cysto-steatonecrosis, idiopathic granulomatous mastitis, inflammatory cysts and galactoceles. Other diagnoses are exceptional and without radiologic specificity: tuberculosis, syphilis, sarcoidosis, hydatism, infarct, reaction to foreign bodies, etc.

In the presence of an inflammatory syndrome, the diagnosis of malignancy should be established rapidly, since these lesions necessitate rapid recourse to chemo- and/or hormone therapy; a short period of observation of a week, during which anti-inflammatory and antibiotic drugs are administered gives time to observe the regression of most cases of non-tumoral mastitis, corticotherapy sometimes proving necessary in case of constituted inflammatory granuloma or granulomatous mastitis. However, in the absence of rapid regression and whatever the cytologic outcome, a histologic examination should be carried out after a 'Tru-cut' or a drill biopsy.

Adenopathies or revealing metastases

An axillary or subclavicular lymph node or a metastasis (lymph node, cutaneous nodule, bone, pulmonary, hepatic or cerebral localization) may reveal breast cancer. The metastatic nature of the lesion then remains to be proved, especially if it is isolated. The essential element is histologic analysis after surgical sampling, or with a trocar, of the most accessible location, and this can eventually be accompanied by an assay of hormone receptors.

When adenocarcinoma of mammary origin is suspected, mammography should be used, even if the physical examination proves negative, since slight signs of malignancy may be present, such as microcalcifications of galactophoric origin, architectural disruption, density gradient. If conjunctive tissue is dense and difficult to analyse, ultrasonography can show any focalized abnormality and thus guide the cytologic puncture.

A negative assessment does not necessarily exclude the mammary origin of a lesion. If histologic examinations suggest this, the patient may benefit from specific treatment, such as chemo- and/or hormone therapy which increases chances of prolonged survival whilst maintaining satisfactory conditions of comfort.

In all cases, extensions should be assessed in search of other metastatic locations.

Special cases

Pregnancy

During pregnancy, the diagnosis of a mammary lesion is difficult, due to the density of the breasts, especially in case of a badly systematized evolutive tumor. Mammography is the initial examination to use in case of suspicious clinical signs, even during the first months of pregnancy. Abdominal protection with a leaded apron should be used and oblique or lateral view radiographs taken, using a high kilovoltage to limit the length of exposure. Coupling ultra-rapid film-screens can be useful. The number of films can be reduced but must be of optimal quality so as not to miss any architectural disruption or small microcalcifications. Ultrasonography may be a determining factor, in view of breast density, and should be carried out systematically if mammography is inconclusive. It helps guide the cytologic puncture and may be used initially if clinical signs appear to indicate a benign lesion in a young woman. It does not however dispense with mammography if it is not conclusive. Because of the difficulties of analysis, assessment which does not indicate any sign of malignancy cannot clear a clinically suspicious lesion and does not dispense with the need for histologic verification with a surgical or trocar biopsy.

Men

In men, the diagnostic work up is based on comparative bilateral mammography, which is almost always possible and is often easy to carry out, in search of the same signs of malignancy as in women; the excentric nature of the lesion in relation to the nipple is evocative since gynecomastia, which is the main differential diagnosis, is always well centered. Ultrasonography may prove useful if mammography is inconclusive, since it can show the same signs of malignancy as in women; it can also be used as a guide for cytologic examinations.

Diagnosis in asymptomatic patients

Mammography is the only supplementary examination indicated in an asymptomatic patient, follow up of dystrophy, for non-specific signs such as mastodynia or galactorrhea, for risk factors such as contralateral cancer or family antecedents, or else systematically in patients over 40 years of age at the request of the GP, the gynecologist or the patient herself. It can show subclinical abnormalities, and the radiologist should then evaluate according to various factors such as age, risk factors, etc., the probability of a malignant infiltrating or in-situ lesion, with the aid of ultrasonography and guided cytologic examinations (ultrasonography, stereotaxy). A diagnostic surgical biopsy can also be proposed.

The radiologist should try to obtain a satisfactory sensitivity/specificity ratio from the quality of the imaging technique, his experience with mammography, his knowledge of elementary lesions and their incidence, according to the age of the patient. He should not miss too many cases of cancer, nor should he request too many unjustified biopsies.

Indications for diagnostic biopsy

Calcifications

Thirty to fifty per cent of subclinical cancers are revealed by microcalcifications.[11,12,20] These are relatively easy to see in view of recent technological progress, but they remain difficult to define: 55–80% of biopsies are benign (fibrocystic disease, secreting ductal ectasia).[9,20]

Calcifications should be carefully analyzed, with geometric magnifications, in order to define those necessitating a biopsy and those which should simply be placed under supervision. Digitalization seems valuable in analyzing their morphology. Other methods, like ultrasound and guided cytology, seem generally to be of little interest.

Decision criteria are summarized in Tables 7.4 and 7.5. The topographic criterion seems to be especially decisive: calcifications, even if they are rounded, pulverulent or not especially numerous, but are situated along the galactophoric axes or in triangular formations, should be investigated by biopsy.

Round masses

Round masses represent 10–20% of subclinical cancers, but at least 50% of those biopsied are not malignant.[9,20] These include not only unnecessary biopsies but also undetected cancers, for, although they are easily distinguished in adipose breasts, they are difficult to identify in dense or nodular breasts. Some are obviously benign and do not necessitate any further investigation:

- opacity containing a single large macrocalcification (adenofibroma) or of the 'egg-shell' type (cyst),
- lenticular opacity with a clear center and external topography (intramammary lymph node),
- low-grade image containing dense fat (hamartoma),
- image identical to that of former mammographies several years previously.

Except for these cases, an ultrasound examination should be carried out, perhaps with puncture cytology guided by ultrasound or using a stereotactic technique, if ultrasound is not reliable. It is thus possible to prove the innocence of a small cyst evacuated with these techniques. A typical image of adenofibroma in a woman under 35 years of age warrants supervision only.

On the other hand, presumption of malignancy may lead to initial biopsy in case of:

- irregular or badly defined outlines,
- associated microcalcifications,
- suspicious findings on ultrasonography,
- recent appearance or increase in size,
- suspicious guided puncture cytology.

Table 7.5 Differential characteristics of lobular and ductal mammary microcalcifications.

Lobular	*Ductal*
Usually benign	Usually malignant
Sclerosing adenosis	Intraductal carcinoma
Sclerocystic disease	Infiltrating ductal carcinoma
Sometimes around lobular carcinoma in situ	

Images may prove difficult to define, for example in a patient with no former mammographies a round regular image of the adenofibroma type which is not visible with ultrasonography or is solid. It is impossible to eliminate completely nodular cancer, which is the cause of 8% of asymptomatic cases, especially the medullary form which can give the same ultrasound result as an adenofibroma or a cyst. But the presumption of benignity (adenofibroma, harmatoma, papilloma, long-known cyst with thick contents) is likely, especially in the case of young patients. It is therefore justifiable to propose follow up, in order to avoid too many biopsies of benign lesions: one or two films every 6 months for 2 years, then once a year for a few more years, perhaps with additional ultrasound examinations. The decision to choose management should be confirmed by puncture cytology guided by ultrasonography or stereotaxy: if the needle is proved to be intralesional, this reinforces the presumption of benignity, even though it is true that cytology is only conclusive when positive. The diagnostic technique is summarized in Diagram 7.3.

Spiculated masses

Spiculated masses represent 20–30% of subclinical cancers, more than 90% of those biopsied being actual cancers. Rare differential diagnoses include sclerosing adenosis, radial scars, scars and some infrequent pathologies. Indications are thus quite unequivocal: all spiculated masses require surgery. Ultrasonography can be useful for presurgical localization, if the mass is visible, but it should not influence the surgical decision.

Focalized distortions

Focalized distortions in structure give an image of stellar convergence without a dense center, and represent 20% of subclinical cancers. They are difficult to distinguish in dense conjunctive tissue and perfect technique is necessary to study them. It is essential to confirm the accuracy of the image, which should be seen on several films and should perhaps be confirmed by oblique views. It is unthinkable to expect the patient to undergo the anguish caused by a biopsy or even follow up because of a constructed image. Cancer is the most common etiology, being present in 50–60% of cases. Others are scars, radial scars and sclerosing adenosis. Criteria of benignity have been described in detail elsewhere[8,20,21] and are:

- different dimensions from one film to another,
- variations in the length and the width of the spicules as opposed to well-centered radiations for cancers,
- curvature of spicules which bend away from contact with the skin instead of attaching themselves to it.

These images leave little doubt as to the course to be taken: after having eliminated scars from partial excision or an abscess, they should always lead to biopsy.

Extensive structural distortions

Extensive structural distortions can be pyramid-shaped, localized to one quadrant, multicentric or diffuse. Perfect technique is necessary for a satisfactory study, perhaps including oblique views with compression, enlargements and systematic comparisons, film by film, with the contralateral breast. After the possibility of a scar (partial excision, plastic surgery or an abscess) has been eliminated, and in the absence of any clinical signs, the decision remains difficult to take: 30% of these images are malignant,[9,20] half being of the infiltrating type; these are often poorly localized multicentric cancers which can rapidly become obvious and bulky.[22] Lobular in-situ carcinoma or atypical epithelial hyperplasia is found in 30% of benign specimens. It is therefore as difficult to propose a follow-up plan as widespread excision. Other techniques are of little practical value but ultrasonography should be tried. Puncture cytology guided by stereotaxy should be considered, but the poorly localized nature of the lesions means that it is of little use if negative. Its use should be considered case by case according to radiologic findings, the presence of other abnormalities such as microcalcifications and age, risk factors, etc. If surgery is not undertaken, follow up should be thorough, with physical examination monthly for 6 months and then every 3 months, and mammograms every 4 months for the first year, every 6 months the following year, then once a year for the next few years.[23]

Presurgical investigations

When a biopsy has been decided upon, surgery is preceded by accurate radiologic localization of the lesion to be excised (Figure 7.15). Many different

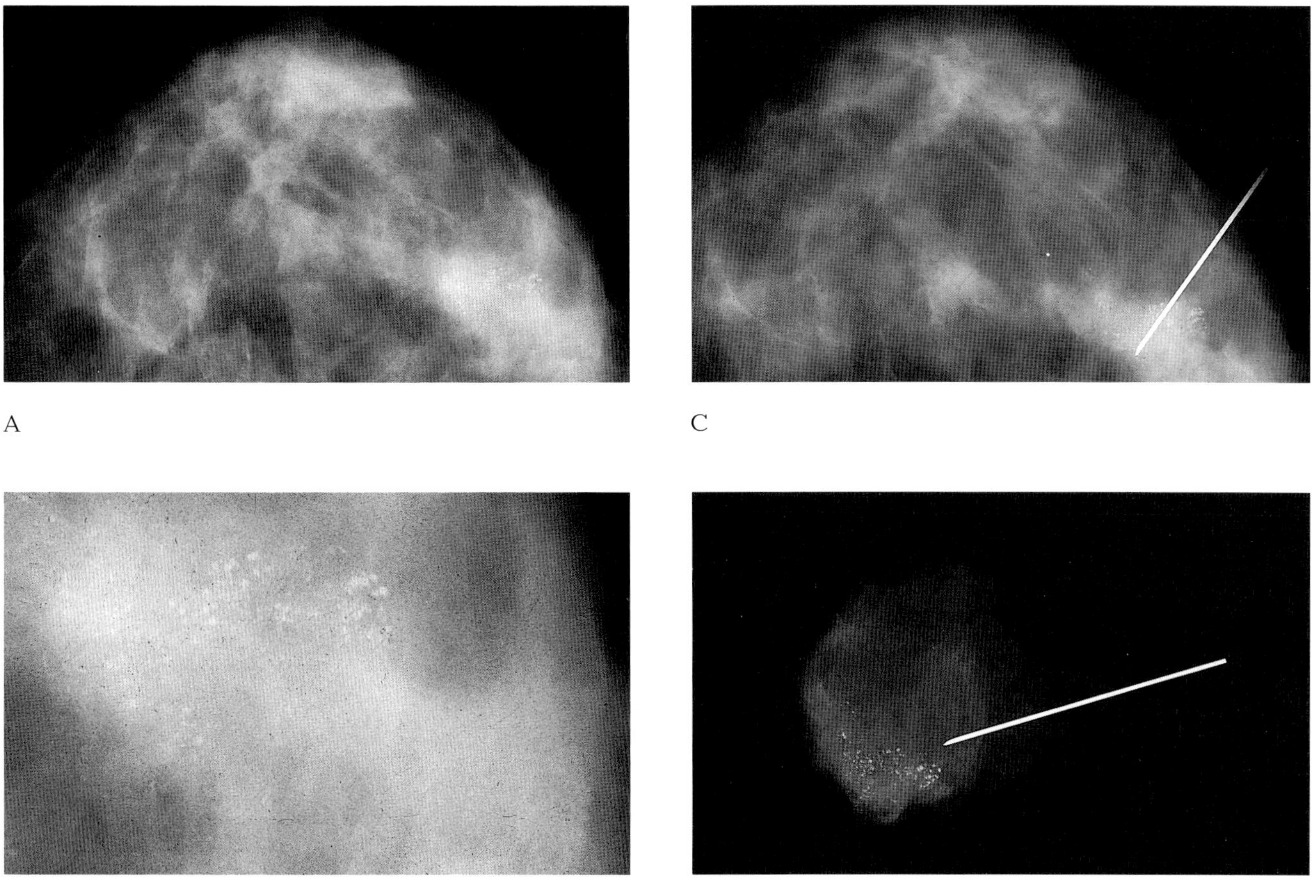

A C

B D

Figure 7.15

Pre-operative radiologic localization.

A,B Mammography in craniocaudal view (**A**) and magnification (**B**) shows clustered microcalcifications.

C Localization with a needle before surgery.

D Microcalcifications on the specimen radiograph.

methods have been suggested, some of which are fairly complicated.[24] The best method to use is that with which the radiologic and surgical teams are most familiar, as interdisciplinary collaboration is the most essential element.

From a practical point of view, if the lesion is visible on ultrasonography, this is the easiest method to use. Otherwise, it can be observed with two-view mammograms, with or without a grid. Stereotaxy is an accurate method but also the longest, the most complicated and the most expensive way of introducing the necessary equipment into the lesion (Figure 7.16).

When localization immediately precedes surgery and there is no need to transport the patient, a simple needle can be left in place. Otherwise a hook can be placed 24 or 48 hours before the operation; the site for introducing the hook should be chosen with the surgeon. It should be fixed correctly to avoid displacement; models with an X-shaped end tend to move less than those with curved ends. Colorings can also be used, such as methylene blue dye or other powders.

In all cases, radiography of the surgical sample should be carried out, if possible using special apparatus (Faxitron) in the surgical unit, in order

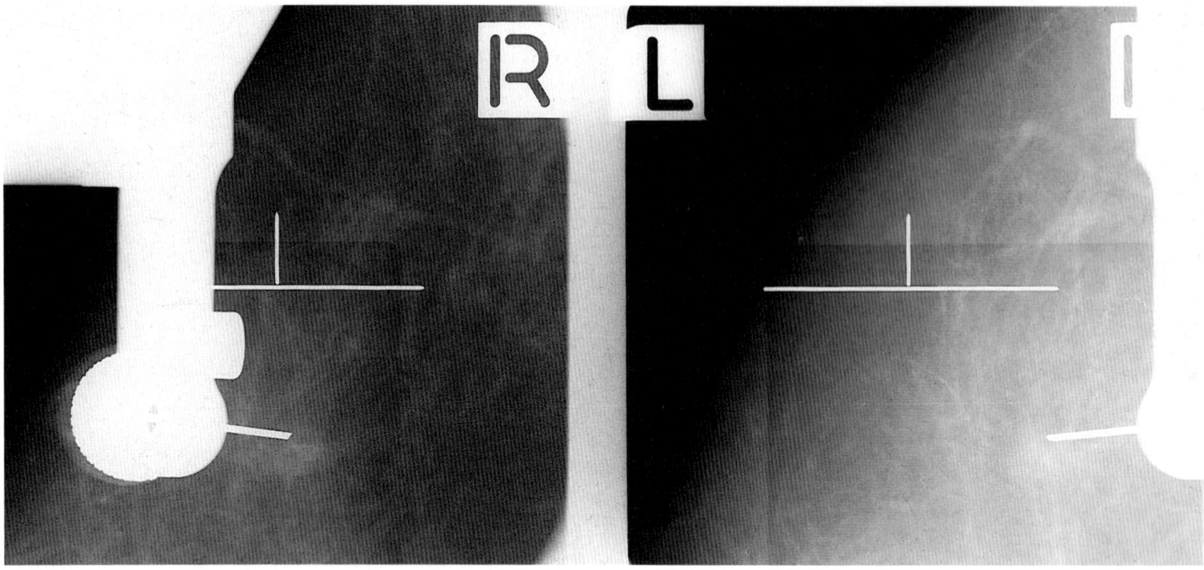

Figure 7.16

Needle biopsy, using a stereotaxic procedure, of a small, impalpable, spiculated opacity. Cytology indicated adenocarcinoma.

to confirm complete excision and to guide the sectioning of the sample for analysis. This necessitates close collaboration of the radiologist, the surgeon and the pathologist.

Results: historadiologic comparison

Several series of diagnostic excisions have been published, of both microcalcifications and infraclinical masses.[8-12,20] From the point of view of specificity, the best give 1.5 benign biopsies (BB) for 1 malignant biopsy (MB), i.e. MB:BB = 1:1.5. For other series, this ratio is 1:5 or even 1:8. The 'return' of biopsies is thus 20–45% of infiltrating or in-situ carcinomas and 55–80% of benign lesions, 30% of which contain atypical hyperplasia or in situ lobular carcinoma.

In our own series of 309 cases, 149 are clustered microcalcifications, 63 infraclinical masses, 97 structural abnormalities. Histologic analysis showed 112 benign lesions (36.2%), 60 'high-risk' mastopathies (atypical epithelial hyperplasia, in-situ lobular carcinoma; 19.5%), and 137 malignant lesions (44.3%), 83 of which were infiltrating carcinoma. The MB:BB ratio is 1:1.2.

In view of the present increase in the systematic examination of asymptomatic women, an MB:BB ratio of 1:1 should be obtained with an improved use of ultrasonography and guided punctures, whilst maintaining sensitivity by stringent follow-up procedures.

The consequences of an unnecessary biopsy are far from negligible, since this necessitates a stay in hospital, pre-surgical localization, a general anesthetic, the occupation of an operating theater for an hour, and the presence of a surgeon, an anesthetist, a radiologist and a pathologist. In the long term, it can have physical consequences such as a deformed breast or a scar and psychological consequences such as anxiety and alteration of the patient's self-image. Finally, the discovery of a 'high-risk' mastopathy does not always lead to a clear-cut line of treatment and does not prevent the patient undergoing anxiety and follow up.

Subclinical cancers are not always small cancers: 10–15% show histologic invasion of the axillary lymph nodes (8 cases in our series). These are poorly localized lesions, which are already widespread and multicentric, and which have a poor prognosis: the diagnosis only slightly precedes clinical recognition in the form of a tumor with a rapid growth.[22] On the other hand, not all subclinical cancers become diseases: some in-situ lesions never become infiltrating, and certain microcarcinomas with a slow evolution would never have become active during the patient's lifetime.

In view of these reservations, the consequences of the mammographic detection of subclinical lesions is generally favorable, as it permits the detection of a maximum number of cancers at a very early stage, which therefore have excellent prognosis. This is the basis for advocating mass screening with mammography.

Mass screening

Breast cancer is an excellent model for mass screening. It corresponds point by point to the criteria defined by the WHO: it is of high frequency, morbidity and mortality; it constitutes a severe risk to public health; treatment is available for patients diagnosed as having the disease; the only test available, which is mammography, is sensitive, specific and acceptable to the general population; the effect of screening on mortality due to the disease has been proved.[4,15,25] A reduction in mortality of approximately 30–40% can be obtained in women aged 50–69 years, provided there is a participation rate of 60%.

The risk of metastases is in close correlation with the size of the tumor and the extent of invasion of the axial lymph nodes,[6] further justification for screening in anticipation of these. The morbidity of breast cancer depends on metastatic recurrences, which can occur late on: the risk of a relapse is constant throughout the first 10 years and persists for 20 years. There is also a correlation between the size of the tumor and the appearance of metastases, with a threshold under which there is little chance of metastases:[26] in patients suffering relapses, 50% of metastases arise in the 2 years preceding diagnosis, which justifies any action taken to anticipate clinical recognition by 1 or 2 years. The reduction in tumoral volume also helps reduce treatment.[25] On the other hand, only minimal residual disease can benefit from general adjuvant treatment in terms of mortality; here again, anticipatory diagnosis can increase effectiveness.

Screening procedures necessitate high quality and permanent quality control. The method of interpretation of mammograms for screening differs from the habits acquired in senological diagnosis. The report is codified and expresses a simple selection which inevitably includes undetected cancers and unnecessary second examinations. The radiologist has to examine rapidly a great number of images, of which 90% are negative and 10% merit further investigation. Training in the reading of examinations for screening and verification with second readings are essential. This permanent evaluation is a necessary safety measure in the difficult task faced by the radiologist, and also helps homogenize and optimize his competence. Quantification of the images should aid realization, since it facilitates teletransmission and gives those interpreting the readings the support of perfected interpretation systems.

The radiation risk of mammography[27] is negligible in view of the advantages of the technique, but with mass screening, all possible efforts must be made to reduce the dose without impairing effectiveness.

Defining the target population

The target population should be accurately defined, since only women of 50–69 years of age seem to benefit from screening. It has not been proved effective for those aged 40–49 years,[4,15,22] and further tests using more energetic plans have still to be analysed. In the meantime, women in this age-group can benefit from examinations on request, or on the advice of their physician (annual physical examination and complete mammography every 2 years).

Women aged 70 years and over do not participate enough to be included in mass screening[4] and it seems probable that the anticipation of diagnosis in this age-group has little influence on mortality. Populations particularly at risk—women with a personal history of breast cancer, suspect mastopathies or a family history of breast cancer—should be followed by the traditional method, which is more sophisticated, and not be included in the screening program.

Generalized invitation of the target population avoids the self-selection involved in any voluntary consultation.[28]

The utmost must be done to obtain a high level of participation, using advertisements, regular information and the use of the media. An essential element in participation is the support of general practitioners.

Effective programming

A period of 2 years between tests seems to give the best cost-effectiveness. From the third year onwards, the rate of cancers which have occurred in the meantime seems to compromise the effectiveness of the program.[29]

A reduction in the number of views reduces the dose and the cost without impairing effectiveness,[4] at least in women whose breasts are fatty. With a single view, sensitivity falls from 95 to 93%.[30] In reducing the number of views from two to one, the rate of second examinations is multiplied by four initially for dense breast but does not change for clear breasts; for subsequent examinations, the existence of reference documents reduces the difference, which suggests two views for the first examination and one thereafter.[31] If a single view is used, an external oblique view gives the best analysis of the whole breast.[32] If two views are used, these should be AP and external oblique views, which are more effective than AP and side views. The effectiveness of a single view in women over 50 years of age has already been proved.[4]

The structure of the program

Participation and cost-effectiveness are influenced by the structure of the program:

- The creation of screening centers[25] represents a high investment initially but facilitates the supervision of quality and cost and the satisfactory follow up of results. These are valid in urban centers.
- Mobile units,[4,30] are less expensive but retain the possibility of supervising quality. They are useful in rural surroundings and can visit work places. However they may be considered as rival structures by local physicians whose cooperation is essential to the program.
- The participation of existing public and private establishments meets with the approval both of patients and physicians, is easily accessible and able to deal with numerous cases. The supervision of quality and cost, as well as the follow up of results, is more difficult but remains essential. Programs at present underway have had to choose one of these methods of evaluation. In the case of a national program, the use of all three types of structure could give the best participation rate.

Pre-treatment assessment

Locoregional assessments

Mammography

Apart from its diagnostic value, mammography plays an important part in locoregional assessment, as it allows an objective and reproducible estimation of the size of the tumor and provides a reference document for following up regression during treatment, if surgery is not used initially. It completes the physical examination in the appreciation of poor prognostic factors such as edema, thickening of the skin and peritumoral edema. However, there does not seem to be any correlation between the mammographic appearance of the tumor, the length of spiculae, and the presence or absence of calcifications and prognosis. Only the nodular type, excluding medullar and colloid forms, can be considered unfavorable.[33]

Mammography may show signs of multifocality (Figure 7.17), such as small close or distant spicular or nodular masses, microcalcifications or structural disorganization. These are especially suggestive when their topography is galactophoric and they arise between the tumor and the nipple. It is important to identify them, since they can make conservative treatment inadvisable. Mammography also permits a study of the contralateral breast in order to diagnose subclinical but eventual synchronous bilateral cancer, and is useful as a basis for subsequent follow up.

Ultrasonography

Ultrasonography can prove a useful supplementary examination in locoregional assessment (Figure 7.18), when mammography is inaccurate, especially for dense breasts. It gives an accurate and reproducible assessment of the three-dimensional size of the tumor.[13] Poorly localized tumors are generally as difficult to measure by ultrasonography as by mammography.

The technique may also show cavitary or necrotic elements within the tumor, confirm or reveal signs of multifocality, show axillary of subclavicular lymph node extensions (Figure 7.19) and guide an eventual cytology puncture.

Assessment of metastatic extensions

Pulmonary radiographs rarely reveal metastases during initial assessment and they are always

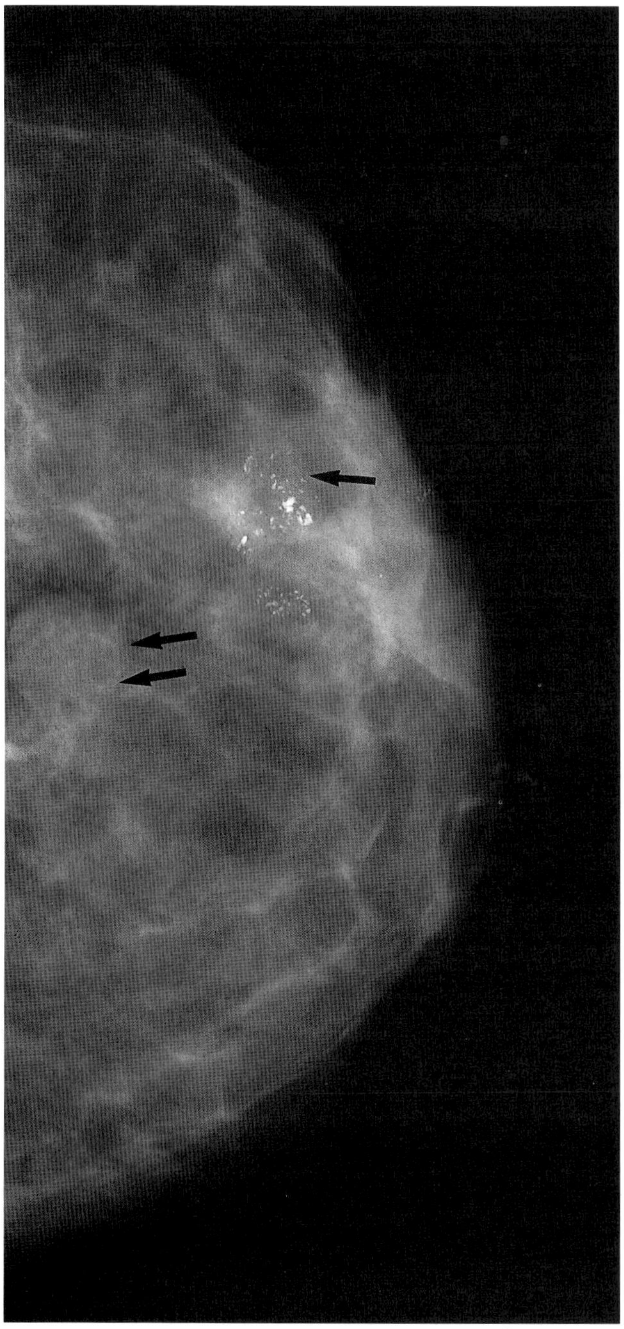

Figure 7.17

Palpable mass. Mammography (lateral view) shows a round poorly limited mass (double arrows) and a cluster of microcalcifications (single arrow). This contraindicates conservative treatment.

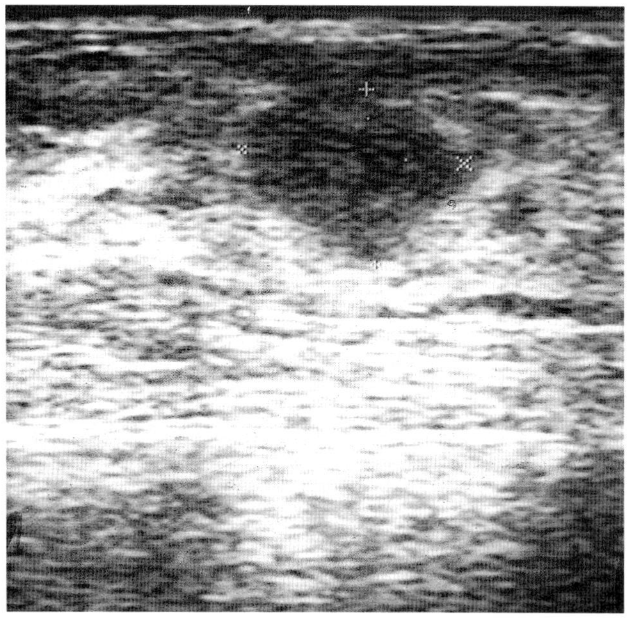

A

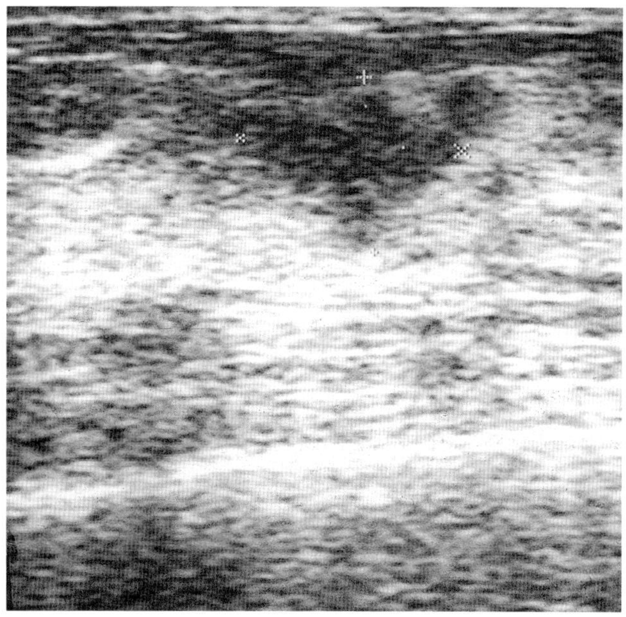

A

Figure 7.18

A,B Ultrasonography in pre-operative evaluation. Lesions were poorly depicted on mammography due to dense parenchyma. Ultrasonography allowed clear delineation of multiple hypoechoic lesions in the breast.

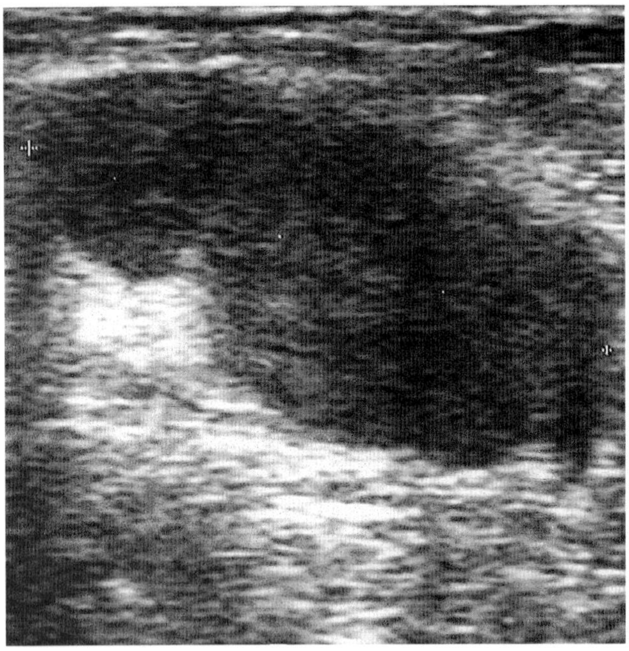

Figure 7.19

Ultrasonography in pre-operative evaluation. Two axillary nodes are clearly visible. The upper one (35 × 20 mm) was hardly palpable.

16% for bulky tumors.[34] Moreover, there exists a significant correlation between the predictive positive value and the stage of the disease, which rises from 22% in stage I to 66.5% in stage III tumors.[35] In order to reduce the cost and morbidity resulting from unnecessary investigation or treatment, scintigraphy should only be used in the assessment of tumors of more than 3 cm or in the presence of symptoms.[34,36]

Systematic brain CT has been evaluated in patients with poor prognosis, in order to treat subclinical brain metastases effectively. It has been shown to have no influence on treatment procedures and survival, and is therefore only indicated in the presence of neurologic signs. It is more and more often replaced by MR with gadolinium injection.

In general, operable tumors of less than 3 cm benefit from locoregional assessment and pulmonary radiographs. If these examinations are normal, and there are no clinical or biological signs, no other examinations are carried out.

Non-operable tumors of more than 3 cm necessitate more detailed assessment, with bone scintigraphy and hepatic ultrasonography. If this proves normal and there are no clinical or biological signs, no other examinations are carried out. This is summarized in Diagram 7.4.

If there are clinical or biological signs of metastases, or if one of the systematic examinations is not normal, the investigations should be continued to confirm metastatic disease and assess all sites.

normal in the case of small tumors;[34] they are, however, carried out systematically, more in general assessment than in search of a specific pathology associated with extensions.

Hepatic ultrasonography rarely reveals clinically and biologically undetected metastases in the initial assessment. It always proves negative in the assessment of small tumors.[34] It is only systematic in patients with a high metastatic risk in the absence of symptoms, i.e. in case of tumors of more than 3 cm or which are inoperable. It constitutes a reference to facilitate follow up, especially in case of benign hepatic lesions such as biliary cysts or angiomas.

A bone scan is the initial examination used in search of bone metastases, the bone being the most common secondary location. It can therefore be included systematically in pre-treatment assessment, but the positivity rate varies according to tumoral size: 4% for tumors of less than 3 cm and

Follow up during treatment

Locoregional follow up

During induction treatment—radiotherapy, chemotherapy or hormone therapy—mammography is an essential addition to the physical examination in order to estimate the degree of tumoral regression and define locoregional treatment.

During initial radiotherapy, mammography is carried out at 45 Gy because, at this dose, radiation sequellae (edema, thickening of the skin) are only slight and do not prevent analysis. Regression can be rather slow and a tumoral 'skeleton' can remain which will continue to regress for 6 or even 12 months.

In initial chemotherapy, the first mammograms are carried out halfway through the course of treatment and the second towards the end. In hormone therapy, they are carried out every 3 or 4 months up to the end of treatment. Sequellae are non-existent and analysis is not therefore affected. Regression can be rapid if the lesion is sensitive; paradoxically, microcalcifications may become more visible because of tumoral regression; they may also become more numerous.

There is a correlation between clinical and radiologic regression; when patients undergo surgery after initial treatment, there is also a good radiologic and histologic correlation in the estimation of tumoral remains.[37] The rare discrepancies are observed when the tumor is poorly localized or slightly radio-opaque, or when there exists a necrotic or colloid component which is not modified by treatment.

If there is difficulty in analysis, ultrasonography is useful to measure objectively the tumor diameter and to identify any necrosis or an eventual cystic component.

Follow up of metastases

If metastases are observed, follow up during treatment is carried out with the most appropriate technique, whilst avoiding unnecessary duplication.

Bone metastases are followed up with scintigraphy every 3–6 months, according to the rate of evolution; with effective treatment, they can show total or partial extinction of areas of hyperfixation. Reactivation or the observation of new sites indicates that treatment is not effective. Between two scintigraphic examinations, films centered on the principal areas confirm consolidation and recalcification, which sometimes shows up former existing lytic lesions which were not previously radiovisible. It can be difficult to differentiate between reconsolidation and aggravation and this necessitates close collaboration between those carrying out physical and isotopic examinations.

Pleuropulmonary and mediastinal metastases are easy to follow up with chest radiographs every 2–4 months, which facilitates objective measurement of well-defined reference elements.

Hepatic metastases should preferably be followed up with ultrasonography, which is the simplest, least restrictive and least expensive method. In the absence of well-defined localizations, which are anatomically observable and reproducible, MR or CT should be used.

Cerebral metastases are followed up with MR or CT, with a direct injection of contrast medium, thus centering on areas already identified.

Follow up of complications

Imaging can prove useful in case of locoregional complications: ultrasonography to verify regression or for the evacuation of hematomas or lymphocysts, mammography for following regression during treatment of post-surgical suppuration.

Follow up after treatment

Follow up after conservative treatment

Mammography is an essential addition to the physical examination, the first being carried out 3 months after radiotherapy as a reference document. The period between two examinations depends on local prognostic criteria, the average being 6 months during the first 2 years, and annually thereafter, unless there are ambiguous images of the post-treatment skeleton.

Mammography shows post-treatment sequellae. Any disorganization resulting from scars, such as thickening of the skin or structural distortion, can cause stellar patterns which are often confluent and may appear ambiguous on certain films. The regression or non-evolution of images tends towards benignity. Ultrasonography can be useful for confirming the absence of a mass syndrome, but fibrous scars can appear doubtful (hypoechoic area with intense posterior absorption). Such sequellae vary from one individual to another and also according to the technique used: they are more intense in case of plastic remodelling of the breast or with complications such as hematoma or sepsis.

Post-radiation sequellae include thickening of the skin and edema, which may vary in intensity and diffusion, mainly in the inferior quadrants, the central area or in areas of superimpression. These regress progressively, leaving fibrosis with thickening throughout the breast which may be more or less marked and a reticulated appearance to subcutaneous tissues. Inflammation may occur long after radiotherapy, and the diagnosis of acute evolutive recurrence or radiodystrophy is difficult, necessitating a Tru-cut or a drill biopsy.

These sequellae are all the more noticeable with high-dose radiotherapy. The reduction of doses in the treatment of small tumors facilitates mammographic follow up, since sequellae are almost non-existent. However, if the dose received is more than 50 Gy (irradiation after initial treatment for bulky tumors, exclusive radiotherapy), mammographic analysis is more difficult.

If there has been no recourse to surgery, mammography aids the follow up of any eventual tumoral skeletons, which may arise in the form of an area of increased density that is more or less stellar and/or microcalcifications. The degree of regression or stability thus shown favors remission. Ultrasonography can be an aid in following and measuring the remains.

Mammography, supplemented by ultrasonography, or punctures guided by ultrasonography or stereotaxy in inconclusive cases, can detect local evolutive relapse,[38–44] which can be rectified by mastectomy (Figure 7.20). Early recurrences occur on the initial tumoral site in 80% of cases, whereas 40% of later recurrences occur outside the treated area and appear to be secondary localizations in the same breast. Relapses are observed because of:

- the appearance of microcalcifications or an increase in residual calcifications,
- the appearance of a tumoral mass or an increase in the residual skeleton, or
- the appearance of or increase in an area of increased density and/or disorganization, edema or thickening of the skin, these phenomena being more difficult to diagnose, since they could be caused by radiodystrophy.

MR seems efficient in characterizing recurrences versus scars (Figure 7.21).

If senological assessment is inconclusive, it is essential to carry out a biopsy, even if guided cytology punctures are negative, in case remedial mastectomy is necessary.

There exist certain predictive criteria of local recurrences[39,41,43] that lead to the intensification of follow up: age under 40 years, tumoral size and axillary lymph-node invasion, a lobular type or the existence of considerable intraductal extension, the histologic state of the edges of the sample, slow initial regression with induction treatment. The radiologist should be in possession of this information, as well as of any reference documents, including those previous to treatment; this necessitates complete interdepartmental collaboration.

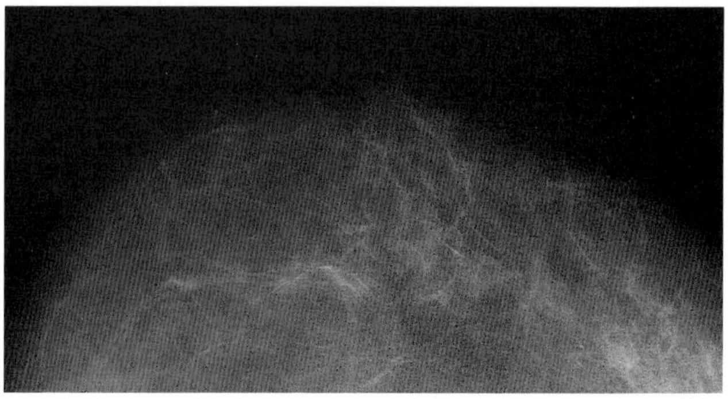

A

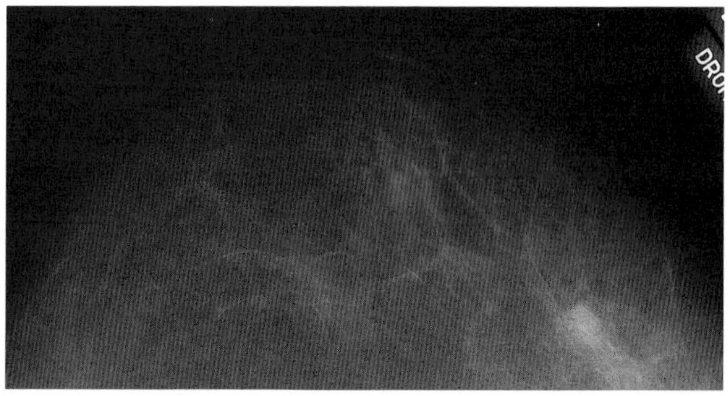

B

Figure 7.20

Post-operative follow up.

A Mammography 6 months after radiotherapy of tumor (craniocaudal view) was normal.

B One year later, a small poorly limited opacity was seen on mammography; clinical examination was normal. The histology was recurrence of previous invasive carcinoma.

Follow up of the contralateral breast

The frequency of synchronous (0.3–1.0%) or asynchronous (accumulated incidence of 1% per year)[45] bilateral localizations justifies mammographic follow up of the contralateral breast in order to detect subclinical lesions which can then benefit from conservative treatment. These high-risk breasts do not benefit from reduced procedure

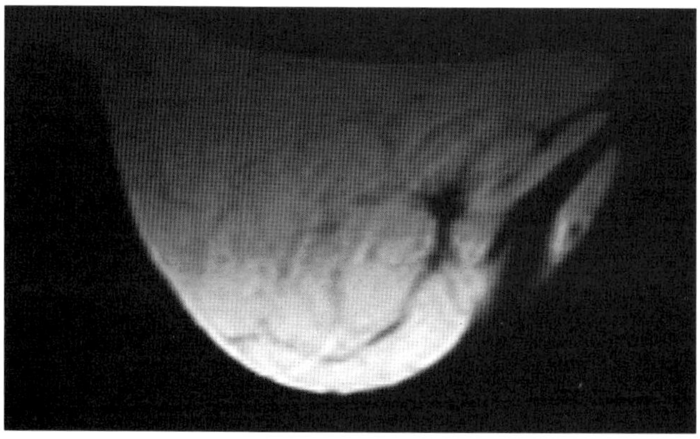

A

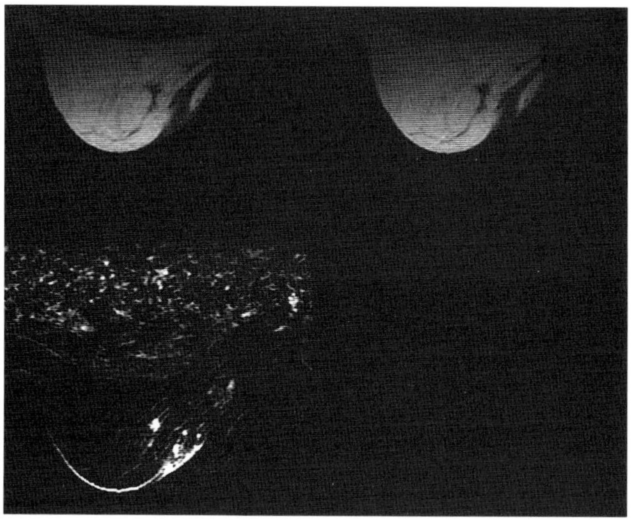

B

Figure 7.21

Suspicion of recurrence of a breast tumor after surgery and radiation therapy: MR with a surface coil.

A T1-weighted imaging shows a spicular mass, and scar.

B After bolus of contrast medium, uptake by the mass was fast (top row: images before and after injection; bottom row: subtraction). The lesion was a recurrence at histology.

of the mass screening type. The procedure used varies according to the difficulties encountered in analysis; the average period between two mammographies is 18 months, and complete mammographic examinations should be carried out.

Follow up of metastatic recurrences

Clinical examination remains of the utmost importance, as does taking into consideration any symptoms. Appropriate additional examinations are necessary at the first sign of modification. Biological examinations, such as phosphatases, alkalines or glutamyl transpeptidase or markers (Carcinogen Antibody (Ca) 15–3) can direct assessment. Diagnostic work up is as described for initial metastatic patients.

Any recent occurrence, metastatic or local recurrence, contralateral localization or other cancer should prompt an intensification of the assessment of extensions in the search for subclinical sites, before any important therapeutic decision: chest radiography, bone scintigraphy and hepatic ultrasonography, in addition to clinical and biological assessment, are used. The same is true when breast reconstruction is decided upon, although subclinical metastases are not necessarily an obstacle to reconstruction if the patient is well-informed and remains motivated.

For asymptomatic patients in clinical remission, their comfort and rehabilitation necessitate reduced follow up procedures, especially as, with present treatments, metastatic mammary carcinoma cannot be cured, even if dissemination is diagnosed early on. The usefulness of early detection of metastatic disease using the markers has still to be proved.

Pulmonary radiographs, which are neither costly nor restrictive and which can identify asymptomatic metastases, are generally carried out every year. This is the only examination used in the assessment of the rare cases of breast sarcoma, because of the pulmonary tropism of their metastases; in these cases, radiographs are far more frequent, every 2 or 3 months during the first few years.

Bone scintigraphy is rarely positive in the absence of symptoms if initial assessment is normal.[34] It does not appear to be of much use in terms of survival or comfort, nor do hepatic ultrasonography or cerebral assessment. These examinations should therefore only be carried out in the presence of clinical or biological symptoms.

Follow up of complications

Imaging can be helpful in the follow up of complications following treatment.

Mammography has proved useful for following the evolution of cytosteatonecrosis which may become encysted and calcified, or in the case of a radiolesion.

In rare cases of conservative treatment with a prosthesis, mammography in addition to a physical examination can evaluate signs of intolerance—thickening of the periprosthetic fatty margins, loss of shape of the prosthesis, appearance of groups of calcifications, etc.

Chest radiographs can be carried out in order to follow thoracic complications resulting from irradiation of the summit, the upper mediastinum or the ribs, sometimes with pathologic fractures of the first axillary homolateral arches. These complications are uncommon at present because of the reduction in and precision of doses. Radiographs of the shoulder can evaluate osteoporosis and/or secondary arthropathies with functional limitations.

Conclusion

The essential role of imaging in diagnosis, assessment, evaluation of prognosis and the follow up of breast cancers is undisputed. It is essential to use existing techniques as efficiently as possible, with no omissions or duplications, as the frequency of breast cancer makes it a public health issue, the management of which can affect the budget and functioning of public or private healthcare establishments. Imaging in breast cancer can only be optimal if there exists intradepartmental collaboration at all levels, in the interest of the patients, as well as permanent evaluation of the quality and results obtained.

References

1. Watherhouse J, Muir C, Correa P et al, eds, *Cancer incidence in five continents* (International Agency for Research in Cancer: Lyons 1982) vol IV.
2. Schraub S, Epidémiologie, coût moral et financier des traitements adjuvants des cancers du sein. In: Serin D, eds, *Cancer du sein, définition du risque métastatique, bilan des thérapeutiques adjuvantes* (Masson: Paris 1988) 69–74.
3. Anderson DE, Breast cancer in families, *Cancer* (1977) **40**:1855–60.
4. Tabar L, Fagerberg L, Gad A, Reduction in mortality from breast cancer after mass screening with mammography, *Lancet* (1985) **1**:829–32.
5. Bloom HJ, Richardson WW, Histological grading and prognosis in breast cancer. *Br J Cancer* (1957) **11**:359–77.
6. Contesso G, Rouëssé J, Genin J, L'envahissement ganglionnaire locorégional des cancers du sein, *Bull Cancer* (1975) **62**:359–72.
7. Feig SA, Mammographic equipment. Principles, features, selection, *Radiol Clin North Am* (1987) **5**:897–911.
8. Silverstein MJ, Gamagami P, Solburn WJ et al, Non palpable breast lesions: diagnosis with slightly overpenetrated screen-film mammography and hook wire-directed biopsy in 1014 cases, *Radiology* (1989) **171**:633–8.
9. Dilhuydy MH, Le Treut A, Guibert JL, Mammography and indications for excisional therapy. In: Le Treut A, Dilhuydy MH, eds, *Mammography: a guide to interpretation* (Mosby Yearbook: St Louis 1991) 182–6.
10. Kopans DB, Swann CA, White G et al, Asymmetric breast tissue, *Radiology* (1989) **171**:639–43.
11. Lanyï M, Microcalcifications of the breast. A blessing or a curse? *Diagn Imaging Clin Med* (1985) **54**:126–45.
12. Le Gal M, Chavanne G, Pellier D, Valeur diagnostique des microcalcifications groupées découvertes par mammographie, *Bull Cancer* (1984) **71**:57–64.
13. Harper AP, Kelly Fry E, Noe J et al, Ultrasound in the evaluation of solid breast masses, *Radiology* (1983) **146**:731–6.
14. Fornage BD, Faraux MJ, Simatos A, Breast masses: US guided fine needle aspiration biopsy, *Radiology* (1987) **162**:409–14.
15. Strax P, Mass screening for control of breast cancer, *Cancer* (1984) **53**:665–70.
16. Dilhuydy MH, Le Treut A, Durand M et al, The importance of thermography in the prognostic evaluation of breast cancers, *Acta Thermographica* (1978) **3**:130–3.
17. Mintun MA, Welch MJ, Siegel BA et al, Breast cancer: PET imaging of estrogen receptors, *Radiology* (1988) **169**:45–8.
18. Hey Wang SH, Hahn D, Schmidt H et al, MR Imaging of the breast using gadolinium DTPA, *J Comput Assist Tomogr* (1986) **10**:199–204.
19. Kaiser WA. Dynamic magnetic resonance breast imaging using a double breast coil: an important step towards routine examination of the breast, *Frontiers Eur Radiol* (1990) **7**:39–68.
20. Sickles EA, Mammographic features of 300 consecutive non palpable breast cancers, *AJR* (1986) **146**:661–3.
21. Tabar L, Dean P, *Teaching atlas of mammography* (G. Thieme: Stuttgart 1985).
22. Buchanan JB, Sprat JS, Meuser LS, Tumor growth, doubling time and the inability of radiologist to diagnose certain cancers, *Radiol Clin North Am* (1983) **21**:115–26.
23. Homer MJ, Non palpable breast abnormalities. Timing the follow-up studies, *AJR* (1981) **136**:923–6.

24. Nordenström B, Zajicek J, Stereotactif needle biopsy and pre-operative indication of non palpable mammary lesions, *Acta Cytol* (1977) **21**:350–3.
25. Baker LH, Breast Cancer Detection Demonstration Project: five years summary report, *CA* (1982) **32**:194–226.
26. Koscielny S, Tubiana M, Valleron AJ, A simulation model of the natural history of human breast cancer, *Br J Cancer* (1985) **52**:515–24.
27. Feig SA, Radiation risk from mammography: is it clinically significant? *AJR* (1984) **143**:469–75.
28. Hobbs P, Factors affecting population participation in breast cancer screening. In: Zient G, ed, *Practical modalities of an efficient screening for breast cancer in the European community* (Elsevier: Amsterdam 1989) 187–95.
29. Tabar L, Fagerberg L, Day NE et al, What is the optimum interval between mammographic screening examinations? An analysis based on the latest results of the Swedish two-county breast cancer screening trial, *Br J Cancer* (1987) **55**:547–51.
30. Sickles EA, Weber WN, Galvin HB et al, Low-cost mammography screening. Practical considerations with emphasis on mobile operation, *Cancer* (1987) **60**:1688–91.
31. Ikeda DM, Sickles EA, Mammography: one versus two views per breast, *Radiology* (1988) **168**:651–6.
32. Lundgren B, Helleberg A, Single oblique-view mammography for periodic screening for breast cancer in women, *J Natl Cancer Inst* (1982) **68**:351–5.
33. Broberg A, Glas U, Gustaffson SA et al, Relationship between mammographic pattern and oestrogen receptor content in breast cancer, *Breast Cancer Res Treat* (1983) **3**:201–7.
34. Durand M, Bonichon F, Wafflart J et al, Bilan préthérapeutique des cancers du sein. In: Rochet Y, Lagarde C, Brémond A, eds, *Cancers gynécologiques et mammaires. Encyclopédie des Cancers* (Flammarion: Paris 1986) 325–47.
35. Khandekar JD, Role of routine bone scan in operable breast cancer: an opposing viewpoint, *Cancer Treat Rep* (1979) **63**:1241–4.
36. Strender LE, Lagergren C, Wallgren A et al, Role of bone scans in the initial assessment of operable patients with breast carcinoma, *Acta Radiol Oncol* (1981) **20**:187–91.
37. Mauriac L, Durand M, Avril A et al, Effects of primary chemotherapy in conservative treatment of breast cancer patients with operable tumors larger than 3 cm, *Ann Oncol* (1991) **2**:347–54.
38. Veronesi V, Saccozi R, Del Vecchio M, Comparing radical mastectomy with quadrantectomy axillary dissection and radiotherapy in patients with small cancers of the breast, *N Engl J Med* (1981) **305**:6–11.
39. Harris JR, Hellman S, Silen W, eds, *Conservative management of breast cancer.* (JB Lippincott: Philadelphia 1983).
40. Durand JC, Poljicak M, Lefranc JP, Wide excision of the tumor axillary dissection and post-operative radiotherapy in treatment of small breast cancer, *Cancer* (1984) **53**:2439–43.
41. Calle R, Pilleron JP, Schlienger P et al, Conservative management of operable breast cancer. Ten years experience at the Foundation Curie, *Cancer* (1978) **42**:2045–53.
42. Fischer B, Redmend C, Poisson R et al, Eight-year results of a randomized clinical trial comparing total mastectomy and lumpectomy with or without irradiation in the treatment of breast cancer, *N Engl J Med* (1989) **320**:822–8.
43. Clarke DH, Le MG, Sarrazin D, Analysis of locoregional relapses in patients with early breast cancers treated by excision and radiotherapy. Experience of the Institut Gustave Roussy, *Int J Radiat Onçol Biol Phys* (1985) **11**:479–83.
44. Mitnick JS, Vasquez MF, Roses DF et al, Recurrent breast cancer: stereotaxic localization for fine-needle aspiration biopsy, *Radiology* (1992) **182**:103–6.
45. MacCredis JA, Inch WR, Alderson M, Consecutive primary carcinoma of the breast, *Cancer* (1975) **35**:1472–7.

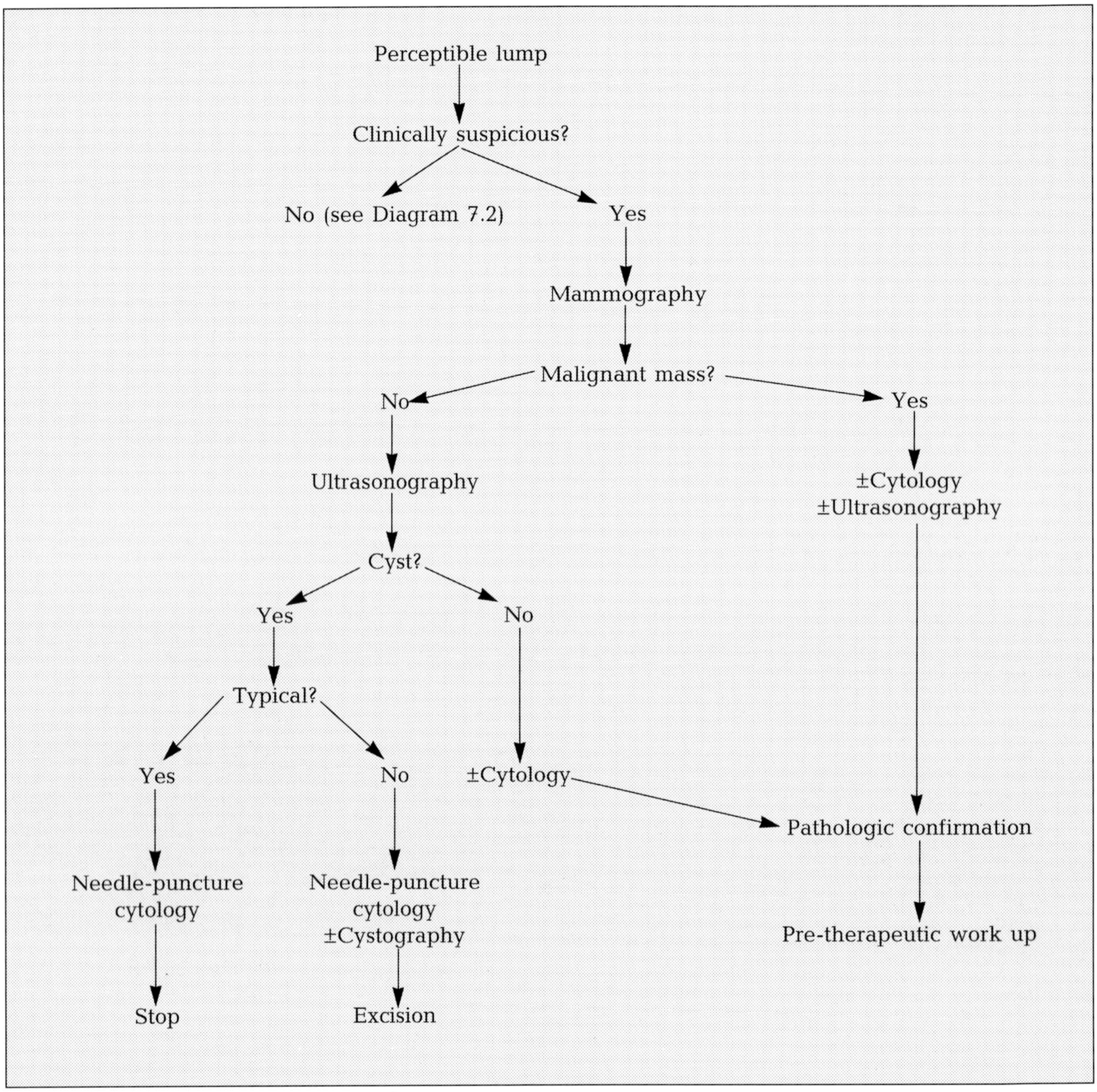

Diagram 7.1

Imaging strategy for diagnosis of a perceptible breast lump that is clinically suspicious.

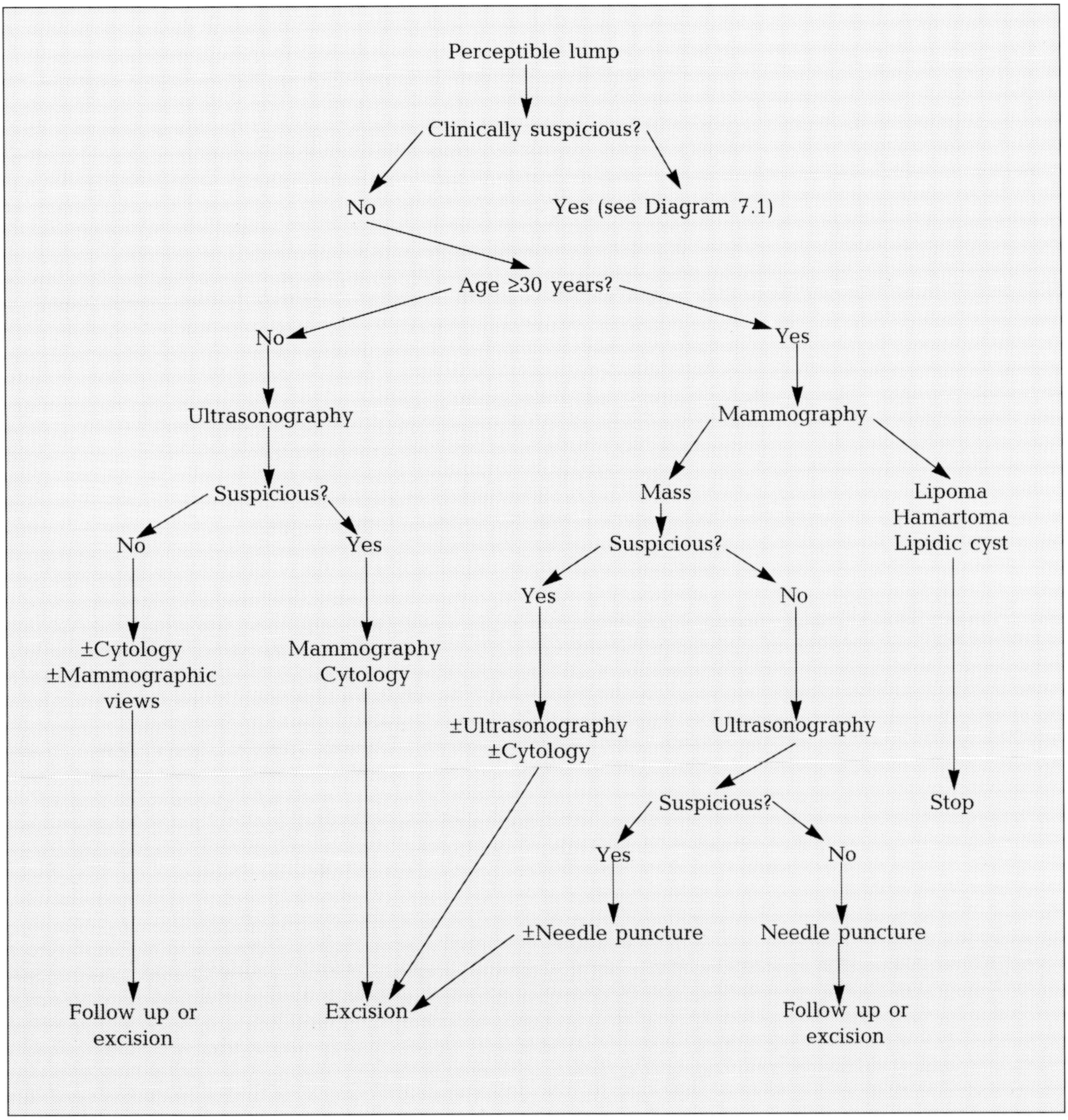

Diagram 7.2

Imaging strategy for diagnosis of a perceptible breast lump that is not clinically suspicious.

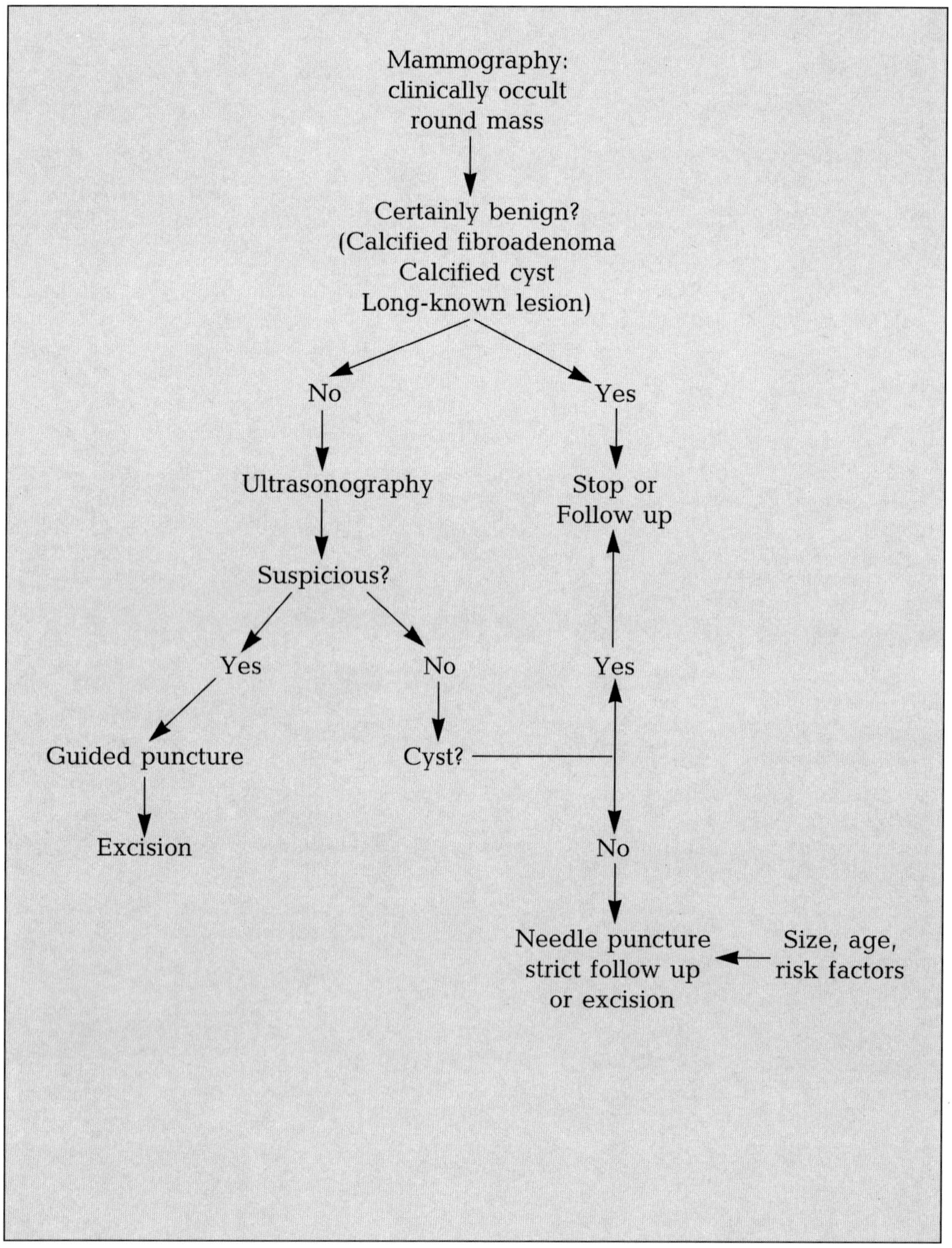

Diagram 7.3

Imaging strategy for diagnosis of a clinically occult round mass on mammography.

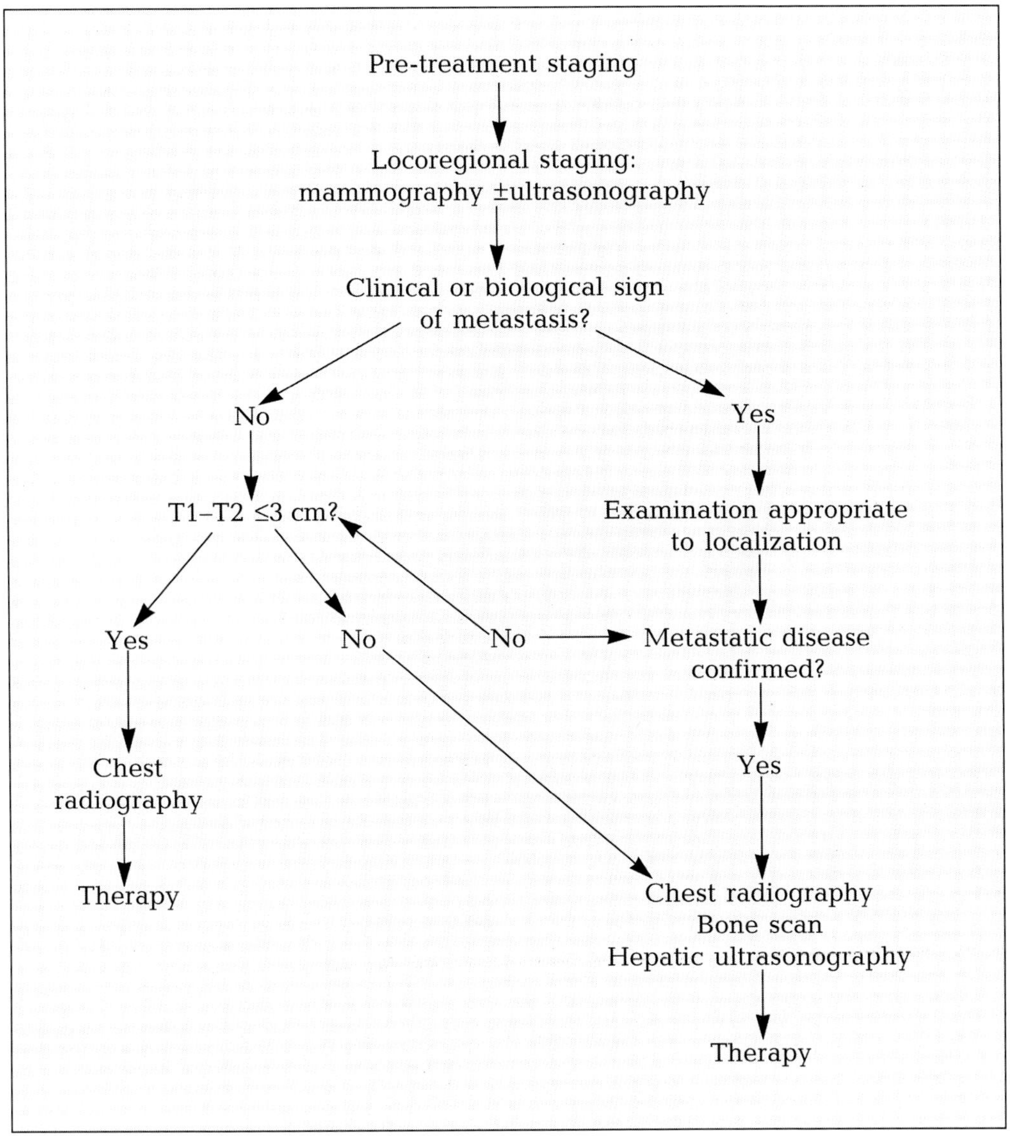

Diagram 7.4

Imaging strategy for pre-treatment staging.

8

The gastrointestinal tract

Jacques Pringot and Bernard Van Beers

The esophagus

Esophageal carcinoma

Epidemiology

The incidence of carcinoma of the esophagus exhibits wide geographic variations. The highest rates are found in parts of Central Asia. In the USA, esophageal carcinoma accounts for about 1% of all cancers. It generally occurs in men older than 50 years of age. High-risk factors are alcohol intake and tobacco use. Also at high risk are patients with chronic esophagitis, Barrett's esophagus, Plummer–Vinson syndrome, lye stricture and long-standing achalasia.[1] Since tobacco and alcohol consumption is related to the development of several malignancies, the frequency of synchronous or metachronous cancers among esophageal cancer patients is high, and they include carcinoma of the mouth, tongue, pharynx and lung, as well as kidney and bladder neoplasms.

Pathology

The majority of esophageal cancers are of squamous-cell origin. Adenocarcinoma involving the esophagus stems from a tumor of the stomach or can arise in the esophagus itself. There is an increased risk of esophageal adenocarcinoma in patients with Barrett's esophagus, a condition in which stomach-like columnar epithelium appears in the lower esophagus and one often associated with gastroesophageal reflux.

The most common appearance of esophageal carcinoma is a fungating mass that obliterates the lumen. Other variants are a raised ulceration or a diffusely infiltrating tumor.[2] Verrucous carcinomas are rare.

Carcinoma of the esophagus is highly malignant. Characteristically, the tumor extends microscopically to the submucosa from substantial distances above and below the area noted to be grossly involved. The peculiar anatomy of the esophagus facilitates rapid spread of tumor cells. For most of its length, the esophagus has a loose adventitia that provides no barrier to tumor spread. An extensive submucosal lymphatic network is also present. Metastases may 'skip' nodes at the same level to invade more distant lymph nodes. In a study of 220 cases of esophageal carcinoma, Akiyama et al[3] found that 32% of patients with carcinoma of the upper third of the esophagus had metastases to subdiaphragmatic lymph nodes.

In the new TNM system for preoperative classification of esophageal carcinoma,[4] criteria of tumor size, circumferential involvement and obstruction have been abandoned in favor of depth of invasion for the assessment of the primary tumor extent (Table 8.1). Early esophageal carcinoma has been defined as T1 carcinoma with no evidence of lymph-node involvement.[5]

Clinical features

Esophageal cancer is a silent tumor in its early stages. Early cancer causes no symptoms in 20–40% of patients.[6] In more advanced disease, the predominant clinical complaint is dysphagia,

Table 8.1 The TNM classification of esophageal carcinoma.

	Stage	*Description*
Primary tumor	Tis	Carcinoma in situ
	T1	Tumor invades lamina propria or submucosa
	T2	Tumor invades muscularis propria
	T3	Tumor invades adventitia
	T4	Tumor invades adjacent structures
Nodal involvement	N0	No regional lymph node metastasis
	N1	Regional lymph node metastasis
Distant metastases	M0	No distant metastasis
	M1	Distant metastasis

often accompanied by weight loss. Other symptoms include regurgitation, vomiting, hoarseness and cough. Pulmonary complications are common. Iron deficiency anemia may develop, and sometimes frank hemorrhage may occur. This may indicate that the tumor is invading the aorta or another major vessel.

Visceral metastases are found in more than half of the patients at autopsy, most frequently in the lungs and liver, less frequently in the adrenal glands, bones and brain. However, local and regional progression of the tumor is the cause of death far more frequently than are distant metastases.

Imaging

Detection

Advanced esophageal cancer is easily depicted on barium esophagograms. Fungating masses, ulcerated flat lesions, or infiltrating lesions may be seen (Figure 8.1).

In early cancer, rather subtle changes such as focal rigidity of the wall, irregularity of the margin and thin barium fleck, may be visible on double-contrast or biphasic (a combination of double-contrast and simple contrast techniques) esophagograms (Figure 8.2). It has been reported that radiographic examination compares favorably with endoscopy in the detection of esophageal carcinoma.[7] However, endoscopy and dye endoscopy are more useful than radiography to detect mucosal esophageal cancer because color changes may be the only anomaly.[6]

Screening

The overall prognosis of esophageal carcinoma is poor, with a 5-year survival rate for only 5–15% of patients.[8] Improvement in patient survival depends on early detection of esophageal carcinoma, when lesions are small and asymptomatic. Once dysphagia is present, the lesion is generally incurable. Mass screening has been proposed in regions where the incidence is high. It is difficult to advocate mass screening for esophageal carcinoma in the Western World.

Staging

Computed tomography (CT) has been the most commonly used technique for the pre-operative staging of esophageal cancer.[9–12] Mediastinal involvement, adenomegaly and direct extension into the tracheobronchial tree, the aorta and the pericardium can be detected by CT (Figure 8.3). Moreover, duration of survival is related to the extraesophageal spread of tumor, as defined by CT.[10]

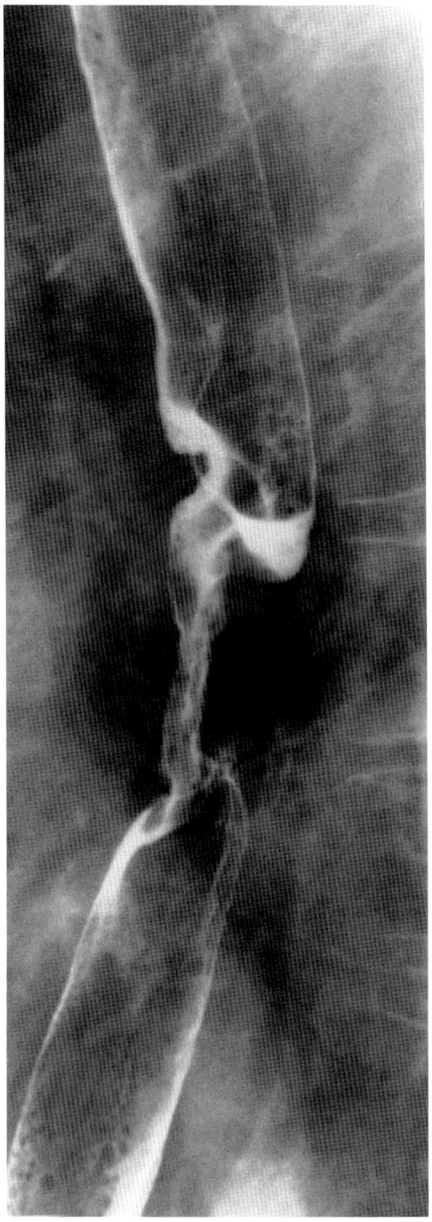

B

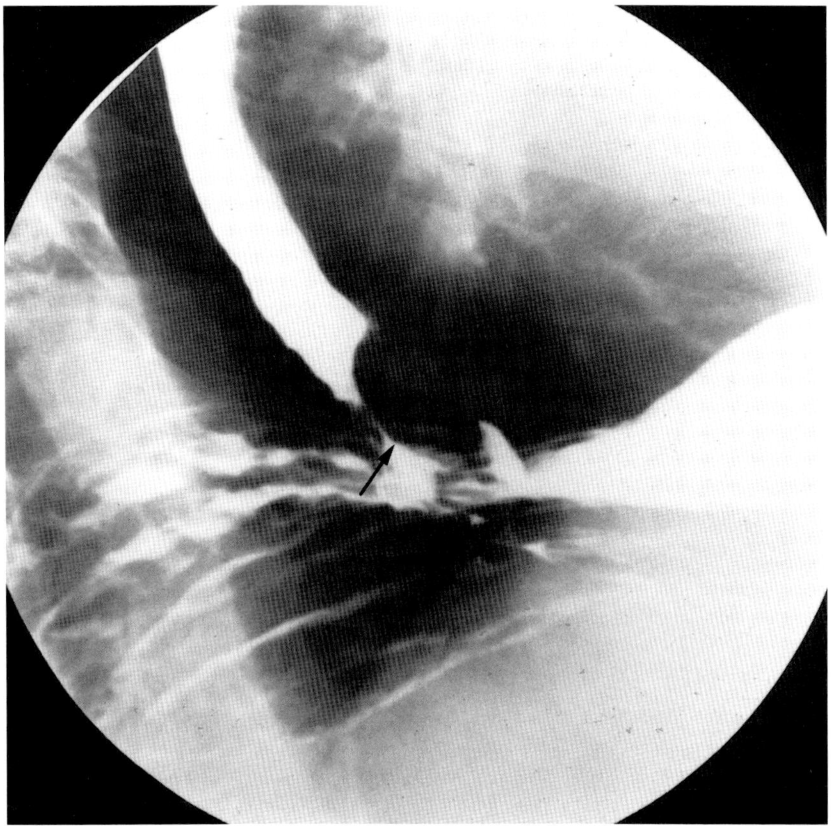

B

Figure 8.1

Two examples of advanced esophageal carcinoma (barium esophagograms).

A Extensive annular mass.

B Eccentric polypoid lesion (arrow).

However, multiple problems remain in staging. The extent of wall invasion cannot be accurately determined by CT. Whatever the threshold size chosen, adenomegaly is not a reliable criterion for lymph-node metastasis. Microscopic metastases to normal size nodes may occur and, conversely, nodes may be enlarged due to benign disease. Peri-esophageal nodes may be difficult to distinguish from contiguous tumor and celiac nodes may be difficult to distinguish from tortuous vessels. Evaluation of peri-esophageal spread may be hampered by the frequent paucity of mediastinal fat.[3] Indentation of the tracheobronchial tree is not a reliable criterion for tumorous invasion, even when scans are obtained in deep inspiration. More specific signs of invasion are encasement and focal irregularity of the tracheobronchial wall, but the most specific signs of invasion include tracheo-esophageal fistula

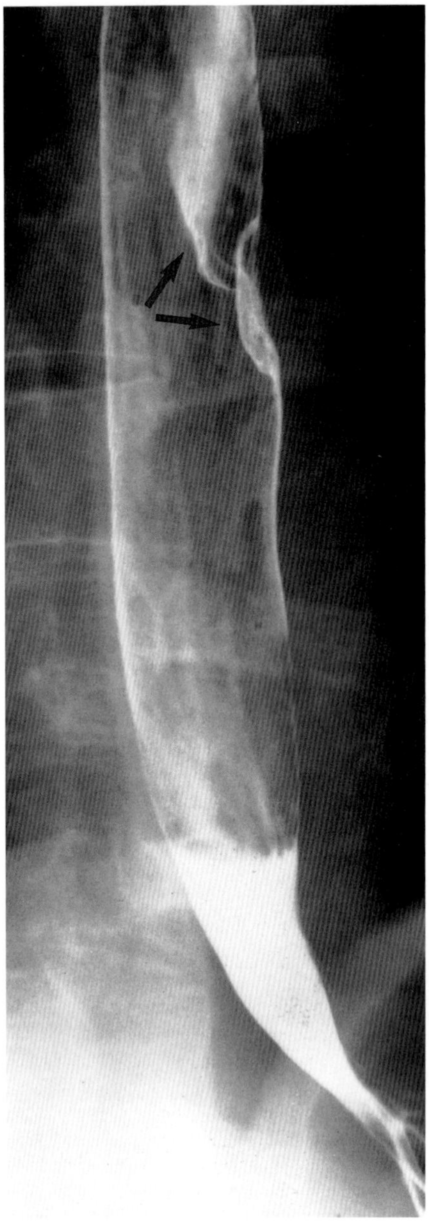

Figure 8.2

Double-contrast esophagogram of an early carcinoma shows two adjacent lesions (arrows).

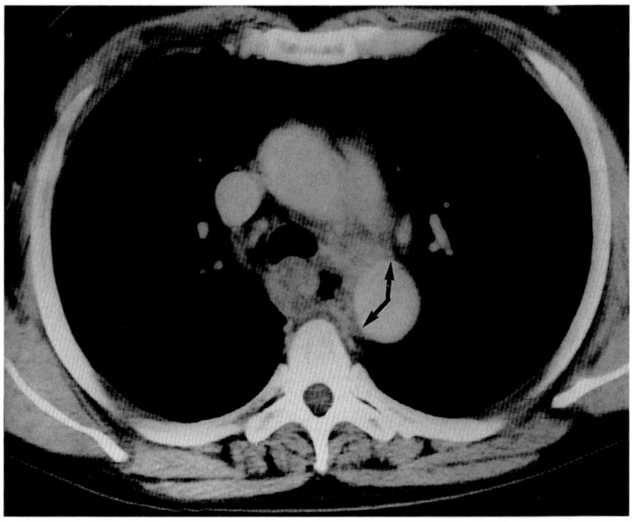

Figure 8.3

CT scan of esophageal carcinoma with aortic invasion. More than 90° of the aortic circumference is in contact with the esophageal tumor (arrows).

or demonstration of tumor tissue within the airway. Uneasy differentiation between compression and invasion by tumor occurs for other mediastinal structures, such as the pericardium, pleura, diaphragm and aorta.

These difficulties explain the great variability in the reported accuracy of CT (from 39 to 100%) for the overall staging of esophageal tumors.[9] Reasons for the wide discrepancy in the results reported by different groups include selection of patient population, relatively limited number of patients and, for some early studies, lack of accurate radiologic–surgical correlation. The role of CT in the pre-operative staging of esophageal carcinoma is thus controversial. Despite limitations, however, CT may be used in predicting resectability. The few contraindications to surgery are related to aortic or tracheobronchial invasion and distant metastases which are detected by CT with a fairly good accuracy.[10]

Endoscopic ultrasonography (US) is a recent technique for staging gastrointestinal neoplasms. Five layers are visible on ultrasound images of the normal gastrointestinal tract and correspond to (1) superficial mucosa, (2) deep mucosa, (3) submucosa, (4) muscularis propria, and (5) serosa and subserosal fat.[12] In patients with esophageal carcinoma, endoscopic US has been shown to be superior to CT in the evaluation of the depth of tumor infiltration, in the diagnosis of mediastinal involvement and in the assessment of regional lymph-nodes metastases[5,13] (Figure 8.4).

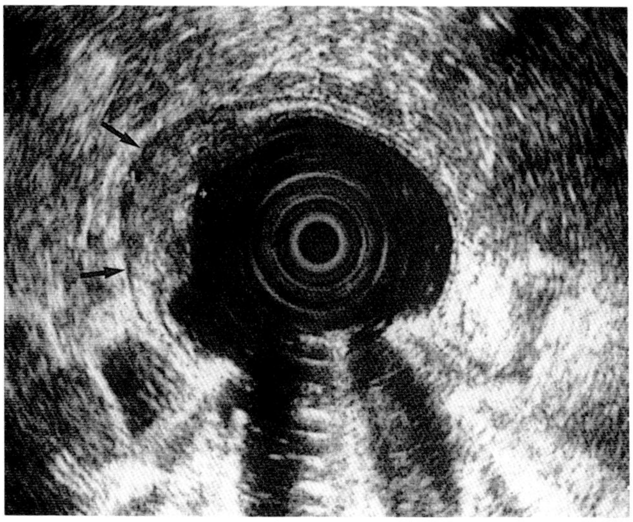

Figure 8.4

Endoscopic US of an early esophageal carcinoma shows a focal thickening of the esophageal wall without invasion of the hypoechoic muscular layer (arrows). The five layers of the digestive wall are easily visible. (Reproduced from Van Beers et al, *J Belge Radiol*, 1989; 72:181–90, with permission.)

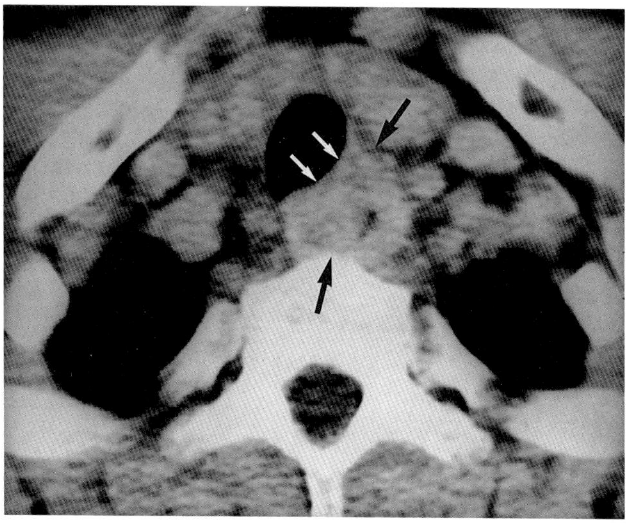

A

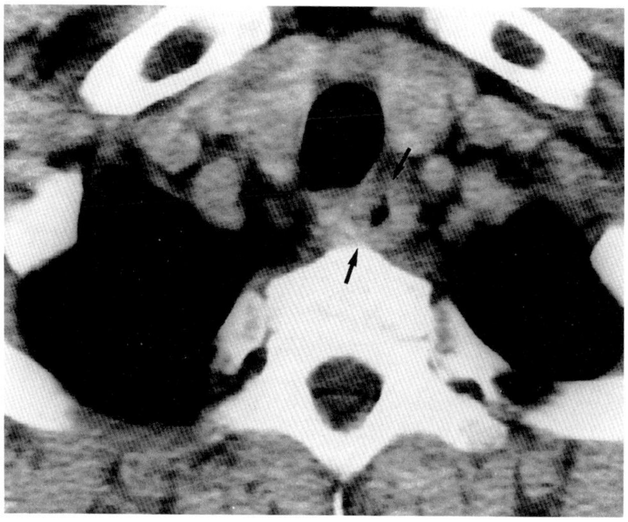

B

Figure 8.5

Follow up of esophageal carcinoma after radiotherapy.

A Initial CT scan shows an esophageal mass (black arrows) with tracheal invasion (white arrows).

B Follow-up CT scan after radiotherapy shows partial regression of the esophageal tumor (arrows).

Sonographic criteria to detect metastases in normal-sized esophageal and gastric lymph nodes have been described. These criteria are based on echogenicity and morphology. Metastatic lymph nodes are usually hypoechoic, round or elliptic structures with well-defined contours.[13,14] However, current criteria for identification of lymph-node metastases by endoscopic US vary somewhat, and false-positive results may occur due to inflammatory changes.[5] The evolving capacity of endoscopic US to enable guided biopsy should further enhance the diagnostic accuracy. Limitations to endoscopic US are severe stenosis, which cannot be passed with the instrument, and the limited penetration of ultrasound, which precludes accurate diagnosis of distant metastases. A combination of endoscopic US for evaluation of local extension and CT for evaluation of distant metastases may provide the highest yield in staging.[13,14]

MR imaging has not proved to be superior to CT in the staging of esophageal cancer.[15] Laparoscopy has also been advocated for abdominal staging of cancer of the esophagus and gastric cardia.[16]

Follow up

Several forms of palliation exist for esophageal tumors, including radiation therapy, chemotherapy, endoprosthetic treatment with tubes or metallic stents, dilation and laser therapy. CT is useful for follow up after palliative therapy (Figure

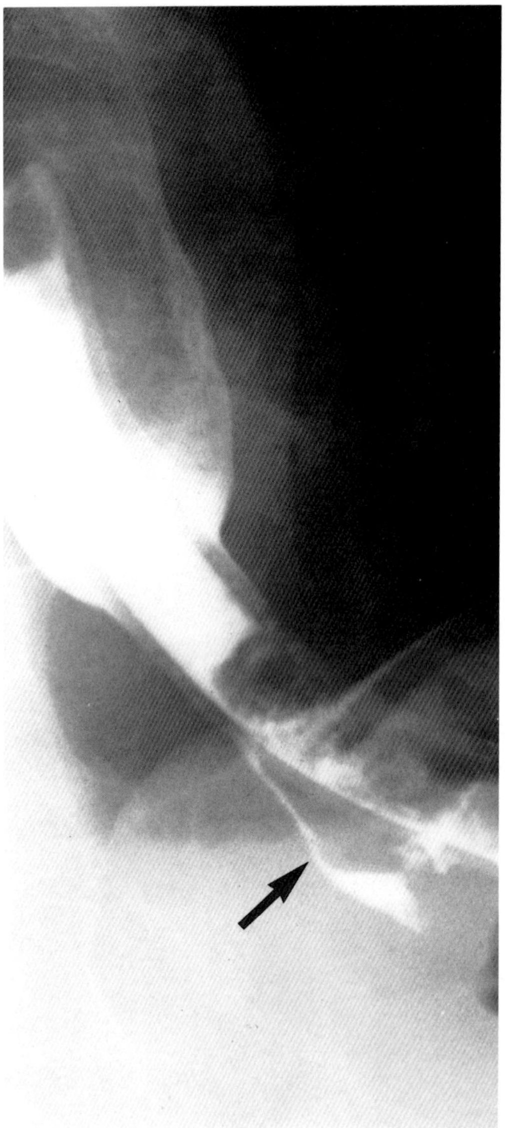

A

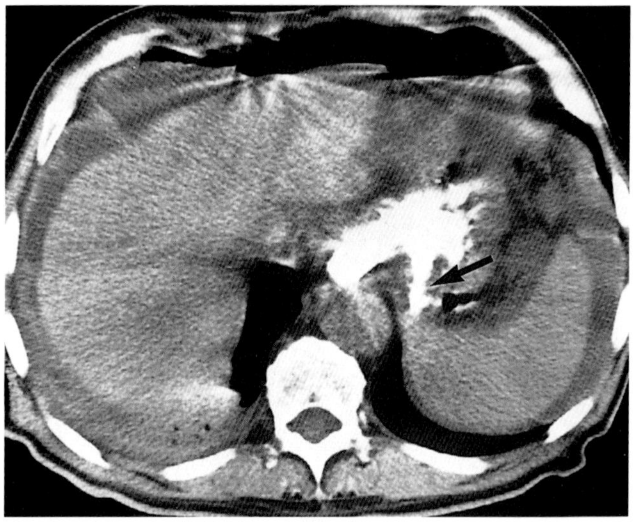

B

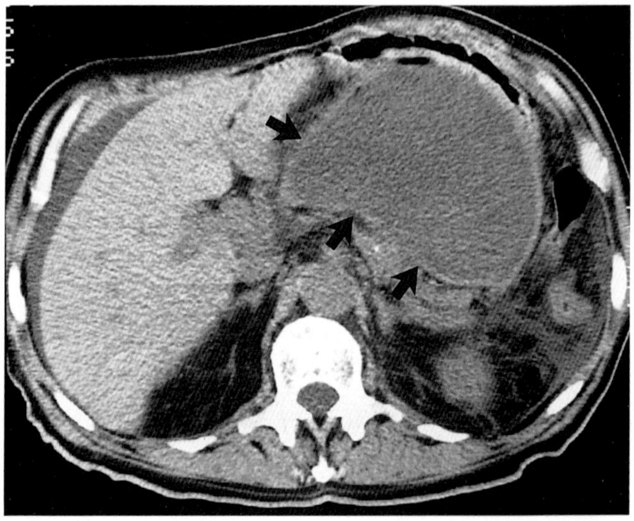

C

Figure 8.6

Complications of esophageal prosthesis.

A Prosthesis placed in the lower third of the esophagus and in the stomach is obstructed by food. A perforation at the gastroesophageal junction is observed with extravasation of contrast material (arrow).

B CT scan confirms the perforation at the gastroesophageal junction (arrow). Ascites and pneumoperitoneum are also seen.

C CT scan at lower level shows large associated retrogastric abscess (arrows).

8.5) and for the diagnosis of complications after surgical or non-surgical treatment such as fluid collections and abscesses. Other complications are better studied by upper gastrointestinal series. These complications include cricopharyngeal incoordination and anastomotic or pyloric stenoses. The exact site of an esophageal perforation may be better demonstrated on an esophagogram than on CT.[17] However, high-quality esophagograms are often uneasy to obtain in seriously ill patients. CT requires minor patient cooperation and allows identification of minute

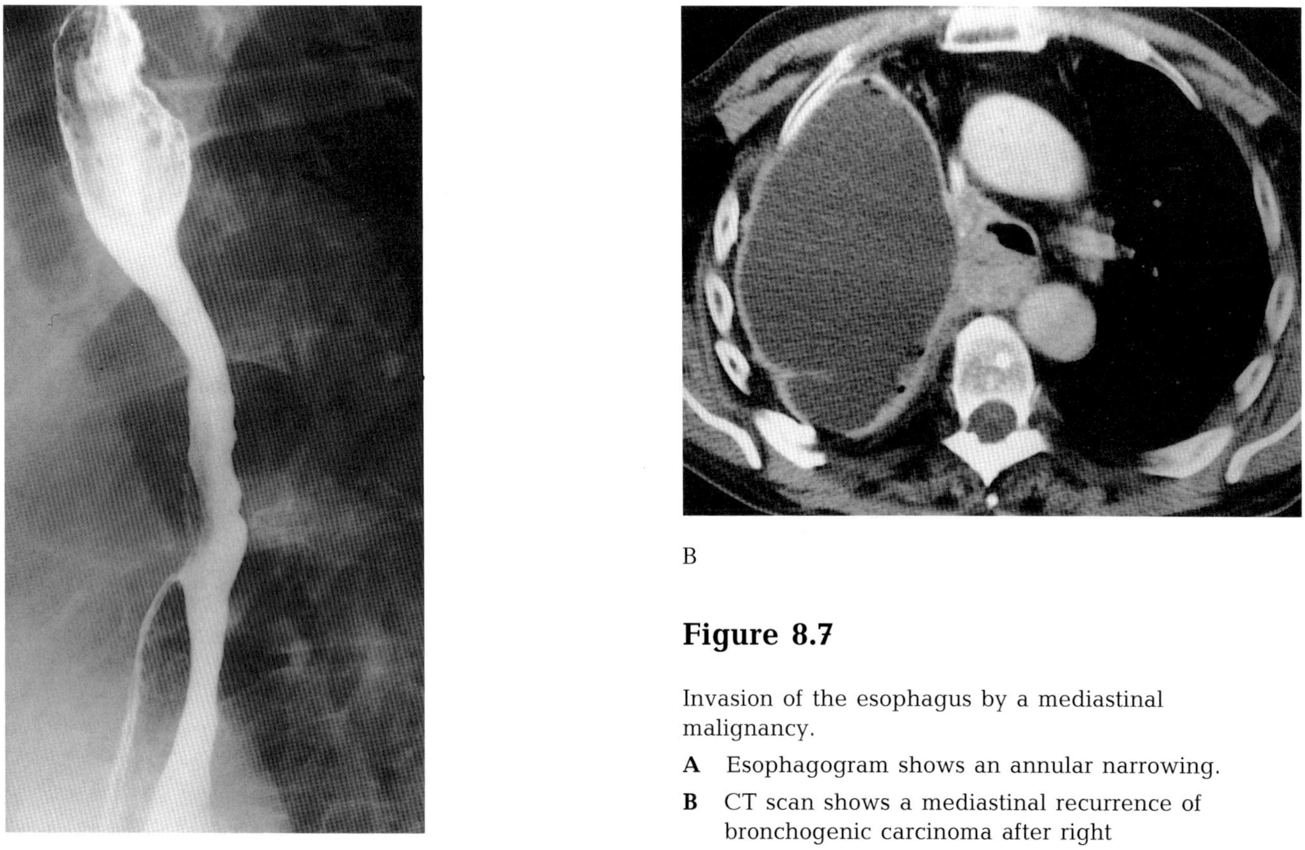

A

B

Figure 8.7

Invasion of the esophagus by a mediastinal malignancy.

A Esophagogram shows an annular narrowing.

B CT scan shows a mediastinal recurrence of bronchogenic carcinoma after right pneumonectomy.

amounts of extradigestive air or contrast material (Figure 8.6).

CT and endoscopic US are also useful for the detection of extrinsic recurrence following surgery of esophageal cancer. Mural recurrence can be detected by endoscopy and barium studies.[18] Diagram 8.1 summarizes the work up of patients with esophageal carcinoma.

Other esophageal malignancies

Primary tumors other than carcinomas and blood-borne metastases are rare in the esophagus. Invasion of the esophagus from adjacent malignancies or malignant mediastinal nodes is more common, especially in case of lung or breast carcinoma (Figure 8.7). As the neoplasm invades the wall it may become impossible to distinguish from a primary carcinoma on esophagograms.

The stomach

Gastric carcinoma

Epidemiology

The incidence of gastric carcinoma varies widely over the world. The highest rates are found in Japan, Chile, Ireland and Finland. The frequency of gastric carcinoma has been declining over the last 50 years, but the relative frequency of gastric carcinoma arising in the cardia is increasing. An emerging concept is that proximal adenocarcinomas, including those arising in the distal esophagus, gastroesophageal junction and cardia, form a distinct group which shares similar epidemiologic features. These features include lower mean age than for other gastric carcinomas and male predominance.[19] Except for the increased risk of esophageal adenocarcinoma in patients with Barrett's esophagus, little is known about the origin of these tumors.[19]

For gastric carcinoma in general, several studies have emphasized the possible role of certain food items and additives, such as starch, polycyclic hydrocarbons and nitrosamines.[20] Atrophic gastritis, pernicious anemia, subtotal gastrectomy, adenomatous polyps and villous tumors are also risk factors.

Pathology

Advanced gastric carcinoma is divided into four gross types, according to the Borrmann classification[20,21] (Table 8.2). The Japanese Research Society for Gastric Cancer has added two types to the Borrmann classification: early cancer (type 0) and lesions unclassifiable in the Borrmann categories (type 5).

Early gastric cancer is defined as a carcinoma limited to the mucosa or submucosa, with or without lymph-node involvement.[22] Early cancer has been divided in three major types and three subtypes[21] (Table 8.3).

The TNM system is used for the assessment of the extent of gastric carcinoma (Table 8.4).[4]

Table 8.2 The Borrmann classification of advanced gastric carcinoma.

Type	*Description*
1	Polypoid lesion
2	Ulcerated tumor with sharp margins
3	Ulcerated tumor that is not sharply circumscribed
4	Infiltrating tumor

Table 8.3 Classification of early gastric carcinoma.

Type	*Description*
I	Protruded lesion (>0.5 cm in height)
II	Superficial lesion
	a Minimally elevated
	b Flat
	c Minimally depressed
III	Excavated lesion

Table 8.4 The TNM classification of gastric carcinoma.

	Stage	*Description*
Primary tumor	Tis	Carcinoma in situ
	T1	Tumor invades lamina propria or submucosa
	T2	Tumor invades muscularis propria
	T3	Tumor penetrates the serosa
	T4	Tumor invades adjacent structures
Nodal involvement	N0	No regional lymph-node metastasis
	N1	Metastasis in perigastric lymph node(s) no more than 3 cm from the edge of the primary tumor
	N2	Metastasis in perigastric lymph node(s) more than 3 cm from the edge of the primary tumor or in lymph nodes along the left gastric, common hepatic, splenic, or celiac arteries.
Distant metastases	M0	No distant metastasis
	M1	Distant metastasis

Clinical features

Symptoms of gastric cancer include weight loss, pain, vomiting, hematemesis, melena and dysphagia. These symptoms are non-specific and explain why gastric cancer, as is the case for esophageal cancer, is often discovered late.

Imaging

Detection

Barium studies and endoscopy are used for the diagnosis of gastric cancer. Barium studies are optimized by the use of double-contrast or biphasic techniques. These techniques are particularly important for the detection of superficial cancers and the distinction between benign and malignant ulcers.[23]

The role of barium studies in the investigation of patients with upper gastrointestinal symptoms is controversial. Some prospective studies have claimed that endoscopy was more sensitive and more specific than double-contrast barium studies.[24] Others have found that both methods had equal merit for the diagnosis of gastric ulcer and cancer.[25] Radiographic examination of the stomach has the advantage of being less expensive and less invasive than endoscopy.[26] On the other hand, endoscopy has the definite advantage of facilitating biopsies. Many authors think that all symptomatic patients should undergo early endoscopy, with immediate biopsy if deemed appropriate.[27] Barium studies are often more reliable than endoscopy and biopsy for the diagnosis of scirrhous carcinoma of the stomach because this tumor is located predominantly in the submucosa and tumor cells are often separated by large areas of fibrosis[28] (Figure 8.8). Endoscopic US has also been shown to be useful for the detection and the diagnosis of scirrhous carcinoma.[29]

Screening

Five-year survival rates higher than 80% have been reported in patients who have undergone surgical treatment of early cancer.[30] This stresses the importance of early detection of gastric cancer. However, most patients with gastric carcinoma already have advanced lesions at the time of clinical presentation, so that early gastric cancer is unlikely to be detected at a high rate on double-contrast barium studies or endoscopic examination as long as these studies are performed predominantly only on symptomatic patients. The incidence of early gastric cancer diagnosed in Japan has risen from 5 to 35% of all gastric cancers. This increase can be attributed primarily to mass screening programs. Lower incidence of gastric cancer in the Western World precludes mass screening,[31] but routine screening should be performed in selected cases: partial gastrectomy is a well-known risk factor of developing late gastric cancer. Patients with a 15-year or longer history of gastric surgery for peptic ulcer should undergo periodic screening by endoscopy, as changes in the anastomotic area may be difficult to interpret on radiographs.[20] Routine surveillance of the stomach and duodenum with endoscopy is also recommended in patients with gastric polyps, pernicious anemia, or a family history of gastric malignancy.[22]

Staging

CT can detect adenomegaly, direct extension to surrounding organs, and distant metastases (Figure 8.8). The detection of tumor invasion by CT may be improved after oral administration of water.[32] However, CT is generally considered not to be very accurate for gastric cancer staging. For example, false-positive results of pancreatic invasion have been reported in emaciated patients and in patients exhibiting a pancreatic inflammatory response to adjacent gastric tumor.[33] False-negative results of pancreatic invasion have also been described because tumor spread to the pancreas may occur not only by contiguity but also by a secondary route, through peripancreatic metastatic lymph nodes. Among distant metastases, hematogenous liver metastases and peritoneal implantations are most frequent. CT is a well-established means of detecting liver metastases, but CT detection of peritoneal implantations may be difficult even with intraperitoneal infusion of contrast material.[34] CT thus has a limited role in staging patients with gastric cancer,[33] especially if surgery, either curative or palliative, is considered as the only treatment. In institutions where surgery is not automatically performed in patients with gastric carcinoma, CT may help to identify patients with definite distant metastases and multiple organ involvement who need palliation.[9,33]

As for the esophagus, endoscopic US of the stomach has been shown to be more accurate to determine the depth of tumor invasion and to assess regional lymph-node metastases.[35] In the future, color-flow imaging and US-guided interventional procedures may further increase the usefulness of endoscopic US.[36]

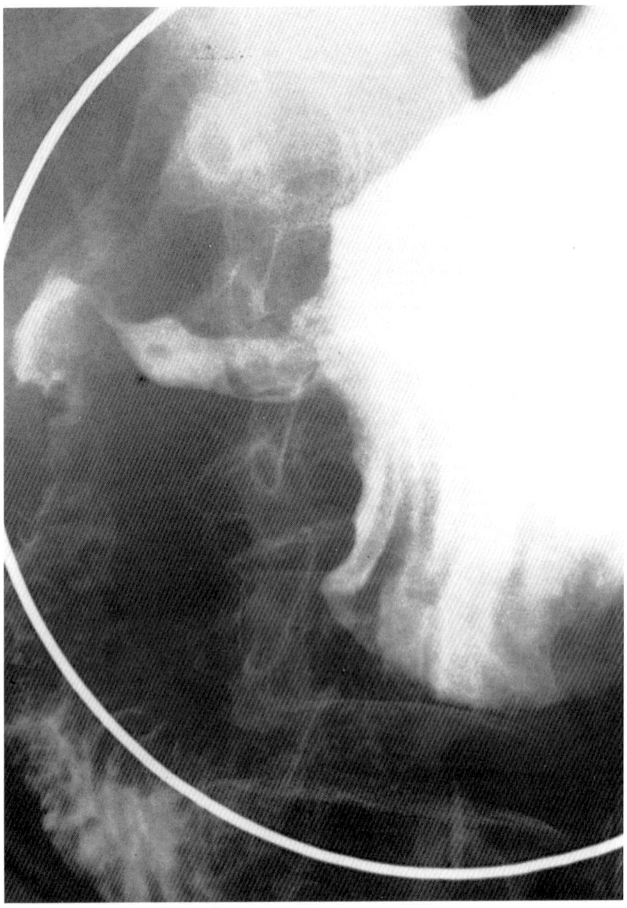

A

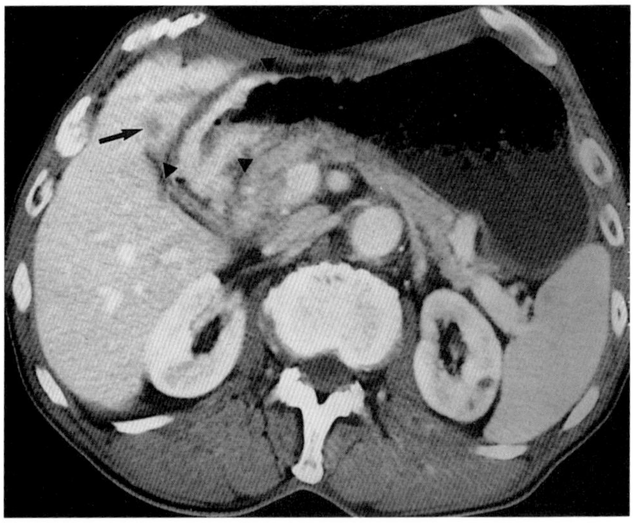

B

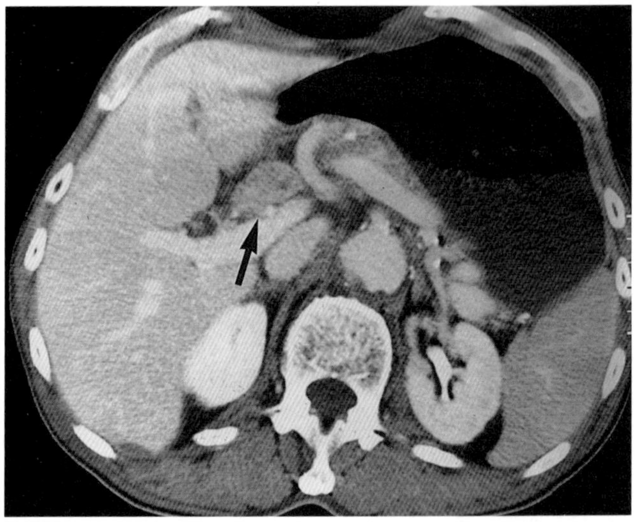

C

Figure 8.8

Linitis plastica (Borrmann type 4 advanced cancer).

A Radiograph shows a severe narrowing of gastric antrum.

B Contrast-enhanced CT scan in same patient demonstrates a hypodense thickening of the gastric wall (arrowheads) and a small hypodense metastasis in the left hepatic lobe (arrow).

C CT scan at higher level shows a metastatic lymph node in the gastrohepatic ligament (arrow).

Follow up

Complications after surgery can be detected by radiologic upper gastrointestinal studies,[37] and recurrence can be diagnosed by endoscopy, barium studies, endoscopic US and CT, according to the site of recurrent tumor.[38] Patient evaluation should include scrutiny of signs and symptoms of second cancer, because gastric cancer is commonly associated with synchronous and metachronous non-gastric malignancies.[22] Diagram 8.1 summarizes the work up of patients with gastric carcinoma.

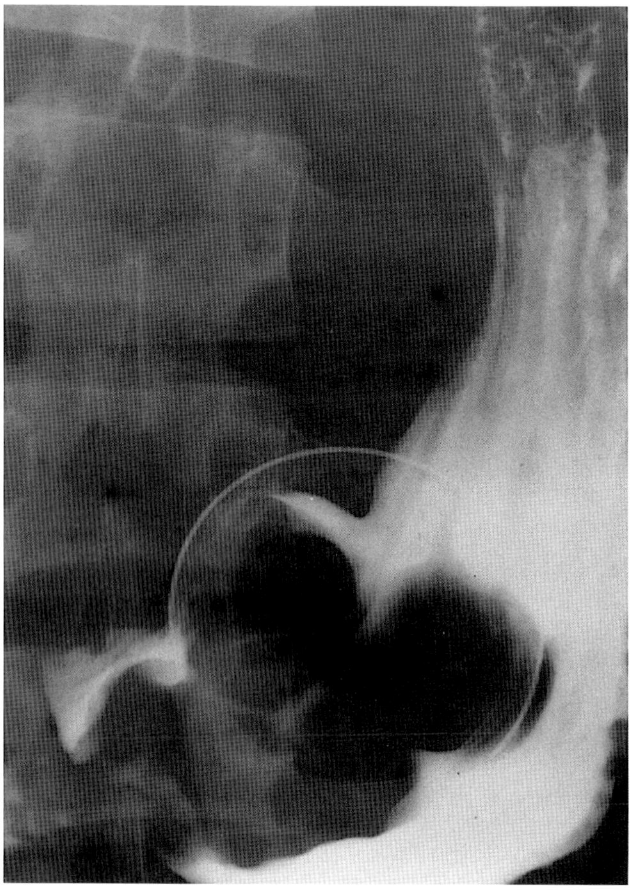

A

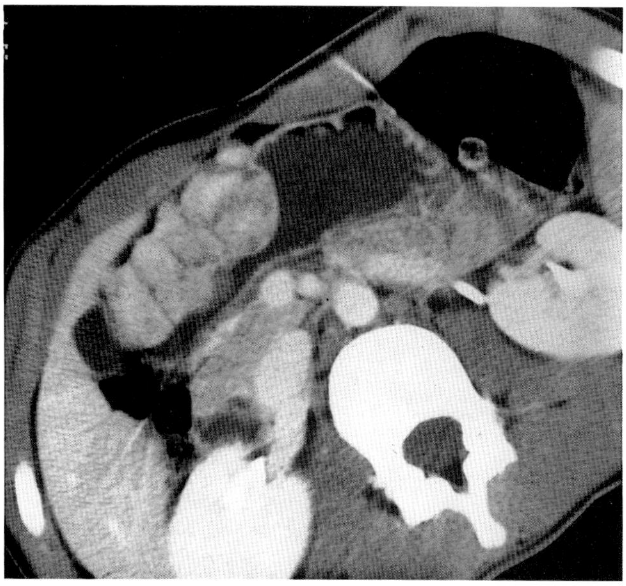

B

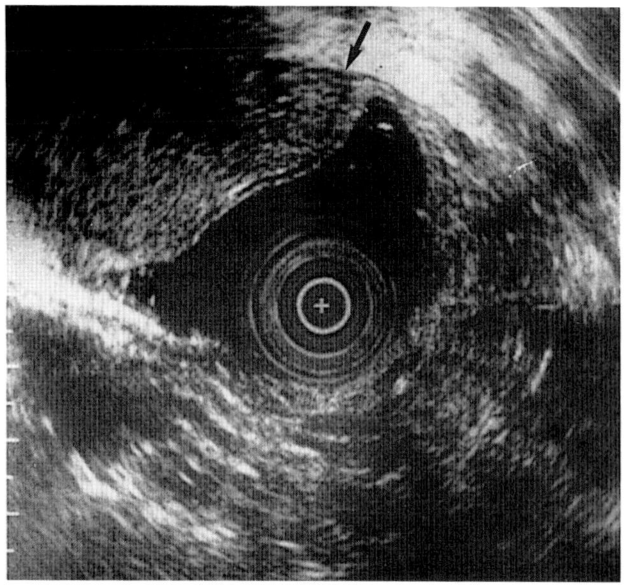

C

Figure 8.9

Gastric leiomyoblastoma.

A Radiograph of gastric antrum shows a multilobular mass.

B CT scan of the stomach filled with water clearly shows the extent of the parietal mass.

C Endoscopic US shows the mass originating from the hypoechoic muscular wall layer (arrow).

Other primary gastric malignancies

Except for lymphomas, gastric smooth-muscle tumors are the most common extramucosal tumors in the stomach.

Pathology

Leiomyoma is the benign form of smooth-muscle tumor while the malignant form is leiomyosarcoma. A more cellular epithelioid tumor is called leiomyoblastoma. It is usually considered as a benign tumor, but may occasionally metastasize.[39]

Clinical features

Leiomyomas are often asymptomatic. Leiomyosarcomas may cause weight loss, abdominal pain, and gastrointestinal bleeding.

Imaging

Endoscopy and barium studies are limited in their ability to detect smooth-muscle tumors. CT and endoscopic US are useful in establishing the relationship of these masses to the wall of the bowel[40,41] (Figure 8.9). On CT scans, smooth-muscle tumors appear as round or oval masses. Leiomyosarcomas are often bulky, lobulated, exophytic masses with central necrosis or liquefaction. When totally liquefied, the tumor may be misdiagnosed as an abscess or pancreatic pseudocyst.[42] Leiomyosarcomas spread to the peritoneum and liver but rarely to lymph nodes.[42] It is not possible to distinguish with certainty between leiomyoma, leiomyoblastoma and leiomyosarcoma by imaging, but leiomyosarcomas tend to be larger and more necrotic than benign smooth-muscle tumors.[40]

Secondary neoplasms

The stomach may be invaded by adjacent neoplasms spreading from the esophagus, transverse colon, pancreas, left kidney or adrenal gland. The stomach may also be involved by blood-borne metastases, usually from melanoma or breast carcinoma. Other distant neoplasms, such as esophageal squamous-cell carcinoma, may also metastasize to the stomach.[43] Gastric metastases primarily involve the submucosa. Metastases from melanoma characteristically produce polypoid masses which frequently show central ulceration. Metastases from breast carcinoma may also produce submucosal nodules or may cause a linitis plastica appearance indistinguishable from a primary gastric cancer.[28]

The small intestine

Small-intestine carcinoma

Epidemiology

The small bowel is the least frequent site of primary malignancies in the gastrointestinal tract, accounting for 3–6% of all gastrointestinal cancers.[44] In the jejunum and ileum, carcinoma, carcinoid tumors, primary lymphomas and leiomyosarcomas are the most common primary lesions, but carcinomas are the commonest primary duodenal malignancies. Small-bowel carcinomas constitute up to 50% of the small-intestinal neoplasms in most series and are usually sited proximally in the duodenum and jejunum and less commonly in the ileum.[45,46] Duodenal carcinoma represents less than 0.4% of all gastrointestinal cancers.[45] The aetiology of small-intestinal cancers is unknown. The highest incidence occurs after the fifth decade of life at an average age of 60 years in large series, and both sexes are equally represented. Certain conditions are associated with a high risk of developing carcinoma: long-standing Crohn's disease, celiac disease, chronic intestinal obstruction and excluded loops associated with bypass operations, and familial polyposis coli.[44,47,48] Villous duodenal adenomas carry a risk of malignant transformation, with a reported rate of approximately 36%.[49]

Recently it has been postulated that the adenoma–carcinoma sequence is as significant in the small as in the large bowel.[50]

Prognosis for malignant small-intestinal tumors continues to be poor. Early diagnosis of these tumors remains a major clinical challenge, as does the development of effective chemotherapeutic agents.[51]

Pathology

Differentiated adenocarcinomas and mucinous adenocarcinomas are the commonest histological types of small-bowel carcinomas.[52] A rare signet-ring type of carcinoma has also been reported, as well as a small number of undifferentiated carcinomas.

Adenocarcinomas arise from the mucosa but rapidly penetrate transversly through the bowel wall and tend to metastasize to the regional lymph nodes and also to the liver.[44] They may be fungating or polypoid and they tend to become annular and constricting. Duodenal carcinomas are most common in the second and third parts of the duodenum.

In contrast to tumor size and grade, depth of tumor invasion or stage at the time of diagnosis do seem to correlate with survival.[53]

Clinical features

Patients may present with acute or chronic obstructive symptoms such as abdominal pain, nausea, vomiting, postprandial fullness, occult or massive hemorrhage, or jaundice in the case of duodenal lesions.[45]

Because symptoms may be vague and nonspecific, tumors in the duodenum or small intestine are often diagnosed at an advanced stage, or even represent unexpected findings at laparotomy. Consequently, the overall prognosis is poor, with a 5-year survival rate of 15–41%.[45,53] Surgical resection—when possible—is the standard management of small-bowel cancers; radiotherapy and chemotherapy have proved to be of little benefit.

Imaging

Detection

Barium examination procedures and duodenoscopy are the primary diagnostic modalities. Barium studies can achieve a high degree of diagnostic accuracy when they rely on carefully performed double-contrast duodenography and detailed small-bowel follow-through or enteroclysis.[54] Detailed per oral small-bowel examination performed with a large volume of low-density barium and frequent compression, possibly complemented with retrograde double-contrast views obtained after insufflation of the colon, is an efficient method for routine examination. However, conventional barium follow-through examination has a much lower sensitivity for tumors than does enteroclysis.[55] Asymptomatic familial polyposis patients should have duodenoscopic screening at regular intervals.[56]

The radiologic features are similar to those of carcinoma elsewhere in the gastrointestinal tract and include polypoid defects, ulceration, rigidity and constriction of the intestinal lumen (Figures 8.10 and 8.11). There may be associated evidence of obstruction with proximal dilatation or, less frequently, presence of an exoenteric mass. In the duodenum, carcinomas are often polypoid or ulcerated.[45] In the jejunum and ileum, they most often appear at presentation as annular constricting lesions that obstruct the lumen, and characteristically show as rigid strictures with destruction of mucosa and overhanging edges.[46] Occasionally, inflammatory stenotic lesions such as those occurring in Crohn's disease or tuberculosis can mimic carcinoma.[54]

At present, enteroscopy is usually not available as a routine endoscopic procedure, consequently only extended duodenoscopy and limited ileoscopy additional to colonoscopy are available for small-bowel endoscopic biopsy.[57]

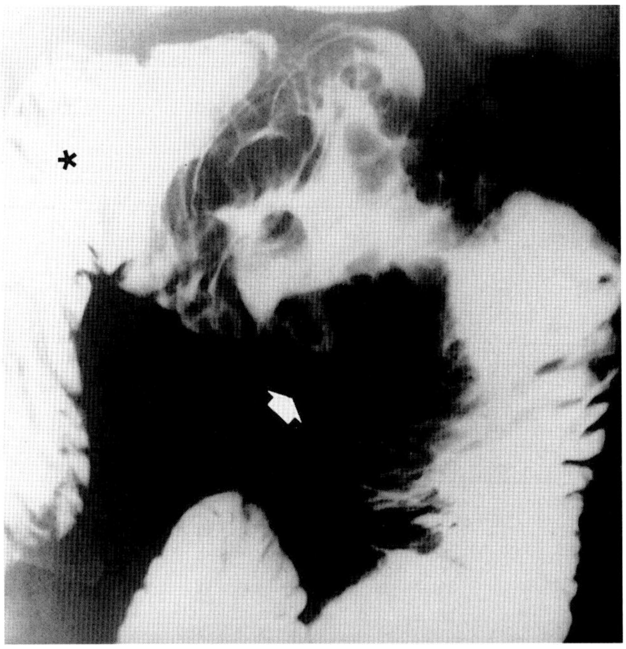

Figure 8.10

Blunt irregular stenosis of the proximal jejunum (broad arrow) a few centimeters distal to the duodenojejunal junction (asterisk) due to a resectable adenocarcinoma.

CT should not be used as a primary diagnostic modality because of its lower degree of diagnostic accuracy despite the fact that, due to improved methods and an increasing number of indications, abdominal CT appears to demonstrate a significant number of small-bowel tumors.[58,59] On CT, carcinoma can be identified as a more than 1.5 cm focal thickening of the intestinal wall, with narrowing of the lumen either concentrically or asymmetrically and dilatation of the proximal bowel. It appears homogeneous or heterogeneous after intravenous contrast, and is possibly associated with an extraluminal mass that is less bulky than that found in lymphoma.[59]

Staging

Small-bowel malignancies often require surgical intervention because of obstruction or hemorrhage, and consequently they are staged surgically. However, CT may be useful to evaluate the

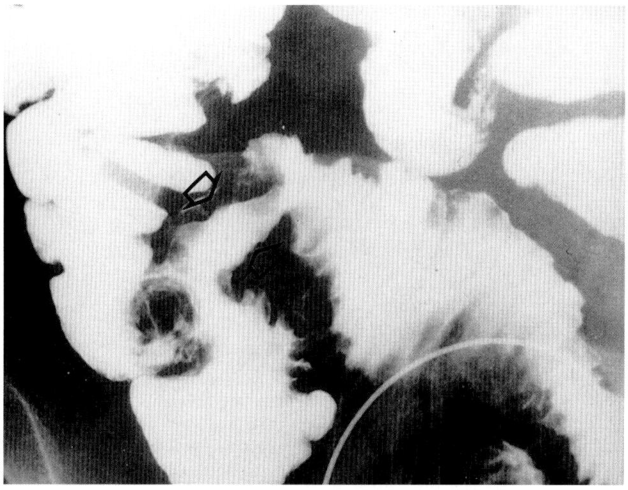

A

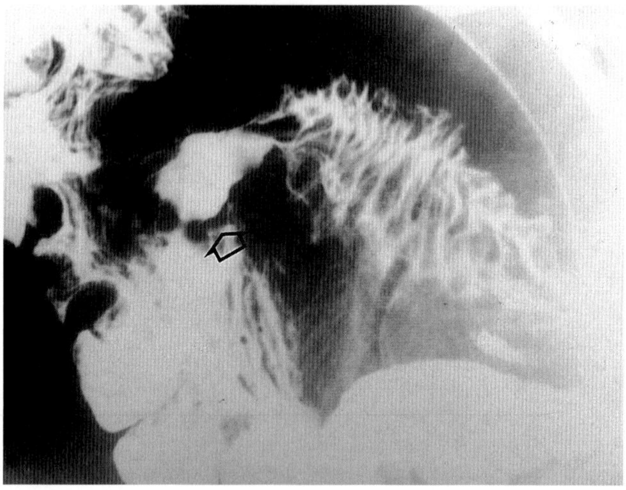

B

Figure 8.11

Small bowel follow-through studies. These are spot films of the opacified ileocaecal region in the filled stage (A) and during compression (B). An ulcerated and stenotic adenocarcinoma is demonstrated (open arrows). Note also the upwards ileal dilatation.

local extent of tumor growth and the presence of metastasis in the mesenteric and retroperitoneal lymph nodes and in the liver, or metastatic implants in the peritoneal cavity. CT may demonstrate large tumors extending beyond the bowel wall, involving the root of the small-bowel mesentery and major blood vessels or neighboring organs, suggesting unresectability.[59] Tumors are usually unresectable when angiographically mesenteric artery branches of the first and second order are invaded.[60] In some duodenal lesions, CT, by showing that the lesion separates clearly from the pancreas, may contribute to the differentiation between the duodenal or pancreatic origin of the cancer.[61] The accuracy of CT examination of the small bowel depends upon optimal filling of the loops with contrast material, which is usually achieved with large volumes (500–1000 ml) of 1–3% barium or water-soluble contrast medium which are drunk at least 1 hour before the examination begins.

Follow up

CT may be of help after surgical resection for following the development of metastasis or recurrence.

Carcinoid tumors

Epidemiology

The small intestine is the most common site for malignant carcinoids, the majority of which occur in the distal part.[62] Carcinoid tumors account for about 20% of malignant small-bowel lesions, and are often invasive when discovered.[63,64] They are rare in the duodenum, accounting for only 3–4% of duodenal neoplasms and being commonly located in the first and second duodenal parts. Despite their variable biologic behavior, all carcinoids are considered to have a malignant potential. Prolonged survival of patients with carcinoids is not uncommon, even in the presence of metastases, if they are adequately managed.[65,66]

Pathology

Carcinoids arise in the intestinal submucosa from enterochromaffin cells. The argyrophilic reaction is the best general stain, but many of the tumors are non-argentaffin.[67] The tumors may be multiple in up to 25% of cases. When smaller than 1.0 cm in diameter, carcinoid tumors may appear histologically benign, but with time all will enlarge, penetrate the bowel wall and tend to invade the mesentery and metastasize to the local lymph nodes and the liver.

Penetration of the bowel wall is present in up to 50% of tumors but occurs less frequently in duodenal tumors than in ileal tumors, which are consistently malignant when greater than 2.0 cm in diameter.[63,64] As they grow through the bowel wall, carcinoid tumors excite an intense hyperplastic response in the muscle layers of the bowel as well as a marked desmoplastic reaction in the adjacent bowel wall and in the invaded mesentery.

The classic carcinoid syndrome is related to serotonin production by the tumor and is almost invariably related to hepatic metastasis.

The World Health Organization (WHO) classification based on 'argentaffinity' of tumors has been replaced by a classification based on immunohistological characteristics.[54]

The topographic site of origin and extent of growth are probably the best predictors of prognosis.

Clinical features

Symptoms are related either to the local development of the carcinoid tumor and may consist of abdominal pain, diarrhea and mediastinal obstruction, or to the carcinoid syndrome, which occurs when serotonin is released in significant quantities into the systemic circulation. In the latter, flushing—particularly following alcohol—and diarrhea, palpitations and intermittent hypertension are the most common manifestations.

Small tumors detected incidentally in the duodenum or in the ileum may be symptomless. The prognosis of invasive tumors is relatively good in the absence of liver metastasis. In the latter case, however, the prognosis is bad, with a 5-year survival of less than 5%.[64]

Imaging

Detection

Duodenoscopy and/or barium studies are the first choice modalities for the demonstration of carcinoid tumors. Small-bowel examinations are significantly successful, even for invasive primary tumors, only if they are performed carefully.[68] In the ileum, the most frequent feature is an intramural or intraluminal filling defect, which may be solitary or multiple (Figure 8.12A and B). Intestinal narrowing, often asymmetrically, thickening of the valvulae conniventes, and separation of adjacent loops with rigidity and fixation may be seen. When fibrosis is associated with a secondary mass in the mesentery, sharp angulation of the involved loop or adjacent loops may be observed.

Angiography has a limited role in detecting the primary neoplasm but angiographic findings are considered quite specific when hypervascular metastases are present in the liver and associated with a stellate configuration, localized kinking and obstruction of small mesenteric arteries, with moderate staining of a tumor mass.[69]

On CT, carcinoid tumors may be seen as homogeneous soft tissue masses involving the intestinal wall and the mesentery. Although in most cases the primary neoplasm is not visualized, the stellate appearance of the mesenteric mass is highly suggestive, particularly when associated with displacement and kinking of adjacent intestinal segments.[70]

Staging

CT can demonstrate the intestine, the mesentery, the lymph nodes and the liver in a single examination and is consequently extremely useful in staging carcinoid tumors (Figure 8.12C). Retractile mesenteritis may be reflected by retraction and kinking of intestinal loops. Mesenteric soft tissue masses with spiculated margins may reflect direct extension or metastasis to the local lymph nodes.[70] Retroperitoneal nodes, ascitis and, of course, hepatic metastases may be present. Hypervascular liver metastases are usually hypodense on precontrast scans and may appear variably on scans obtained after intravenous bolus contrast.[71] They are not always associated with a carcinoid syndrome.

MRI can demonstrate liver metastases which may produce a hyperintense signal on T2-weighted images (Figure 8.12D).

Angiography is more useful for the palliative management of liver metastases by selective embolization than for staging.[65,66]

In vivo somatostatin receptor imaging of carcinoid tumors is opening a new era in identification of primary tumors or metastases.[72]

Follow up

CT is also useful for the follow up of patients after surgery and for monitoring the effect of

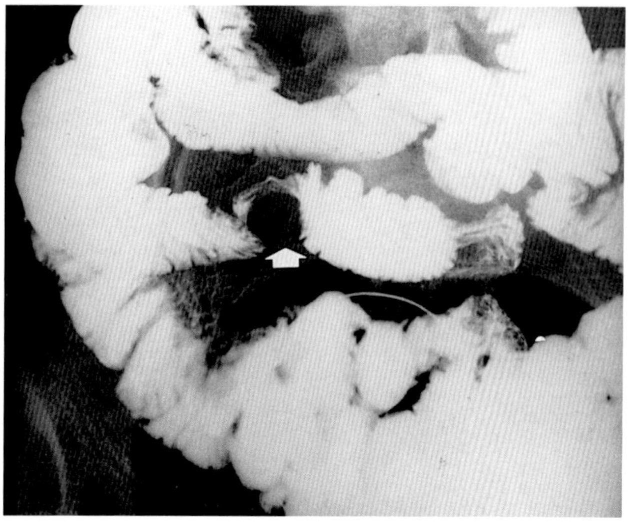

A

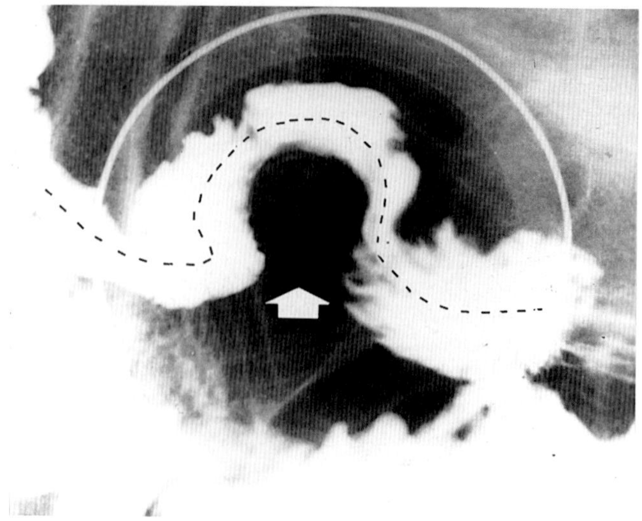

B

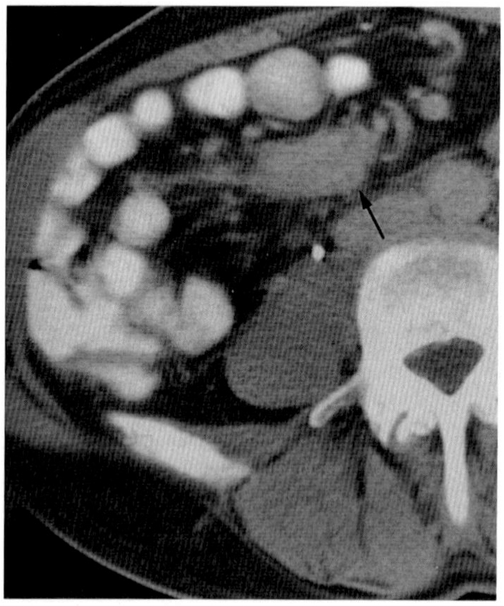

C

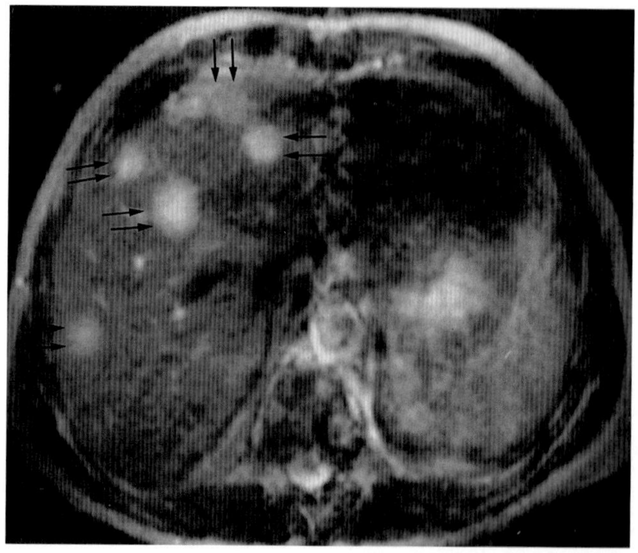

D

Figure 8.12

Primary small carcinoid tumor in the ileum demonstrated by barium follow-through studies.

A Detected filling defect on overview film (broad arrow).

B Compression studies showing a pattern suggestive for carcinoid tumor (mainly submucosal filling defect (broad arrow) on the concave border of an omega-shaped loop (dots)).

C Mesenteric involvement demonstrated on CT as conglomerating enlarged nodes (arrow) around mesenteric vessels, associated with streaks radiating towards adjacent intestinal loops.

D Liver metastases imaged more conspicuously on MR than CT and showing as hypersignal on T2-weighted images (double arrows).

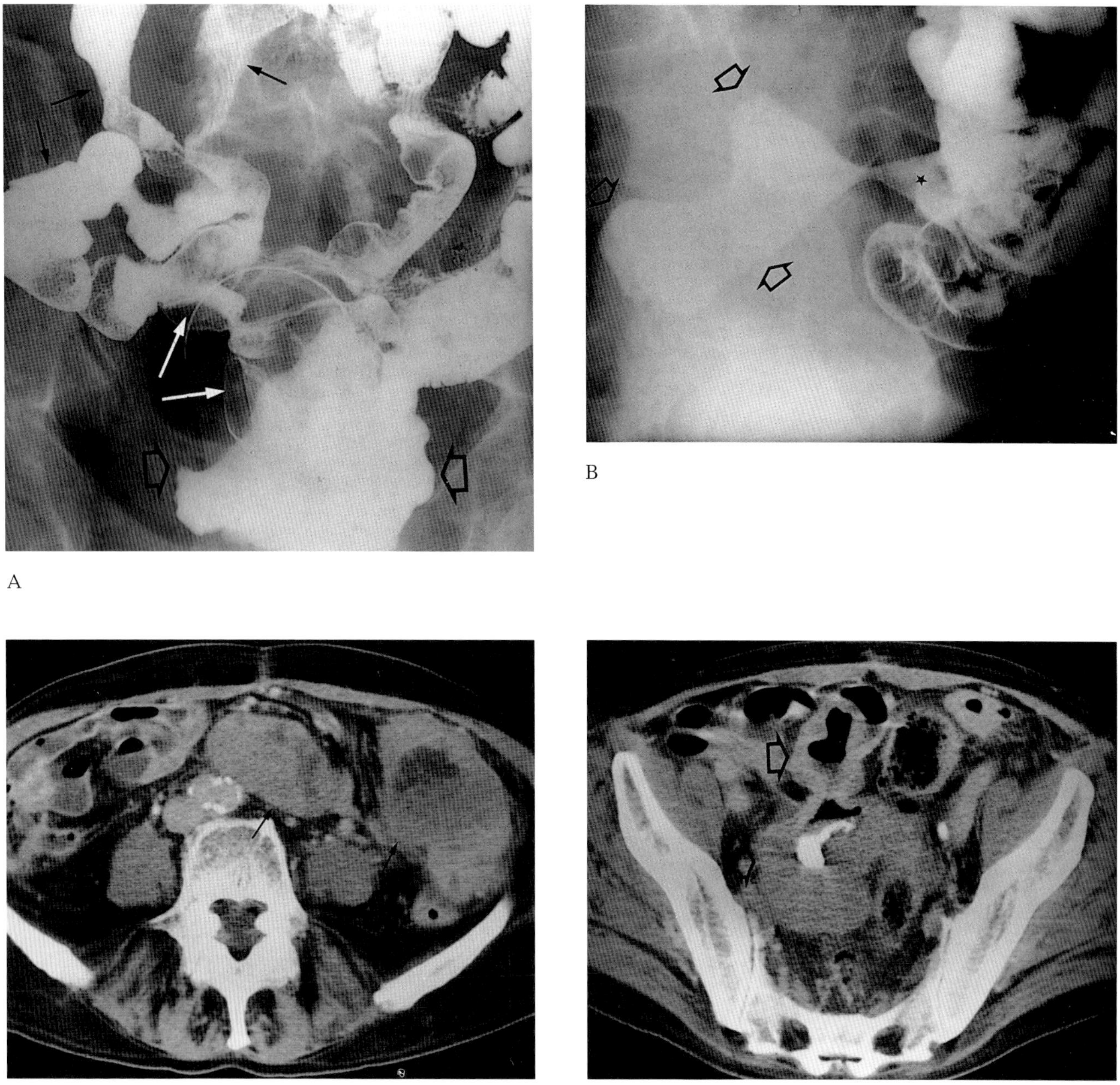

A

B

C

D

Figure 8.13

Small-bowel leiomyosarcoma with peritoneal metastases. Barium studies demonstrated (A, B) an excavated pelvic mass (open arrows) communicating with an adjacent intestinal loop (asterisk on **B**) as well as many impressions on intestinal loops (arrows). (B) On the AP view, the excavated mass (open arrows) superimposes over the lower intestinal loops. CT (C) demonstrated several more or less necrotic soft tissue masses (arrows) as well as (D) two excavated masses (open arrows).

chemotherapy on the disease or of hepatic artery embolization on the liver metastases. After resection of the intestinal lesion, the carcinoid tumor may recur locally with similar signs of mesenteric fibrosis.

Other primary malignancies

Of all gastrointestinal leiomyosarcomas, 90% arise in the small bowel, and leiomyosarcomas are the most common small-intestinal sarcomas.[73] Angiosarcomas and liposarcomas are seen only rarely. Neurofibrosarcomas occur occasionally in association with neurofibromatosis. Kaposi's sarcoma occurs in relation with acquired immune deficiency syndrome (AIDS) and chronic immunosuppressive therapy.[74]

Leiomyosarcomas

Leiomyosarcomas arise from the muscular layers of the intestine or more rarely from the muscularis mucosae. They grow extraluminally and eccentrically, displacing adjacent loops or organs, and tend to become large and necrotic by outgrowing their blood supply. The most important gross finding indicating malignancy—apart from metastasis—is the size of the mass.[75] Intestinal bleeding is the most common presenting symptom.

On barium studies, the main feature is frequently a large extrinsic mass displacing adjacent intestinal loops or organs, possibly associated with a filling defect or evidence of ulceration, cavitation, or fistula formation[76] (Figure 8.13A and B).

Leiomyosarcomas are highly vascular and tend to be visible on angiography even if the study is done at a time when active bleeding is not occurring.[73]

CT can accurately demonstrate the size and extent of the usually large eccentric primary mass as well as the peritoneal and liver metastases, which show a marked enhancement following intravenous contrast.[77] Hypodense areas of central necrosis are usually identified within the primary tumor or metastases (Figure 8.13C and D). Intratumoral gas or oral contrast material can also be seen when the tumor is ulcerated.[59] A large size and a low attenuation center are unreliable CT findings for suggesting the malignant nature of a tumor.[59,61]

Largely excavated leiomyosarcomas should be differentiated from aneurysmal lymphomas and excavating metastatic melanomas.

Secondary neoplasms

The duodenum is involved more commonly by direct spread from a tumor of an adjacent organ than by lymphatic or blood-borne metastases.[78] Carcinoma of the pancreas, right colon, kidney, gall bladder or common bile duct, breast, and teratoma of the testes can cause secondary duodenal involvement.[79] Sometimes patients present with duodenal symptoms before the primary neoplasm has been identified or many years after it has been surgically resected. Clinically, the patients present with obstruction, intussusception, bleeding or, less frequently, perforation.

Secondary neoplasm of the duodenum frequently produces stenotic or ulcerating lesions that appear similar to those of primary carcinoma on barium studies. Invasion of the small bowel occurs most frequently by direct extension from adjacent organs or peritoneal implants and is most common from primary carcinomas of the ovary, colon, uterus and kidney.[78,80]

Blood-borne metastases to the small intestine are rare, and the commonest are from malignant melanoma and primary carcinoma of the breast, lung, kidney and genital tract.[78]

Metastases from carcinoma of the breast result in infiltration with narrowing and stricture formation, while metastases from carcinoma of the lung produce large associated mesenteric masses.[78]

Approximately 50% of patients with AIDS and cutaneous Kaposi's sarcoma have gastrointestinal involvement occurring in the form of multiple nodules.[74]

Characteristic radiologic features consist in a tapered narrowing with intact mucosa, tethering of the mucosal folds and separation of intestinal loops.

Barium studies characteristically show metastatic melanoma as multiple submucosal polypoid lesions, frequently with central ulceration, or as cavitating masses.[81] (Figure 8.14C).

On CT, the major portion of metastatic deposits often appears located in the mesentery, next to the wall of the small bowel (Figure 8.14A and B).[82] CT may demonstrate more clearly the size and extent of lesions when they are secondary to peritoneal carcinomatosis associated with ascitis or macro-

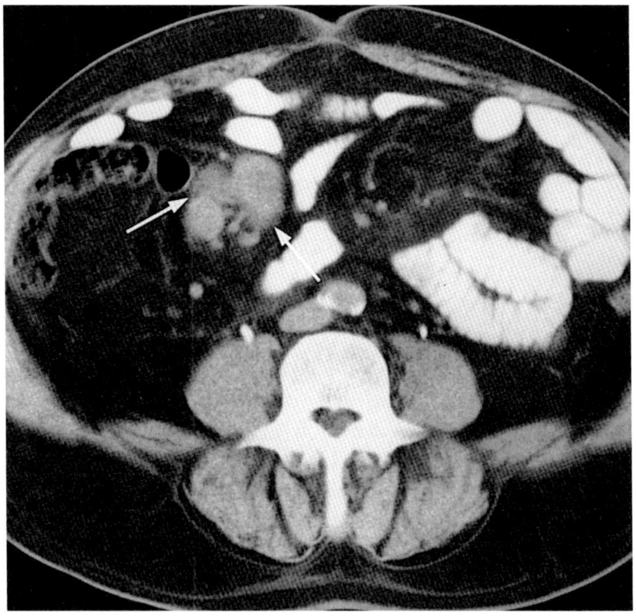

A

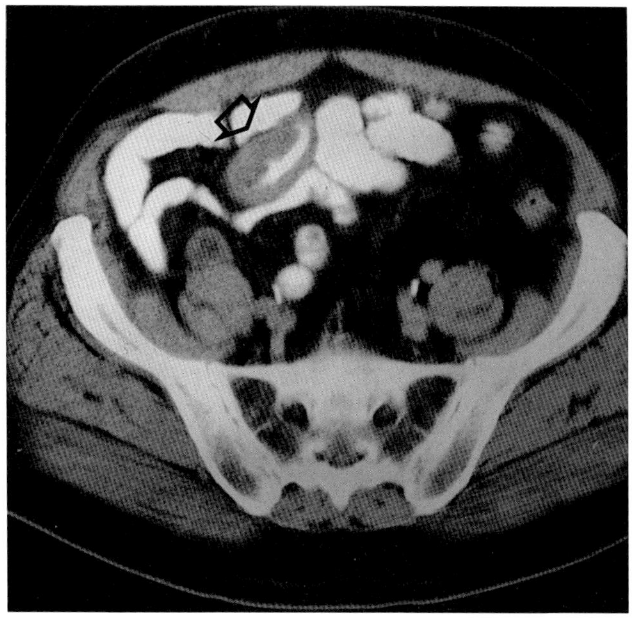

B

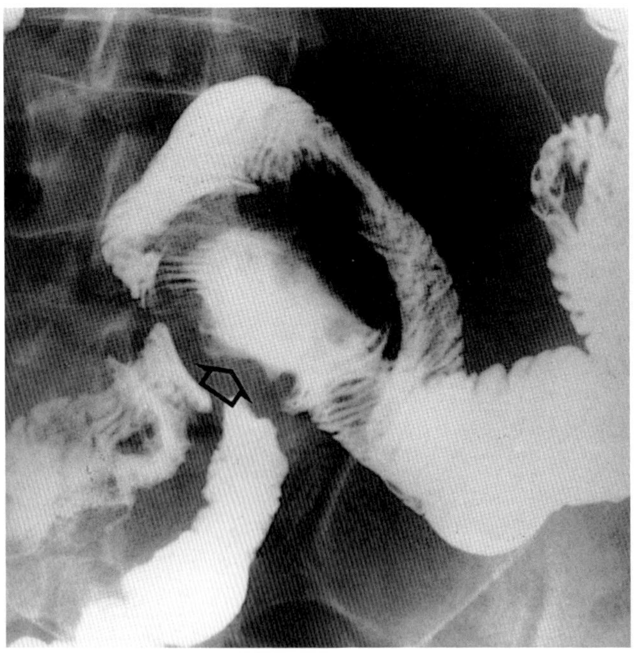

C

Figure 8.14

Skin melanoma resected 1 year earlier. At the time of imaging, the patient had anemia due to surgically proved small bowel metastasis. CT demonstrated (A) enlarged mesenteric nodes (arrows) and (B) a focal small bowel mass (open arrow) which appeared on barium studies (C) as a largely excavated lesion (open arrow).

scopic peritoneal implants. CT is not advocated as a screening method for detecting metastatic disease to the small bowel, but it may provide unique information about the extent and location of lesions detected by other diagnostic techniques.[58]

The work up of patients with small bowel malignant tumors is summarized in Diagram 8.2.

The colon and rectum

Colorectal cancer

Epidemiology

Over 100 000–150 000 new cases of colorectal carcinoma occur in the USA each year, with an almost equal incidence in both sexes.[83] In France 25 000 new cases occur each year.[84] According to the American Cancer Society, the incidence and mortality rate of colorectal cancer in the USA is second after lung cancer in men and third in women; its incidence increased by 9.4% between 1973 and 1986. Colorectal cancer affects primarily the elderly, the risk increasing dramatically above 40 years of age.[83,85] The cancer develops more frequently in the colon than in the rectum, but the distribution of sites has shifted more proximally over recent decades.[84,85]

The differences in incidence between different geographic locations is related to differences in the degree of economic development. The highest rates of colorectal cancer are found in North America, New Zealand and Europe. Within the same geographic area, there are racial differences in incidence; for example, in North America, rectum cancer is less frequent among Blacks and colorectal cancer is less frequent among Hispanics than among Whites.[83] The effects of diet on the incidence are still being studied. Eating higher-fiber food and vegetables seems to reduce risk, whereas eating meat and fatty food tends to increase risk. Environment and life-style factors also seem to play a part in the incidence, for example, the incidence is higher among urban residents than among rural residents and the risk increases rapidly after migration from a low-incidence to a high-incidence area. Predisposing factors for colorectal cancer include a genetic tendency and a medical history of polyps, ulcerative colitis or, to a lesser extent, Crohn's disease or breast or endometrial tumors.[86]

In the majority of patients, development of colorectal cancer usually follows the development of adenomatous polyps and is due to an inherited susceptibility to colonic adenomatous polyps and colorectal cancer, even when the polyp or cancer is apparently isolated.[87] The risk for direct descendants of colorectal cancer patients is three to five times higher than that of the general population.[88] In familial adenomatous polyposis and its variants, polyps of the colon usually arise in the first and second decade, and colorectal cancer develops in almost 100% of untreated patients.[48] In North America and Europe, 5–19% of the general population have one or more adenomatous polyp(s) of the large intestine.[89]

Pathology

The vast majority of colorectal cancers are well-differentiated adenocarcinomas and their histologic variants.[4] The latter are the less frequent and include mucinous adenocarcinomas and linitis plastica of the colon, both very aggressive lesions which grow circumferentially through the wall of the colon, usually with regional lymph-node metastasis.[90]

On resected specimens, the majority of well-differentiated adenocarcinomas are polypoid, fungating or ulcerating masses sharply separated from surrounding normal mucosa. Cecal carcinomas tend to present as bulky masses with a tendency for central necrosis and ulceration. In the sigmoid colon and rectum, the tumors tend to grow into the wall and become annular and constricting. The sigmoid colon and rectum are still more common locations than the cecum, but tumors are becoming more frequent in the right part of the colon.[85]

The development of the colorectal carcinoma is considered to be a multistage process spanning a considerable period of time, sometimes many years.[83] There is a progression from dysplastic or adenomatous changes from apparently normal mucosa to non-invasive microadenoma or microcarcinoma, which by further growing reaches the size required for invasion to begin. Invasion is usually directly into the submucosa but occasionally into the lamina propria mucosae. A minority of colorectal cancers develop in the absence of any intervening adenomatous changes. In those following the adenoma–carcinoma sequence, there is a direct correlation between large dysplastic villous adenomas and invasiveness of the tumor. Invasive colorectal tumors tend to grow perpendicularly to the wall rather than longitudinally.

Lymphatic or hematogenous metastases rarely occur before the carcinoma has spread by direct continuity through the muscularis propria into the extracolonic tissues. Lymphatic spread follows an orderly and predictable course.[58] The first nodes to receive metastases usually are those adjacent to the primary tumor. The next nodes to be affected are those located in the corresponding regional lymphatic chain. Colon tumors metastasize primarily to the liver through the portal vein and subsequently to the lung. Rectal tumors may metastasize directly to the lung because of venous drainage from inferior hemorrhoidal veins to iliac veins, and directly into the inferior vena cava through the liver. Consequently, it is unusual to find lung metastases in a patient with colon cancer above the rectum whose liver is free of metastases.

The prognosis of primary colorectal cancer is clearly linked to the stage of the disease, as is the risk of recurrence after curative surgery.[91]

There are many different classifications for separating patients with colorectal cancer into prognostic groups in order to make decisions about treatment.[58] The system described by Dukes in 1932 and its modification by Astler and Coller in 1954 are largely used in the surgical literature, but these do not segregate patients with remote metastases.[58,92]

In the Dukes' system, tumor limited to the wall is classified stage A, tumor extending directly through pericolorectal tissue is stage B, tumor spreading to regional lymph nodes is stage C. In the Astler and Coller classification, stage A according to Dukes is subdivided into stage A, tumor extending into the submucosa, and stage B1, tumor extending into but not through the muscularis. Further, the stage C of Dukes is subdivided into stage C1, tumor extending into the muscularis with regional lymph-node involvement, and stage C2, tumor extending through the muscularis with regional lymph-node involvement.

The classification proposed by the International Union against Cancer (UICC) is based on the TNM staging system for colorectal cancer (Tables 8.5 and 8.6).[4] The TNM system allows a precise histopathologic staging but has found only limited practical application for pretreatment staging, mainly because of the inability of the available imaging methods to correctly classify colorectal tumors by this system. Imaging cannot detect tumors in normal-sized lymph nodes, and enlarged lymph nodes may not contain tumors.

Table 8.5 Comparison of staging systems.

Dukes' system	*TNM (UICC) system*	
Stage	*Stage*	*Grouping*
A	I	T1/T2, N0, M0
B	II	T3/T4, N0, M0
C	III	Any T, Any N, M0
D[a]	IV	Any T, any N, M1

[a]Stage D, tumor with peritoneal seeding or distant metastases added by Turnbull et al, 1967 (see Thoeni [92]).

Table 8.6 The TNM classification of colorectal cancer.

	Stage	*Description*
Primary tumor	T1	Tumor invades submucosa
	T2	Tumor invades muscularis propria
	T3	Tumor invades directly into subserosa or into non-peritonealized pericolonic/perirectal tissues
	T4	Tumor perforates the visceral peritoneum or invades directly organs or structures
Nodal involvement	N1	Spread in 1–3 pericolonic/perirectal nodes
	N2	Spread in 4 or more pericolonic/perirectal nodes
	N3	Spread in any lymph node along a named vascular trunk
Distant metastases	M0	No distant metastases
	M1	Distant metastases present

Clinical features and screening

Few patients are asymptomatic when their colon or rectal cancer is found, and the great majority have one or more symptoms. The most commonly recorded symptoms are melena, constipation and diarrhea occurring often intermittently, tenesmus and abdominal pain. A feeling of incomplete evacuation or of rectal mass is also fairly common in patients with rectal cancer.[93] Cecal carcinoma tends to cause insidious bleeding often leading to anemia as the presenting symptom. Some colon cancers even present with acute obstruction.

The diagnosis of colorectal cancer is based on a thorough clinical history and physical examination, digital rectal examination, protosigmoidoscopy and barium enema to detect synchronous lesions. Digital rectal examination will generally enable identification of one-third of the colorectal cancers. Visualization of the tumor by protosigmoidoscopy is required to establish the diagnosis by biopsies.

The reported incidence of synchronous primary cancers in the colorectum ranges from 2–8%, and benign polyps have been found in 12–62% of patients with single cancer and 38–86% of patients with synchronous cancers.[94]

Tumors sited higher in the rectum or in the colon are classically demonstrated first by barium enema and subsequently visualized by endoscopy and biopsies taken.[83] More recently, however, colonoscopy has been more and more frequently performed as the initial morphological investigation of the colon in patients with suspected or known tumor.[92,95] A comparison of both techniques shows that each has some advantages that the other does not (Table 8.7). In particular double-contrast barium enema is less expensive, less invasive and has a higher success rate for examination of the entire colon than colonoscopy, which may be unable to pass through a narrowed colonic lumen or to reach the cecum. For these reasons, colonoscopy is probably not an optimal primary technique for routine examination. Colonoscopy, however, represents a major breakthrough in diagnosis and treatment of colon cancer because most adenomas and small cancers can be removed via colonoscope on an outpatient basis. Barium enema and colonoscopy may be complementary, as endoscopy has been shown to miss 10–20% of the lesions that are seen on radiologic examinations.[88] Barium enema is not generally necessary to evaluate cancers demonstrated by an endoscopic examination but, in case of partial colonoscopy, the remainder of the colon must be assessed to identify other possible colorectal pathologies.

Curative surgery remains the best form of treatment of colorectal carcinoma. However, pretreatment assessment of local invasion and perirectal

Table 8.7 Barium enema compared with colonoscopy in the examination of colorectal cancer.[a]

	Barium enema[b]	*Colonoscopy*
Success rate for examination of entire colon	High(?)	64–90%
Sensitivity for cancer	65–99% DCE ± 95%	70–95%
Sensitivity for polyps larger than 7–10 mm	SCE 80% DCE 90%	95%
Sensitivity for polyps smaller than 5 mm	Lower than endoscopy	Higher than DCE
Multireading capability	Yes	No
Tissue removal	No	Yes
Patient acceptabilty	SCE good DCE fair	Good
Perforation rate	0.01%	0.2%
Mortality rate	0.002%	0.02%
Cost		2 to 10 times higher

[a]Data summarized from Whalen [83]
[b]SCE = single-contrast enema; DCE = double-contrast enema

lymph-node involvement may guide more accurately the choice of individual surgical procedures as well as the selection of patients who would be suitable for adjuvant therapy.[92,96] The detection of distant metastases may be achieved with varying degrees of accuracy by biochemical and imaging techniques, particularly CT and chest radiograph. This topic is addressed in Chapter 9.

The prognosis of patients with colorectal cancer is closely related to the stage of the disease. Under the Dukes' classification, the 5-year survival rate decreases from 81–85% for stage A, to 64–78% for stage B, 27–33% for stage C, and 5–14% for stage D.[92] The risk of local recurrence after an apparent curative resection is related both to disease extension beyond the bowel wall and to nodal involvement. Local recurrence occurs in 20–25% of patients with tumors confined to the wall but with nodal involvement, compared with 30–35% of patients with tumors that extend through the wall without nodal involvement. The local recurrence rate in patients with both tumor extension through the bowel wall and nodal metastases doubles to 50–70%.[58,97,98]

Earlier detection of locally recurring disease is another area in the management of colorectal cancer where surgical decision making could benefit from more precise anatomic information.[91]

Population screening for symptoms of colorectal cancer is not 'profitable', and the only practical methods of population screening are tests to detect blood in the feces, but these have many limitations. In the population as a whole, the only risk factor that is helpful for selection is the age of the patient, so that screening a population below the age of approximately 45 years is unlikely to be cost-effective. Endoscopic methods of screening, which do have a high accuracy, are practical only in high-risk groups.[99]

The hemoccult test, the most commonly used fecal occult blood test (FOBT), remains a significant method for cancer detection. Because most colonic carcinomas bleed intermittently, FOBT has shown a relatively low sensitivity for cancer detection: 50–70% with a specificity of 90–94%. However, the test successfully detects a large proportion of early cancers.[100] The FOBT provides us with at least a reasonably effective, safe and inexpensive screening test. In general, only 2–6% of FOBTs produce positive results, which means that the number of positive studies that warrant further evaluation is not excessive. Of patients with positive FOBT, 5-10% will have colorectal cancer, and most of these cancers will be Dukes' stage A or B. An additional 13–40% of patients with a positive FOBT will have adenomatous polyps in the colon or rectum.[101] An asymptomatic patient screening strategy based on 60 cm flexible sigmoidoscopy, having a 80% success rate for examination of the entire sigmoid colon, has been suggested to be able to detect 90% of patients with colorectal polyps: it is followed by barium enema in patients who do not have adenomas detected by sigmoidoscopy, and by colonoscopy in patients in whom adenomas are found on sigmoidoscopy.[100]

In many institutions, flexible sigmoidoscopy combined with a well-performed barium enema, is used in place of colonoscopy alone for safe, cost-effective, complete and accurate examination of the colon in patients with a positive FOBT.[100,102]

Colonoscopy also causes more complications than barium enema, which has a similar detection rate for cancer, and therefore it is impractical as a routine screening tool.

Imaging

Detection

Imaging the abdomen by US and CT can be useful for detecting colonic tumors that are clinically suspected in patients with non-specific symptoms or are still undiagnosed at the time the patient is imaged (Figure 8.15). The sensitivity of CT for detecting primary carcinoma of the colon varies betwen 68 and 95%, depending on the size of the lesion and the quality of the examination.[103] However, CT cannot be used as a primary modality in diagnosing colorectal tumors because of its low sensitivity for small lesions and the low specificity of its findings.[58]

Double-contrast barium enema (DCE) of optimal quality is considered by expert radiologists to be as accurate as colonoscopy for the detection of colorectal cancer in symptomatic patients.[88,99,104] It is considered less accurate than colonoscopy for the detection of polyps smaller than 1.0 cm, the difference in their detection rates being 5% for polyps larger than 5 mm. On the other hand, in the non-radiologic literature mainly, DCE is considered less accurate than colonoscopy for the detection of polyps as well as cancer.[105] Despite a high accuracy rate, both modalities have limitations in sensitivity for colorectal tumors, but the fact that limitations are different for each technique makes the techniques potentially complementary.[106] Single-contrast enema (SCE)—requiring low density barium (20% w/v), effective compression and high kilovoltage filming—is almost as accurate as DCE for the detection of advanced cancer, and

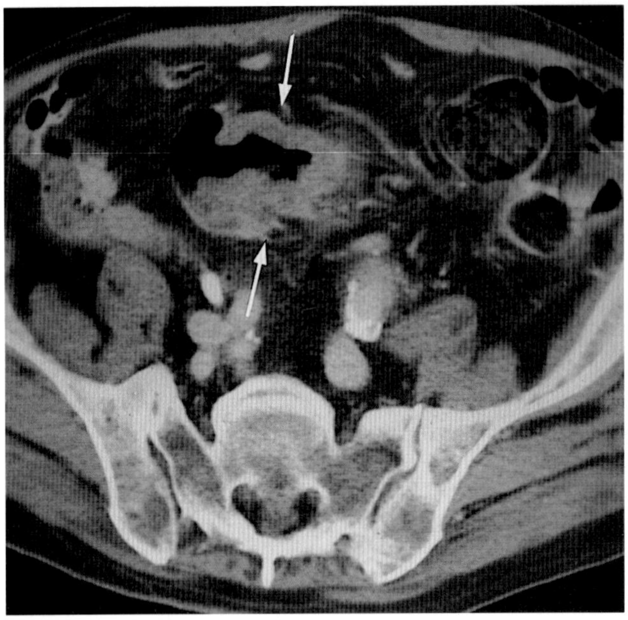

A

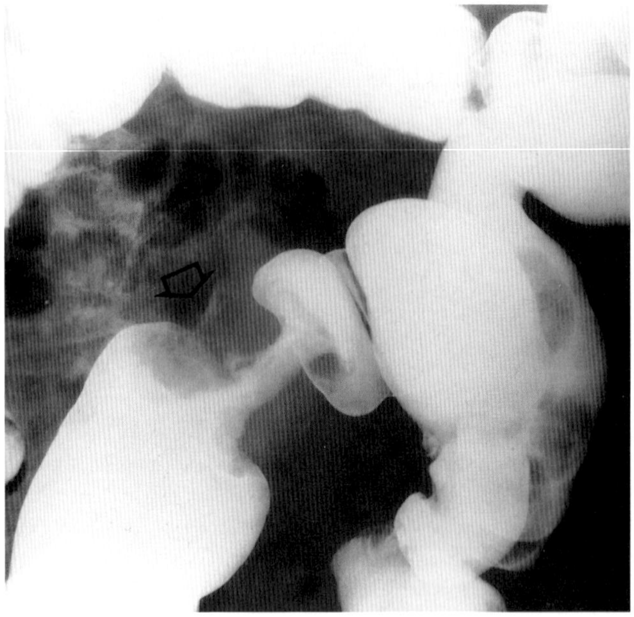

B

Figure 8.15

Occasionally imaging studies suggest a bowel neoplasm before the lesion has been diagnosed by barium enema or endoscopy.

A CT findings suggested a mass lesion in the sigmoid (arrows).

B The findings were subsequently confirmed by contrast enema (open arrow).

significantly less accurate for the detection of polyps and tumors smaller than 1–2 cm in size.[97,104]

DCE should be performed in patients with clinical signs who are at risk for colon neoplasm—predominantly patients over 40 years of age—unless they are too old, insufficiently mobile or cooperative or if preparation is less than ideal.[104]

In most cases of small polypoid filling defects in the colon, it is not possible on the basis of radiologic information to tell whether the tumor is benign or malignant.[107] The only helpful criterion is size: polyps less than 1 cm in diameter harbor carcinoma in 1% of cases, polyps 1–2 cm have a 10% incidence of malignancy, and polyps over 2 cm are malignant in 33–46% of cases.[108] However, as tumors grow, they assume the more classical appearance of fungating intraluminal masses or constricting lesions—more or less circumferential—with overhanging margins and mucosal destruction, and the differential diagnosis is usually not difficult (Figure 8.16).

Because of the risk of synchronous primary cancers and polyps, the entire colon should be carefully examined when a primary tumor is found. In most cases, contrast enema is possible even when the tumor is severely obstructing.

Staging

Accurate pre-operative staging of rectal carcinoma has taken an increased importance with the implementation of localized resection for superficial non-invasive tumors, the sphincter-saving operation for localized malignancies and pre-operative radiation therapy for more advanced lesions. Clinical evaluation has not proved sufficiently reliable, and digital examination of rectal cancers, with an overall accuracy of 50–70% and a sensitivity for

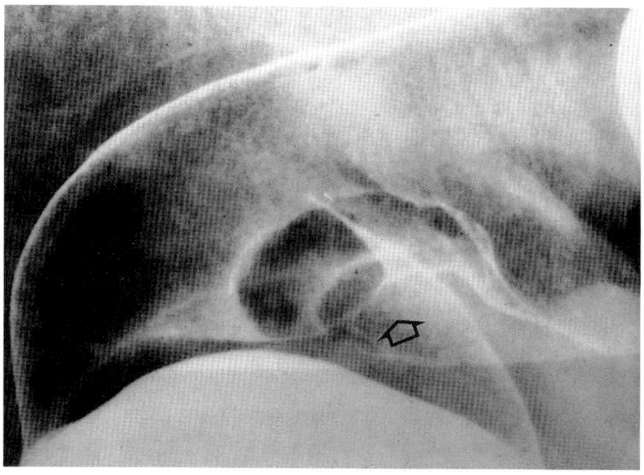

Figure 8.16

Ulceration of an elevated small-colon carcinoma often correlates with invasion outside the submucosa layer. This close-up view of the rectosigmoid shows a small invasive carcinoma (open arrow).

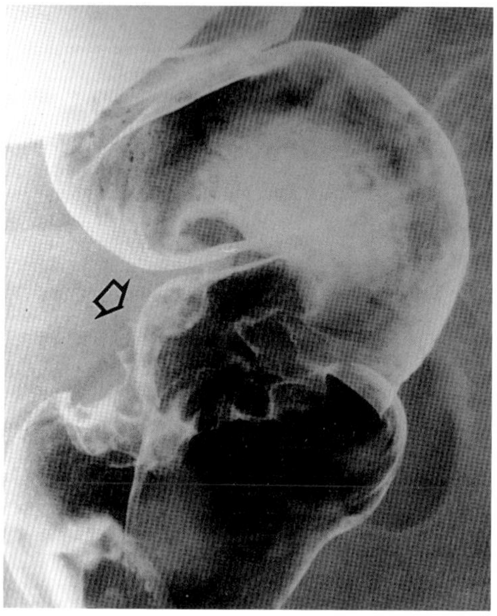

A

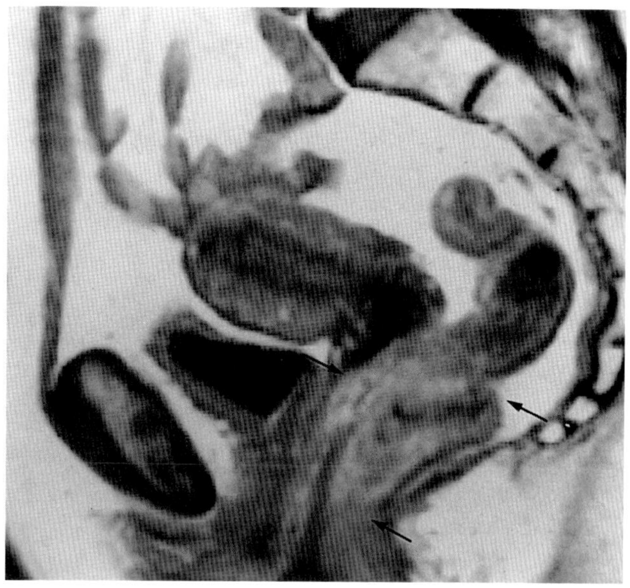

C

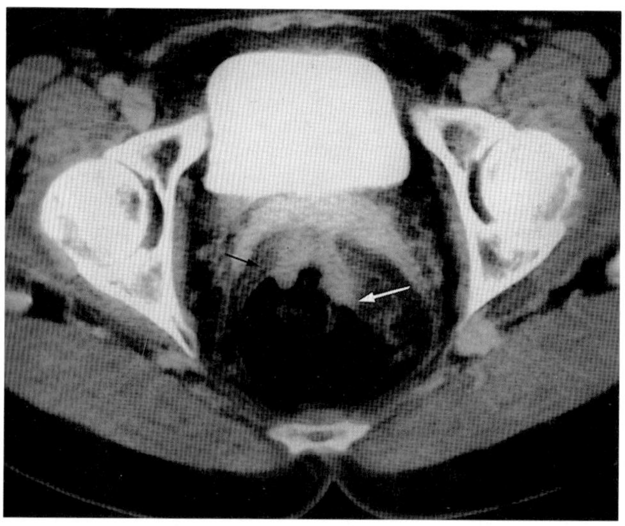

B

Figure 8.17

Rectum carcinoma detection and staging.

A Barium enema shows an ulcerated rectal mass (open arrow).

B The ulcerated mass and infiltration of anterior perirectal fat is demonstrated on CT (arrows).

C T1-weighted SE image after intravenous gadolinium delineates the mass in the sagittal plane (between arrows) from the vagina and the muscle levator ani and shows its extension into the anal canal.

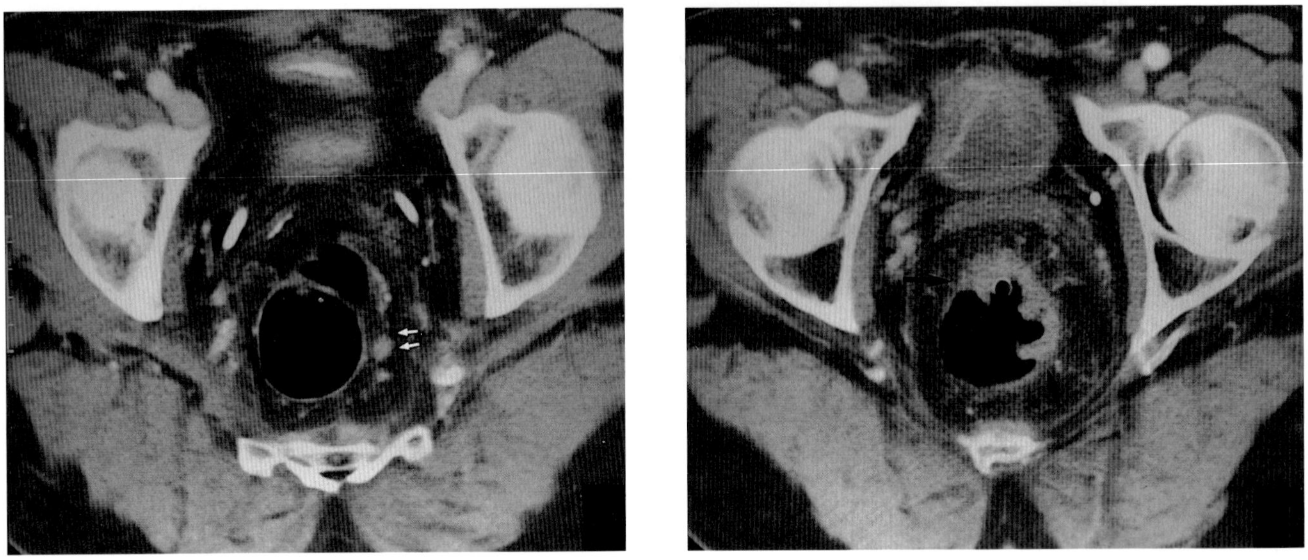

A B

Figure 8.18

CT staging of rectum carcinoma.

A Normal rectal wall thickness, but enlarged lymph node in perirectal fat (double arrow).

B A more caudal slice shows an ulcerated rectal carcinoma invading through the rectal wall in the perirectal fat (between arrows).

enlarged lymph nodes of 50%, is only reliable for clinical stage I non-invasive rectal tumors.[109]

Barium enema and colonoscopy cannot assess the local, regional and distant extent of a cancer. However, fungating intraluminal tumors of the colon have a higher 5-year survival rate of 83% compared with the 28% rate for ulcerating tumors. Ulcerating tumors invariably have tumor extension through the entire thickness of the wall and are associated with a high incidence of lymph-node metastasis[110] (Figure 8.17). On rare occasions, barium enema is helpful in staging colorectal cancer by demonstrating pericolonic peritoneal metastasis or, more rarely, distant colon metastasis.

At present, CT together with transrectal endosonography (TES) is more accurate for local staging and allows appropriate treatment planning before surgery.[92,96,111,112] CT may image colorectal cancer as a discrete mass of focal-wall thickening and demonstrate direct extension of disease in adjacent fat and structures as well as local, regional and distant enlarged lymph nodes, but it is unable to assess precisely the cancer extent in the wall (Figures 8.17 and 8.18). A CT staging method was introduced in 1981 to correlate the CT findings with Dukes' classification[92] (Table 8.8). Early in the 1980s enthusiastic reports showed high correlation of accuracy of CT findings and surgical pathologic findings.[58] Subsequent — more ctitical — studies showed a lower correlation of accuracy of CT and pathologic findings and questioned the sensitivity of CT for the detection of invaded lymph nodes below 1.5 cm (22–73%) and for the detection of local tumor extent in pericolonic/rectal fat (57–77%).[58,92] However, the accuracy of CT increases in relation with the increase in the Dukes' stage of the lesions, reaching 81% for Dukes' stage D lesions.[103] Consequently, CT staging is not recommended routinely for primary colorectal tumors, due to its poor sensitivity in detecting possible lymph-node involvement. CT should be reserved for those patients in whom locally extensive or widespread or even complicated disease is suspected and in whom the resectability of the lesion is questionable.

MR imaging is becoming an important modality for evaluating the pelvis but shows similar limitations to those of CT in predicting TNM classification of rectal cancer, and it has a 40% sensitivity

Table 8.8 CT staging of primary recurrent colorectal tumor.[92]

Stage	*Description*
I	Intraluminal mass without thickening of wall
II	Thickened wall (>0.6 cm) or pelvic mass; no invasion or extension to side walls
IIIa	Thickened wall or pelvic mass, with invasion of adjacent structures but not the pelvic side walls or abdominal wall
IIIb	Thickened wall or pelvic mass with extension to pelvic side walls and/or abdominal wall without distant metastases
IV	Distant metastases with or without local abnormality

for detecting metastatic spread to pelvic lymph nodes.[113] MR is slightly superior to CT in determining the distance of the lower tumor edge from the levator ani.[113] Improvement in imaging technique by special surface coils may enable accurate staging of local extent of rectal carcinoma, but it fails to improve the sensitivity for the detection of lymph nodes.[114] Fat suppression sequence and contrast enhanced images may also improve MR resolution[115] (Figure 8.17). Specimen studies with surface coils and preliminary clinical studies with endorectal coils have shown great promise for the assessment of local tumor extent.[116,117]

Transrectal endosonography performed with a non-optic ultrasonic instrument or, more recently, with an echoendoscope, is able to display the normal layers of the rectum and colon wall (Figure 8.19). Colorectal cancer has a hypoechoic appearance on the sonogram; by comparing the changes caused by a tumor with the normal sonogram, the depth of tumor invasion in and beyond the wall can be assessed (Figures 8.19 to 8.21). An endosonography (ES) staging method was introduced in 1985 to correlate the ES findings with TNM classification[118] (Table 8.9). ES allows accurate staging of all tumors except T2 carcinomas, which tend to be overstaged as UT3 due to the non-specific inflammation that often surrounds the tumor.[112,119] The overall accuracy of tumor staging with ES varies between 78 and 93% in rectal carcinoma, and is 93% in colon carcinoma.[112,119] ES may detect enlarged lymph nodes of 4.0 mm or more in diameter that result from non-specific inflammation or metastasis (Figure 8.22). The overall accuracy of lymph-node staging with ES varies between 70 and 73%, with a sensitivity varying between 68 and 74%, and a specificity varying between 55 and 77%.[112,119] In comparison with CT and MR, ES is the most accurate imaging method for staging of local rectal cancer.[120] It has also been suggested that ES is accurate for detecting the degeneration of villous adenomas.[96]

ES could have an impact on therapy, in particular for tumors confined to the mucosa and submucosa and possibly also for tumors confined to the muscularis propria without nodal involvement in selected elderly patients who could be treated by local excision.[119]

Follow up

In the early postoperative period, early after curative resection of colorectal cancer, contrast and imaging radiography essentially serve to evaluate complications such as leak of the anastomosis or fluid collections and abscesses. In the longer term, these investigations serve to evaluate for evidence of local recurrence, distant metastases, and metachronous polyps and cancers in the remaining colon.

The major risk of tumor recurrence occurs during the first 5 years following treatment; 70% of recurrences are detected during the first 2 years in most series.[101, 121] Two patterns of local recurrent disease are recognized after cancer resection: suture-line recurrence, representing a minority; and extraluminal recurrence, occurring in most instances near the anastomosis or in the operative bed. The latter is the usual site of local recurrence after abdominoperineal excision.[122]

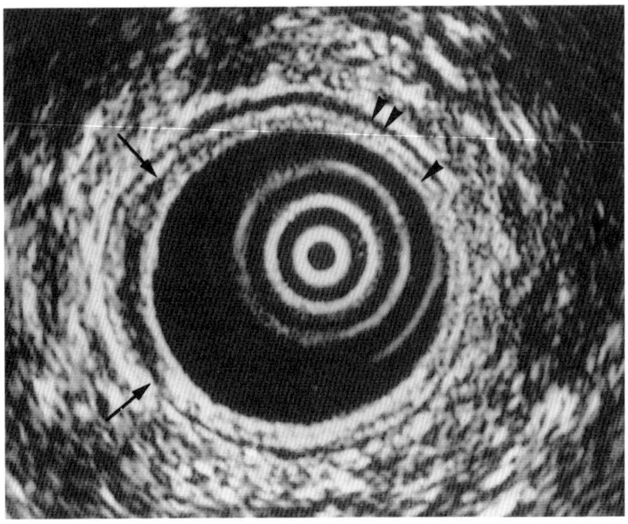

Figure 8.19

Endoechographic demonstration of the normal rectal wall as a five-layer structure: three hyperechoic and two hypoechoic layers. The inner hypoechoic layer corresponds to the mucosa (single arrowhead) and the outermost one to the muscularis propria (double arrowhead). UT1 tumor limited to the mucosa is demonstrated on the right side of the endoechogram as a hypoechoic thickening of the mucosa layer (between arrows), the lesion being separated from the muscularis propria by a normal hyperechoic layer.

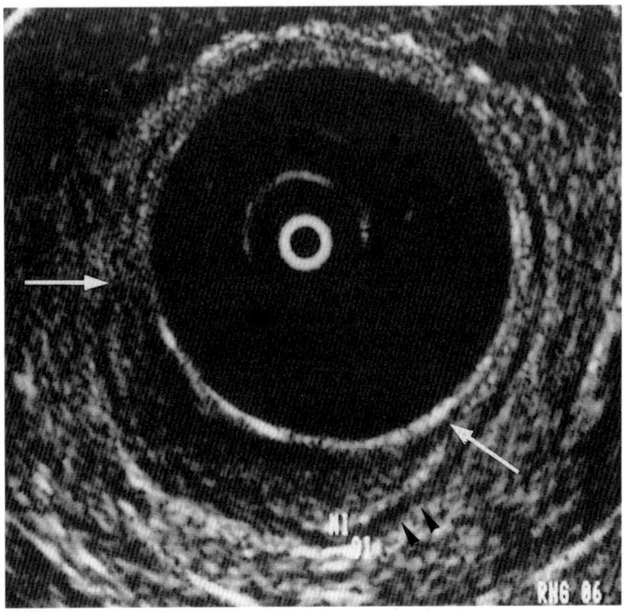

Figure 8.20

Stage UT2 adenocarcinoma (between arrows) extending into the muscularis propria (double arrowhead).

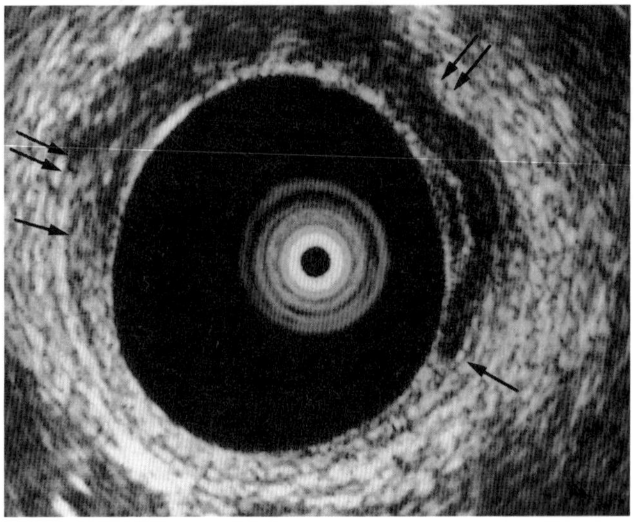

Figure 8.21

Large UT3 adenocarcinoma of the anterior half circumference of the rectum (between arrows) extending into and partly beyond the muscularis propria (between double arrows).

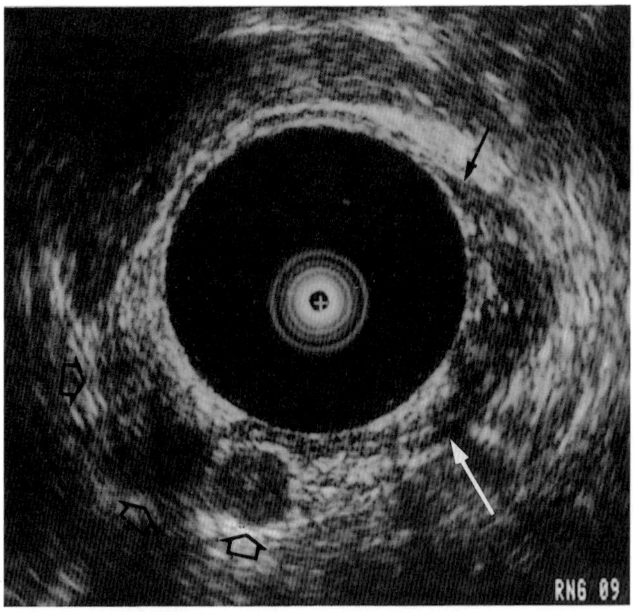

Figure 8.22

UT3 adenocarcinoma on the left side of the rectum (between arrows). Enlarged metastatic perirectal nodes are also demonstrated (open arrows).

Table 8.9 Transrectal endosonography staging of primary rectal tumor.[118]

	Stage	*Description*
Primary tumor depth	UT1	Tumor invades mucosa and submucosa
	UT2	Tumor invades into the muscularis propria
	UT3	Tumor invades through the muscularis propria
	UT4	Tumor invades directly adjacent organs
Lymph node involvement	UN0	Absence of involvement
	UN1	Involvement present

Routine postoperative sigmoidoscopy or barium enema and colonoscopy should detect suture-line recurrence but, as true anastomotic recurrence is rare, these investigations are unlikely to have a major impact on the early diagnosis of recurrent disease. Because most recurrences, including anastomotic ones, are initially extramucosal, imaging is the most sensitive method. Furthermore, imaging has a distinct advantage: identification of possible local recurrence in patients who have undergone an abdominal perineal excision.

Recurrence is suggested clinically by new symptomatology, rising carcinoembryonic antigen or physical examination. Carcinoembryonic antigen (CEA), an antigen marker, has become useful principally in following the absence and detecting recurrence of colorectal cancer.[123] A progressive elevation is characteristic of local recurrence if distant metastasis can be ruled out. But even in proved recurrence, imaging methods have to demonstrate the exact extent of tumorous mass to allow planning of further treatment. A substantial number of patients who develop pelvic recurrence also have concomitant or subsequent systemic metastases, which are at least as great a problem as local recurrence in determining survival.[124] However, the symptoms from local recurrence tend to dominate whenever it occurs.

Early diagnosis and treatment of local recurrent colonic carcinoma has been associated with an improved prognosis.[91] This implies detection before the development of clinical evidence, including laboratory studies such as CEA.

CT has been the most frequently performed study in assessing recurrent carcinoma after surgery for tumors in the sigmoid or rectum and is more sensitive than CEA values.[125–129] Its main role in evaluation of local recurrence has been for the detection of pelvic tumor after abdominoperineal resection.[125,130] The accuracy of CT in evaluating patients with suspected recurrent colorectal cancer is significantly better than it is for the pre-operative staging of these patients. CT is accurate in detecting local recurrence as well as lymph-node metastases, with an overall accuracy for recurrent rectosigmoid cancer of 87%, a sensitivity of 91% and a specificity of 72%.[58] In symptomatic patients, CT demonstrates soft tissue masses of 3–5 cm in size, appearing solid, centrally hypodense or, rarely, as gas-containing masses (Figures 8.23 and 8.24). In the absence of invasion of adjacent structures or bone, differentiation between local recurrent cancer and postoperative change (hematoma, abscess, fibrosis and normal pelvic structures) cannot be based on visual criteria alone or on a single CT examination[127,129,131,132] (Figure 8.25).

Percutaneous CT-guided fine-needle biopsy, which is the most sensitive method, and serial CT follow-up studies are common approaches to the problem of detecting recurrences, but both have limitations due to false-negative biopsy results and no change in CT findings over time[127,131,132] (Figure 8.26). To detect minor changes that may represent early asymptomatic recurrence, all patients who have undergone resection for rectal or sigmoid carcinoma should have a baseline CT 2–4 months after surgery, and subsequently every 6 months for 2 years. CT should then be performed at yearly intervals for 3 years. A CT-guided biopsy should be performed on any new or enlarged presacral mass or enlarged lymph node not present on a previous study.[132]

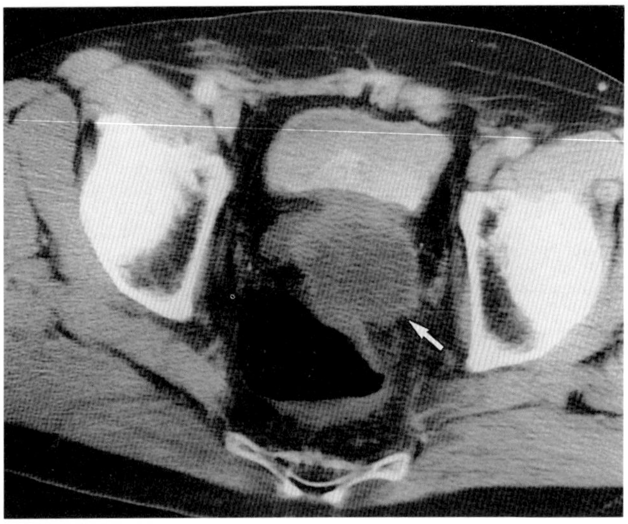

A

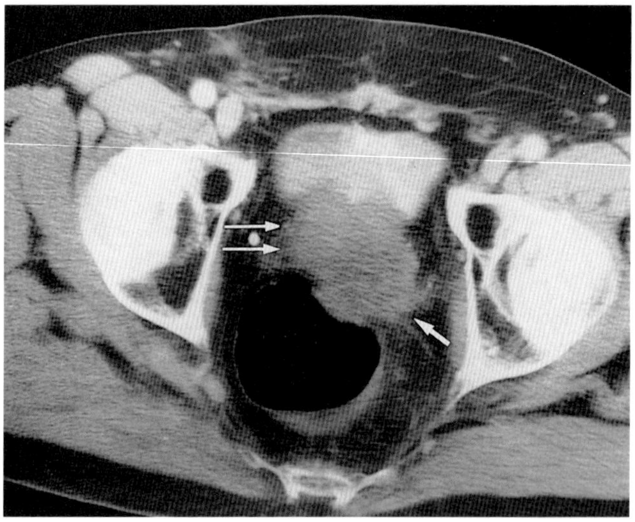

B

Figure 8.23

Extracolonic recurrence of sigmoid carcinoma after surgery.

A Hypodense mass outside the lumen of the rectum (arrow).

B Mass (arrow) invading the prostate (double arrow).

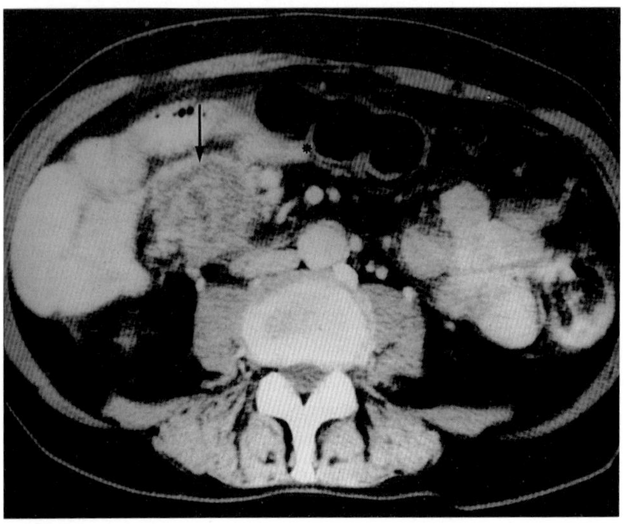

Figure 8.24

Mesenteric recurrence of carcinoma after right hemicolectomy (arrow); normal ileocolic anastomosis (asterisk) is seen.

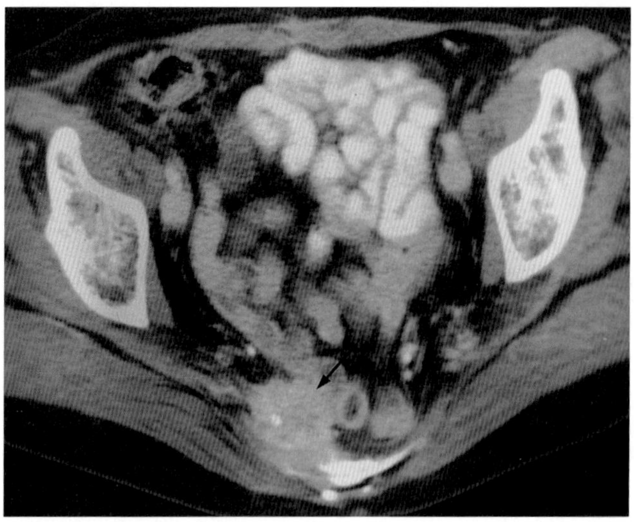

Figure 8.25

Recurrent carcinoma after rectal amputation invading pelvic soft tissues and right part of sacrum is seen on CT (arrow).

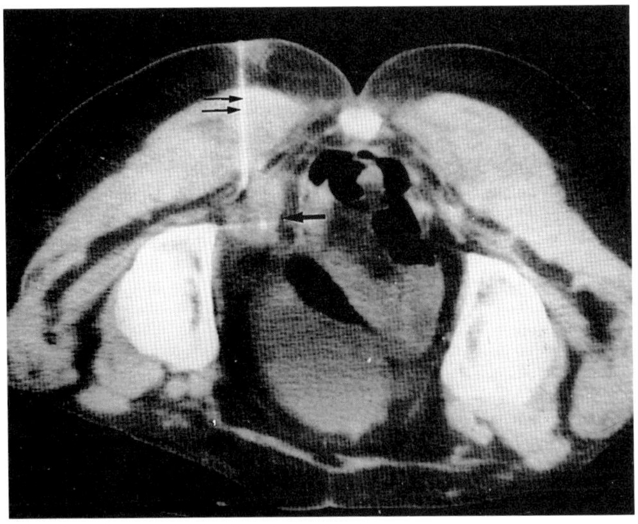

Figure 8.26

After rectal amputation, recurrence of carcinoma in pelvic lymph nodes (arrow) is seen and cytologic diagnosis is established by percutaneous CT-guided fine-needle aspiration biopsy (double arrow).

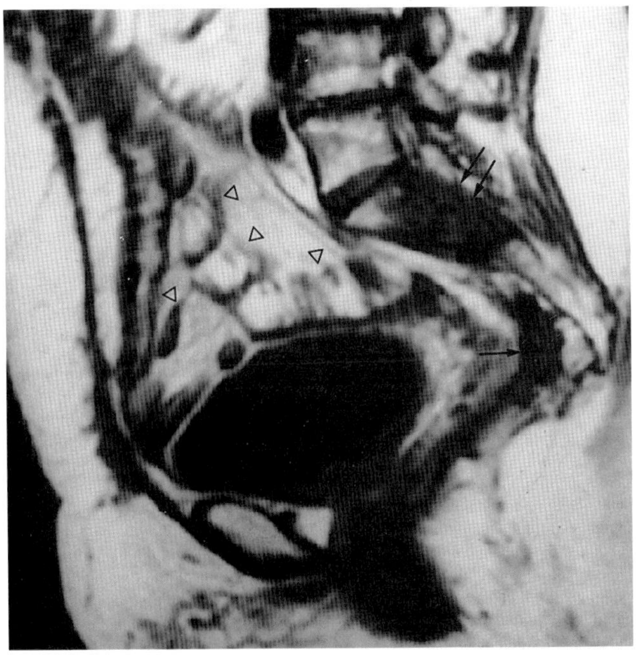

A

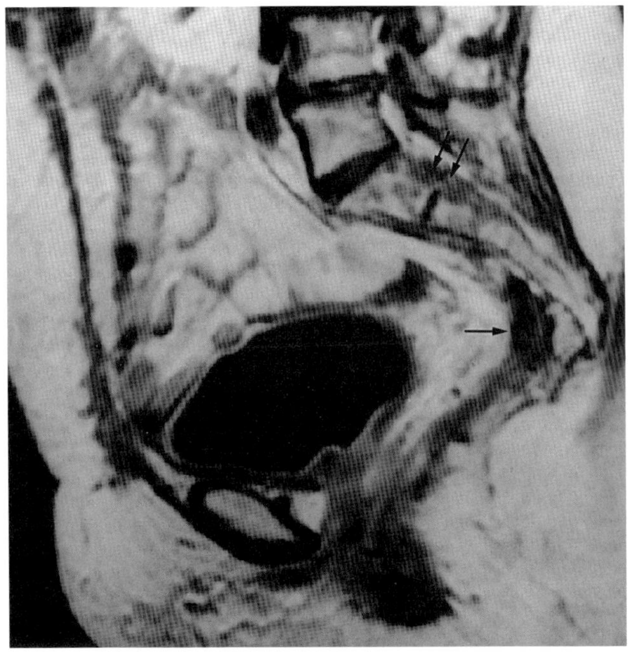

B

Figure 8.27

Follow-up MR studies after rectal amputation and radiotherapy.

A T1-weighted SE image: the content of the small-bowel loops is enhanced by oral gadolinium (arrowheads). An abnormal amount of hypointense tissue is present in the presacral space (arrow) and a hypointense lesion is also demonstrated in the sacrum (double arrow). Note the wall thickening of small bowel loops due to radiation side-effects.

B T1-weighted SE image after intravenous gadolinium shows no enhancement of presacral tissue, suggesting its fibrous nature (arrow), and shows enhancement of the sacral lesion, suggesting its metastatic nature (double arrow).

Initial reports suggested that MR imaging might provide accurate discrimination between tumor and fibrotic tissue, on the basis of signal intensity.[133] A low signal intensity on T2-weighted images will often be found in fibrotic tissue with low cellular and water content; on the other hand, a high signal intensity is considered suggestive of recurrent tumor.[134] However, it was demonstrated that malignant and benign masses may be indistinguishable by MR due to the presence of fibrosis and inflammatory cells within tumor or the presence of microscopic tumor regions in fibrotic tissue.[135] Early postoperative cases with possible inflammatory reaction or early postradiation fibrosis must especially be interpreted with caution. In some other cases, correct diagnosis can be impaired by artifacts due to metallic suture material. MR imaging may be of value and probably more accurate than CT in assessing the extent of proven recurrences and invasion of pelvic structures and bone.[132] Using an intravascular contrast agent (gadolinium-DTPA) (Figure 8.27) improves the delineation of recurrent cancer on T1-weighted images, increasing the overall accuracy of MR to 93%.[132,136] For an overall abdominal screening to detect non-local recurrence, CT or US may be more valuable, though the efficacy of MR for this purpose remains to be determined. Evaluation of the anastomosis or bowel wall may be more accurate with CT, as suture material can produce artifacts at high magnetic field strength.

Endosonography can be used per rectum following restorative resection or per vaginam in female patients after abdominoperineal excision. Only a small number of clinically suspected recurrent extraluminal lesions are detected by US alone, but the routine use of ES may be a more efficient method to detect local recurrence at an early stage, especially when combined with conventional methods of clinical examination and rectosigmoidoscopy.[111] It was recently reported that ES demonstrated an accuracy of 97% with specificity, sensitivity and negative predictive value between 94 and 99% and positive predictive value of 85%.[137]

Local recurrence has an appearance similar to that of primary rectal cancer (Figure 8.28). It is hypoechoic but not always homogeneous and may have either a sharp or a blurred edge. Islands of recurrent tumor as small as 5 mm can be detected. The pitfalls in diagnosis are collection of fluid, granulation tissue or a loop of small bowel. For these reasons, detection of early extraluminal lesions is not diagnostic of recurrence; these must be biopsied under US control or carefully documented, and the examination repeated after an interval of time.[111]

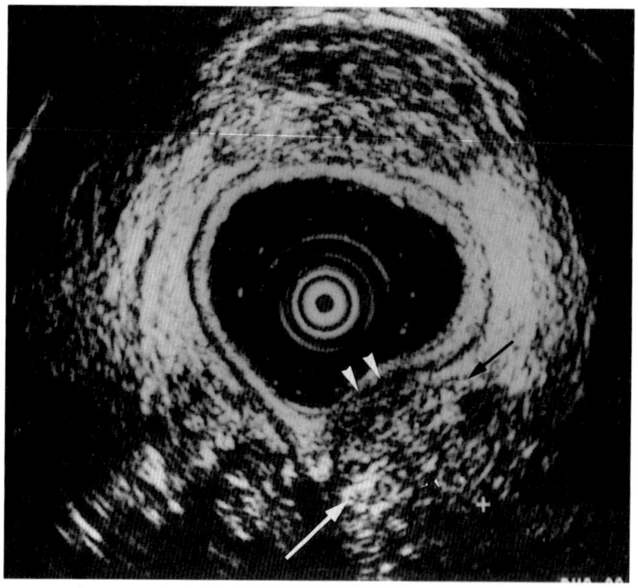

Figure 8.28

Rectal carcinoma (between arrows) recurring outside the mucosa and impressing on the muscularis propria (double arrowhead).

Nuclear medicine, in particular immunoscintigraphy and positron emission tomography after fluorine deoxyglucose injection (FDG-PET), appears to have potential to detect local and distant tumor recurrence[138,139] and to differentiate recurrent cancer from scars, by showing an increased uptake of FDG in tumorous tissues.[140]

Finally, CT and MR may play a role in imaging locally advanced rectal carcinoma after pre-operative irradiation, in determining the impact of treatment on the resectability of a lesion initially considered non-resectable. Recent studies suggest that MR and FDG-PET may be useful in determining the reduction in tumor size after radiotherapy and perhaps in downstaging the tumor.[140,141]

Other primary malignancies

Carcinoids are rarer in the large bowel than in the small intestine and are somewhat more common in the rectum than in the colon. They tend to be

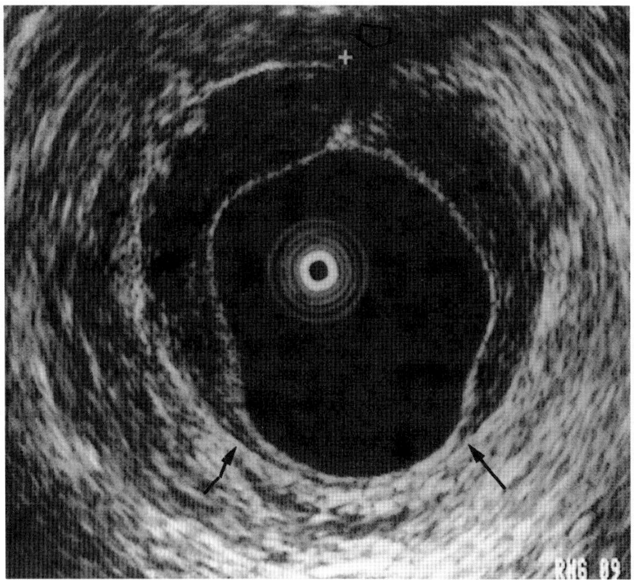

Figure 8.29

UT4 melanosarcoma of the rectum extending into nearly three-quarters of its circumference (between arrows) and infiltrating all the layers of the rectal wall as well as the prostate (open arrow).

solitary and are more aggresive than elsewhere in the gastrointestinal tract, invading the bowel wall and spreading to adjacent lymph nodes even when the primary lesion is small.[63,64] The risk of metastasis increases rapidly as the tumor grows beyond 1.0 cm in size.[142] Leiomyosarcomas are, with lymphomas, the most common non-epithelial tumors in the colon and rectum. Leiomyosarcomas are more common than their benign counterparts and do not differ significantly in their pathologic characteristics from those found elsewhere in the gastrointestinal tract.[77] Symptomatic lesions arising from the muscularis propria are usually large even when they occur in the rectum.[143]

Primary melanoma is rarer in the rectum than in the anal region and is similarly aggressive (Figure 8.29).

Secondary neoplasms

Metastatic spread can occur from a variety of sites, including primary malignancies of the colon itself. Gastric, breast and ovary carcinomas have a tendency to intra-abdominal spread, with peritoneal seeding and creation of a colonic or rectal shelf.[78] Direct extension from prostatic, cervical or left ovary carcinoma may simulate a stenotic rectal primary tumor.

The work up of patients with colorectal cancer is summarized in Diagram 8.3.

Anal canal carcinoma

Epidemiology

Carcinomas of the anal canal are not only oncologically different from colorectal cancers but, due to their particular anatomic location, they also pose special problems in imaging.[144] Anal carcinomas constitute 1–4% of large bowel cancers.[145] They are more common in women than men and have a higher prevalence in patients with perianal Crohn's disease or other chronic benign anal conditions, in homosexual males, and in patients with renal transplants or of lower social status.[144,146]

Pathology and classification

Most lesions are located within 1.0 cm from the mucocutaneous line and are variants of epidermoid carcinomas; usually they respond to radiation therapy.[144] Most tumors are fungating, ulcerating or excavating, with an average size of 4.2 cm.[147]

The tumors spread locally to sphincter muscles, perineal soft tissues and upward to the rectum. The vagina is the most common site of extension of tumors located anteriorly in the canal. Lymphatic spread occurs frequently in perirectal, mesocolic and inguinal nodes, the first of these being involved in 75% of the cases.[148]

The frequency of hematogenous spread varies in different series but remains low.

Anal cancer is classified according to the TNM system[4] (Table 8.10).

Diagnosis and clinical staging

In patients presenting with local symptoms, the diagnosis of anal canal cancer is usually suggested by the digital and anuscopic examination and is established histologically by biopsy.

Table 8.10 The TNM classification of anal carcinoma.

	Stage	*Description*
Primary tumor	Tis	Carcinoma in situ
Anal canal	T1	Tumor 2 cm or less in greatest dimension
	T2	Tumor more than 2 cm but not more than 5 cm in greatest dimension
	T3	Tumor more than 5 cm in greatest dimension
	T4	Tumor of any size invades adjacent organ(s), e.g. vagina, urethra, bladder (involvement of the sphincter muscle(s) alone is not classified T4)
Nodal involvement	N1	Metastasis in perirectal lymph node(s)
	N2	Metastasis in unilateral internal iliac and/or inguinal lymph node(s)
	N3	Metastasis in perirectal and inguinal lymph nodes and/or bilateral internal iliac and/or inguinal lymph nodes
Distant metastases	M0	No distant metastasis
	M1	Distant metastasis

Local extension of the tumor to the perianal tissues and organs, in particular to the sphincter muscles, the posterior vaginal wall and the prostate, and to the perianal and inguinal nodes, is detected by digital examination. Combined digital examination with a fine-needle biopsy of perianal or pelvic nodes by a transrectal or transvaginal approach can verify the presence of metastatic disease.[144,145] However, clinical staging may be problematic in patients with advanced disease, and there may therefore be limitations in detecting pelvic nodes.

Imaging

CT has been used with some success for the staging and follow up of anal canal carcinoma. From a limited number of reports, it appears that CT can demonstrate anal masses and detect invasion of the anorectal musculature, perirectal and para-aortic nodes.[144,149] On CT scans performed after intravenous contrast, primary necrotic tumors may be directly visualized as hypodense masses, sometimes containing gas. Non-necrotic tumors remain isodense to the surrounding muscular sphincter and may be suspected indirectly on asymmetric appearance of the perineal structures (Figure 8.30A).

Direct extension to the vagina or prostate may be difficult to recognize at an early stage. Perirectal nodes located a few centimeters above the anorectal junction appear often larger than those associated with rectal cancer. Although enlarged perirectal nodes are in most cases easily palpated, CT is helpful in their detection in obese patients or in advanced disease with stenosis of the anal canal. CT is also helpful in identifying lymphatic spread along the pelvic chains, but there is no precise criterion of tumoral invasion. Consequently, CT performed before treatment is helpful in evaluating pelvic nodes, especially in obese patients and when digital examination is impossible because of anal stenosis or pain. In patients with advanced disease, CT is helpful for assessing visceral involvement and distant metastasis.

MR imaging may be more accurate than CT for the delineation of tumor masses on T2-weighted images and provides a higher anatomic resolution on T1-weighted images after intravenous gadolinium-DTPA (Figure 8.30B and C).

Anal ES can demonstrate the anal canal layers and the internal and external sphincter, and

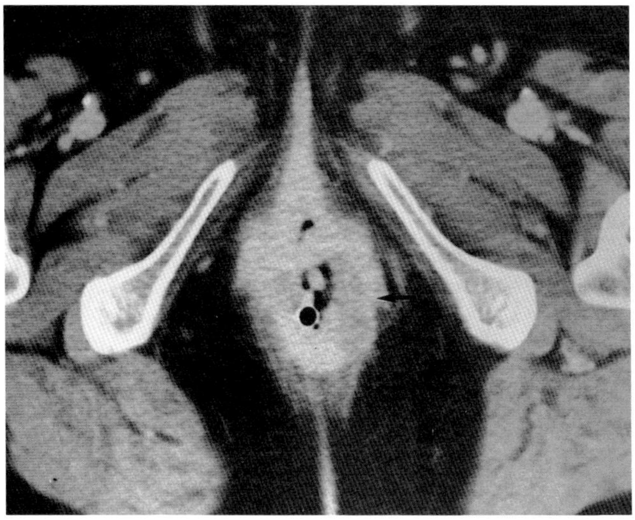

A

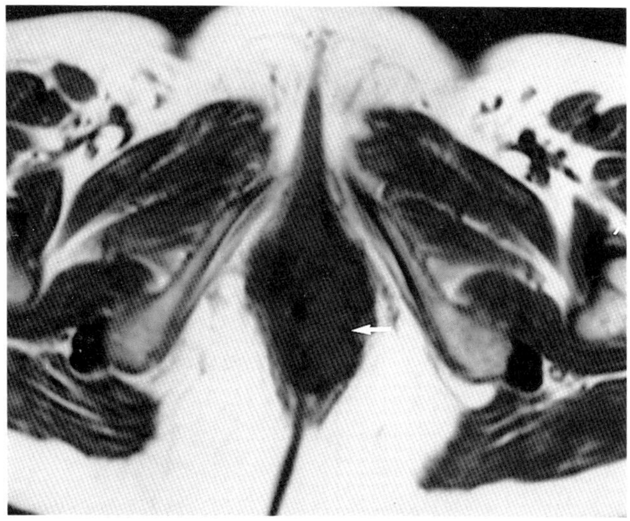

B

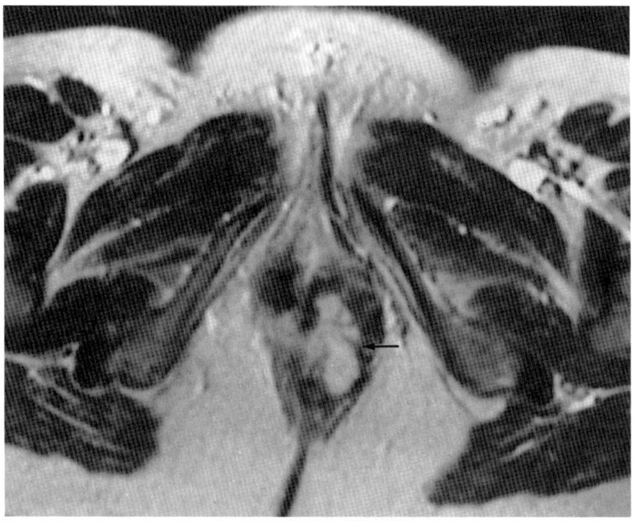

C

Figure 8.30

Invasive carcinoma of the left part of the anal canal comparatively imaged by CT and MR. On CT images (A), precise delineation of the lesion is difficult (arrow), but it is easy on T1-weighted SE images (B) and even easier on gadolinium-enhanced T1-weighted SE images (C), in which the lesion appears as a hyperintense area (arrow).

consequently it may have a role in assessing the depth of invasion of anal cancers.[150] Rectal ES may be useful for the assessment of pararectal nodes and rectal invasion.[119] After curative radiation therapy, CT is useful for visualizing regression of perirectal nodes, local complications of irradiation, or metachronous metastases to the inguinal nodes.[144] Postoperative and/or postradiation scanning has also been found to be useful in detecting locally or distant recurrent disease.[149]

After curative surgery, local recurrence occurs sooner than distant recurrence, with a rate of 26% in large series.[148] It occurs usually within a period of 2 years in inguinal nodes, soft pelvic tissues or the sacrum.

The work up of patients with anal cancer is summarized in Diagram 8.4.

Acknowledgments

We are grateful to our colleague R. Detry, Clinical Professor of Surgery, for providing us with a fine selection of endosonographic material.

References

1. Livstone EM, Skinner DB, Tumors of the esophagus. In: Berk JE, ed, *Gastroenterology*, 4th edn (WB Saunders: Philadelphia 1985) 818–50.
2. Dodds WJ, Radiology of the esophagus and esophagogastric region including diaphragm. In: Margulis AR, Burhenne HJ, eds, *Alimentary tract radiology*, 4th edn (Mosby: St Louis 1989) 427–500.
3. Akiyama H, Tsurumaru M, Kawamura T, et al, Principles of surgical treatment for carcinoma of the esophagus. Analysis of lymph node involvement, *Ann Surg* (1981) **194**:438–46.
4. Hermanek P, Sobin LH, *TNM classification of malignant tumours*, 4th edn (Springer-Verlag: Berlin 1987).
5. Tio TL, Coene PP, Schouwink MH, et al, Esophagogastric carcinoma: peroperative TNM classification with endosonography, *Radiology* (1989) **173**:411–17.
6. Misumi A, Harada K, Murakami A, et al, Early diagnosis of esophageal cancer. Analysis of 11 cases of esophageal mucosal cancer, *Ann Surg* (1989) **210**:732–9.
7. Op den Orth JO, Use of barium in the evaluation of disorders of the upper gastrointestinal tract: current status, *Radiology* (1989) **173**:601–8.
8. Ellis FH, Treatment of carcinoma of the esophagus or cardia, *Mayo Clin Proc* (1989) **64**:945–55.
9. Halvorsen RA, Thompson WM, Computed tomographic staging of gastrointestinal tract malignancies. Part I. Esophagus and stomach, *Invest Radiol* (1987) **22**:2–16.
10. Lefor AT, Merino MM, Steinberg SM, et al, Computerized tomographic prediction of extraluminal spread and prognostic implications of lesion width in esophageal carcinoma, *Cancer* (1988) **62**:1287–92.
11. Gayet B, Frija J, Cahuzac J, et al, Intérêt de la tomodensitométrie dans le cancer de l'oesophage. Etude prospective et aveugle, *Gastroenterol Clin Biol* (1988) **12**:23–8.
12. Kimmey MB, Martin RW, Haggit RC, et al, Histologic correlates of gastrointestinal ultrasound images, *Gastroenterology* (1989) **96**:433–41.
13. Botet JF, Lightdale C, Zauber AG, et al, Preoperative staging of esophageal cancer: comparison of endoscopic US and dynamic CT, *Radiology* (1991) **181**:419–25.
14. Ziegler K, Sanft C, Zeitz M, et al, Evaluation of endosonography in TN staging of oesophageal cancer, *Gut* (1991) **32**:16–20.
15. Takashima S, Takeuchi N, Shiozaki H, et al, Carcinoma of the esophagus: CT vs MR imaging in determining resectability, *AJR* (1991) **156**: 297–302.
16. Watt I, Stewart I, Anderson D, et al, Laparoscopy, ultrasound and computed tomography in cancer of the esophagus and gastric cardia: a prospective comparison for detecting intra-abdominal metastases, *Br J Surg* (1989) **76**:1036–9.
17. Merandi SF, Quinn SF, Clark RA, Complications of esophageal prostheses: roentgeonologic manifestations, *South Med J* (1989) **82**:1365–9.
18. Becker CD, Barbier PA, Terrier F, et al, Patterns of recurrence of esophageal carcinoma after transhiatal esophagectomy and gastric interposition, *AJR* (1987) **148**:273–7.
19. Blot WJ, Devesa SS, Kneller RW, et al, Rising incidence of adenocarcinoma of the esophagus and gastric cardia, *JAMA* (1991) **265**:1287–9.
20. Kurtz RC, Sherlock P, Carcinoma of the stomach. In: Berk JE, ed, *Gastroenterology*, 4th edn (WB Saunders: Philadelphia 1985) 1278–1304.
21. Shirakabe H, Maruyama M, Neoplastic diseases of the stomach. In: Margulis AR, Burhenne HJ, ed, *Alimentary tract radiology*, 4th edn (Mosby: St Louis 1989) 595–625.
22. Farley DR, Donohue JH, Early gastric cancer, *Surg Clin North Am* (1992) **72**:401–21.
23. Levine MS, Rubesin SE, Herlinger H, et al, Double-contrast upper gastrointestinal examination: technique and interpretation, *Radiology* (1988) **168**:593–602.
24. Dooley CP, Larson AW, Stace NH, et al, Double-contrast barium meal and upper gastrointestinal endoscopy. A comparative study, *Ann Intern Med* (1984) **101**:538–45.
25. Shaw PC, Van Romunde LK, Griffioen G, et al, Peptic ulcer and gastric carcinoma: diagnosis with biphasic radiography compared with fiberoptic endoscopy, *Radiology* (1987) **163**:39–42.
26. Colin-Jones DG, Endoscopy and radiology for upper gastrointestinal symptoms? *Lancet* (1986) **i**:1022–3.
27. Lawrence M, Shiu MH, Early gastric cancer: twenty-eight-year experience, *Ann Surg* (1991) **213**:327–34.
28. Levine MS, Kong V, Rubesin SE, et al, Scirrhous carcinoma of the stomach: radiologic and endoscopic diagnosis, *Radiology* (1990) **175**:151–4.
29. Fujishima H, Misawa T, Chijiiwa Y, et al, Scirrhous carcinoma of the stomach versus hypertrophic gastritis: findings at endoscopic US, *Radiology* (1991) **181**:197–200.
30. Carter KJ, Schaffer HA, Ritchie WP, Early gastric cancer, *Ann Surg* (1984) **199**: 604–9.
31. White RM, Levine MS, Enterline HT, et al, Early gastric cancer. Recent experience, *Radiology* (1985) **155**:25–7.
32. Hori S, Tsuda K, Murayama S, et al, CT of gastric carcinoma. Preliminary results with a new scanning technique, *Radiographics* (1992) **12**:257–68.
33. Sussman SK, Halvorsen RA, Illescas FF, et al, Gastric adenocarcinoma: CT versus surgical staging, *Radiology* (1988) **167**:335–40.
34. Nelson RC, Chezmar JL, Hoel MJ, et al, Peritoneal carcinomatosis: preoperative CT with intraperitoneal contrast material, *Radiology* (1992) **182**:133–8.
35. Botet JF, Lightdale CJ, Zauber AG, et al, Preoperative staging of gastric cancer: comparison of endoscopic US and dynamic CT, *Radiology* (1991) **181**:426–32.

36. Baker MK, Kopecky KK, Endoscopic US in the staging of esophageal and gastric cancer, *Radiology* (1991) **181**:342–3.
37. Levine MS, Fisher AR, Rubesin SE, et al, Complications after total gastrectomy and esophagojejunostomy: radiologic evaluation, *AJR* (1991) **157**:1189–94.
38. Mullin D, Shirkhoda A, Computed tomography after gastrectomy in primary gastric carcinoma, *J Comput Assist Tomogr* (1985) **9**:30–3.
39. Van Steenbergen W, Kojima T, Geboes K, et al, Gastric leiomyoblastoma with metastases to the liver. A 36-year follow-up study, *Gastroenterology* (1985) **89**:875–81.
40. Megibow AJ, Balthazar EJ, Hulnick DH, et al, CT evaluation of gastrointestinal leiomyomas and leiomyosarcomas, *AJR* (1985) **144**:727–31.
41. Yasuda K, Nakajima M, Yohisda S, et al, The diagnosis of submucosal tumors of the stomach by endoscopic ultrasonography, *Gastrointest Endosc* (1989) **35**:10–15.
42. Choi BI, Ok ID, Im JG, et al, Exogastric cystic gastric leiomyoblastoma with unusual CT appearance, *Gastrointest Radiol* (1988) **13**:109–11.
43. Glick SN, Teplick SK, Levine MS, et al, Gastric cardia metastasis in esophageal carcinoma, *Radiology* (1986) **160**:627–30.
44. Adotey JM, Primary malignant tumours of the small intestine, *Br J Clin Pract* (1985) **39**:54–8.
45. Nix GA, Wilson JH, Dees J, Primary malignant tumours of the duodenum, *RÖFO* (1985) **142**: 385–90.
46. Papadopoulos VD, Nolan DJ, Carcinoma of the small intestine, *Clin Radiol* (1985) **36**:409–13.
47. Riddell RH, Dysplasia and cancer in inflammatory bowel disease, *Br J Surg* (1985) **72**(Suppl):83–6.
48. Harned RK, Buck JL, Olmsted WW, et al, Extracolonic manifestations of the familial adenomatous polyposis syndromes, *AJR* (1991) **156**:481–5.
49. Hessler PC, Braustein E, Adenocarcinoma of the duodenum arising in a villous adenoma, *Gastrointest Radiol* (1978) **2**: 355–7.
50. Sellner F, Investigations on the significance of the adenoma–carcinoma sequence in the small bowel, *Cancer* (1990) **66**:702–15.
51. Koretz M, Graham R, Primary adenocarcinoma of the jejunum, *Am Surg* (1989) **55**: 539–42.
52. Lien GS, Mori M, Enjoji M, Primary carcinoma of the small intestine, *Cancer* (1988) **61**:316–23.
53. Lioe TF, Biggart JD, Primary adenocarcinoma of the jejunum and ileum: clinicopathology review of 25 cases, *J Clin Pathol* (1990) **43**:533–6.
54. Pringot J, Bodart P, Inflammatory diseases of the small bowel. In: Margulis AR, Burhenne HJ, eds, *Alimentary tract radiology*, Vol I, 4th edn (Mosby: St Louis 1989) 786–90.
55. Bessette JR, Maglinte DDT, Kelvin FM, et al, Primary malignant tumors in the small bowel: a comparison of the small bowel enema and conventional follow-through examination, *AJR* (1989) **153**:741–4.
56. Domizio P, Talbot IC, Spigelman AD, et al, Upper gastrointestinal pathology in familial adenomatous polyposis: results from a prospective study of 102 patients, *J Clin Pathol* (1990) **43**:738–43.
57. Lewis BS, Waye JD, Chronic gastrointestinal bleeding of obscure origin: role of small bowel enteroscopy, *Gastroenterology* (1988) **94**:1117–20.
58. Thompson WM, Halvorsen RA, Computed tomographic staging of gastrointestinal malignancies. Part II. The small bowel, colon, and rectum, *Invest Radiol* (1987) **22**:96–105.
59. Laurent F, Raynaud M, Biset JM, et al, Diagnosis and categorization of small bowel neoplasms: role of computed tomography, *Gastrointest Radiol* (1991) **16**:115–9.
60. Ekberg O, Ekholm S, Radiology in primary small bowel adenocarcinoma, *Gastrointest Radiol* (1980) **5**:49–53.
61. Farah MC, Jafri SZH, Schwab RE, et al, Duodenal neoplasms: role of CT, *Radiology* (1987) **162**:839–43.
62. Jeffree MA, Barter SJ, Hemingway AP, et al, Primary carcinoid tumours of the ileum: the radiologic appearances, *Clin Radiol* (1984) **35**:451–55.
63. Balthazar EJ, Carcinoid tumors of the alimentary tract. I. Radiographic diagnosis, *Gastrointest Radiol* (1978) **3**:47–56.
64. Antoniades J, Carcinoid tumors of the gastrointestinal tract. In: Antoniades J, ed, *Uncommon malignant tumors* (Masson: New York 1982) 162–72.
65. Allison DJ, Embolization of liver tumours. In: Blumgart LH, ed, *Surgery of the liver and biliary tract* (Churchill Livingstone: Edinburgh 1988) 1201–7.
66. Carrasco CH, Charnsangavej C, Ajani J, et al, The carcinoid syndrome: palliation by hepatic artery embolization, *AJR* (1986) **147**:149–54.
67. Yang K, Ulich T, Cheng L, et al, The neuroendocrine products of intestinal carcinoids, *Cancer* (1983) **51**:1918–26.
68. Jeffree MA, Nolan DJ, Multiple ileal carcinoid tumours. Case report, *Br J Radiol* (1987) **60**:402–3.
69. Kinkhabwala M, Balthazar EJ, Carcinoid tumors of the alimentary tract. II. Angiographic diagnosis of small intestinal and colonic lesions, *Gastrointest Radiol* (1978) **3**:57–61.
70. Cockey BM, Fishman EK, Jones B, et al, Computed tomography of abdominal carcinoid tumor, *J Comput Assist Tomogr* (1985) **9**:38–42.
71. Bressler EK, Alpern MB, Glazer GM, et al, Hypervascular hepatic metastases: CT evaluation, *Radiology* (1987) **162**:49–51.
72. Lamberts SWJ, Bakker WH, Reubi JC, et al, Somatostatin-receptor imaging in the localization of endocrine tumors, *N Eng J Med* (1990) **323**:1246–9.
73. Hansen CP, Colstrup H, Mogensen AM, Recurrent gastrointestinal bleeding due to leiomyosarcoma of the small intestine, *Eur J Surg Oncol* (1991) **157**:227–9.

74. Wall SD, Friedman SL, Margulis AR, Gastrointestinal Kaposi's sarcoma in AIDS: radiographic manifestations, *J Clin Gastroenterol* (1984) **6**:165–70.
75. Starr GF, Dockerty MB, Leiomyomas and leiomyosarcoma of the small intestine, *Cancer* (1955) **8**:101–11.
76. Martin JF, Leiomyosarcoma of the small intestine: report of three cases and review of the literature, *AJR* (1955) **74**:1081–8.
77. McLeod AJ, Zornoza J, Shirkhoda A, Leiomyosarcoma: computed tomographic findings, *Radiology* (1984) **152**:133–6.
78. Meyers MA, McSweeney J, Secondary neoplasms of the bowel, *Radiology* (1972) **105**:1–11.
79. Diamond RT, Greenberg HM, Boult IF, Direct metastatic spread of right colonic adenocarcinoma to duodenum—barium and computed tomographic findings, *Gastrointest Radiol* (1981) **6**:339–41.
80. Meyers MA, Intraperitoneal spread of malignancies and its effect on the bowel, *Clin Radiol* (1981) **32**:129–46.
81. Beckley DE, Alimentary tract metastases from malignant melanoma, *Clin Radiol* (1974) **25**:385–9.
82. Kawashima A, Fishman EK, Kuhlman JE, et al, CT of malignant melanoma: patterns of small bowel and mesenteric involvement, *J Comput Assist Tomogr* (1991) **15**:570–4.
83. Whalen E, Colon cancer: diagnosis in an era of cost containment, ACR conference, November 8, 1989. Meeting news, *AJR* (1990) **154**:875–81.
84. Blery M, Valleur P, Chagnon S, et al, Apport de la radiologie au bilan du cancer du rectum, *Feuillets Radiol* (1991) **31**:107–17.
85. Ahlquist DA, Epidemiology, etiology, diagnosis, and screening of colorectal neoplasia, *Curr Opin Gastroenterol* (1991) **7**:18–24.
86. Mecklin JP, Frequency of hereditary colorectal carcinoma, *Gastroenterology* (1987) **93**:1021–5.
87. Cannon-Albright LA, Skolnick MH, Bishop T, et al, Common inheritance of susceptibility to colonic adenomatous polyps and associated colorectal cancers, *N Engl J Med* (1988) **319**:533–7.
88. Gelfand DW, Ott DJ, Methodologic considerations in comparing imaging methods, *AJR* (1985) **144**:1117–21.
89. Winawer SJ, Miller DG, Sherlock P, Risk and screening for colorectal cancer. In: Stollerman GH, ed, *Advances in internal medicine* (Year Book Medical: Chicago 1984) 471–96.
90. Symonds DA, Vickery AL, Mucinous carcinoma of the colon and rectum, *Cancer* (1976) **37**:1891–1900.
91. Wanebo HJ, Gaker DL, Whitehill R, et al, Pelvic recurrence of rectal cancer, *Ann Surg* (1987) **205**:482.
92. Thoeni RF, Colorectal cancer: cross-sectional imaging for staging of primary tumor and detection of local recurrence, *AJR* (1991) **156**:909–15.
93. Postlethwait RW, Malignant tumors of the colon and rectum, *Ann Surg* (1949) **129**:34–6.
94. Langevin JM, Nivatvongs S, The true incidence of synchronous cancer in the large bowel. A prospective study, *Am J Surg* (1984) **147**:330–3.
95. Warden MJ, Petrelli NJ, Herrera L, et al, Endoscopy versus double-contrast barium enema in the evaluation of patients with symptoms suggestive of colorectal carcinoma, *Am J Surg* (1988) **155**:224–6.
96. Glaser F, Schlag P, Harfarth C, Endorectal ultrasonography for the assessment of invasion of rectal tumours and lymph node involvement, *Br J Surg* (1990) **77**:883–7.
97. Heald RJ, Ryall RD, Recurrence and survival after total mesorectal excision for rectal cancer, *Lancet* (1986) **i**:1479–82.
98. Benotti PN, Bothe A, Eyre RC, et al, Management for recurrent pelvic tumors, *Arch Surg* (1987) **122**:457–60.
99. Hardcastle JD, Symposium: screening for colorectal cancer, *Int J Colorect Dis* (1986) **1**:63–78.
100. Rice RP, Lowering death rates from colorectal cancer: challenge for the 1990s, *Radiology* (1990) **176**:297–301.
101. Stevenson GW, Robertson A, Hecker R, Barium enema in colonic cancer: a retrospective audit, *Aust Clin Rev* (1984) **13**:13–18.
102. Barry MJ, Richter JM, Effect work-up strategy on the cost effectiveness of fecal occult blood screening for colorectal cancer (abstr), *Gastrointest Endosc* (1984) **30**:141.
103. Balthazar EJ, Mejibow AJ, Hulnick D, et al, Carcinoma of the colon detection and preoperative staging by CT, *AJR* (1988) **150**:301–6.
104. Gelfand DW, Chen YM, Ott DJ, Radiologic detection of colonic neoplasms: benefits of a systems-analysis approach, *AJR* (1991) **156**:303–6.
105. Parithival VS, Pandya GP, Gerst PH, Which one first? Barium enema or colonoscopy, *Am Surg* (1989) **55**:417–20.
106. Glick SN, Teplick SK, Balfe DM, et al, Large colonic neoplasms missed by endoscopy, *AJR* (1989) **152**:513–17.
107. Skucas J, Spataro RF, The radiographic features of small colon cancers, *Radiology* (1982) **143**:335–40.
108. Muto T, Bussey HJR, Morson BC, The evolution of cancer of the colon and rectum, *Cancer* (1975) **36**:2251–70.
109. Nicholls RJ, York Mason A, Morson RC, et al, The clinical staging of rectal cancer, *Br J Surg* (1982) **69**:404–9.
110. Grinnell RS, The grading and prognosis of carcinoma of the colon and rectum, *Ann Surg* (1939) **109**:500–33.
111. Beynon J, Mortensen NJM, Foy DMA, et al, The detection and evaluation of locally recurrent rectal cancer with rectal endosonography, *Dis Colon Rectum* (1989) **32**:509–17.
112. Tio TL, Coene PPLO, Van Delden OM, et al, Colorectal carcinoma: preoperative TNM classification with endosonography, *Radiology* (1991) **179**:165–70.
113. Guinet C, Buy JN, Ghossain MA, et al, Comparison of magnetic resonance imaging and computed tomography in the preoperative staging of rectal cancer, *Arch Surg* (1990) **125**:385–8.

114. De Lange EE, Fechner RE, Edge SB, et al, Preoperative staging of rectal carcinoma with MR imaging: surgical and histopathologic correlation, *Radiology* (1990) **176**:623–8.
115. Aisen AM, Body MR imaging and the local staging of neoplasm, *Radiology* (1990) **176**: 617–19.
116. Imai Y, Kressel HY, Saul SH, et al, Colorectal tumors: an in vitro study of high-resolution MR imaging, *Radiology* (1990) **177**:695–701.
117. Chan TW, Kressel HY, Milestone B, et al, Rectal carcinoma: staging at MR imaging with endorectal surface coil, *Radiology* (1991) **181**:461–7.
118. Hildebrandt U, Feifel G, Preoperative staging of rectal cancer by intrarectal ultrasound, *Dis Colon Rectum* (1985) **28**: 42–6.
119. Beynon J, Mortensen NJMcC, Foy DMA, et al, Preoperative assessment of mesorectal lymph node involvement in rectal cancer, *Br J Surg* (1989) **76**:276–9.
120. Rifkin MD, Ehrlich SM, Marks G, Staging of rectal carcinoma: prospective comparison of endorectal US and CT, *Radiology* (1989) **170**:319–22.
121. Carlsson U, Lasson A, Ekelund G, Recurrence rate after curative surgery for rectal carcinoma, with special reference to their accuracy, *Dis Colon Rectum* (1987) **30**:431–4.
122. Detry R, Detection and treatment of locally recurrent rectal cancer, *Adv Coloproctol* (1987) 495–502.
123. Putzki H, Student A, Jablonski M, et al, Comparison of the tumor markers CEA, TPA, and CA 19–9 in colorectal carcinoma, *Cancer* (1987) **59**:223–6.
124. Gerard A, Berrod JL, Pene F, et al, Interim analysis of a phase III study on preoperative radiation therapy in resectable rectal carcinoma, *Cancer* (1985) **55**:2373–9.
125. Husband JE, Hodson NJ, Parsons CA, The use of computed tomography in recurrent rectal tumors, *Radiology* (1980) **134**:677–82.
126. Freeny PC, Marks WM, Ryan JA, et al, Colorectal carcinoma evaluation with CT: preoperative and postoperative CT staging and detection of postoperative recurrence, *Radiology* (1985) **158**:347–53.
127. Kelvin FM, Korobbin M, Heaston DK, et al, The pelvis after surgery for rectal and rectosigmoid carcinoma: serial CT observations with emphasis on nonneoplastic features, *AJR* (1983) **141**:959–64.
128. Lee JKT, Stanley RJ, Sagel SS, et al, CT appearance of the pelvis after abdominoperineal resection for rectal carcinoma, *Radiology* (1981) **141**:737–41.
129. Grabbe E, Winkler R, Local recurrence after sphincter-saving resection for rectal and rectosigmoid carcinoma, *Radiology* (1985) 155:305–10.
130. Zaunbauer W, Haertel M, Fuchs WA, Computed tomography in carcinoma of the rectum, *Gastrointest Radiol* (1981) **6**:79–84.
131. Butch RJ, Wittenberg J, Mueller PR, et al, Presacral masses after abdominoperineal resection for colorectal carcinoma: the need for needle biopsy, *AJR* (1985) **144**:309–12.
132. Mathias K, Hasse FM, Theophil B, et al, Diagnostische und therapeutische Strategie beim lokal rezidivierenden Rektumkarzinom, *Radiologe* (1992) **32**:60–7.
133. Rafto SE, Amendola MA, Gefter WB, MR imaging of recurrent colorectal carcinoma versus fibrosis, *J Comput Assist Tomogr* (1988) **12**:521–6.
134. Krestin GP, Steinbrich W, Friedmann G, Recurrent rectal cancer: diagnosis with MR imaging versus CT, *Radiology* (1988) **163**:307–11.
135. De Lange EE, Fechner RE, Wanebo HJ, Suspected recurrent rectosigmoid carcinoma after abdominoperineal resection: MR imaging and histopathologic findings, *Radiology* (1989) **170**:323–8.
136. Balzarini L, Ceglia E, D'Ippolito G, et al, Local recurrence of rectosigmoid cancer: what about the choice of MRI for diagnosis? *Gastrointest Radiol* (1990) **15**:338–42.
137. Mascagni D, Corbellini L, Urcivoli D, et al, Endoluminal ultrasound for early detection of local recurrence of rectal cancer, *Br J Surg* (1989) **76**:1176–80.
138. Strauss LW, Clorius JH, Schlag P, et al, Recurrence of colorectal tumors: PET evaluation, *Radiology* (1989) **170**:329–32.
139. Bishof-Delaloye A, Delaloye B, Buchel F, et al, Clinical value of immunoscintigraphy in colorectal carcinoma patients: a prospective study, *J Nucl Med* (1989) **30**:1646–56.
140. Ito K, Kato T, Tadokoro M, et al, Recurrent rectal cancer and scar: differentiation with PET and MR imaging, *Radiology* (1992) **182**:549–52.
141. De Lange EE, Fechner RE, Spaulding CA, et al, Rectal carcinoma treated by preoperative irradiation: MR imaging and histopathologic correlation, *AJR* (1992) **158**:287–92.
142. Nauenheim KS, Zeitels J, Kaplan EL, et al, Rectal carcinoid tumors—treatment and prognosis, *Surgery* (1983) **94**:670–6.
143. Walsh TH, Mann CV, Smooth muscle neoplasms of the rectum and anal canal, *Br J Surg* (1984) **71**:597–9.
144. Scherrer A, Reboul F, Martin D, et al, CT of malignant anal canal tumors, *Radiographics* (1990) **10**:433–53.
145. Quan SHQ, Anal and para-anal tumors, *Surg Clin North Am* (1978) **58**:591–602.
146. Slater G, Greenstein A, Aufses AH Jr, Anal carcinoma in patients with Crohn's disease, *Ann Surg* (1984) **199**:348–50.
147. Welch JP, Malta RA, Appraisal of the treatment of carcinoma of the anus and anal canal, *Surg Gynecol Obstet* (1977) **145**:837–41.
148. Klotz RG, Pamukcoglu T, Souilliard DH, Transitional cloacogenic carcinoma of the anal canal, *Cancer* (1967) **20**:1727–45.
149. Cohan RH, Silverman PM, Thompson WM, et al, Computed tomography of epithelial neoplasms of the anal canal, *AJR* (1985) **145**:569–573.
150. Law PJ, Bartram CI, Anal endosonography: technique and normal anatomy, *Gastrointest Radiol* (1989) **14**:349–53.

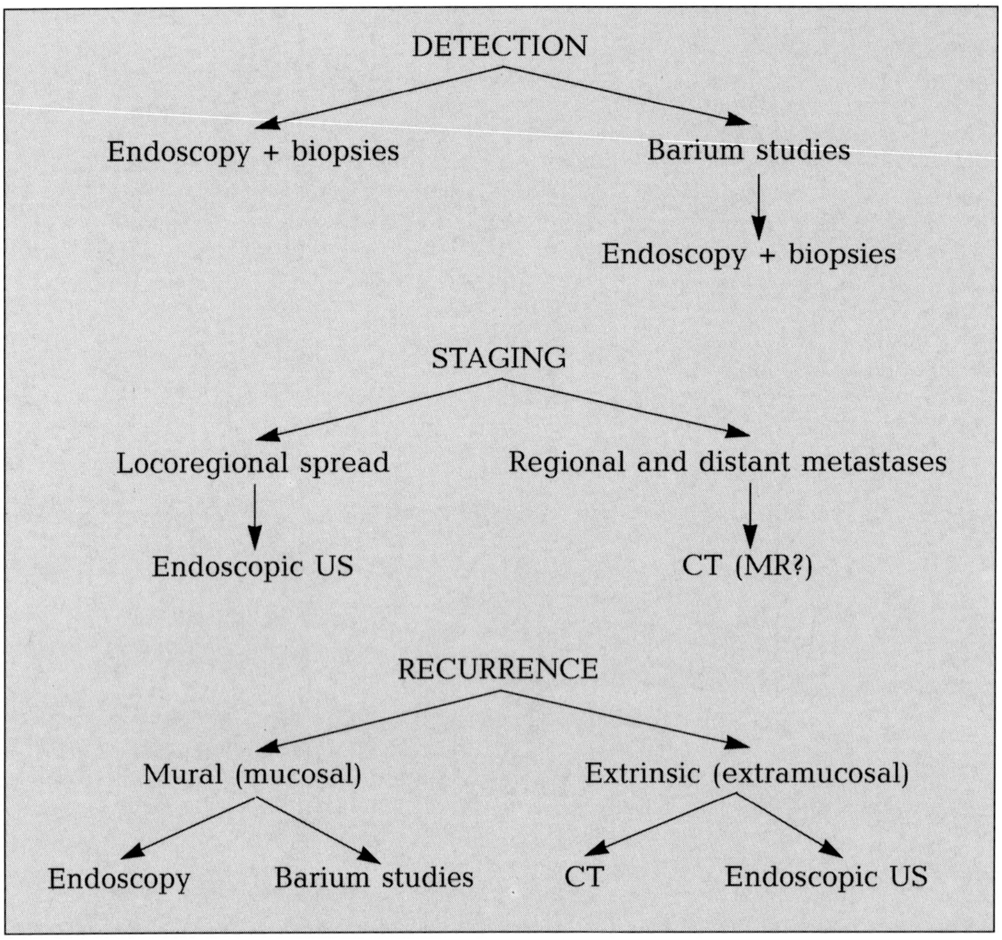

Diagram 8.1

Algorithm for the work up of patients with esophageal or gastric carcinoma.

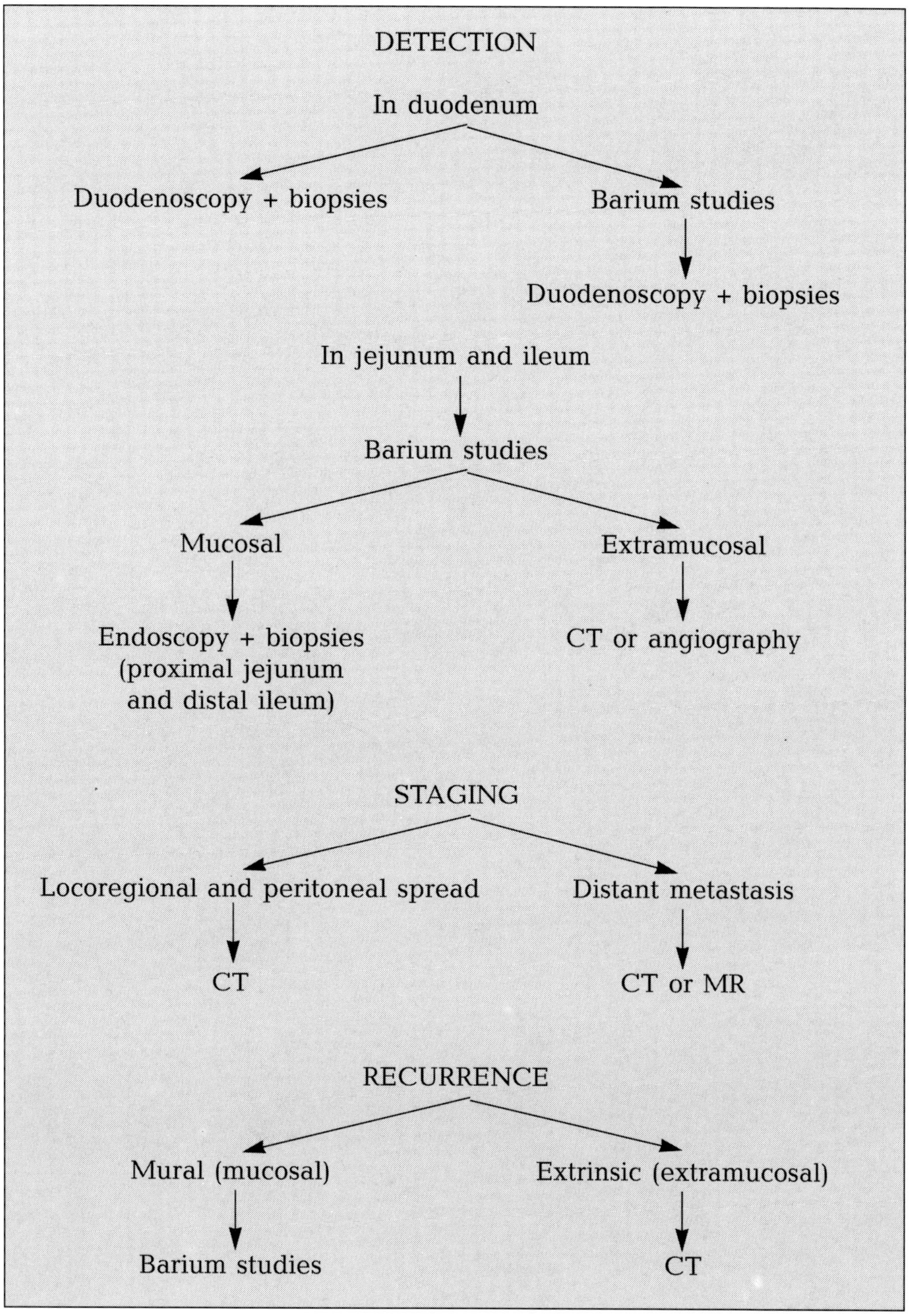

Diagram 8.2

Algorithm for the work up of patients with malignant small-bowel tumors.

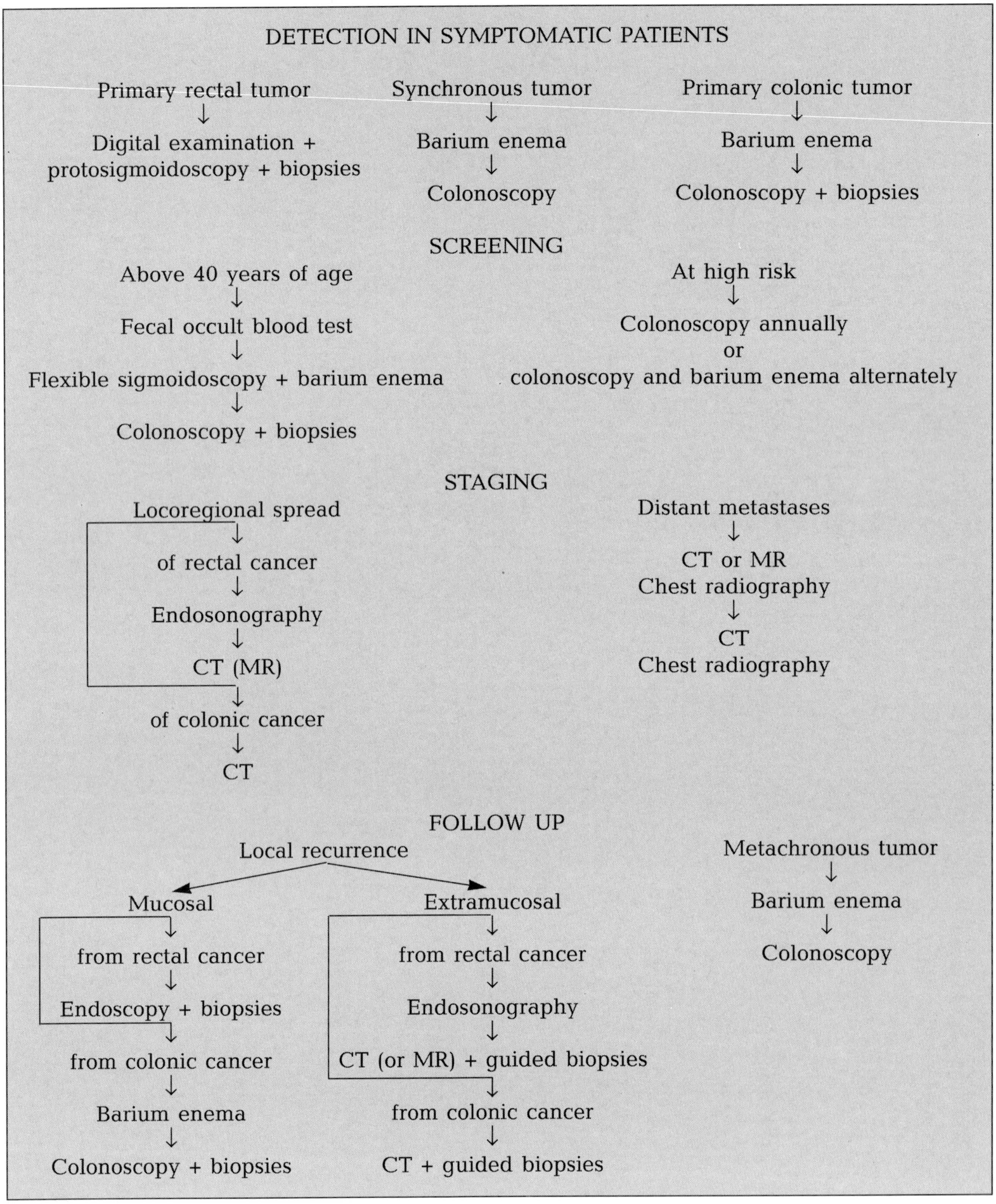

Diagram 8.3

Algorithm for the work up of patients with colorectal cancer.

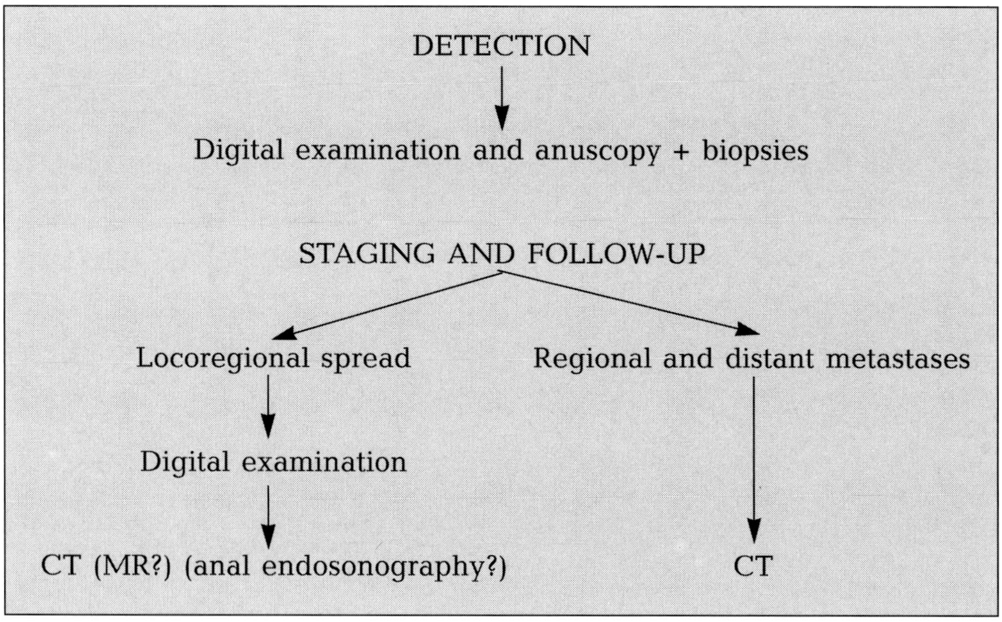

Diagram 8.4

Algorithm for the work up of patients with anal canal cancer.

9

The liver, biliary system, pancreas and spleen

Ashley Davidoff, François Aubert, Yves Menu and David Stark

Introduction[1–4]

The upper abdomen presents unique diagnostic challenges as numerous organs with diverse physiological functions are in close proximity with each other, abut the cardiopulmonary system through a thin diaphragm and have open contact with the dependent organs of the pelvis. Thus, tumors, inflammatory disease and other pathology of the upper abdomen may present clinically with symptoms attributable to an organ involved only secondarily, or they may appear to arise from the thorax or pelvis, leading the clinician away from the primary problem.

Imaging of the abdomen is confounded by its large anatomic area, mobility of its organs and their fluids, and the presence of tissues of varying imaging characteristics.

This chapter will briefly introduce the advantages and limitations of different physical imaging methods as applied to the evaluation of abdominal cancer. After the technical introduction, which provides an understanding of the physics and philosophy of probing the abdomen by various techniques for known or unknown disease, the remainder of our discussion will review imaging characteristics of the major upper abdominal neoplasms.

Virtually all diagnostic medicine and certainly diagnostic imaging is guided by three hierarchical objectives:

- Detection of disease
- Characterization of disease
- Staging of disease.

Detection itself is the most important challenge as it begins with the patients themselves deciding whether a symptom is sufficiently abnormal to warrant a visit to the doctor. After several clinical steps, imaging is most commonly used to determine whether an anatomic area (head, neck, chest, abdomen, pelvis or musculoskeletal system) or physiologic organ system (e.g. hepatobiliary system) is normal or abnormal. This simple, binary decision is critical to selecting patients for more intensive investigation at considerable expense and no small risk of iatrogenic complications.

Characterization of disease commences once an abnormality is found. In the abdomen, nearly all patients develop benign masses if they live long enough (e.g. renal cyst or nodular hyperplasia of the prostate). Where imaging for other reasons causes us to detect these benign masses, imaging must also solve the diagnostic dilemma it created and, at low cost, identify these lesions as benign and of no clinical significance.

Staging is essential to determine prognosis and therapy once treatable disease has been characterized. In many ways, staging is a subset of detection as it is the process by which multiple lesions are discriminated from a single abnormality, and the extent of disease within an organ or spread to adjacent areas is measured. Since staging often involves monitoring of treatment, it presents unique problems because the background normal structures may be altered by surgery, radiation or progression of the disease itself. As society raises ethical and economic questions concerning the merit of treating various conditions, imaging becomes more important as a non-invasive low-cost method of determining which treatments are appropriate and effective.

Imaging techniques

Most of the major abdominal techniques involve the use of ionizing radiation, either in the form of X-rays (radiographs, angiography, CT) or nuclear medicine (scintigraphy). The latter method is unique in that a pharmaceutical is indispensable to the imaging process and the energy form used to create the image is placed within the body.

Cross-sectional images may also be created using reflected sound waves (ultrasound, US) or absorbed and transmitted radiowaves (nuclear magnetic resonance, MR). Ultrasonography, CT and MR were developed, historically in this chronological order. This order also reflects increasing cost of the procedure and decreasing availability of the technology in the USA and world-wide. It also reflects the increasing sophistication and versatility of the three cross-sectional methods.

As a consequence of the limitations of the various imaging methods and their complementary strengths, clinicians can rely on the general rule that the evaluation of suspected abdominal pathology begins with the plain radiograph and, as further diagnostic investigation is justified by clinical findings, the historical ladder of non-invasive radiology unfolds for each patient. Contrast radiography (barium or iodine) US, CT and MR may all be used in the long-term management of complex neoplastic conditions. Angiography is increasingly restricted due to its invasiveness and expense. Furthermore, angiography performed by MR now offers an alternative in the abdomen for many common conditions (e.g. aortic and portal venous disease).

Ultrasonography

Cost, availability and versatility make US the procedure of choice for evaluating suspected biliary and renal disease and a host of poorly defined symptoms that may produce a clinical request to 'take a look' at the upper abdomen.

Machines costing less than US$10 000 can effectively screen for the presence or absence of ascites and gallstones. More expensive equipment and operator training is required to detect biliary obstruction or neoplasms impinging on the biliary system. Machines intended for general use in the abdomen must have transducers operating at a range of frequencies, including 3.5 and 5.0 MHz. Higher frequency transducers offer improved spatial resolution but suffer from decreased penetration, reducing anatomic coverage. The imaging characteristics of sound waves are quite tricky and US is plagued by blind spots as well as artifacts mimicking disease. Therefore, as with many things, a little knowledge of US is dangerous. The temptation to treat it as the 'modern stethoscope' should be tempered by the naive practitioner's propensity to diagnose surgical conditions where none exist and to miss significant lesions due to intervening bone, bowel gas and other difficulties that can be overcome by a more sophisticated practitioner and better equipment.

Technological advances relevant to abdominal imaging and ultrasound include the availability of Doppler techniques to determine flow direction and velocity. This information may be displayed either as numerical values with statistical analysis or as color representing flow, superimposed on the black and white anatomic background. Transducers may also be configured for endoscopic and intraoperative use, providing unique access to critical, small structures. In close proximity to the anatomy of interest, extremely high resolution US images can be obtained; for example, intraoperative US (IOUS) allows a surgeon to place a transducer directly on the liver and detect resectable lesions not visible or palpable, even during laparotomy.

Computed tomography

A major advantage of CT scanning over US is its full, cross-sectional field of view unimpeded by bowel gas or bone. Second, CT is not operator dependent and therefore the risk of an inexperienced practitioner failing to recognize pathology is minimized. The film record of a stack of contiguous transverse sections of the abdomen documents completely the information available through CT. This has further importance in providing a baseline for subsequent lesion characterization, staging or treatment planning.

The principal limitation of CT is its restriction to the transverse plane in the abdomen. Where organs having complex shapes form boundaries oblique to the transverse plane of the CT image, the structures overlap and their attenuation values are averaged into a single dot (picture-element; pixel) on the image. This commonly occurs where a rounded organ surface is tangential to the image section. The experienced radiologist can use many clues to discern true anatomic relationships: this is known as 'volume averaging'. Nevertheless, volume averaging obscures tissue boundaries and quite often US or MR may be preferred to section the structures in a more optimal plane. For example, in unusual or large adrenal or retroperitoneal masses, US or sagittal MR may better distinguish a plane between the liver and the mass, excluding the diagnosis of a primary hepatic neoplasm and showing a tissue plane that provides a 'road map' for surgical excision. However, in the vast majority of cases, the transverse plane alone is sufficient for diagnostic imaging of the abdomen, and therefore the advantages of CT establish it as a work-horse for the investigation of suspected abdominal cancer.

While the fundamentals of CT scanning have not changed in 15 years, improved mechanical arrays of the detectors and engineering of the gantry or ring that orbits the patient has significantly reduced scan times and improved image quality. For example, slip-ring technology is now widely available, allowing scanning of the entire abdomen in a single, screw-like procedure ('spiral CT') with the patient table moving continuously. This method, combined with sophisticated computer reconstruction techniques, allows faster and simpler acquisition of thin sections covering a large anatomic area.

Contrast media

X-Ray attenuation is fundamentally unable to discriminate diseased from normal tissue except in unusual circumstances where the disease causes the accumulation of calcium, gas or fat. CT relies upon morphologic distortions of high-contrast tissue planes, including invasion of fat or destruction of bone, to diagnose mass lesions. The fundamental weakness of X-ray based techniques has required an intensive search for pharmaceutical-based strategies to improve image contrast. Thus, Roentgen himself introduced X-ray attenuating substances which outlined normal and abnormal anatomy.

CT scanning of the upper abdomen can be performed without any contrast agent. However, in nearly all cases enteric and parenteral contrast agents, or both, are used. Orally administered barium or iodine is administered over a period of time to cause opacification of the lumenal contents, allowing reliable identification of stomach, small intestine and large bowel. This is essential because loops of normal bowel otherwise mimic pathologic masses or fluid collections.

Parenchymal tissue contrast is enhanced by intravenous or arterial administration of iodinated agents. Commonly diatrizoate or the newer nonionic contrast agents, such as iohexol or iopamidol are given by the intravenous route. These agents are designed for rapid excretion and do not significantly interact with body physiology. Binding to blood proteins or cells is negligible. Excretion is by passive glomerular filtration. Thus, these agents, introduced to the blood stream, will penetrate capillaries in the body and have an extracellular distribution, although in the brain they are limited to the vascular space by the blood–brain barrier. It is the molecular weight of these agents (less than 1000 Da) that determines their diffusion into the extracellular space of the abdominal organs.

Intravenous contrast marks normal kidney as the agents are concentrated in the renal tubules, distinguishing normal functioning kidney tissue from all but the most vascular renal tumors. Unfortunately, in the liver, spleen and pancreas, the blood supply, capillary permeability and capacity of the extracellular space of tumors is quite variable. The kinetics and degree of enhancement of the tumors is described in generalities such as 'hypovascular' or 'hypervascular'. Unfortunately, enormous biological variation exists, and tumors of a common cell type (e.g. colon adenocarcinoma) may show widely varying enhancement characteristics.

Efforts to selectively enhance liver parenchyma and improve the contrast between normal liver and cancer include rapid intravenous infusion of iodine to exploit the dual (portal venous and hepatic arterial) vascular supply of normal liver as opposed to cancers, which may have fewer vessels. Dissatisfaction with this 'dynamic intravenous bolus technique' has stimulated attempts to administer contrast at angiography via selective cannulation of the hepatic artery or via the superior mesenteric artery, looking at the portal venous phase of contrast circulation. This latter approach has generally greater contrast and some authors have claimed improved sensitivity for detecting liver lesions. However, due to variations in the portal venous perfusion of the liver, non-neoplastic perfusion inhomogeneities create numerous false-positive diagnoses of cancer, limiting the value of this technique for planning therapy.

For more than a decade, investigators have attempted to adapt cholegraphic agents excreted into the biliary system, to the detection of liver cancer. Similarly, emulsions or particulate iodinated agents have been used to target the normal hepatic Kupffer cells in an attempt to contrast these areas against cancer, which does not show phagocytic uptake of particulate iodine. Unfortunately, these attempts to target iodinated agents in bulk to normal liver have been complicated by toxic side-effects. Newer agents under development may show improved safety profiles; however, none as yet is in clinical trials.

Magnetic resonance imaging

MR is similar to CT in providing a full field of view of the entire body area, a permanent record of the entire examination, and similar anatomic detail (spatial resolution). MR has the further advantage of allowing selection of sagittal, coronal or oblique planes of section. It excels in high-resolution images, which can be acquired as a three-dimensional volume. However, as yet, MR of the abdomen is technically underdeveloped and suffers from motion artifacts similar to the problems CT faced in the 1970s. Until the problem of motion is solved, MR will be applied only in selected cases to solve specific imaging problems. Notably, MR, like CT, is getting faster, and speed solves the problem of motion. Furthermore, MR appears more robust and its technical evolution has outlasted that of CT. Clinically useful non-invasive angiography by MR has already impacted the management of abdominal disease. The ability to identify normal flow and measure flow velocities is already affecting the work up of neurovascular disease, and, in the near future, cardiothoracic and abdominal vascular applications will become routine.

Briefly, motion is a major source of contrast on MR images and moving tissue or blood protons can be magnetically 'tagged' without use of a catheter or administration of a pharmaceutical. Furthermore, microscopic motion within tissue, either at the capillary level or brownian motion of extracellular and intracellular water, may even allow assessment of perfusion. Naturally, this is of greatest interest in organs where ischemia is the principal disease, such as the brain and heart. Perfusion studies have already been applied to the characterization of liver masses, and further refinement and broadened applications are expected.

Angiography

Invasive catheter angiography, also known as contrast angiography, remains the procedure of choice for defining vascular anatomy in preparation for resection of many abdominal neoplasms. As yet, MR cannot reliably identify replaced right hepatic arteries, the presence of multiple renal arteries or the major branches supplying tumor neovascularity. While advances in MR may well assume these applications in the future, catheter techniques for interventional radiology will undoubtedly continue to grow. Therapeutic radiology is beyond the scope of this chapter; however, it is evident that a catheter can be used to deliver locally high concentrations of chemotherapeutic agents or to embolize malformations or tumor growths.

Scintigraphy

The fundamental advantage of scintigraphy in the diagnosis of abdominal neoplasia is the selectivity of physiologically targeted radiopharmaceuticals. The method has inherently high sensitivity and can detect nanomolar (10^{-9} local concentrations of pharmaceuticals, allowing selective targeting of low-density receptors and sensitive metabolic processes. However, the use of pharmaceuticals as the energy source for imaging and problems with diffuse vascular distribution of the radiopharmaceutical undermine image quality by providing a diffuse signal source. Thus, the statistics of sparse and dispersed gamma emissions, combined with problems of scatter of the emitted energy by intervening tissues, and the use of low-resolution imaging devices (Geiger counters or photomultiplier tubes) result in grossly inferior spatial resolution.

Scintigraphy is best applied where low spatial resolution can be turned to advantage. For example, low resolution is equated with larger fields of view and thus whole-body scanning is reasonable. The bone scan, searching for active metabolism indicative of metastatic disease, is perhaps the most natural and best application of scintigraphy.

In the abdomen, scintigraphy is occasionally applied to functional studies of bile flow and cystic duct obstruction. Particles can be used to probe reticuloendothelial function, producing functional but low spatial resolution 'liver–spleen scans'. Unfortunately, scintigraphy has little or no advantage over US, CT and MR in evaluating suspected abdominal neoplasms. Perhaps in the future pharmaceuticals will be targeted to metabolic processes of interest, or immunologic targeting of cancer may resurrect scintigraphy. However, with currently available radiopharmaceuticals, efforts to improve spatial resolution such as single photon emission CT (SPECT) and positron emission tomography (PET) have not significantly changed the approach to the management of abdominal cancer, even in the most specialized academic centers.

The liver

Metastases

The liver is the most common organ in the body to which cancer spreads from primary disease elsewhere. Gastrointestinal neoplasms, including those in the pancreas, nearly always involve the liver before metastasizing to other organs. In addition, breast, lung, renal and ovarian and other common malignancies spread hematogenously, lymphatically or transperitoneally to the liver. Indeed, liver failure is one of the most common causes of death in cancer patients, and liver metastases serve as a basis for determining prognosis and monitoring therapy.

Liver enzymes that leak into the blood stream when the liver is injured (serum glutamic oxaloacetate transaminase, SGOT; serum glutamic pyruvic transaminase, SGPT; alkaline phosphatase) have such poor sensitivity and specificity that they cannot be justified as an independent diagnostic test. When metastatic cancer to the liver is suspected or a reasonable risk exists, imaging must be performed. Unfortunately, imaging also has its limitations and pitfalls.

Metastatic spread of cancer is thought to begin as a single cell or a small cluster of cells, well below the resolution limit of imaging. Indeed, imaging cannot reliably detect liver lesions smaller than 5 mm in size. Since a metastasis grows exponentially it is submillimeter in size for the vast majority of its 'lifecycle' before it enlarges to the point of causing symptoms and ultimately killing the patient. Therefore, it is obvious that the majority of metastases present in an individual, or epidemiologically the majority of metastases present in a population, are below the threshold size for detection by any means.

Imaging

Detection

Liver cancer detection does offer clinically useful information because most patients with metastatic cancer have multiple lesions, some of which are sufficiently large (greater than 1 cm diameter) to be reliably detected. The accuracy of imaging for detecting liver metastases is the subject of endless disputes and revision of the radiological literature. The major problem with our literature is the lack of suitable 'gold standards'. It is simply impossible to collect a large series of patients with autopsy and histologic confirmation of imaging findings. Thus, radiologists frequently resort to comparative studies where one modality is compared to another and a third technique, such as surgery, or a third imaging modality, is used as the arbiter of 'truth'. Such comparative studies consistently establish a higher hierarchy of overall accuracy for detection of liver lesions.

It is now generally accepted that MR is the best test, followed by CT, US and then angiography. CT angioportography (CTAP) techniques are equal to or slightly better than MR; however, the angiographic CT methods are generally not available and are nearly 10 times more expensive. Therefore, when the clinician is able to focus the diagnostic question of the detection of liver metastases, MR is now the preferred technique. Unfortunately, such clarity is rarely present. If a clinician also requests inspection of the adrenals, retroperitoneum and other abdominal organs, then CT is a preferred modality, as its combined capabilities presently exceed those of MR.

Verification of the accuracy of imaging requires hepatectomy or major hepatic resection proximate to imaging with a state-of-the-art technique. In 1989,[5] dynamic intravenous bolus iodine-enhanced CT was compared with thin histologic sections of resected liver. Not surprisingly, given the best gold standard to date, the former gave the lowest numbers for imaging accuracy. Only 38% of individual metastases were detected by contrast-enhanced CT. This study is in sharp contrast to earlier publications claiming accuracy rates as high as 98% for CT. It also calls into question all previous, poorly controlled studies of US and nuclear medicine. It can be inferred from numerous comparative studies, which showed US and nuclear medicine to be significantly inferior to CT, that no more than 30% of lesions in the liver are detected by these alternative methods. The good news is that CT, properly performed, rarely causes false-positive examinations. And finally, because the biology of metastatic cancer is such that lesions

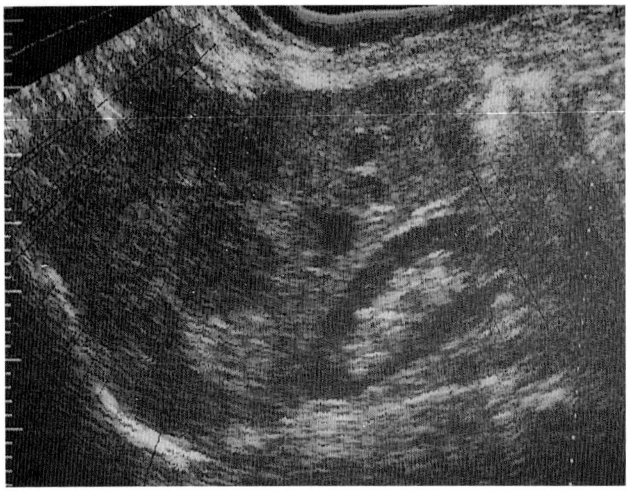

A

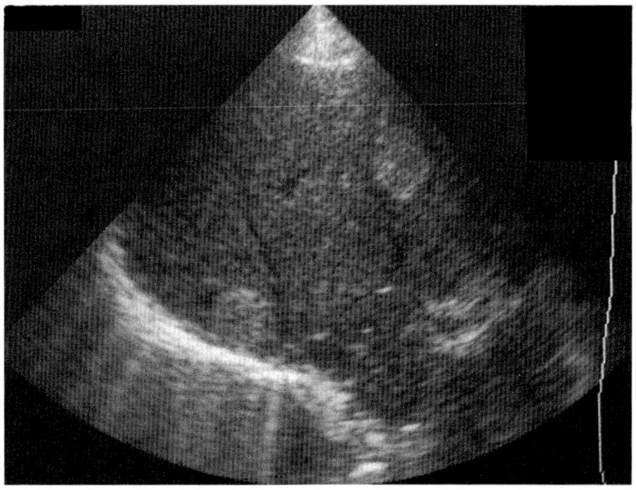

B

Figure 9.1

Hepatic metastases. US shows multiple hypoechoic metastases of breast origin (**A**) and a purely echogenic metastasis of neurendocrine origin (**B**).

tend to be multiple and at various stages of growth, most patients with any metastatic liver cancer have a sufficient tumor burden to allow detection of at least one lesion. Thus, CT has an accuracy in excess of 80% for distinguishing abnormal patients (i.e. those with one or more metastases) from those patients having entirely normal livers. Again, given the biology of metastatic disease, it is this simpler task which influences therapy.

The lack of an effective blood test for metastatic cancer and the poor performance of imaging for identifying individual metastases may explain the confusion concerning the efficacy of resective surgical treatment of metastatic disease. If many patients thought to have solitary lesions and successful resections were in fact understaged, many treatment failures were in fact staging errors. Thus, it may not be possible to determine whether resection of isolated metastases is effective until improved staging methods are used in therapeutic trials.

In summary, for patients at risk for metastatic cancer it is an economic and public policy issue whether the best test, MR, is made available. Given the cost of misdirected cancer therapy in patients with undiagnosed metastases, it is likely that diagnostic imaging pays for itself. Setting aside humanitarian and economic issues, as a practicality MR and even CT are not available to all patients. Therefore, we must accept the insensitivity of this method and cost of false-negative and false-positive examinations when US is used as the primary screening test.

The dominant world-wide use of US for liver imaging may in fact be cost-effective, as this rapid and inexpensive method does reliably identify the majority of patients having metastatic cancer; and in those cases having a solitary or questionable lesion at US, CT should be made available. Setting aside economic issues, state-of-the-art oncologic practice in the abdomen requires use of either CT or MR to screen for liver metastases.

Lesion characterization

US shows most metastatic lesions as hyperechoic (60%), with 20% being hypoechoic and 20% heterogeneous (Figure 9.1). Purely cystic, anechoic lesions are uncommon and may be seen in ovarian,

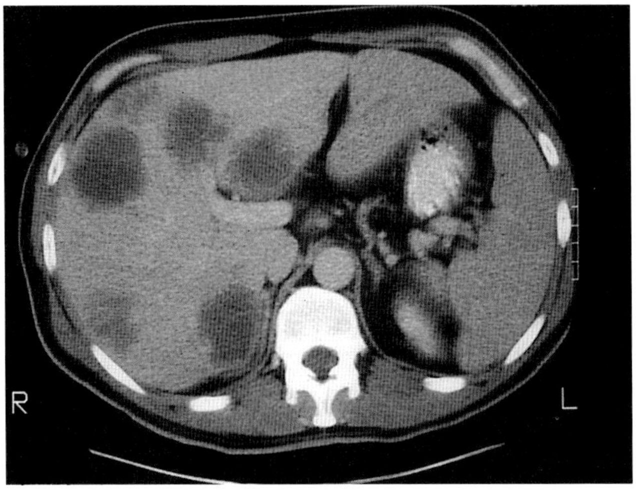

A

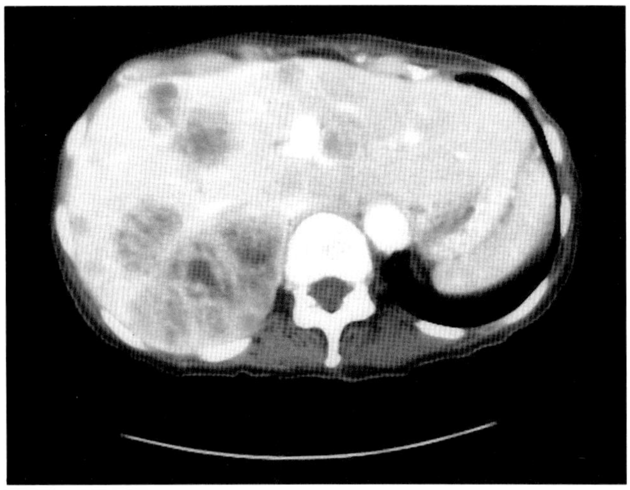

B

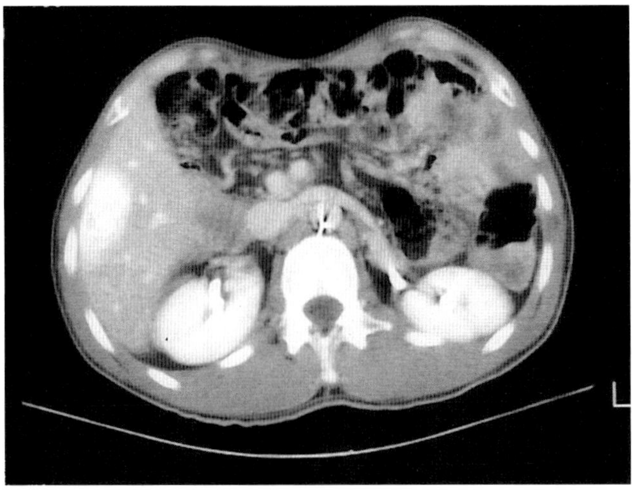

C

Figure 9.2

Hepatic metastases: CT scans.

A Multiple hypodense metastases of colonic origin.

B Heterogeneous colonic metastases, with secondary hypertrophy of the left lobe of the liver.

C Homogeneous hypervascular metastasis of malignant islet cell origin.

cystic pancreatic and carcinoid metastases. Necrotic tumor may appear cystic or echogenic, mimicking solid tissue.

CT may demonstrate calcifications which occur uncommonly, most often in mucinous carcinomas, such as metastatic colon cancer. Low-density areas may correlate with necrosis on unenhanced as well as iodine-enhanced scans (Figure 9.2). The morphologic pattern of contrast enhancement, demonstrating heterogeneity (Figure 9.2) or rings is a useful finding that distinguishes solid neoplasms from cysts or cavernous hemangiomas (discussed later).

MR is more likely than CT to demonstrate internal nodular structure, rings and hemorrhage (Figure 9.3). In particular, T2-weighted MR images are useful as they show edema at the border active lesions which may be manifested as rings or as geographic zones of increased signal intensity. T1-weighted images are less sensitive to edema; as a result metastases are virtually always the same size or larger on T2-weighted images.

All three sectional modalities can detect vascular invasion; however, MR is the most sensitive due to its greater soft-tissue contrast, as well as its ability to image flowing blood (Figure 9.4).

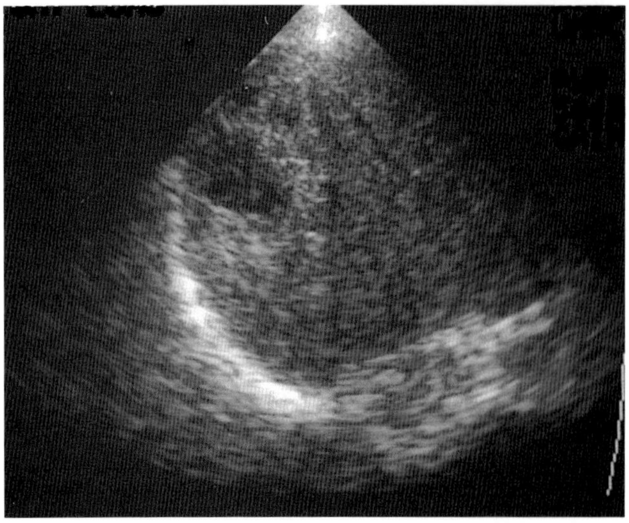

A

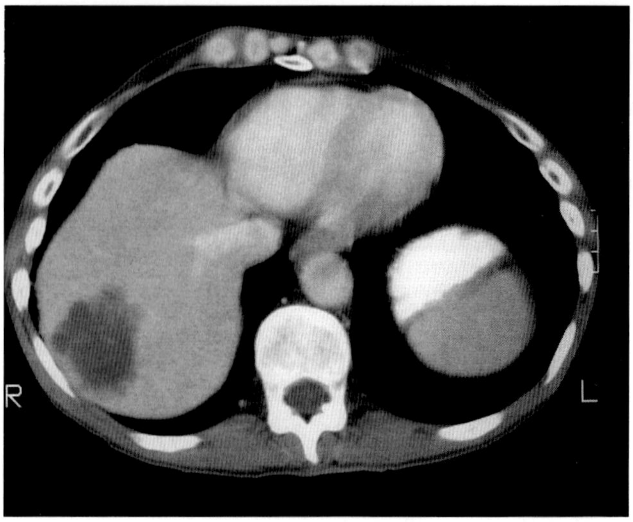

B

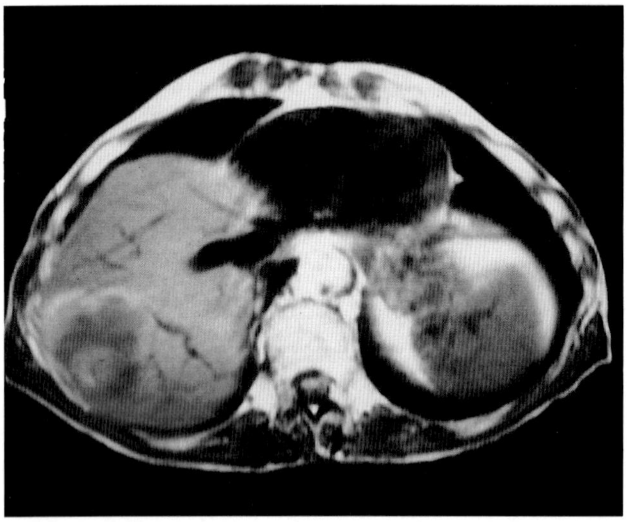

C

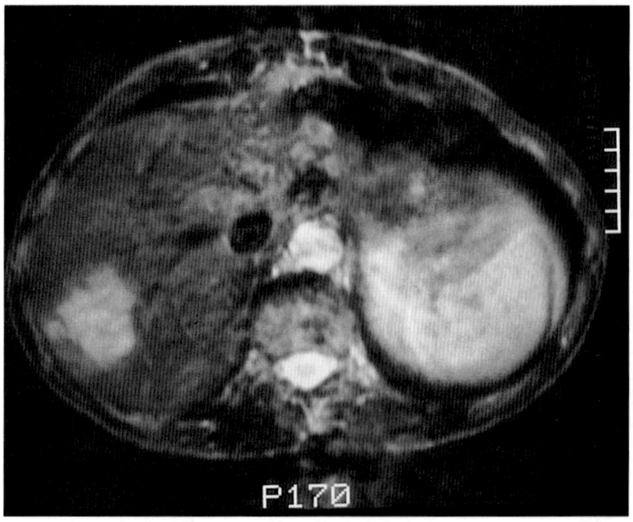

D

Figure 9.3

Hepatic metastases.

A US shows a mass with a central hypoechoic region, probably representing fluid, and a peripheral echogenic rim.

B CT shows a predominantly low density, but heterogeneous mass.

C,D MR, with a central bright area on T1 (C), and persistance of this brightness on T2 (D) with additional brightening of the whole lesion, suggests hemorrhage and a fluid-containing mass.

This patient had a surgically proven hemorrhagic mucin containing metastasis of colonic origin. This is an exemplary case demonstrating the strength of MR in characterizing lesions.

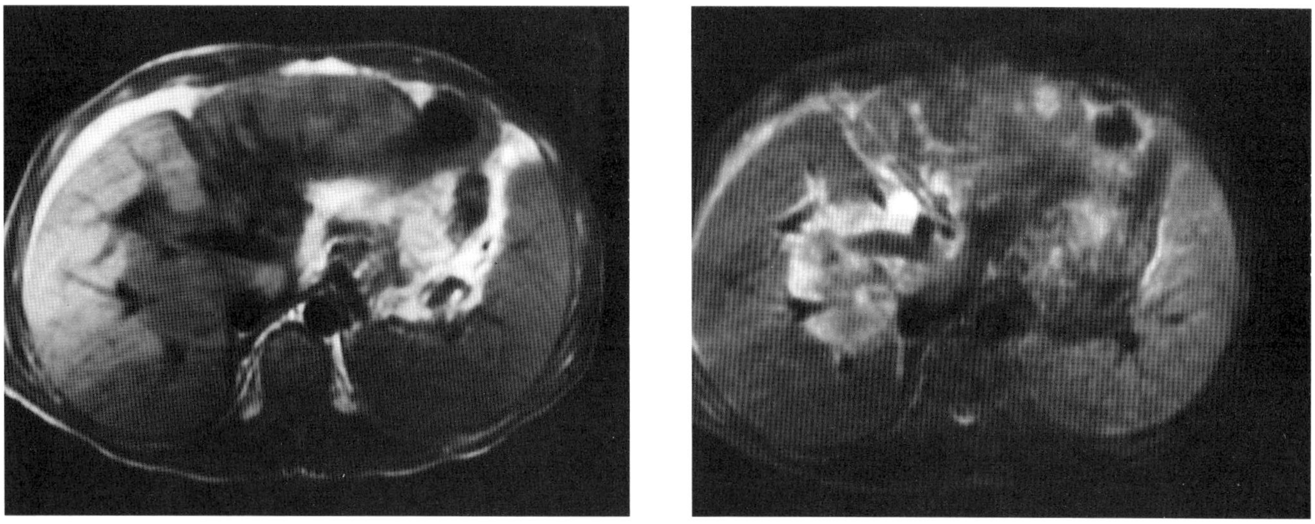

A B

Figure 9.4

Hepatic metastases: MR demonstrating mass effect.

A The T1-weighted image shows a central lesion (adenocarcinoma of unknown primary) with a peripheral wedge-shaped area of high intensity.

B The proton density image shows a faint persistance of the wedge-shaped defect.

These findings suggest a central solid lesion with mass effect on central vessels, resulting in ischemia and fatty change distal to the obstruction.

Staging

Staging of hepatic neoplasms involves principally identifying the lobe and segment of disease. Patients with larger tumor burdens and receiving chemotherapy can be monitored by scan-to-scan comparison of tumor diameters or estimates of tumor volume.

Surgical approaches to hepatic metastases depend primarily on confidence that all of the tumors have been identified. If there is reason to believe that a solitary metastasis exists or that a cohort of a few similar-sized lesions represent the only disease in the liver, then the question of resection depends upon the functional hepatic reserve and technical ability to remove the lesions. Lesions invading adjacent structure, such as the diaphragm or inferior vena cava, or lesions in difficult areas, such as the porta hepatis, make surgery challenging and risky. Undoubtedly, the greatest risk to resective therapy is the undiagnosed residual disease.

Hepatocellular carcinoma (HCC)

Also known as hepatoma, primary malignancy of hepatocytes, i.e. HCC, comprises 1% of all cancers in the USA. World-wide, variation in nutritional factors and the incidence of viral hepatitis[10,11] account for major differences in the incidence and nature of HCC. It is far more common in Japan, the rest of Asia and sub-Saharan Africa in association with chronic viral hepatitis. The epidemiology may be shifting from hepatitis B to hepatitis C now that effective vaccination is available for the former. In countries with a high incidence of viral hepatitis and hepatoma, the male to female ratio is 1:1 and the average age of incidence is 30–40 years. In the USA and Europe, where alcoholic cirrhosis is relatively more common, the male to female ratio is 5:1 and the average age of incidence is increased to 60–70 years.

Serologic testing is useful in the detection of hepatoma, because α-fetoprotein (AFP) levels above 400 ng/mg are present in 25% of small lesions and 60% of medium-sized lesions, and because AFP is rarely encountered in benign hepatic disease.[12] In fetal life this protein is produced by both the fetal liver and the yolk sac. After the age of 2 years AFP is barely detectable in normal individuals (less than 30 ng/ml). Interestingly, hepatoma patients in the USA are less likely to have elevated AFP levels than patients in Africa.

Nonspecific elevation of AFP may occur in patients with other tumors of embryonic nature. In a variety of non-malignant conditions, such as normal pregnancy, or fetal abnormality, such as neural tube defects, AFP rises. Unfortunately, AFP may also be abnormal in patients without cancer but with cirrhosis or chronic hepatitis. AFP levels greater than 10 000 ng/ml are considered pathognomonic for the presence of cancer. However, certain subtypes of hepatoma, such as fibrolamellar carcinoma, may show normal levels.

Imaging

Detection

Cross-sectional imaging is fundamental to the detection and management of hepatocellular carcinoma. Articles can be found in the literature citing a wide range of sensitivity, specificity and overall accuracy for US, CT and MR.[13,14,15] It is evident that hepatocellular carcinoma is more difficult to detect with any of the imaging methods than is metastatic cancer. The principal reason for this difficulty is that hepatoma most often occurs against a background of chronic hepatitis, fatty liver and cirrhosis.

Ongoing regeneration and areas of nodular hyperplasia serve to mask or mimic hepatoma. Bands of scar tissue in the liver have increased water content, and the long T1/T2 signal intensity characteristics are very similar to hepatoma.

Lesion characterization

Characterization of hepatoma and discrimination from metastatic cancer or benign hepatic masses is rarely possible with US, CT, or scintigraphy. MR, however, has the ability to detect three features characteristic of hepatoma. Each of these features is present in approximately 30% of hepatomas, and therefore one or more features can be found in a majority of cases.

First, a capsule[11,16–18] of compressed liver or scar tissue may create a sharp boundary with adjacent liver tissue. The capsule has long T1/long T2 signal intensity characteristics, and is usually best seen on T1-weighted images. The capsule must be distinguished from low signal intensity blood vessels on T1-weighted spin echo images. Hepatic adenoma may also show peripheral capsules indistinguishable from those of hepatoma. However, hepatic adenoma is an unusual tumor with different demographics. Tumor capsules can be distinguished from the rings of metastases, as the latter are better seen on T2-weighted images and are not well seen at all on T1-weighted images.

Second, hepatomas accumulate intracellular triglyceride (Figure 9.5).[16,19,20] Fatty accumulation can be detected using a variety of chemical shift methods such as phase-contrast frequency-selective imaging. Although fatty accumulation may occur in injured hepatocytes in other conditions, including adenoma, focal nodular hyperplasia, hepatitis and dietary disturbances, it is usually possible to distinguish focal fatty infiltration from fat within a mass, as the latter displaces normal blood vessels while focal fat infiltration usually does not.

Third, hepatoma has a propensity to grow into hepatic and portal veins (Figures 9.6 and 9.7), and MR is able to demonstrate this morphology to advantage. Certainly US also has this capability; however, the ability of US to distinguish the solid tumor from adjacent liver makes it more difficult to follow the tumor into vessels.

The hypervascularity of the lesion sometimes leads to spontaneous hemorrhage that can be characterized both by CT and MR (Figure 9.8).

Angiography is also useful for characterization of hepatoma as most tumors are quite hypervascular with neovascularity and arteriovenous shunting. Portal or hepatic venous thrombosis may also be confirmed angiographically.

Hepatocellular carcinoma is a surgical disease with well-encapsulated lesions showing a better prognosis than diffuse tumors or those with satellite nodules (intrahepatic metastases). Patients who had a single lesion removed, had survival rates at 1, 3, and 5 years of 81, 41 and 41%, respectively. When satellite nodules were identified in the region of a resected lesion, survival rates were 65, 33 and 20%, respectively.[21] The superior ability of MR to visualize the capsule and demonstrate tumor–liver interfaces has established it as the procedure of choice in Japan, where surgical and alternative therapies are most highly developed. Japanese radiologists also perform arterial contrast enhanced CT using Lipiodol which stains tumors selectively due to their capillary endothelial defects.

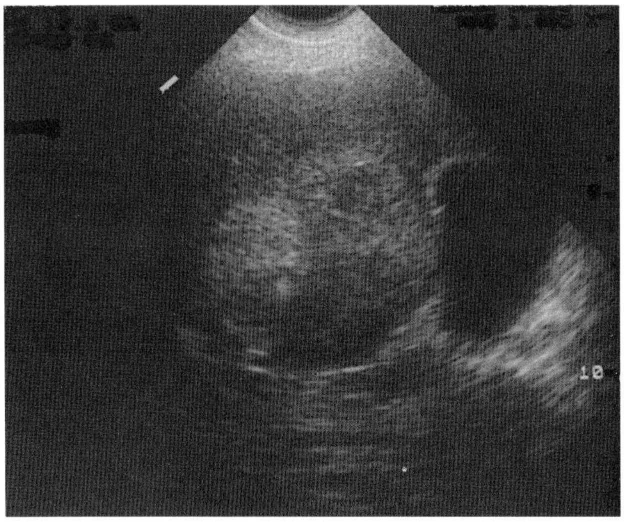

A

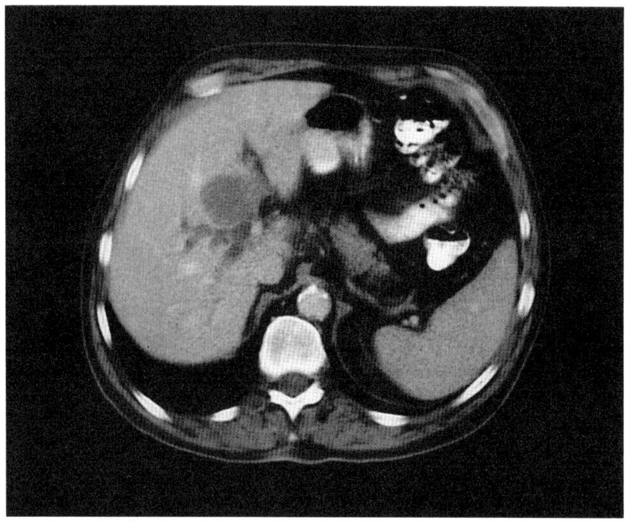

B

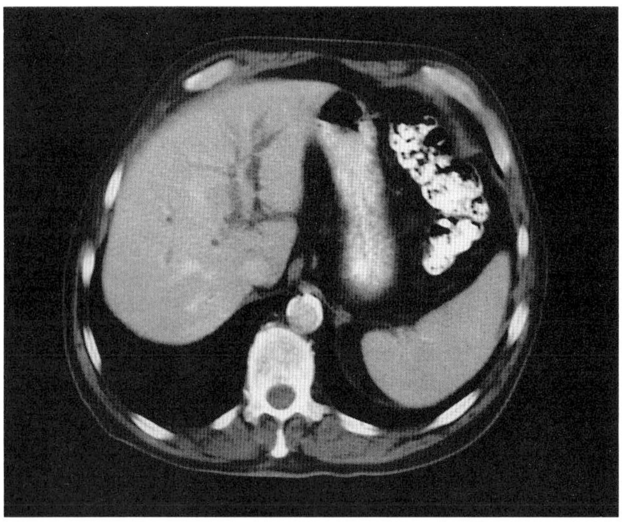

C

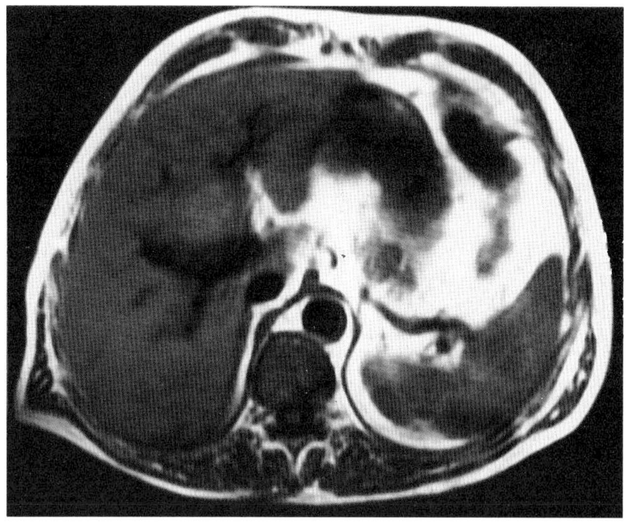

D

Figure 9.5

Hepatocellular carcinoma (HCC).

A US shows a single predominantly echogenic mass.

B CT confirms the central single mass.

C CT also shows obstruction of the left-sided bile ducts.

D MR shows a subtle area of relatively high intensity on the T1-weighted image, in this case found to be fat, and characteristic for HCC.

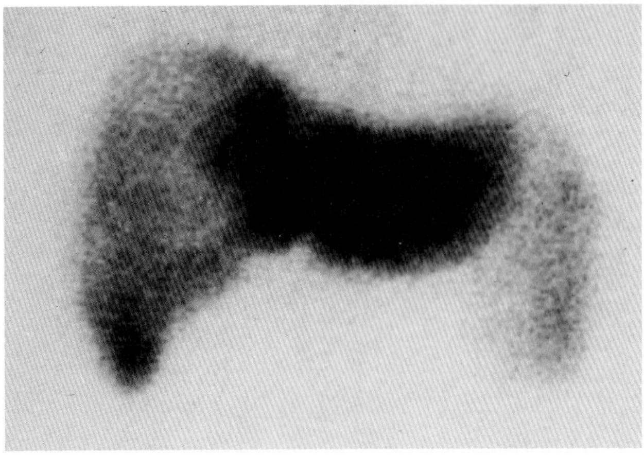

A

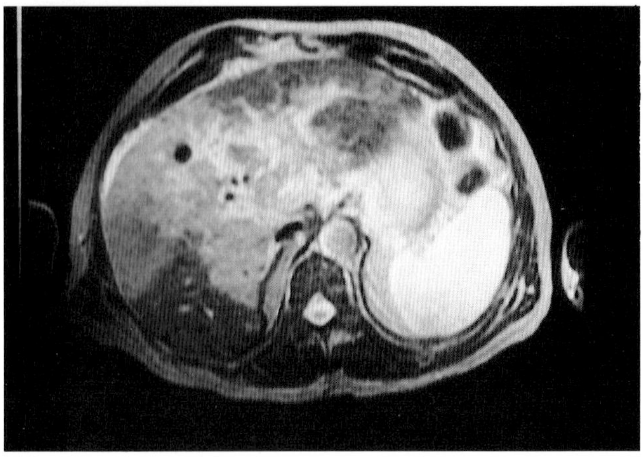

B

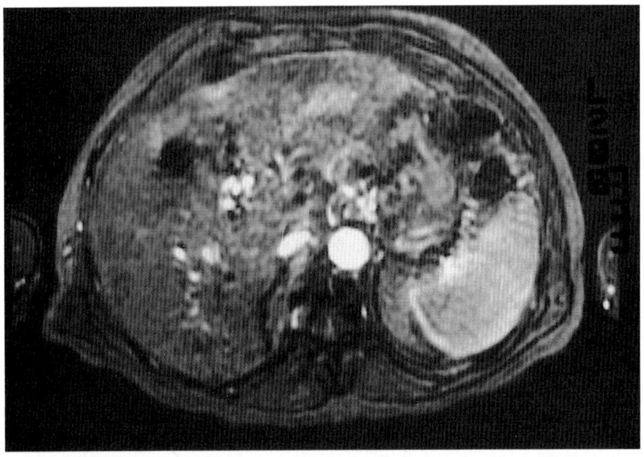

C

Figure 9.6

Hepatocellular carcinoma (HCC).

A The sulfur colloid scan shows non-specific infiltrative lesions in the right lobe of the liver.

B The proton density image reveals a similar geographic involvement, and in addition fails to demonstrate the portal vein. Rather, three small flow void vessels are seen in its place, representing cavernous transformation of the portal vein.

C This is confirmed by gradient echo technique.

The diagnosis of HCC was made and confirmed by biopsy.

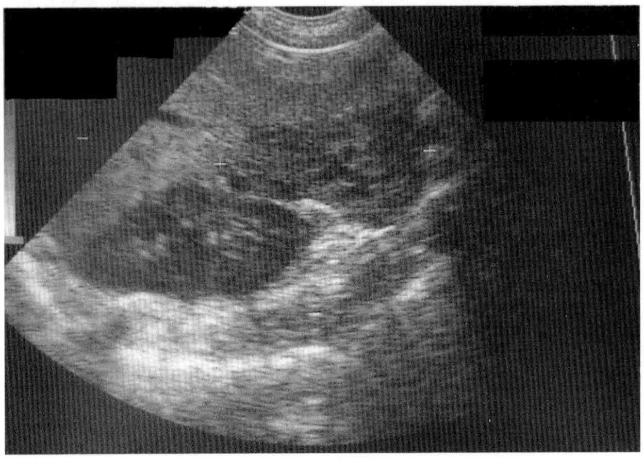

A

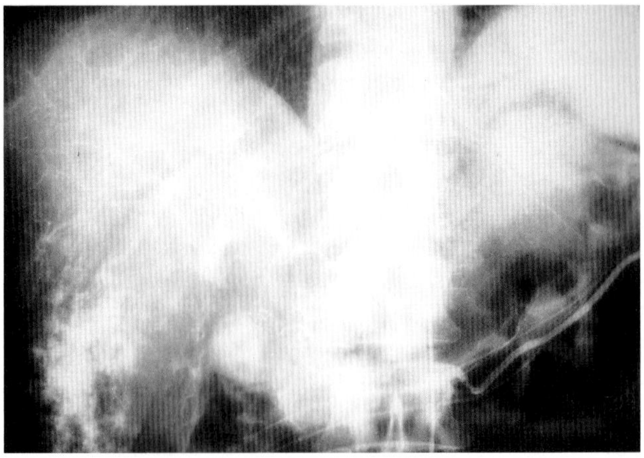

B

Figure 9.7

Hepatocellular carcinoma (HCC): US.

A A predominantly hypoechoic mass, with heterogeneity and central tubular defects, is shown in this US.

B Obstructed hepatic veins are shown on the venous phase of a hepatic angiogram.

Invasion and obstruction of the veins by HCC is characteristic.

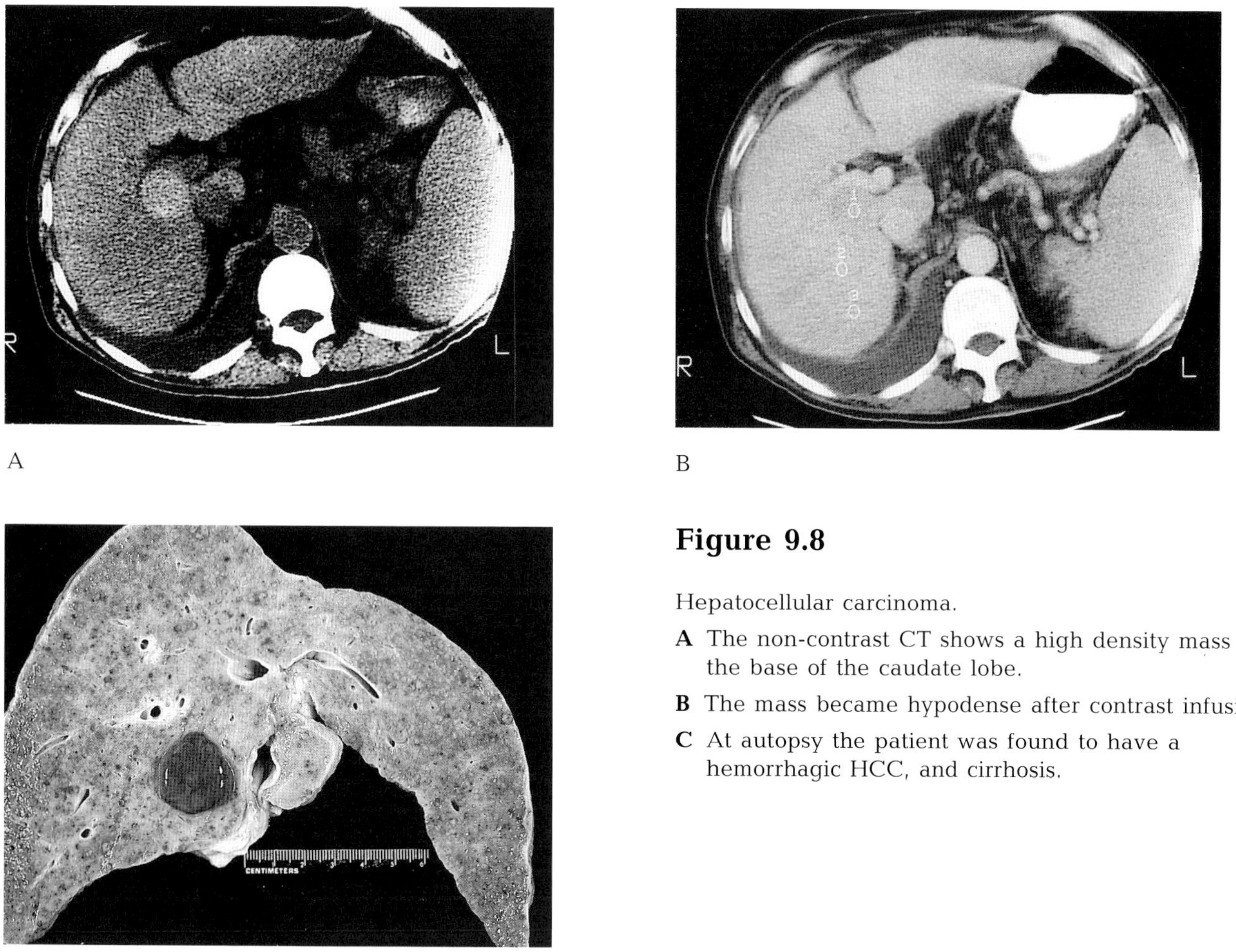

A

B

C

Figure 9.8

Hepatocellular carcinoma.

A The non-contrast CT shows a high density mass at the base of the caudate lobe.

B The mass became hypodense after contrast infusion.

C At autopsy the patient was found to have a hemorrhagic HCC, and cirrhosis.

Benign disease

Cavernous hemangiomas

Hemangioma is a vascular malformation characterized by a cavernous collection of blood spaces. Blood flow is very slow and virtually undetectable except for occasional peripheral site of venous entry. Hemangioma is exceedingly common in both sexes and all races around the world. Approximately 15–20% of the adult population has such a lesion.[22–24] As nearly all these lesions are asymptomatic and of no clinical significance, it is the incidental finding of a liver mass in the patient undergoing imaging for another purpose that creates a diagnostic dilemma.

Detection

The oncologic patient undergoing imaging for the purpose of detecting a liver mass has a higher probability of harboring a malignancy. In this population, the pre-test probability of liver cancer is obviously increased, and there coexists a 15% probability of a cavernous hemangioma. Indeed, cancer and hemangioma are commonly found side by side. Therefore, while we do not seek to detect cavernous hemangiomas, we unfortunately do find them. Indeed, given their fluid content they are high-contrast lesions readily seen by US, CT, MR, scintigraphy and angiography.

Lesion characterization

Characterization of hemangiomas has been attempted with all of the foregoing modalities. US and MR often display tissue features that suggest a greater likelihood of cavernous hemangioma than malignancy. For example, US displays cavernous hemangiomas as uniformly echogenic lesions with sharp margins and increased acoustic transmission. Unfortunately, 10–20% of tumors may have this appearance and conversely 40% of cavernous hemangiomas do not have this 'typical' appearance (Figure 9.9).[25–28] The remaining cavernous hemangiomas may be hypoechoic or heterogeneous.

MR has been remarkably successful in identifying the fluid content of cavernous hemangiomas by its long T2 relaxation time (Figure 9.9).[18,24,29,30] Long TE spin-echo images, which reduce the signal intensity of solid tissue relative to fluid, show cavernous hemangiomas, cerebral spinal fluid, bile and gastric contents as extremely bright structures. Properly performed with TE in excess of 120 ms and successful suppression of motion artifact, cavernous hemangiomas are homogeneous and sharply circumscribed. Tumors, on the other hand, are ill defined, heterogeneous and lower in signal intensity due to their gelatinous (solid) makeup.

Contrast-enhanced blood-pool studies provide an alternative method to identify hemangiomas and other vascular lesions. CT uses iodine based diagnostic pharmaceuticals, scintigraphy uses technetium-labeled red blood cells, and MR uses the paramagnetic agent gadolinium (Gd-DTPA). In addition, iron oxide particles and other magnetic contrast media have been shown to be effective blood pool markers. The concept behind these studies depends principally on the kinetics and distribution of the vascular agents. Similar findings are seen with all three modalities, in that cavernous hemangiomas enhance uniformly over 5–30 min and may retain contrast longer than the circulating blood pool. Tumors show more rapid wash-in and wash-out of the contrast agent and usually show less peak enhancement than cavernous hemangiomas. As these findings depend upon the cardiac output, circulation time, timing of contrast administration and specifics of the vascular malformations perfusion pattern, contrast-enhanced studies are less predictable than plain T2-weighted MR. Nevertheless, MR is capable of both methods.

Controlled studies have shown that MR can discriminate cavernous hemangioma from solid neoplasm with an overall accuracy of 90%. If, in addition to this T2-weighted technique, a contrast study is added, accuracy increases further. With MR one can perform both an unenhanced and enhanced scan within a single 1-hour examination.

Scintigraphy is still widely practised due to tradition amongst radiologists and familiarity with referring clinicians. However, scintigraphy with technetium-labeled red cells is often one of a series of tests performed on separate days and therefore is more expensive than MR alone. Furthermore, scintigraphy with SPECT is unable to diagnose lesions smaller than 2 cm in size, while MR techniques are reliable for lesions as small as 1 cm,' and is still improving.

Hepatocellular adenoma

Hepatocellular adenoma is a benign neoplasm of heptocytes occurring almost exclusively in women taking oral contraceptives. The usual clinical presentation is one of minimal epigastric discomfort. Acute abdominal pain classically accompanies hemorrhage into an adenoma (Figure 9.10).

Adenomas are large vascular masses ranging between 5 and 15 cm in size, and often contain necrosis and hemorrhage. They are occasionally surrounded by a capsule, and occasionally multiple.

Adenomas are characterized microscopically by proliferation of hepatocytes and loss of the lobular architecture of the liver. The involved hepatocytes are high in glycogen and uncommonly contain fat, and the support structure lacks Kupffer cells. [31,32]

Detection and lesion characterization

The mass, mostly by virtue of its size, is readily detected by all modalities.[33] A solid liver mass in an asymptomatic female is a perplexing problem, often defying characterization. Because of the risk of bleeding following biopsy of an adenoma, together with difficulty in cytologic interpretation, the clinical options are either to follow conservatively or to resect completely. The diagnosis of adenoma is likely, however, if the patient is taking contraceptive pills and the lesion decreases in size with discontinuation of the pill (Figure 9.11), or if

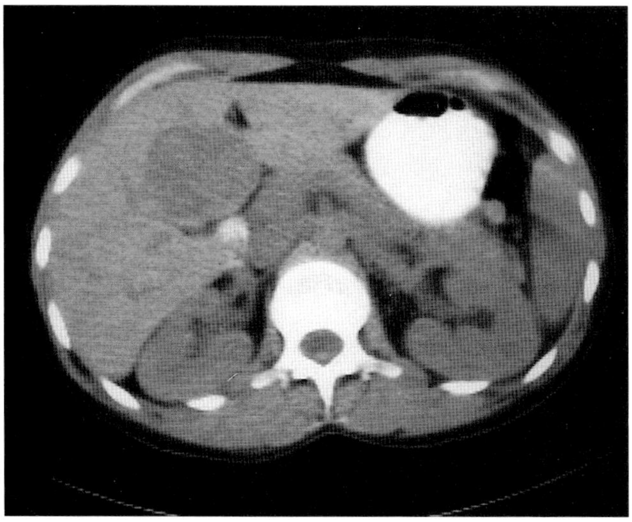

A

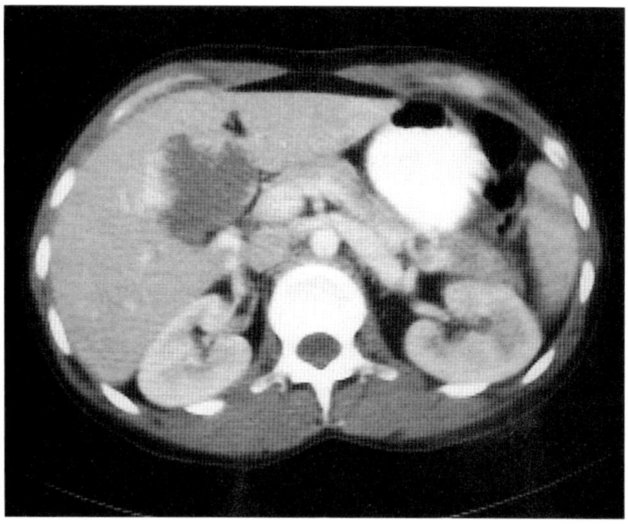

B

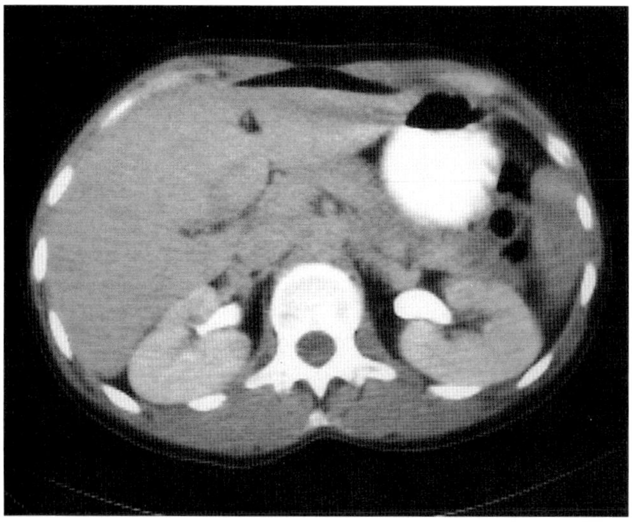

C

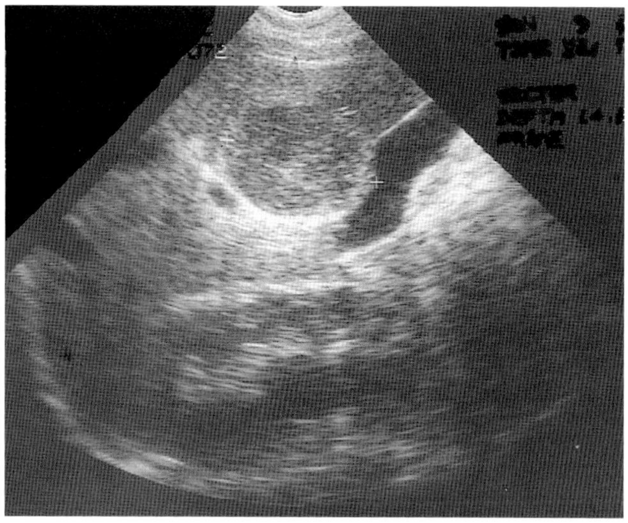

D

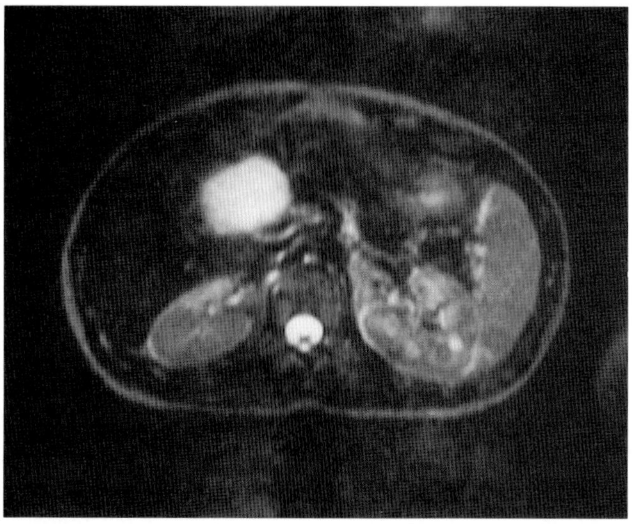

E

Figure 9.9

Hemangioma.

A The non-contrast CT shows a hypodense lesion with minimal heterogeneity.

B CT scan: peripheral puddling with contrast is characteristic.

C The lesion failed to become isodense on the delayed CT scan.

D US was atypical for hemangioma in that the lesion is heterogeneous and predominantly hypodense.

E The T2-weighted sequence shows the lesion to have a prolonged T2, characteristic of benign disease, in this case a hemangioma. The diagnosis of hemangioma was confirmed at autopsy.

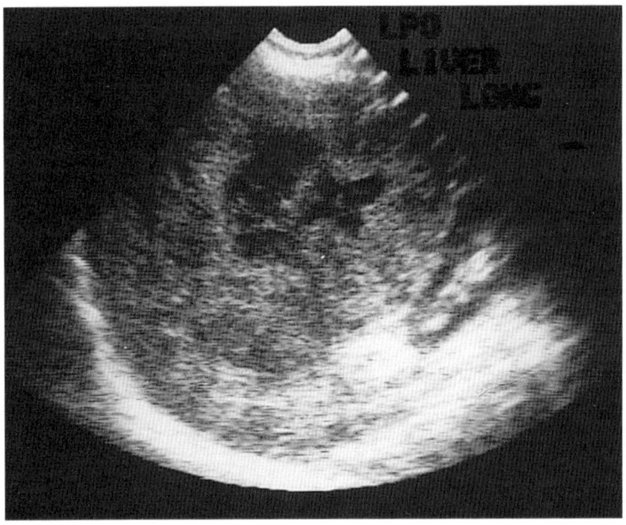

A

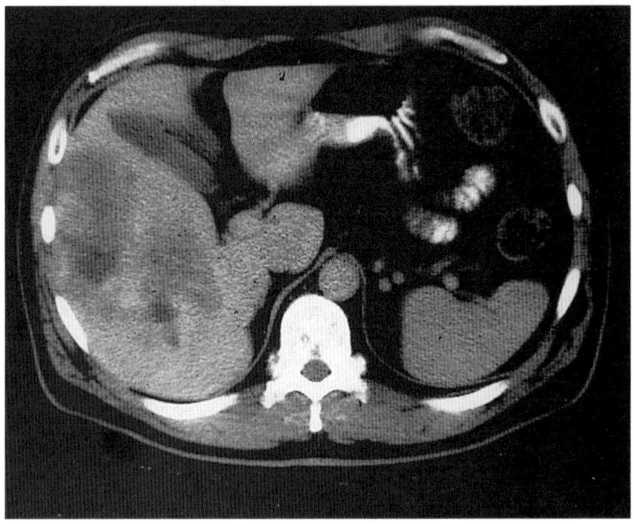

B

Figure 9.10

Adenoma.

A US: a heterogenous lesion with a fluid center is identified in this patient with acute right upper quadrant pain.

B CT does not add significant additional information, other than defining the limits of the mass.

The diagnosis of acute hemorrhage into an adenoma was made.

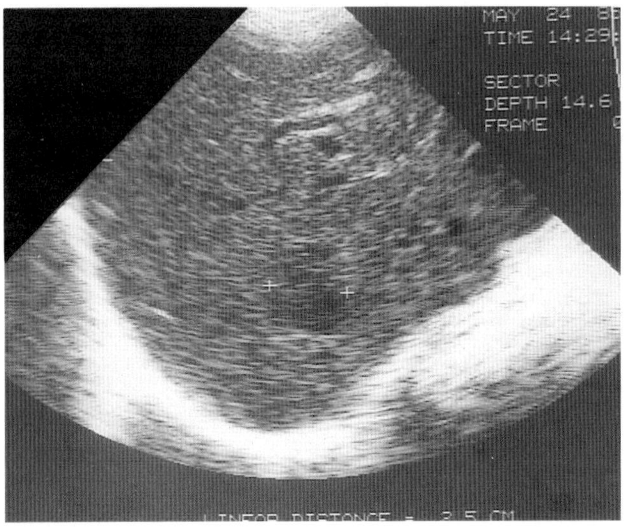

A

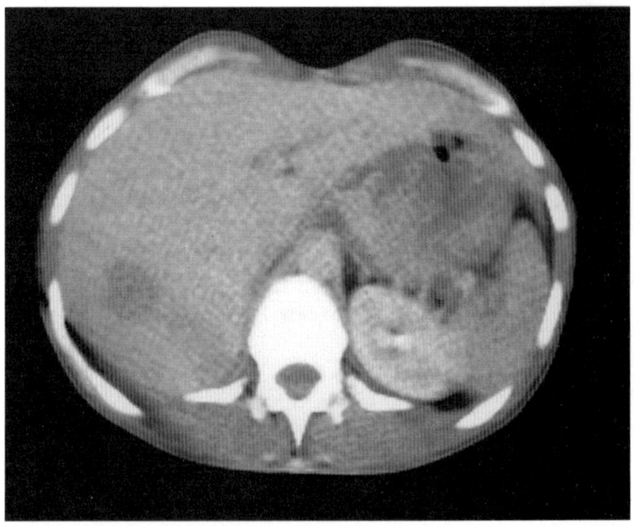

B

Figure 9.11

Adenoma.

A US: a 2.5 cm hypoechoic lesion is seen in the posterior segment of the right lobe of the liver, in a patient using oral contraceptives.

B The non-contrast CT confirms this nonspecific finding.

Serial follow-up CT scans after discontinuation of the drug showed resolution of the mass, suggesting the diagnosis of adenoma.

it shows a propensity to bleed (Figure 9.10), shows no activity on the colloid scan and contains no central scar.

Focal nodular hyperplasia

Focal nodular hyperplasia (FNH) is a tumor-like malformation that occurs mostly in patients between the ages of 20 and 50, with a 2:1 female preponderance. No definite etiologic factor has been isolated, but a relationship with contraceptive hormones has been noted.[34]

These lesions tend to be slightly smaller than adenomas, are well circumscribed, occur predominantly in the left lobe and rarely hemorrhage.[35] They are characterized by a typical central stellate scar in 50%.[36] Microscopically, the scar contains abnormal central arteries, fibrous bands, and inflammatory infiltrate. Proliferating hepatocytes, with sinusoids, Kupffer cells, portal triads, and central veins compose the surrounding lesion.

Detection and lesion characterization

Focal nodular hyperplasia is readily detected by cross-sectional imaging. The presence of a scar in the right clinical setting aids in the diagnosis of FNH, although it can be seen in other conditions, such as fibrolamellar carcinoma and giant hemangiomas.

On US the scar is characteristically echogenic,[37] and CT shows a low-density central abnormality (Figure 9.12). The scar has characteristic features on MR: its high water content leads to brightening on T2-weighted images. This finding is unfortunately not pathognomonic, but is nevertheless very helpful.[38]

Miscellaneous tumors of the liver

Liver cysts are common lesions that are easily characterized by US or MR and can be diagnosed definitively, though with the remote possibility of cystic metastatic disease. This reservation can be

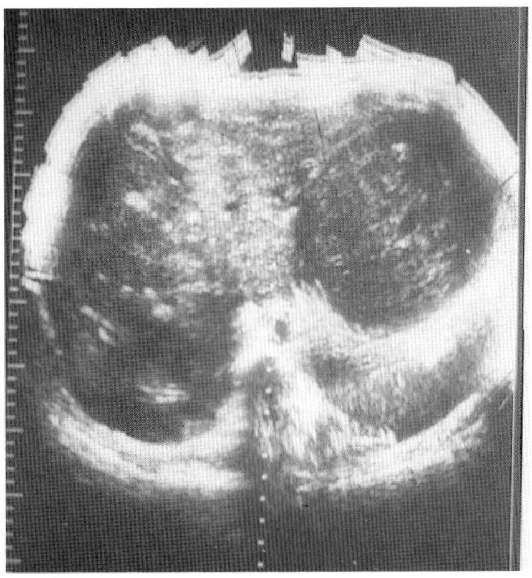

A

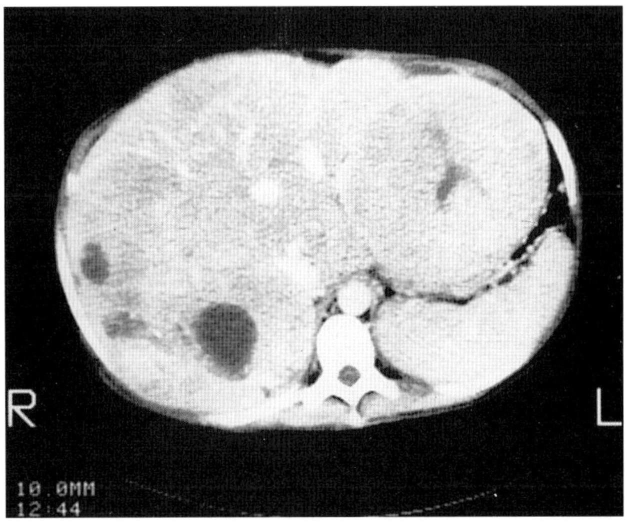

B

Figure 9.12

Focal nodular hyperplasia (FNH).

A A large, hypoechoic, well-marginated mass situated in the left lobe of the liver, as seen in this US, cannot be characterized as FNH.

B The finding of a central stellate scar by CT characterizes this lesion.

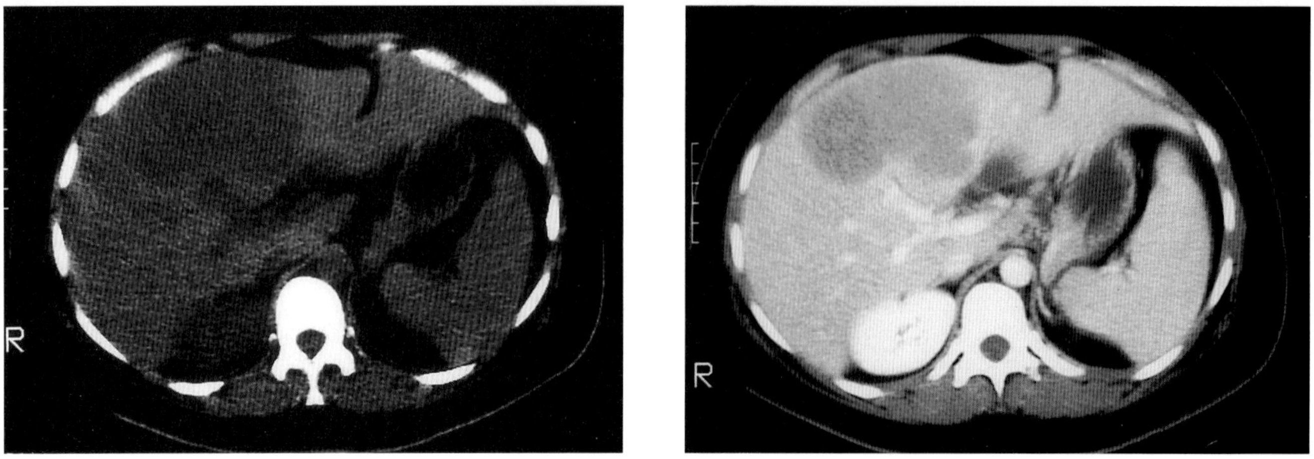

A B

Figure 9.13

Lymphoma. A lobulated mass seen as hypodense on both the non-contrast (**A**) as well as the contrast study (**B**) with enhancing rim was biopsy-proven primary lymphoma of the liver, in an HIV-positive patient.

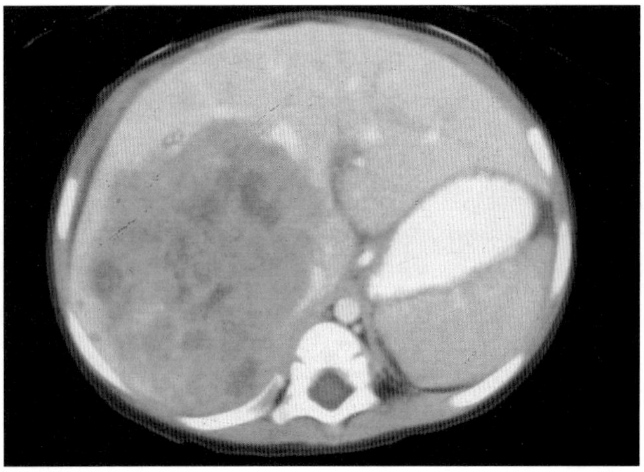

Figure 9.14

Hepatoblastoma. CT shows a heterogenous mass with some lobulation of the border of the lesion. No coarse calcification was identified. The diagnosis was confirmed at surgery.

made in the presence of a known primary with preponderance to cystic change (carcinoid, ovary and pancreas).

Primary lymphoma of the liver (Figure 9.13) is rare but is becoming increasingly more common in the AIDS population. Lymphomatous deposition in the liver as a systemic manifestation of the cancer is rarely seen with current imaging.

Benign hemangioendothelioma is a relatively common neoplasm occurring in the pediatric population, consisting of proliferation of vascular endothelial cells. This tumor is usually between 0.5 and 3.0 cm in diameter, but can be as large as 15 cm. It is characterized by its multinodularity and involvement of other organs. Most lesions involute spontaneously. The radiologic appearance depends on the dominance of the vascular component. US may show a hypoechoic, cystic or echogenic mass, and CT may show findings similar to those of hemangioma in the adult.

Hepatoblastoma is a malignant tumor of embryonic hepatocytes, usually affecting children under the age of 3 years. It is characteristically large (3–20 cm), and most commonly affects the right lobe. The presence of coarse calcification on radiologic imaging is suggestive of the diagnosis. The imaging is otherwise that of a non-specific vascular mass (Figure 9.14).[39]

Embryonal cell sarcoma, or mesenchymal sarcoma, is the third most common malignant liver tumor in children, characterized by hemorrhage, necrosis and a gelatinous matrix. Cross-sectional imaging shows a complex mass with cystic and solid components, and thick septations (Figure 9.15). Distinction from mesenchymal hamartoma is difficult.

Cholangiocarcinoma

Cholangiocarcinoma is a malignant adenocarcinoma arising from the intrahepatic bile ducts. It is less common than hepatocellular carcinoma, accounting for 8–10% of primary liver tumors.[40,41] Parasites, hepatolithiasis and Thorotrast have been causally linked to the disease. Additionally, there is a high incidence of cholangiocarcinoma in patients with sclerosing cholangitis and inflammatory bowel disease. The incidence of cholangiocarcinoma in patients with ulcerative colitis is about 0.4%.[42] There are a number of cystic diseases of the bile ducts which are associated with cholangiocarcinoma. These include Caroli's disease, choledochal cysts and congenital hepatic fibrosis.

This disease is seen mostly in patients over the age of 50 years, without a significant gender bias. Clinically, peripheral lesions remain asymptomatic until far advanced, and patients may present only with an elevated alkaline phosphatase. The Klatskin tumor, referred to as such by virtue of its position at the bile-duct bifurcation, presents relatively early with obstructive jaundice.

Serum AFP can be increased in bile duct carcinoma.[43]

The prognosis is generally poor, with a 5-year survival of 5%. Polypoid lesions tend to have a better prognosis than the diffuse sclerotic type.[44] The patients usually die of complications relating to the local obstructive process—-cholangitis, liver abscess, periportal fibrosis and portal hypertension.

The most common tumor type is infiltrative, nodular or papillary types being less common. The papillary type is the only form that presents as an intraluminal mass.

Metastases spread most commonly to the local lymph nodes (50%), the lungs (43%), serosa (23%) and bone (17%).[41]

Microscopically, the most outstanding feature of this tumor is its associated desmoplasia.

Imaging

Detection and lesion characterization

US and CT both have limited capability of identifying the infiltrative type, and are only able to detect larger lesions. Initially the lesion is low density; 5–8 min after administration of contrast it becomes diffusely hyperdense.[45] The presence of intrahepatic bile duct obstruction is readily identified by US. Thus, with abrupt obstruction without obvious stone or mass, particularly when at the bifurcation of the main right and left common hepatic duct, cholangiocarcinoma should rank high in the differential diagnosis.[46–49]

MR may be able to detect infiltrative lesions surrounding the portal triad and bile duct, but current experience is limited.

Cholangiography has the resolution required to identify small ductal abnormalities, and is the single best test for this purpose. Nodules and strictures are readily identified. The lesions of cholangiocarcinoma are usually short and irregular, but pathognomonic findings are still lacking. Metastatic disease to the porta, and less commonly HCC in this location, may give similar findings.

Staging

Although the primary lesion is difficult to identify, the desmoplastic complications of obstruction of bile ducts and portal vein, and the secondary effects of atrophy of involved lobes and hypertrophy of uninvolved lobes, can be evaluated by US, CT and MR.

Endoscopic retrograde cholangiopancreatography (ERCP)

The single best method of defining ductal architecture is cholangiography, whether performed endoscopically or percutaneously. The endoscopic technique offers the advantages of direct visualization, easier access for biopsy and ability to evaluate the pancreatic duct. Both techniques offer the advantage of therapeutic intervention, and

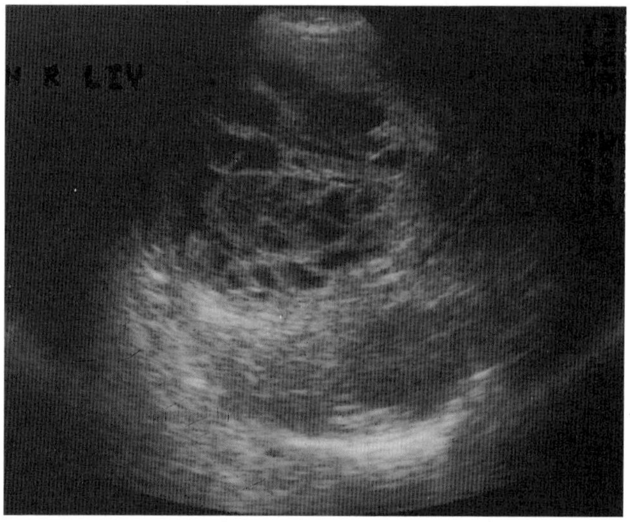

A

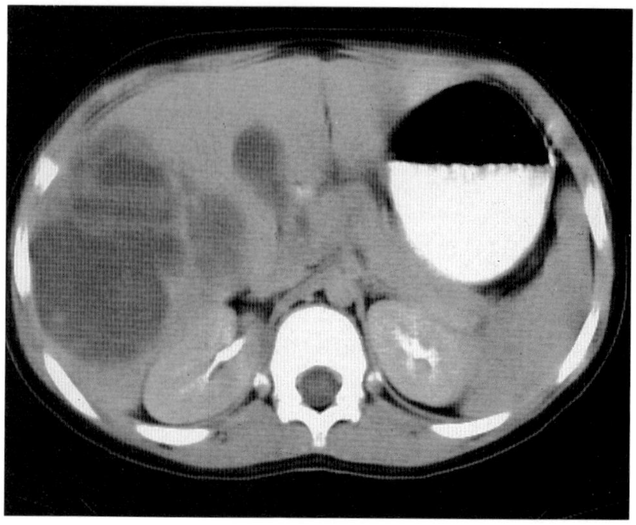

B

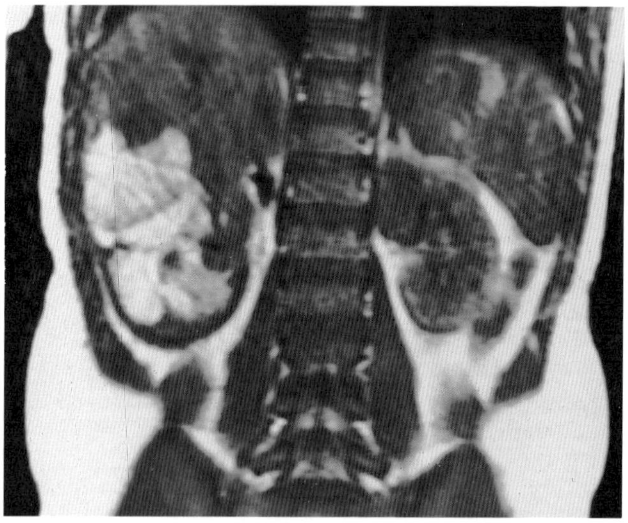

C

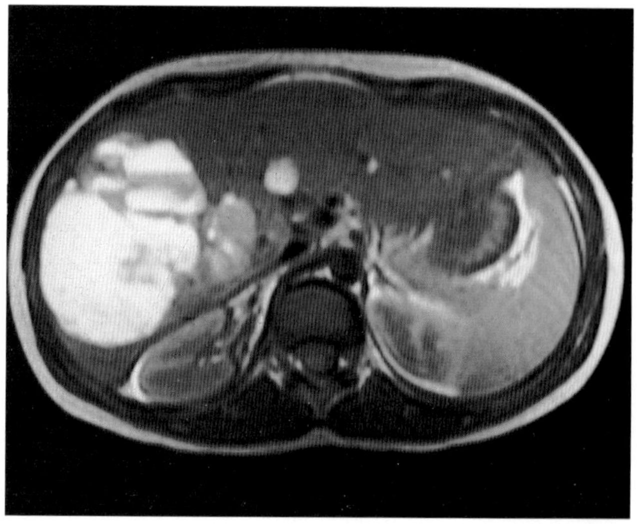

D

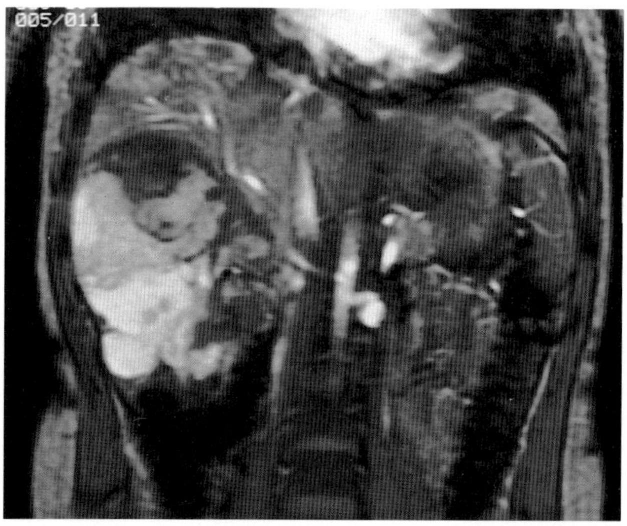

E

Figure 9.15

Embryonal cell sarcoma.

A US shows a septated cystic lesion with some solid components in the liver of an 8-year-old boy.

B CT confirms the findings and suggests two fluid–fluid levels, the most dependent of which are of high density. Hemorrhage into a multiloculated, and predominantly cystic mass was suspected.

C,D The T1 proton density (D), and gradient echo (E) sequences show the fluid–fluid levels, confirming the cellular dependent portions of a hemorrhage.

Additionally, MR suggested that the lesion was predominantly hemorrhagic due to the high signal intensity of the mass on all sequences. An embryonal cell sarcoma was found at surgery.

sometimes both may be needed to accomplish a successful decompression.

The indications for the use of ERCP are many, but the most common oncologic settings include suspicion of pancreatic neoplasia, benign or malignant papillary stenosis, and neoplasia of the intrahepatic biliary tree.

Endoscopic US offers an exquisite window to the pancreas, and small lesions inaccessible to other modalities are within the realm of the endoscopic transducer. Improved staging of pancreatic neoplasia will follow.

Cholangitis and acute pancreatitis are relative contraindications to this procedure, and complications include pancreatitis and sepsis. Aggressive therapeutic endoscopy has increased the risk of these complications.

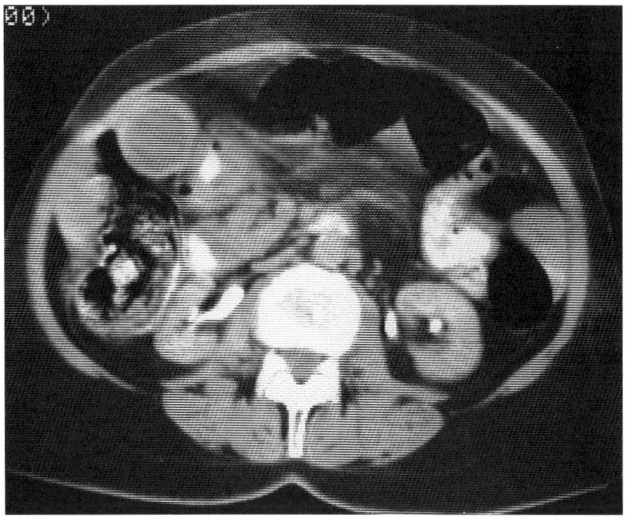

Figure 9.16

CT: thickening of the gallbladder wall, accompanying a distended gallbladder without focal irregularity. Surgery confirmed adenocarcinoma of the gallbladder.

The gallbladder

Malignancy of the gallbladder is uncommon, occurring in 1–3% of autopsy series. Patients are usually between the ages of 60 and 65 years, with a four-fold female predominance. The associations with cholelithiasis (60–95%), chronic cholecystitis and porcelain gallbladder are well known.

Adenocarcinomas are the most common type, with uncommon instances of squamous cell or adenosquamous cell, and rare cases of sarcoma. The tumor may grow intralumenally, obliterating the lumen (most common), as a polypoid mass (least common), or it may spread into the wall of the gallbladder. It invades locally into the liver and surrounding structures, causing only vague symptoms until far advanced. The 5-year survival is less than 5%, partly due to the late presentation of the disease.

Imaging

Detection

When far advanced, the disease is easy to detect. Difficulty arises when the gallbladdeer wall is thickened in the presence of stones, and distinction between the common entity of chronic cholecystitis and carcinoma is virtually impossible to make (Figure 9.16). Focal irregularity is a significant clue to the diagnosis, and is best evaluated by US.

The other forms (endophytic mass or polypoid mass) are easier to diagnose but have to be distinguished from tumefactive bile. Stimulation of the gallbladder with a fatty meal or cholecystokinin will not empty it of a mass, nor will it significantly affect its configuration. A porcelain gallbladder will shadow the interrogating sound waves, making optimal visualization of the gallbladder and tumor difficult. Under these circumstances CT is preferable.

Staging

Once the tumor extends beyond the gallbladder, the diagnosis of carcinoma can be made with certainty, and the diagnostic challenge is then to define its extent. The most common sites of extension are the liver, colon and duodenum (Figure 9.17). The latter two, particularly when air-containing, present well-known shadowing difficulties for US.

MR and nuclear scintigraphy have played little role in the diagnosis and staging of this tumor, and angiography has served only to map the hepatic arterial anatomy when surgery is contemplated.

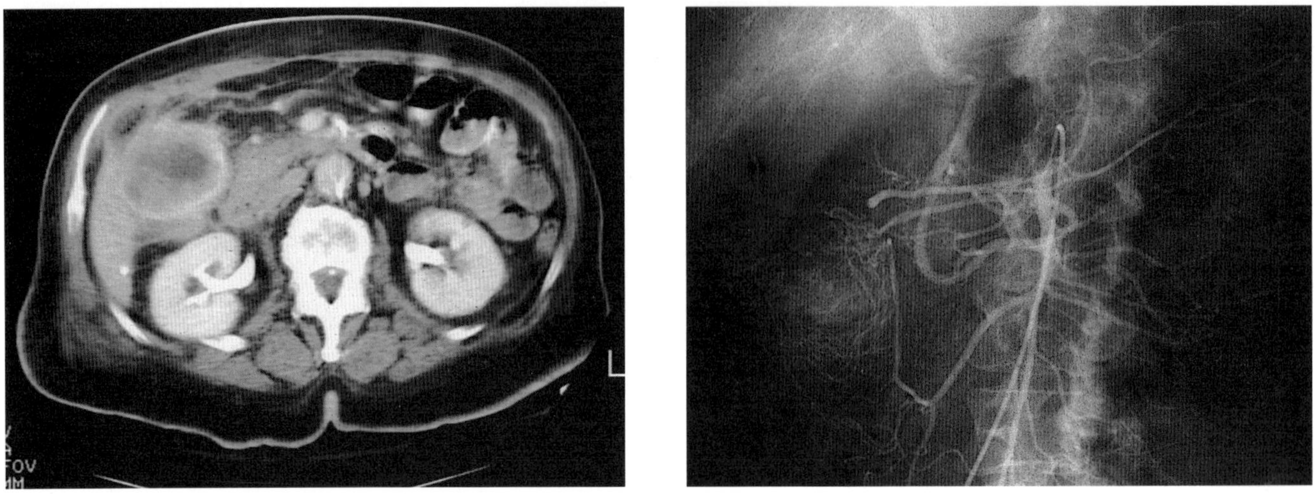

A

B

Figure 9.17

Gallbladder cancer.

A The CT angiogram reveals a necrotic mass at the fundal portion of the gallbladder, with an enhancing rim and a central fluid center. Anterolateral to this is a small focal collection of fluid and air representing an abscess, probably following perforation.

B Angiography confirmed the presence of a hypervascular mass with some central puddling, supplied by the superior mesenteric artery. The question as to whether this arose from the colon and invaded the gallbladder or vice versa was raised. At surgery a primary neoplasm of the gallbladder invading the colon was identified.

The pancreas

Pancreatic adenocarcinoma paints a dismal picture, reflective of the absence of a screening test, lack of symptoms early in the disease, and the aggressive and scirrhous nature of the disease that goes unimpeded in its growth beyond the non-encapsulated organ. We therefore see the disease at a late stage when therapeutic hopes for a cure are small (5%).

Adenocarcinoma

Adenocarcinoma is a malignant mucinous neoplasm of the pancreas that arises from the ductal epithelium. It is the fourth most common cause of death from cancer in the USA and accounts for 3% of all cancers.[50] Adenocarcinoma represents 75% of non-endocrine pancreatic malignancies. The disease usually affects people over the age of 70 years, with a male to female ratio of 1.5:1.0. Proposed etiologic factors include cigarette smoking and coffee consumption,[51–53] alcohol consumption and dietary intake of fat, protein and high calories.[53,54]

Disease states of the pancreas that are reportedly associated with the development of pancreatic carcinoma include diabetes mellitus and familial pancreatitis.[54,55] The etiologic association with chronic pancreatitis is not clear.

Because the pancreas is not encased by a capsule, early spread into the surrounding retroperitoneal fat is common. Local structures then become involved, including the portal vein, superior mesenteric vein, splenic vein, gastroduodenal artery, bile duct and duodenum. Local lymph-node involvement and hematogenous spread to the liver via the portal vein are also seen. Transperitoneal spread is less common. Stage I disease is confined to the pancreas, stage II involves regional nodes, and stage III describes spread beyond the nodes and the pancreas. Only 5% of patients are in the stage I group.[54]

Pain, weight loss, anorexia, malaise and jaundice are the common modes of presentation. A new onset of depression has also been well described in patients with pancreatic cancer. Painless jaundice and an enlarged gallbladder are classical findings in lesions of the head of the pancreas. An associated hypercoagulable state can lead to thrombus formation. Elevated alkaline phosphatase, elevated fasting blood sugar and anemia are present in the majority of patients. Although every patient has microscopic pancreatitis, only a minority have an elevated amylase level.

Prognosis is extremely poor, with a median survival time of 4 months and 5-year survival rate of less than 1%.[56]

Grossly, the tumor is usually small, but it can be as large as 8–10 cm. Lesions in the head of the pancreas tend to be smaller because they present at an earlier stage; conversely, those in the body and tail are larger on diagnosis. The mass is most commonly situated in the head of the pancreas (60%), with lesions in the body (5%), tail (5%), both body and tail (10%) and whole pancreas (10%) being less common presentations.[54] Dense fibrosis is characteristic. Macroscopic evidence of focal pancreatitis is present in 25–40% of cases.[54,57] Hemorrhage, necrosis and calcification are uncommon features.

Microscopically, the features are of malignant glandular or ductal cells, sometimes with papillary formation. Focal areas of pancreatitis are almost always present.

Imaging

Detection

Lesions in the head of the pancreas are generally visualized by both US and CT. The former is limited by surrounding bowel gas or obesity in about 30% of patients. Maneuvers such as altering respiration, filling the stomach with water, placing the patient in the upright position and repeat scanning are helpful. Lesions in the tail of the pancreas are difficult to detect by US, but visualization can be improved by using the spleen as a window. With CT, tail and body lesions are sometimes obscured by partial volume artifact from bowel not filled with contrast. Intraoperative US scanning is very sensitive to small and impalpable tumors, particularly for small functioning tumors such as insulinomas.[58,59]

Characterization

Most lesions are hypoechoic by US and hypodense by CT (Figure 9.18). It is extremely difficult to differentiate between neoplasia and pancreatitis, which may occur simultaneously (Figure 9.19). ERCP is used as an accessory procedure to differentiate the two. The 'double-duct' sign (Figure 9.20), revealing obstruction of approximate bile and pancreatic ducts, is specific if the obstructions are short, abrupt or irregular.[60] Although ERCP is reportedly 95% specific, distinction from pancreatitis still remains difficult.[61] If there is a large mass in the head of the pancreas and no obstruction, lymphoma involving peripancreatic nodes is a strong consideration. MR is currently limited by surrounding bowel motion and lack of tissue contrast. The pancreas is readily accessible to biopsy, usually performed under CT guidance through the stomach.

Staging

CT is the study of choice for staging. It lacks the sensitivity of US for early bile duct and pancreatic duct obstruction, but more importantly it is superior in evaluating extension into perivascular fat, peripancreatic fat, duodenum and local lymph nodes. Angiography is sometimes utilized to show the extent of vascular encasement, giving the surgeon a better idea of the disease in the anatomic plane. MR angiography will soon replace this function of angiography. ERCP has little place in staging the disease, but endoscopic US is promising for this purpose, with its ability to visualize immediate extent.

Because liver metastases occur in about 50% of patients at the time of presentation, an intensive search should be made at the initial evaluation.[62] CT is therefore overall a superior study for identification and staging.

The important prognostic question for imaging is the resectability of the lesion, and therefore of extrapancreatic extension. Optimistic evaluation commonly reveals inoperable disease in the operating room. The 5% resectability, and a median survival time measured in months, give patients little hope.

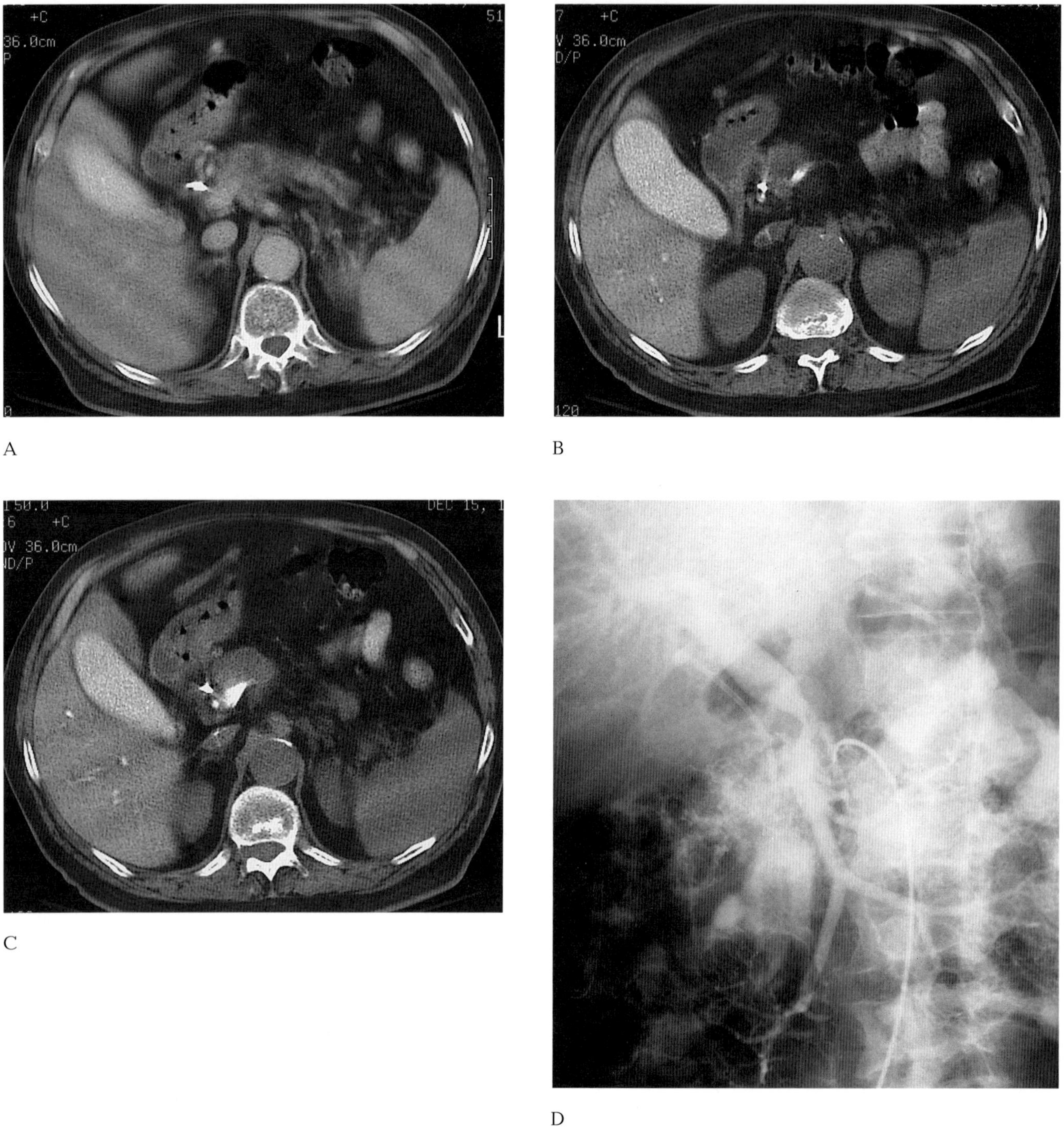

Figure 9.18

Pancreatic adenocarcinoma.

A A mass in the neck, body and head of the pancreas is seen, with obstruction of the pancreatic duct and common bile duct.

B,C CT angiography shows effacement of portomesenteric confluence.

D Angiography shows the venous phase of superior mesenteric arterial injection showing a smooth extrinsic impression of the superior mesenteric vein/portal vein confluence.

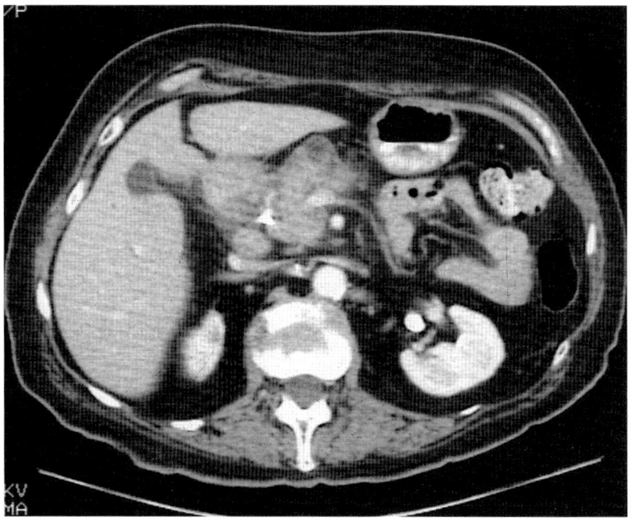

Figure 9.19

Pancreatic adenocarcinoma. This CT scan shows a mass in the head of the pancreas with a focal cystic lesion situated anteriorly, representing either a pseudocyst or a cystic component of the mass.

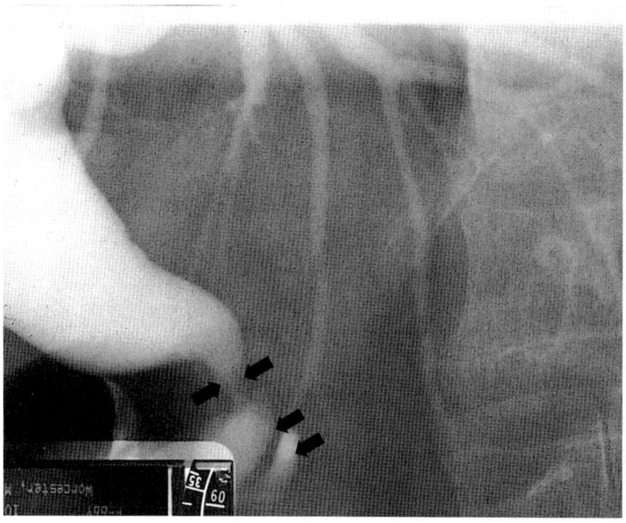

Figure 9.20

Pancreatic carcinoma. ERCP reveals the 'double-duct' sign with encasement and obstruction of the common bile duct and the pancreatic duct (arrows). This finding is suggestive of pancreatic carcinoma, which was confirmed at surgery. (Courtesy of Dr J. Colby, University of Massachusetts Medical Center.)

Cystic tumors

Microcystic adenoma is a glycogen-rich benign neoplasm occurring in patients over the age of 60 years, more commonly in females. The lesion is large (10–12 cm), lobulated with a thick fibrous capsule and contains occasional central stellate calcification. US reveals cysts of varying sizes, without focal thickening of the walls, and CT best visualizes the characteristic central stellate calcification seen in a minority of patients (Figure 9.21).

Mucinous lesions are of two types: cystadenoma and cystadenocarcinoma. Cystadenoma is a 'benign' abnormality, with atypical cells in slightly less than half of the lesions.[63] These lesions affect patients between 20 and 80 years old, and females predominate by a small margin. Both forms are large (2–20 cm), encapsulated, smoothly lobulated, thick-walled, and often contain wall or peripheral calcification. They may be unilocular or multilocular.

On US, the presence of solid internal soft tissue excrescences within the cysts is characteristic. A poorly circumscribed mass with amorphous peripheral calcification is the typical CT appearance.

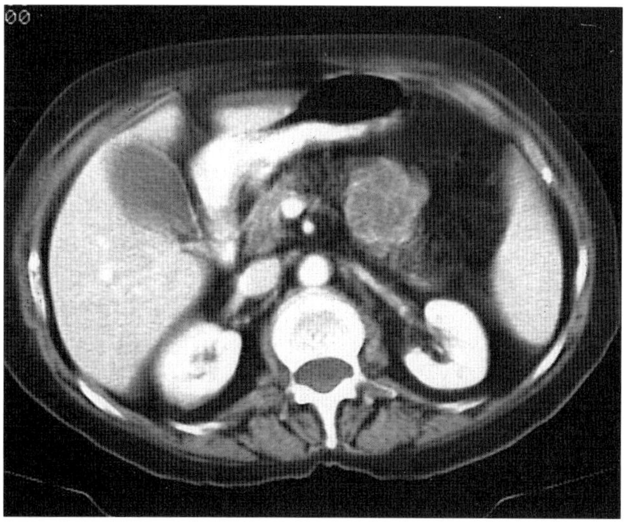

Figure 9.21

CT: pancreatic mass in the body/tail of the pancreas. This mass was stable over 2 years and had an enhancing rim and lobulated border, thought to represent a microcystic adenoma in an 88-year-old female. Biopsy showed 'atypical' cells without malignancy.

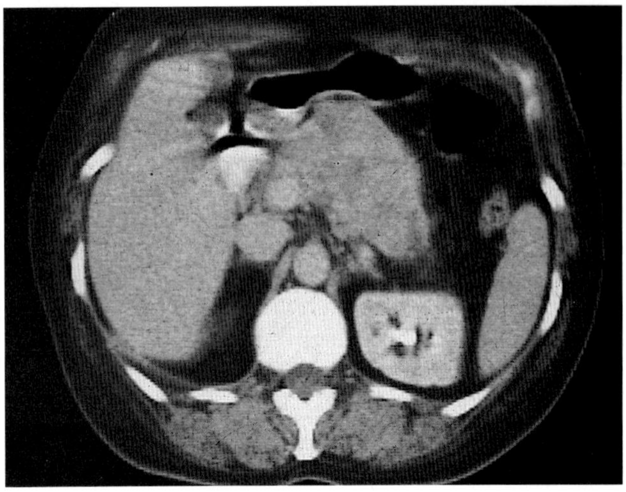

A

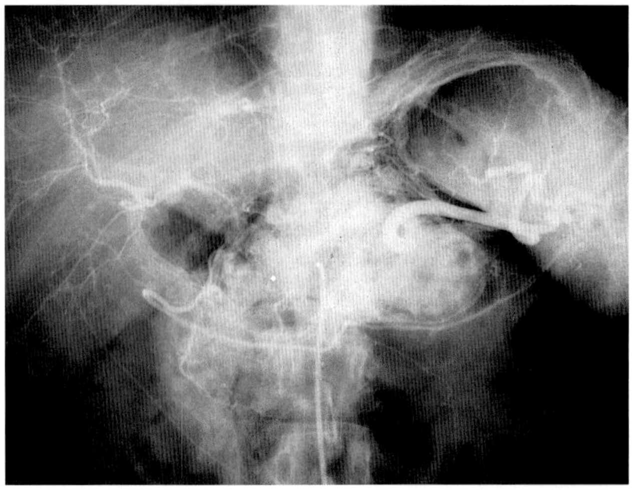

B

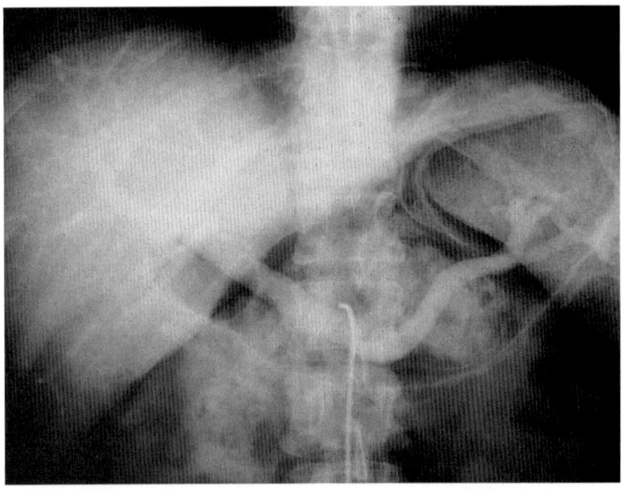

C

Figure 9.22

Microcystic adenocarcinoma.

A This is a rare case of a hypervascular malignant neoplasm seen by CT as a large mass in the body of the pancreas that is isodense with liver.

B,C The mass is characteristically hypervascular on angiogram, with a focal round or low-density area in its superolateral margins, and a patent splenic vein despite the large mass.

There is a very rare malignant microcystic adenocarcinoma that is large and shows no evidence of desmoplasia and has a larger component of necrosis (Figure 9.22).[56]

Endocrine tumors

The islet cells of the pancreas can give rise to functioning tumors that may be benign, malignant or indeterminate. Insulinomas, glucagonomas, gastrinomas, VIPomas and somatostinomas are examples.

The role of radiology is to isolate these small and commonly multiple lesions. Preoperative localization techniques, including selective angiography of the gastroduodenal artery, subselection of the pancreatic arteries, and sampling of the portal vein and its branches, may fail to localize the lesion. Intraoperative US combined with palpation at surgery is very effective.[64]

The distinction between benign and malignant disease is sometimes made only when metastatic disease is identified (Figure 9.23); the radiologist may be the only one to make this distinction.

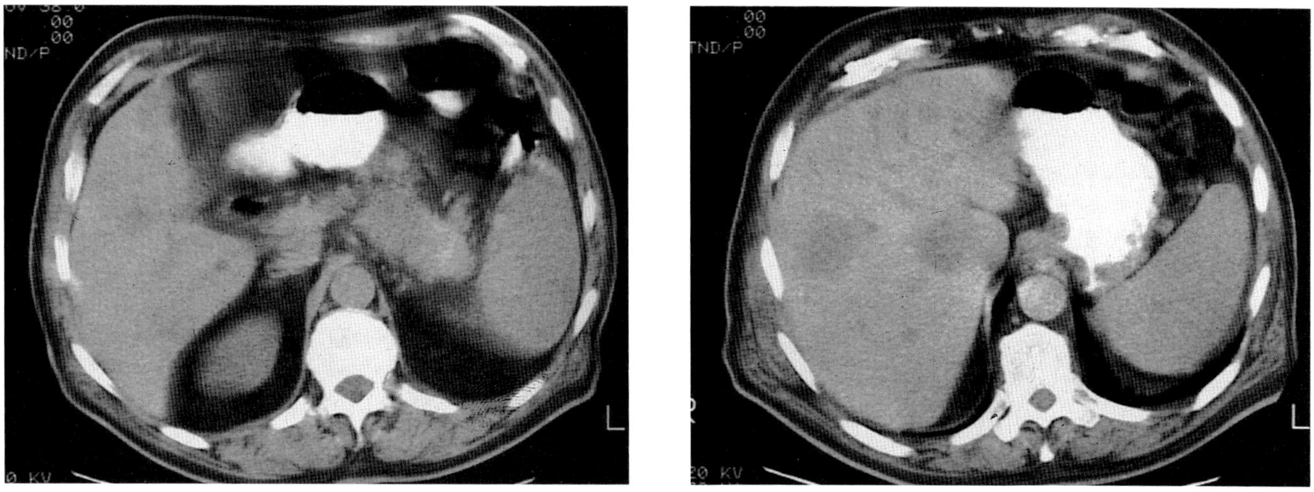

A B

Figure 9.23

CT: VIPoma. A large mass seen in the tail of the pancreas (**A**) is hyperdense with respect to the liver, associated with metastatic disease to the liver and wall of the stomach (**B**). (Courtesy of Dr J. Colby, University of Massachusetts Medical Center.)

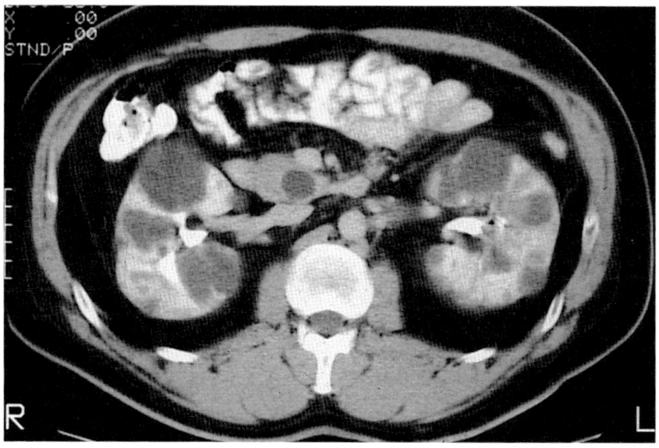

Figure 9.24

Pancreatic cyst. A single simple pancreatic cyst in the uncinate process of the pancreas is seen on CT in a patient with polycystic kidney disease.

Miscellaneous tumors of the pancreas

Pancreatic cysts are associated with polycystic kidney disease (Figure 9.24) and von Hippel–Lindau disease. Cystic neoplasia is also associated with the latter.

Metastases to the pancreas and peripancreatic nodes arise from primary tumors of the lung, breast, kidney and prostate, as well as lymphoma and melanoma (Figure 9.25). They cannot be distinguished from primary pancreatic carcinoma. Lymphoma, when situated in the head of the pancreas, may not cause bile-duct obstruction; a large mass in the head of the pancreas without obstruction is unlikely to be adenocarcinoma and most likely to be lymphoma.

Rare tumors include leiomyosarcoma, liposarcoma, fibrosarcoma and schwannoma (Figure 9.26).

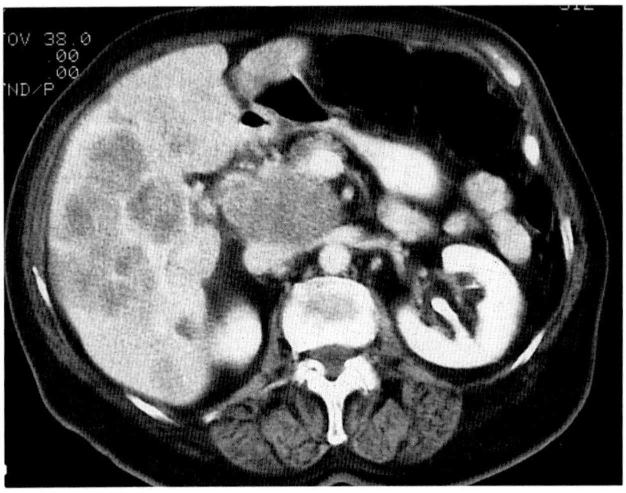

Figure 9.25

Metastases: large metastatic melanoma in the head and uncinate process of the pancreas, masquerading as a primary pancreatic lesion. No overt dilatation of the common bile duct or radicles was apparent on CT.

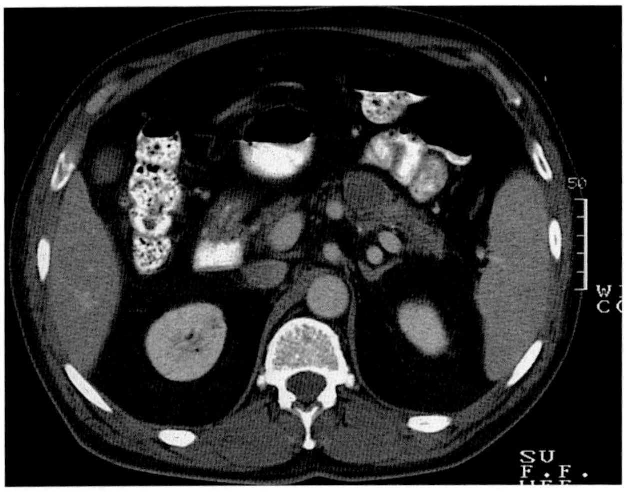

A

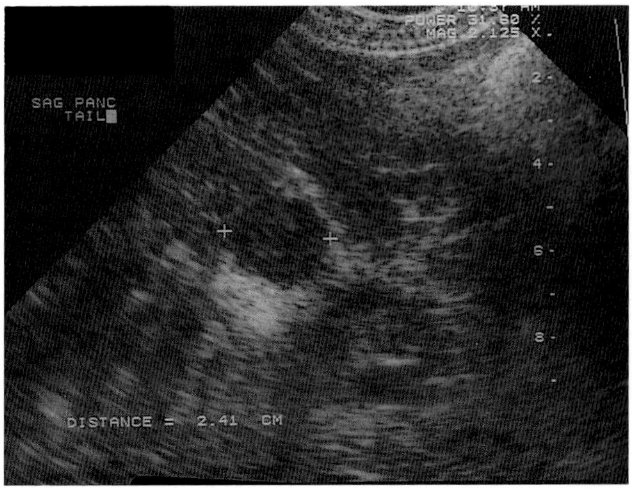

B

Figure 9.26

Schwannoma.

A CT shows a rounded low-density lesion in the body of the pancreas.

B US confirmed that the lesion was 'cystic'.

Surgical pathology revealed a schwannoma.

The spleen

Oncologic disease within the spleen is infrequently identified, even though more than half of patients with widespread malignancy may have splenic involvement at autopsy.[65] Melanoma probably accounts for most of the metastases found in the spleen, although various studies have described the origin of metastases, in decreasing order of frequency, as lung, prostate, colon, stomach, melanoma, ovary and pancreas.[68–69]

Lymphoma

Imaging of lymphoma has traditionally been insensitive to splenic involvement. Splenic size is unreliable, as one-third of patients with splenomegaly do not have lymphomatous involvement, and one-third of patients without splenomegaly have involvement. In patients with aggressive disease, such as the poorly differentiated nodular type, involvement becomes probable, but not necessarily visible.

US, CT and scintigraphy have unsatisfactory accuracy rates, ranging between 54 and 75%.[70,71] Imaging by MR is beginning to show some promise. When the water content of lymphoma is high, such as in the large lesions of histiocytic lymphoma, they become detectable on T2-weighted sequences. MR using super-paramagnetic iron oxide is showing promise in demonstrating splenic involvement,[72] but the findings need further verification.

References

1. Freeny PF, Lawson TL, *Radiology of the pancreas* (Springer-Verlag: Berlin, New York 1982).
2. Friedman AC, *Radiology of the liver, biliary tract, pancreas and spleen* (Williams and Wilkins: Baltimore 1987).
3. Mitchell DG, Stark DD, *Hepatobiliary MRI* (CV Mosby: St Louis 1992).
4. Okuda K, Ishak KG, *Neoplasms of the liver* (Springer-Verlag: Berlin, New York 1987).
5. Heiken JP, Weyman PJ, Lee JK et al, Detection of focal hepatic masses: prospective evaluation with CT, delayed CT, CT during arterial portography, and MR imaging, *Radiology* (1989) **171**(1):47–51.
6. Hahn PF, Stark DD, Saini S et al, The differential diagnosis of ringed hepatic lesions in MR imaging, *AJR* (1990) **154**:287–90.
7. Rummeny E, Saini S, Wittenberg J et al, MR imaging of liver neoplasms, *AJR* (1989) **152**:493–9.
8. Wittenberg J, Stark DD, Forman BH et al, Differentiation of hepatic metastases from hepatic hemangiomas and cysts by using MR imaging, *AJR* (1988) **151**:79–84.
9. Outwater E, Tomaszewski JE, Daly JM et al, Hepatic colorectal metastases: correlation of MR imaging and pathologic appearance, *Radiology* (1991) **180**(2):327–32.
10. Ebara M, Watanabe S, Kita K et al, MR imaging of small hepatocellular carcinoma: effect of intratumoral copper content on signal intensity, *Radiology* (1991) **180**:617–21.
11. Itoh K, Nishimura K, Togashi K et al, Hepatocellular carcinoma: MR imaging, *Radiology* (1987) **164**:21–5.
12. Sawabu N, Hattorri N, Serological tumor markers in hepatocellular carcinoma. In: Okuda K, Ishak KG, eds, *Neoplasms of the liver* (Springer-Verlag: Berlin, New York 1987) 227–37.
13. Inamoto K, Tanaka S, Yamazaki H et al, Computed tomography in the detection of small hepatocellular carcinomas, *Gastrointest Radiol* (1983) **8**(4):321–6.
14. Ebara M, Ohto M, Kondo F, Strategy for early diagnosis of hepatocellular carcinoma (HCC), *Ann Acad Med Singapore* (1989) **18**(1):83–9.
15. Ryu M, Watanabe Y, Ozaki M et al, The indication of hepatic resection from medical imaging techniques for hepatocellular carcinoma, *Nippon Geka Gakkai Zasshi* (1983) **84**(9):904–7.
16. Ebara M, Ohto M, Watanabe Y et al, Diagnosis of small hepatocellular carcinoma: correlation of MR imaging and tumor histologic studies, *Radiology* (1986) **159**:371–7.
17. Ros PR, Murphy BJ, Buck JE et al, Encapsulated hepatocellular carcinoma: radiologic findings and pathologic correlation, *Gastrointest Radiol* (1990) **15**:233–7.
18. Yoshida H, Itai Y, Ohtomo K et al, Small hepatocellular carcinoma and cavernous hemangioma: differentiation with dynamic FLASH MR imaging with Gd-DTPA, *Radiology* (1989) **171**:339–42.
19. Rummeny E, Weissleder R, Stark DD et al, Primary liver tumors: diagnosis by MR imaging, *AJR* (1989) **152**:63–72.
20. Yoshikawa J, Matsui O, Takashima T et al, Fatty metamorphosis in hepatocellular carcinoma: radiologic features in 10 cases, *AJR* (1988) **151**:717–20.
21. Okamoto S, Yamanaka A, Toyosaka A et al, Current status of hepatic resection in the treatment of hepatocellular carcinoma. In: Okuda K, Ishak KG, eds, *Neoplasms of the liver* (Springer-Verlag: Berlin, New York 1987) 353–65.
22. Itai Y, Ohtomo K, Furui S et al, Noninvasive diagnosis of small cavernous hemangioma of the liver: advantage of MRI, *AJR* (1985) **145**:1195–9.
23. Glazer GM, Aisen AM, Francis IR et al, Hepatic cavernous hemangioma: magnetic resonance imaging, *Radiology* (1985) **155**:417–20.

24. Stark DD, Felder RC, Wittenberg J et al, Magnetic resonance imaging of cavernous hemangioma of the liver: tissue specific characterization, *AJR* (1985) **145**:213–20.

25. Bree RL, Schwah R, Glazer GM et al, The varied appearances of hepatic cavernous hemangiomas with sonography, computed tomography, magnetic resonance imaging and scintigraphy, *RadioGraphics* (1987) **7**:1153–75.

26. Gibney RG, Hendin AP, Cooperberg PL, Sonographically detected hepatic hemangiomas: absence of change over time, *AJR* (1987) **149**:953–7.

27. Itai Y, Ohtomo K, Araki T et al, Computed tomography and sonography of cavernous hemangioma of the liver, *AJR* (1983) **141**:315–20.

28. Takayasu K, Moriyama N, Shima Y et al, Atypical radiographic findings in hepatic cavernous hemangioma: correlation with histologic features, *AJR* (1986) **146**:1149–53.

29. Birnbaum BA, Weinreb JC, Megibow AJ et al, Blinded retrospective comparison of MR imaging and Tc-99m-labeled red blood cell SPECT for definitive diagnosis of hepatic hemangiomas, *Radiology* (1989) **173**(P):270.

30. Vlachos L, Trakadas S, Gouliamos A et al, Comparative study between ultrasound, computed tomography, intra-arterial digital subtraction angiography, and magnetic resonance imaging in the differentiation of tumors of the liver, *Gastrointest Radiol* (1990) **15**:102–6.

31. Kerlin P, Davis GL, McGill DB et al, Hepatic adenoma and focal nodular hyperplasia: clinical, pathologic, and radiologic features, *Gastroenterology* (1983) **84**:994–1002.

32. Itai Y, Ohtomo K, Kokubo T et al, CT and MR imaging of fatty tumors of the liver, *J Comput Assist Tomogr* (1987) **11**(2):253–7.

33. Gabata T, Matsui O, Kadoya M et al, MR imaging of hepatic adenoma, *AJR* (1990) **155**:1009–11.

34. Schild H, Kreitner KF, Thelen M et al, Focal nodular hyperplasia of the liver in 930 patients, *RöFo* (*Forttschr Geb Rontgenstr Nuklearmed*) (1987) **147**(6):612–8.

35. Brady MS, Coit DG, Focal nodular hyperplasia of the liver, *Surg Gynecol Obstet* (1990) **171**(5):377–81.

36. Kreft B, Steudel A, Harder T et al, [Qualitative and quantitative NMR tomographic findings in focal nodular hyperplasia of the liver] *RöFo* (*Fortschr Geb Rontgenstr Nuklearmed*) (1990) **152**(6):649–53.

37. Scatarige JC, Fishman EK, Sanders RC, The sonographic "scar sign" in focal nodular hyperplasia of the liver, *J Ultrasound Med* (1982) **1**(7):275–8.

38. Rummeny E, Stark DD, Compton CC et al, Central scars in primary liver tumors: MR features, specificity, and pathologic correlation, *Radiology* (1989) **171**:323–6.

39. Dachman AH, Pakter RL, Ros PR et al, Hepatoblastoma: radiologic–pathologic correlation in 50 cases, *Radiology* (1987) **164**(1):15–9.

40. Craig JR, Peters RL, Edmonson HA, Primary malignant epithelial tumors. In: *Tumors of the liver and intrahepatic bile ducts* (Washington DC: Armed Forces Institute of Pathology 1988) 123–214.

41. Okuda K and the Liver Cancer Study Group of Japan, Primary liver cancers in Japan, *Cancer* (1980) **45**:2663–9.

42. Ritchie JK, Allan RN, Macartney J et al, Biliary tract carcinoma associated with ulcerative colitis, *QJ Med* (1974) **43**:263–79.

43. Okuda K, Kubo Y, Okazaki N et al, Clinical aspects of intrahepatic bile duct carcinoma including hilar carcinoma. A study of 57 autopsy-proven cases, *Cancer* (1977) **39**:232–46.

44. Warren KW, Tan EGC, Disease of the gallbladder and bile ducts. In: Schiff L, ed. *Diseases of the liver* (JB Lippincott: Philadelphia 1975) 1278–335.

45. Takayasu K, Ikeya S, Mukai K et al, CT of hilar cholangiocarcinoma: late contrast enhancement in six patients, *Am J Roentgenol* (1990) **154**(6):1203–6.

46. Levine E, Maklad NF, Wright CH et al, Computed tomographic and ultrasonic appearances of primary carcinoma of the common bile duct, *Gastrointest Radiol* (1979) **4**:147–51.

47. Subramanyam BR, Raghavendra BN, Balthazar EJ et al, Ultrasonic features of cholangiocarcinoma, *J Ultrasound Med* (1984) **3**:405–8.

48. Schnur MJ, Hoffman JC, Koenigsberg M, Ultrasonic demonstration of intraductal biliary neoplasms, *J Clin Ultrasound* (1982) **10**:246–8.

49. Bondestam S, Kivilaakso EO, Standertskjold-Nordemstam CM et al, Sonographic diagnosis of a bile duct polyp, *AJR* (1980) **135**:610–11.

50. Hermann RE, Cooperman AM, Current concepts in cancer. Cancer of the pancreas, *N Engl J Med* (1979) **301**:482–5.

51. McMahon B, Yen S, Trichopolous D et al, Coffee and cancer of the pancreas, *N Engl J Med* (1981) **304**:630–3.

52. Goldstein HR, No association found between coffee and cancer of the pancreas [letter], *N Engl J Med* (1982) **306**:997.

53. Benarde MA, Weiss W, Coffee consumption and pancreatic cancer: temporal and spatial correlation, *Br Med J* (1982) **284**:400–2.

54. Cubilla AL, Fitzgerald PJ, Pancreas cancer (non-endocrine): a review—-part II, *Clin Bull* (1978) **8**:143–55.

55. Schultz RE, Finkler NJ, Pancreatic calcification and pancreatic carcinoma: the relationship reconsidered, *Mt Sinai J Med* (1980) **47**:622–6.

56. Cubilla AL, Fitzgerald PJ, Cancer (non-endocrine) of the pancreas. A suggested classification, *Monogr Pathol* (1980) **21**:82–100.

57. Frantz VK, Tumors of the pancreas. In: *Atlas of tumor pathology* (Washington DC: Armed Forces Institute of Pathology 1959) Sect. 7, Fasc. 27 & 28:36–75.

58. Sigel B, Coelho JCU, Nyhus LM et al, Detection of pancreatic tumors by ultrasound during surgery, *Arch Surg* (1982) **117**:1058–61.

59. Galiber AK, Reading CC, Charboneau JW et al, Localization of pancreatic insulinoma: comparison of

pre- and intraoperative US with CT and angiography, *Radiology* (1988) **166**(2):405–8.
60. Plumley TF, Rohrmann CA, Freeny PC, Silverstein FE, Ball TJ, Double duct sign: reassessed significance in ERCP, *AJR* (1982) **138**(1):31–5.
61. Pomerri F, Pittarello F, Muzzio PC, Pancreatic carcinoma, diagnostic ERCP, *Int J Pancreatol* (1988) **3**(suppl 1):S131–6.
62. Weinstein DP, Wolfman NT, Weinstein BJ, Ultrasonic characteristic of pancreatic tumors, *Gastrointest Radiol* (1979) **4**:245–51.
63. Compagno J, Oertel JE, Mucinous cystic neoplasms of the pancreas with overt and latent malignancy (cystadenocarcinoma and cystadenoma). A clinicopathologic study of 41 cases, *Am J Clin Pathol* (1978) **69**:289–98.
64. Norton JA, Cromack DT, Shawker TH et al, Intraoperative ultrasonographic localization of islet cell tumors. A prospective comparison to palpation, *Ann Surg* (1988) **207**(2):160–8.
65. Warren S, Davis AH, Studies on tumor metastasis. V. The metastases of carcinoma to the spleen, *Am J Cancer* (1934) **21**:517–33.
66. Anderson WAD, Kissone JM, eds, *Pathology*, 7th edn, vol 2, (CV Mosby: St Louis 1977) 1504.
67. Federle M, Moss AA, Computer tomography of the spleen, *CRC Crit Rev Diagn Imaging* (1983) **19**:1–16.
68. Warren S, Davis AH, Studies on tumor metastasis: the metastases of carcinoma to the spleen, *Am J Cancer* (1934) **21**:517.
69. Marymont JH Jr, Gross S, Patterns of metastatic cancer in the spleen, *Am J Clin Pathol* (1963) **40**:58–66.
70. Marglin SI, Castellino RA, Selection of imaging studies for the initial staging of patients with Hodgkin's disease, *Semin Ultrasound CT MR* (1985) **7**:2–8.
71. Silverman S, DeNardo GL, Glatstein E et al, Evaluation of the liver and spleen in Hodgkin's disease. II. The value of splenic scintigraphy, *Am J Med* (1972) **52**:362–6.
72. Weissleder R, Elizondo G, Stark DD et al, The diagnosis of splenic lymphoma by MR imaging: value of superparamagnetic iron oxide, *AJR* (1989) **152**(1):175–80.

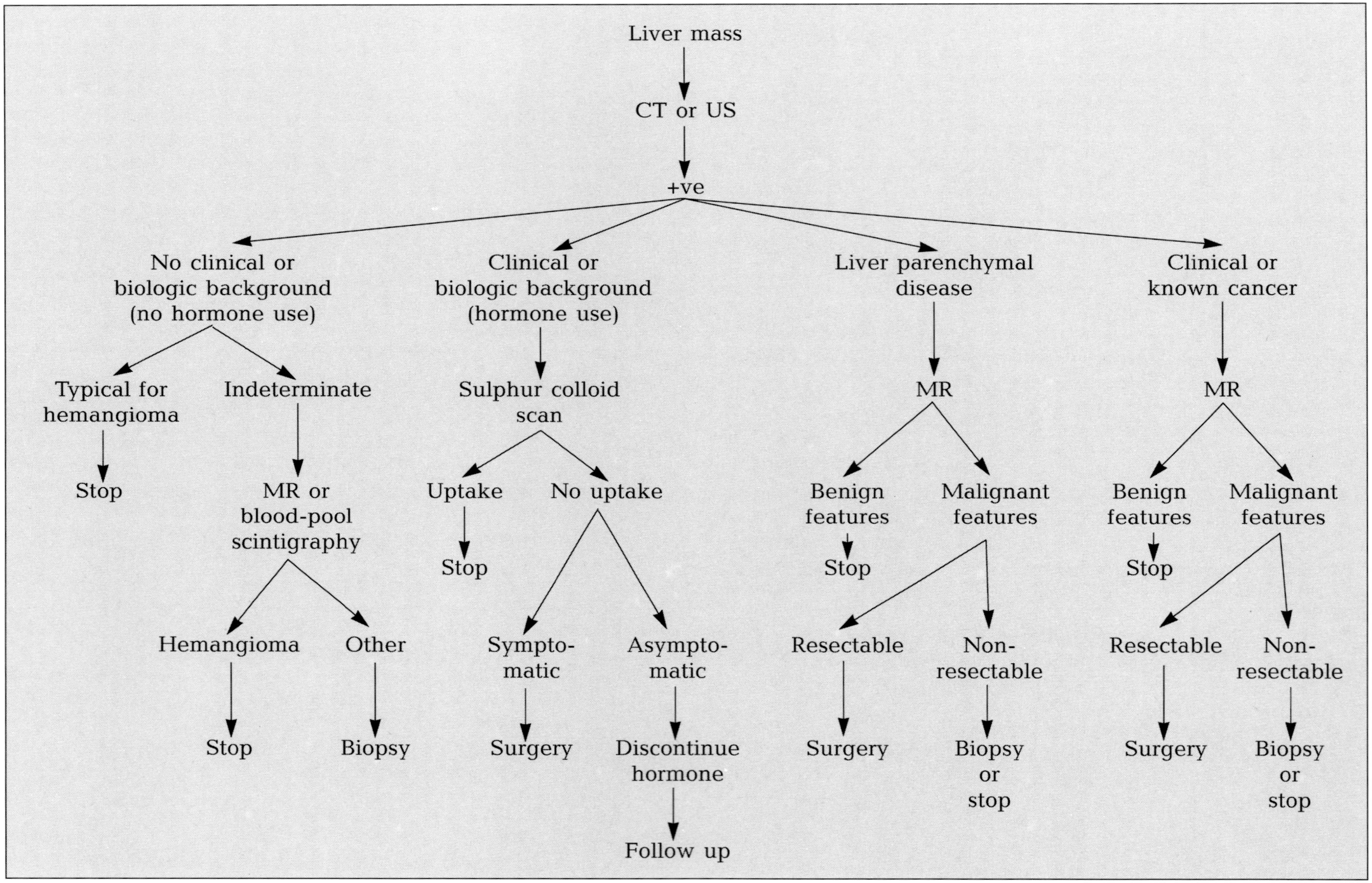

Diagram 9.1

Strategy for diagnosis of a liver mass.

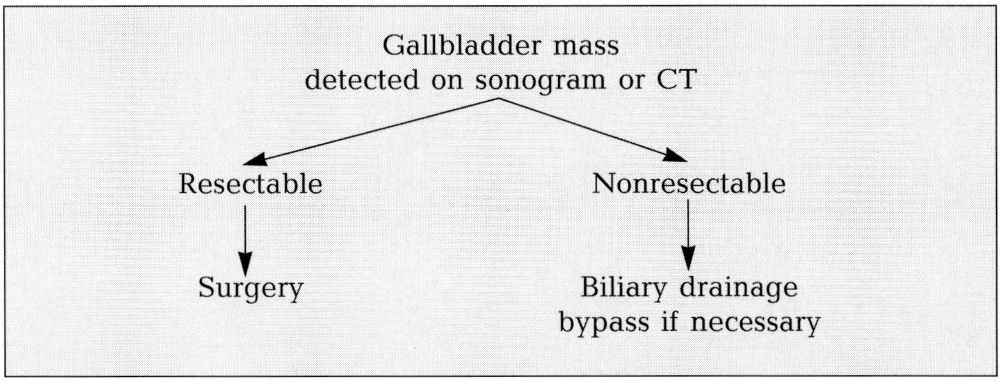

Diagram 9.2

Strategy for diagnosis of a gallbladder mass.

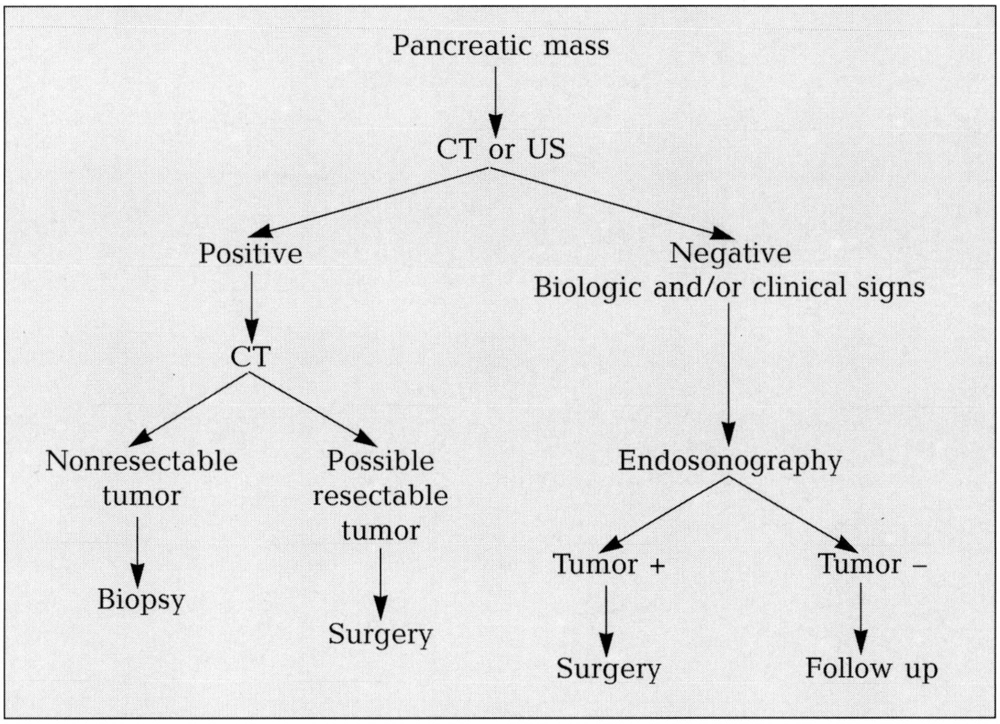

Diagram 9.3

Strategy for diagnosis of a pancreatic mass.

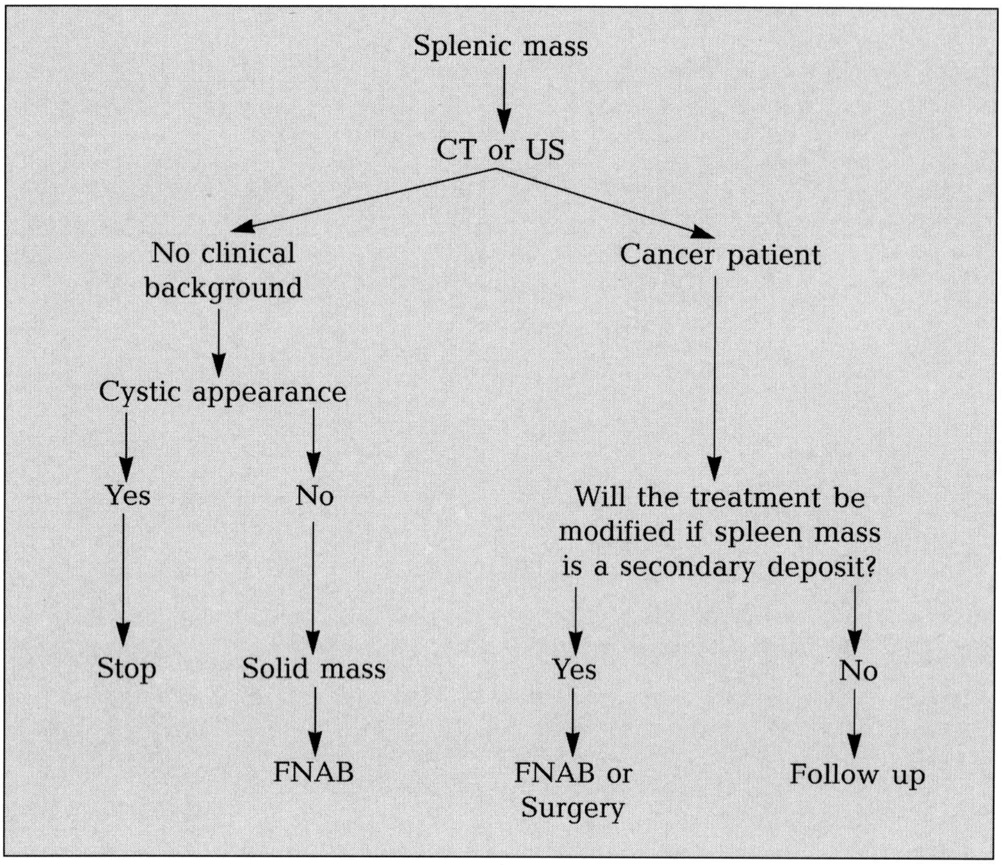

Diagram 9.4

Strategy for diagnosis of a splenic mass. FNAB = fine-needle aspiration biopsy.

10

The kidney

Peter McCarthy, Parvati Ramchandani and Howard Pollack

Renal-cell carcinoma

Renal-cell carcinoma accounts for 86% of all primary malignant renal parenchymal tumors and 3% of adult malignancies, making it a common malignant tumor in adults.[1] There is a 2:1 male to female ratio and an increasing frequency with advancing age. Patients most commonly present between 50 and 60 years and the classical 'triad' of symptoms described in these patients is flank pain, gross hematuria and a palpable renal mass. However, this constellation is seen in only 4–9% of patients at presentation[2] and is an ominous sign, as 47% of such patients have metastases.[3] More commonly, patients present with fever, malaise and anemia, without signs or symptoms specific to the kidney. Gross hematuria occurs in approximately 20% of patients and microscopic hematuria in 50–60%. Thus, renal-cell carcinoma is often not diagnosed early in its course.

However, the widespread use of CT and ultrasound for all manner of medical problems is leading to the frequent serendipitous discovery of small, asymptomatic renal-cell carcinomas during examinations performed for reasons other than suspected kidney tumor.[4] In one study, 0.3% of patients undergoing abdominal CT scanning were found to have occult renal-cell carcinoma.[4] These incidentally discovered tumors are usually of a lower stage and may have a better prognosis than those presenting with clinical symptoms, as tumor stage and histologic grade are the most important prognostic indicators in renal-cell carcinoma. Other recent reports suggest that 64–97% of tumors measuring 3 cm or less are discovered incidentally.[5,6] Renal cortical tumors measuring less than 3 cm in diameter have been referred to as renal adenomas in the past. Ample reports are now available in the literature to support the theory that size alone is not a valid criterion for excluding a diagnosis of renal-cell carcinoma. There are no microscopic or histochemical features that reliably distinguish between the so-called cortical adenomas and renal carcinoma that has not yet metastasized.[7] It is probably more accurate to consider these small neoplasms as carcinomas of low metastatic potential which should be treated in the same fashion as larger tumors. Widely disseminated metastases have in fact been described in patients whose primary renal neoplasms were 3 cm or less.

Papillary varieties constitute 5–15% of renal-cell carcinomas and have a better prognosis than non-papillary tumors. They tend to be more slowly growing, are relatively avascular, and frequently have extensive necrosis and cystic degeneration. They often have peripheral calcification.[8]

Detection and diagnosis

The initial imaging performed will be determined by the patient's symptoms. An intravenous urogram, being performed for urinary tract symptoms such as hematuria, may detect a renal mass. Alternatively, a renal mass may be found on CT or ultrasound as an incidental finding, as discussed earlier.

Excretory urography

Tomography is considered an essential component of the excretory urogram (EU) in adults. Masses, especially those protruding anteriorly or posteriorly, often can be detected in no other way. Unfortunately, the nature of a renal mass cannot be determined with certainty on an EU unless a smooth, extremely thin wall, seen throughout the entirety of the mass periphery, is discernable by tomography and indicates the presence of a cyst. The presence of certain signs would suggest the diagnosis of carcinoma, as follows. Contour abnormalities caused by peripherally located masses (Figure 10.1) and distortion of the collecting system due to centrally located masses can be seen in both cysts and renal-cell carcinoma; a CT or ultrasound is required to make the distinction. Invasion of the renal pelvis and calyces, causing filling defects in the collecting system, is suggestive of carcinoma (Figure 10.2) and is unlikely to occur with cysts, as is the presence of a thick-wall and heavy central calcification.

Calcification is the most helpful sign – central calcification strongly suggests malignancy and 87% of such lesions are malignant (Figure 10.3).[9] A mass with peripheral calcification apparent on an EU should be further evaluated by CT to confirm that the calcification is truly peripheral. Approximately 20–30% of peripherally calcified masses are malignant.[9,10]

EU is relatively insensitive in detecting masses less than 3 cm in diameter. A recent report by Warshauer et al compared the relative sensitivities of EU and ultrasonography in detecting CT-confirmed renal masses.[11] EU detected only 10% and ultrasound 26% of masses less than 1 cm, 21% and 60% of masses less than 2 cm, 52% and 82% of masses 2–3 cm, and 85% and 85% of masses 3 cm or more in diameter, respectively. Warshauer et al go so far as to recommend CT evaluation of the kidneys not only in cases which are questionable on urography and sonography, but also whenever clinical suspicion of a lesion is high, even in the face of an apparently negative urogram.

Excretory urography remains the mainstay of urologic diagnosis as it is the most effective way of evaluating the renal collecting system and the renal parenchyma simultaneously. It is best suited to detection of large, contour-deforming tumors and is relatively insensitive in detecting deep-seated intraparenchymal lesions or small tumors. Thus, the initial urogram may miss up to 6% of renal-cell cancers.[12]

Computed tomography

CT scanning, when combined with bolus contrast injection for enhancement and thin sectioning (≤5 mm or less slice thickness with continuous slices) is extremely sensitive in the detection of renal masses. Over 94% of renal masses less than 3 cm in diameter are detected by CT;[7] tumors of this size constituted 14% of all renal-cell carcinomas in one series.[13] CT also plays a primary role in pre-operative staging – this will be discussed further in the next section.

Lesions smaller than 1 cm in diameter are often too small to characterize with certainty on CT, due to partial volume averaging with adjacent tissues. Small lesions located at the polar regions are also more difficult to evaluate and may be missed due to respiratory motion.

It is important to emphasize that the most commonly encountered renal masses are benign cysts, estimated to occur in over 50% of the population over 50 years old. Benign cysts can vary in size but meet the following criteria: (1) they are sharply demarcated from adjacent surrounding renal parenchyma, (2) they have a thin, imperceptible or barely perceptible smooth wall, (3) they are of water density with attenuation values of 0–20 Hounsfield units (HU) and (4) they do not enhance after contrast administration. If a cyst does not meet these criteria, it is considered to be a complicated cyst, which must be differentiated from a cystic neoplasm.

Unenhanced scans should be performed first during evaluation of a renal mass, primarily to look for tumor calcification (which may be obscured once contrast is given), and also to determine whether a renal mass enhances after contrast administration.

Calcification

As with plain films, non-peripheral calcification in a soft tissue mass is strongly suggestive of carcinoma. Fine, peripheral calcification is usually a sign of benignity but can also be seen in carcinoma. Thick, irregular, wall calcification may be present in complicated, benign cysts (such as hemorrhagic renal cysts) or in cystic renal-cell carcinoma.[14] Attenuation values in both these lesions may be identical. Cystic carcinomas, especially papillary cystadenocarcinomas, can have densities in the fluid range (-10 to 20 HU) and hemorrhagic benign cysts may have attenuation values much higher than those usual for benign cysts. Contrast administration, and even

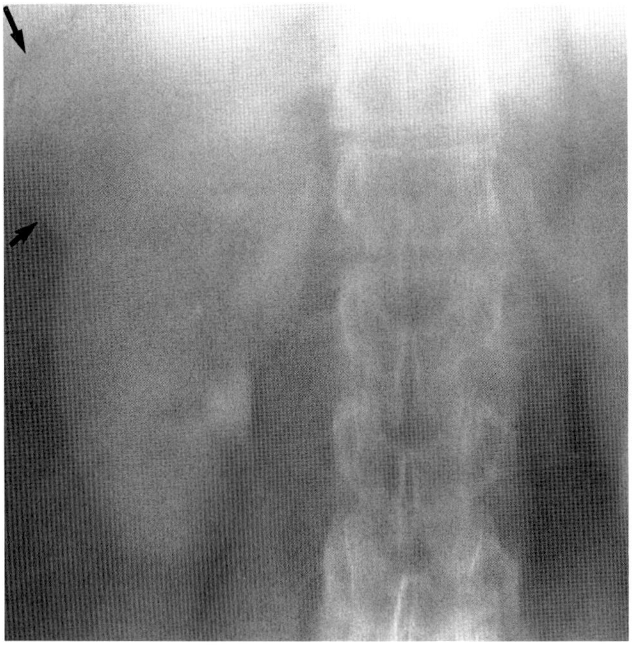

A

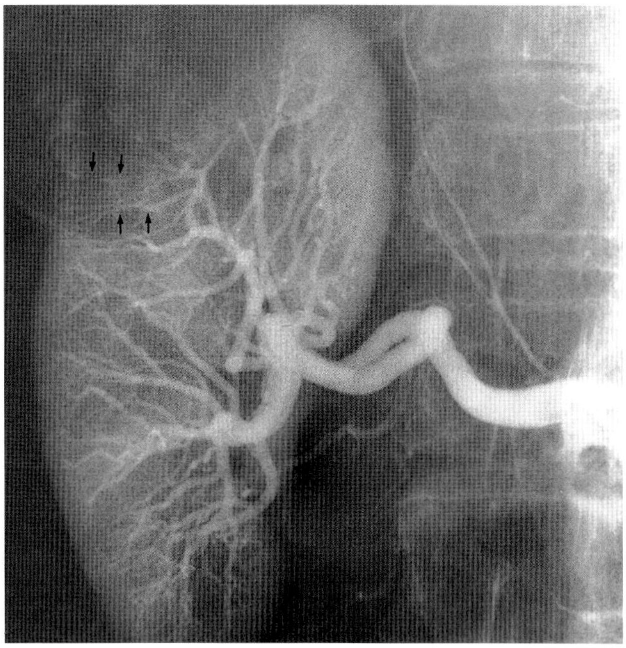

C

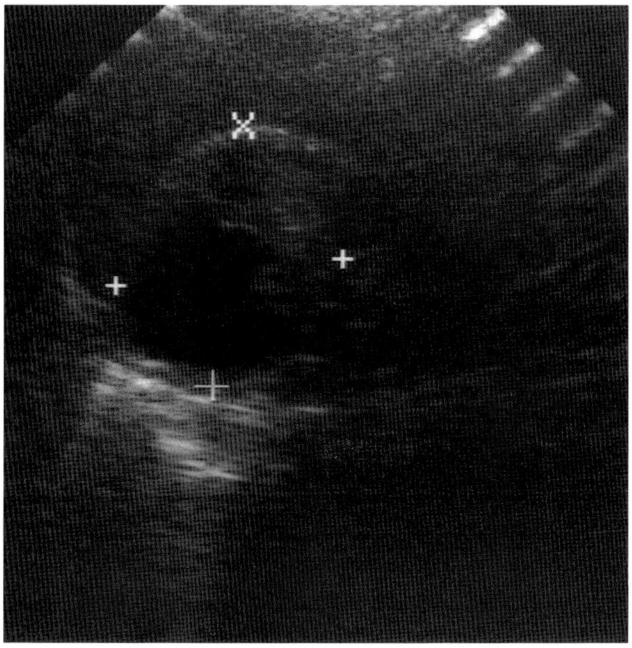

B

Figure 10.1

Papillary cystadenocarcinoma.

A Excretory urography demonstrates a large mass in the upper pole of the right kidney (arrows). The lesion appears to be thin walled.

B Sonography demonstrates the mass to be complex with only a small cystic component and a large echogenic, solid component.

C Selective renal arteriography demonstrates the relative hypovascularity of these lesions as compared to the usual clear cell carcinoma (compare with Figure 10.3). Encasement of small arterial branches within the tumor is seen (arrows).

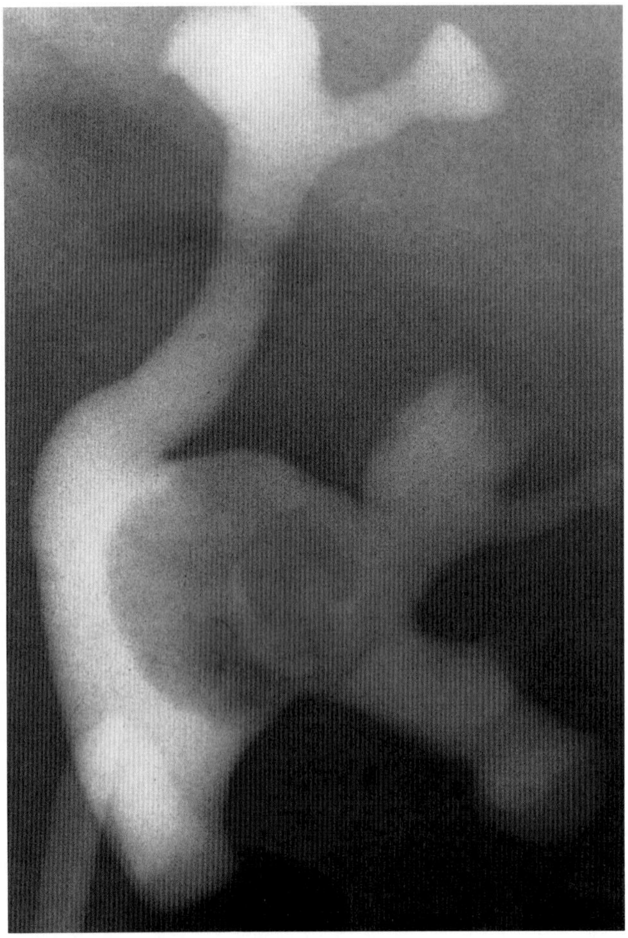

A

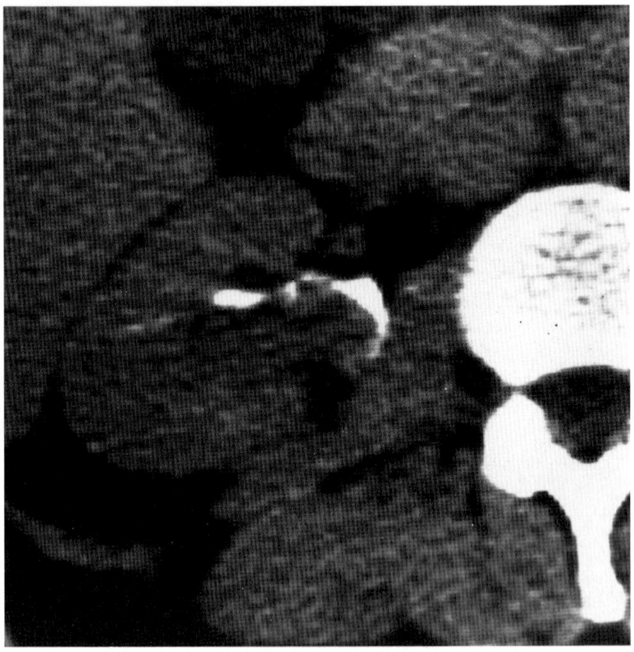

B

Figure 10.2

Excretory urography (**A**) and CT (**B**) demonstrate invasion of the renal pelvis by a renal-cell carcinoma.

angiography, may be unhelpful as cystic renal carcinomas are typically hypovascular and may not enhance. Percutaneous aspiration biopsy has not proven to be definitive in separating these two lesions since some cystic renal carcinomas have clear fluid with no malignant cells detectable by cytology. The instillation of contrast material will sometimes be helpful in showing mural irregularities, but more often than not ultrasonography will be the most valuable discriminator (see Figure 10.1). Surgical exploration is the only alternative in indeterminate cases, due to the significant risk of renal carcinoma in masses with dense peripheral calcification.

Contrast enhancement

On the unenhanced scan, renal carcinomas are seen as non-homogeneous masses of variable attenuation. They are usually isodense or slightly hypodense, less often they are hyperdense. Areas of cystic degeneration or necrosis appear as low-density areas. Areas of high density may be seen if recent hemorrhage has occurred or if the tumor contains calcification. Small tumors may not be apparent on unenhanced scans.[15]

Contrast administration should optimally be performed with bolus technique. Subsequent dynamic scanning (multiple scans obtained at one level to evaluate the arterial, venous and

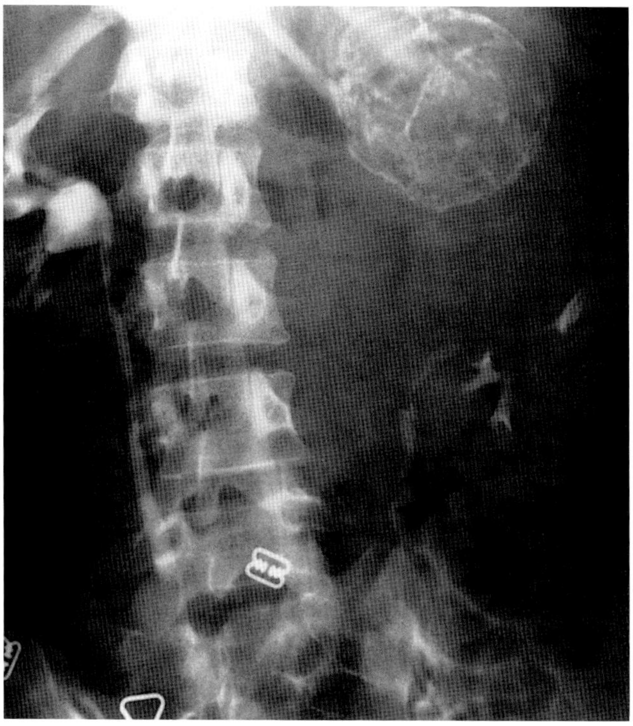

A

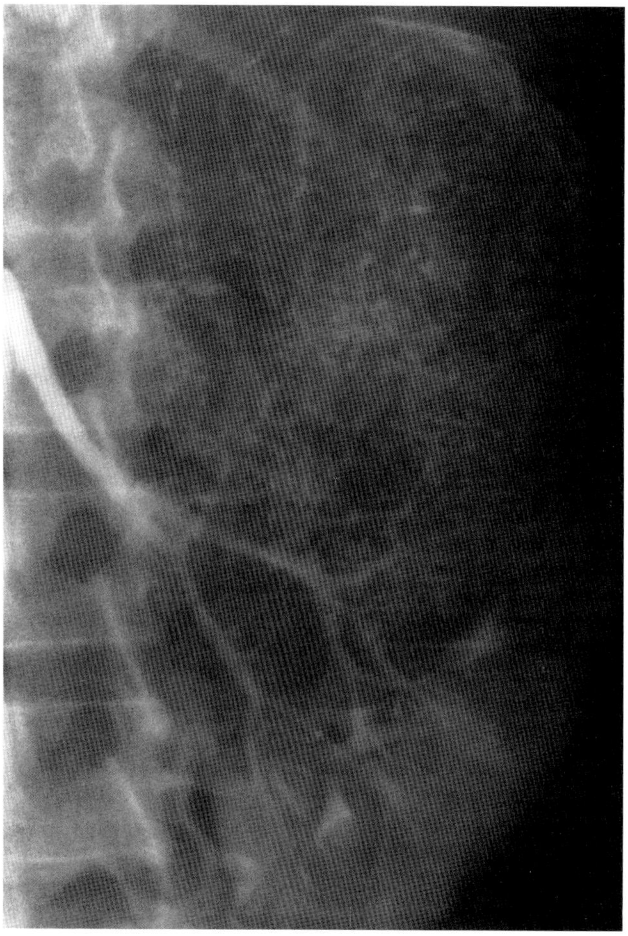

B

Figure 10.3

Calcified renal-cell carcinoma.

A Excretory urography demonstrates a large calcified left renal mass in a 24-year-old female. Note the caudal displacement of the pelvicalyceal system.

B Selective renal arteriography depicts the tumor extent well. Tumor is replacing the upper half of the left kidney and is extending towards the renal hilus.

nephrographic phases) helps in depicting the renal vein and inferior vena cava more consistently than does standard CT scanning.[16] The vascularity of a tumor can also be quantified by comparing the serial changes in attenuation value of the mass relative to the aorta and plotting these values on a graph. This technique can be useful in demonstrating minimal vascularity in a mass of perplexing nature and in confirming the presence of a pseudotumor.

Renal-cell carcinomas usually enhance after contrast administration but they do so to a lesser degree than normal renal parenchyma and therefore become easier to detect. The degree of enhancement is dependent on the vascular perfusion; thus, vascular tumors demonstrate marked enhancement, but hypovascular lesions (such as papillary carcinoma) may not enhance significantly. Lesions with necrosis and cystic degeneration also demonstrate little or no enhancement.[16]

True enhancement is indicated by an increase in attenuation value of at least 20 HU - lesser increases may simply represent partial volume averaging with adjacent enhanced normal renal parenchyma. Papillary carcinomas may show little or no contrast enhancement.

The pattern of enhancement is usually non-homogeneous and the tumors may be poorly demarcated from adjacent parenchyma. Contrast administration facilitates the evaluation of wall thickness: cystic carcinomas have thick walls which may not be irregular; benign cysts have imperceptible walls and are sharply demarcated from the adjacent parenchyma. Spontaneous perinephric (subcapsular and/or extracapsular) hematomas may be the initial manifestation of renal-cell carcinomas; such tumors are often small, cortical lesions. The hematoma appears as high density fluid in the subcapsular or extracapsular location. The underlying tumor itself may not be identified on pre-operative studies such as CT or angiography. Surgical exploration may sometimes be unavoidable if other causes of spontaneous bleeding, such as vasculitis or a bleeding diathesis, have been excluded; but if serial CT studies after reabsorption of the hematoma fail to show a neoplasm, surgery might be put off.

Hyperdense cysts

These are benign cysts which are denser than the normal renal parenchyma on unenhanced scans, with CT numbers 40–240% higher than renal parenchyma.[17] After contrast administration, there is no significant enhancement, and attenuation values increase less than 6% relative to normal cortex. Morphologically, these cysts are akin to the usual benign renal cyst in that the walls are smooth and imperceptible and the lesions are sharply demarcated from the adjacent kidney. The exact etiology of the high density is uncertain; it may be related to a high protein content or the presence of old blood or calcific material. The cysts often contain a firm coagulum which cannot be aspirated, thus rendering percutaneous aspiration useless. They may be multiple and bilateral.

Magnetic resonance imaging

Initial reports about the use of MR in the diagnosis and staging of renal neoplasms were extremely optimistic and suggested a 100% detection rate and 82–96% accuracy in staging. However, as experience has accumulated, it has become clear that MR has significant limitations in the detection of solid renal neoplasms; at present, it should not be used as the conclusive examination to exclude renal-cell carcinoma.[18,19] The usefulness of MR may be greatly expanded by the advent of paramagnetic contrast media and technical modifications such as fat saturation and surface coil imaging; but, for now, the impact of these adjuvants on the MR assessment of renal-cell carcinoma is unclear.[20]

On spin-echo (SE) imaging, renal-cell carcinomas have varied appearances, ranging from hypointense to hyperintense with respect to the normal renal parenchyma. Most commonly, the lesions have a signal intensity (SI) intermediate between the renal cortex and the medulla on T1-weighted images and are hyperintense on T2-weighted images (Figure 10.4). In a recent study,[18] four of seven solid tumors were isointense with surrounding normal renal parenchyma at all pulse sequences using a 0.35 T unit. No correlation was found between signal intensity and specific tissue or histologic type. Fourteen per cent of the tumors were isointense at all pulse sequences.[20] Initial reports suggest that most renal-cell carcinomas enhance after gadolinium administration.[21] Even without contrast enhancement, MR is superior to unenhanced CT for detection of non-calcified solid renal masses because MR has better contrast resolution (20–225%, compared to less than 5% for non-enhanced CT).

Renal cysts

Simple renal cysts are easily diagnosed and detected by MR as the cyst fluid has long relaxation times. On T1-weighted SE images, typical simple cysts are very hypointense compared to normal parenchyma and equally hyperintense on T2-weighted images. As on CT scans, they have imperceptible walls and are sharply defined; unfortunately, though, many of them present signal patterns that depart from the stereotype, for reasons which are unclear.[22]

Complicated cysts, whether due to infection or hemorrhage, cannot be reliably separated from solid or cystic renal neoplasms as signal intensities may overlap. Some authors[19] have found that many cystic renal cell carcinomas have intensities identical to those of simple cysts, but others[22] have found that cystic lesions with intensities equal to urine were benign, regardless of the presence of morphologic characteristics such as a thick lobulated wall or septa.

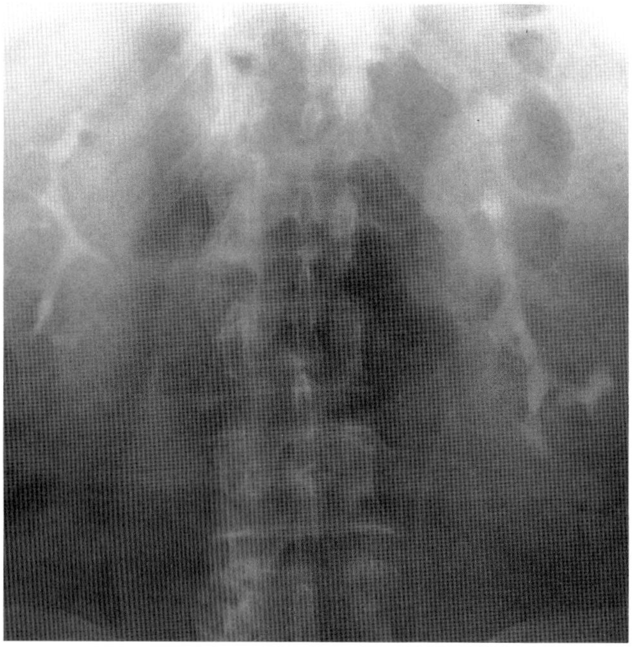

A

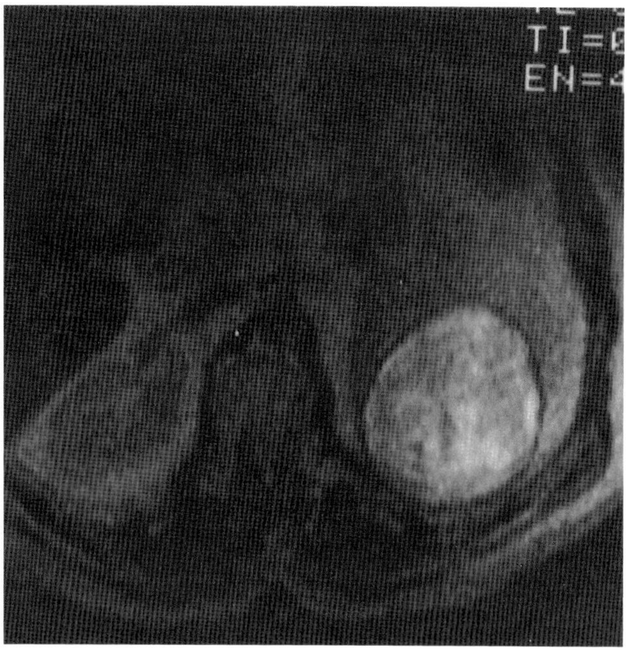

C

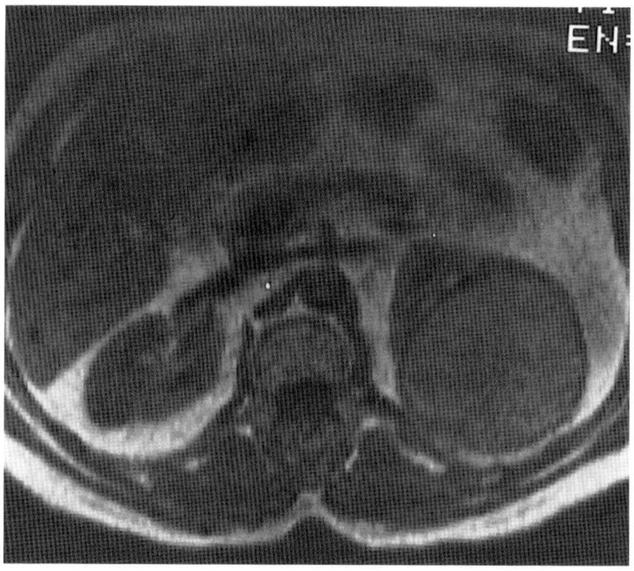

B

Figure 10.4

Renal-cell carcinoma.

A Excretory urography shows a large left renal upper polar mass with compression of the pelvicalyceal system.

B Axial T1-weighted MR (TR 600/TE 20) shows the mass to be of intermediate signal intensity between cortex and medulla.

C Axial T2-weighted MR (TR 2500/TE 80) shows the mass to be hyperintense.

At present, assessment of morphologic features is important in differentiating benign cysts from malignant ones, even on MR. The signal intensity of the cyst fluid is an unreliable indication of benignancy. Another serious limitation of MR in the evaluation of cystic lesions is its inability to reliably depict and detect calcification in lesions.

Ultrasonography

Ultrasonography, like CT, may detect small renal carcinomas incidentally during scans performed for other reasons. However, it is less sensitive than CT for small masses; it detected only 60% of 1–2 cm lesions in one series.[11] A more common indication for ultrasonographic evaluation is characterization of a mass found on urography or CT.

With respect to normal renal cortex, 86% of renal-cell carcinomas are isoechoic.[23] However, the echo pattern is often heterogeneous with mixed hyper- and hypoechoic areas which distinguish it from the adjacent normal tissue. If the echo texture is uniform and the lesions are small enough that there is no contour abnormality or distortion of the renal sinus echo complex, the lesions may be overlooked.

Ten per cent of renal carcinomas are hypoechoic and, rarely, they may be anechoic. Hyperechoic echo pattern occurs in 4% of cancers. There is poor sound transmission through the carcinomas in most cases, but there may be good acoustic transmission if liquefactive necrosis has occurred in the lesion (reported in 13% of renal-cell carcinomas).[24] However, even these lesions will usually exhibit nodular or thickened walls and some irregular echoes within the mass—these signs indicate that the lesion is not a benign cyst (Figure 10.5). Mural calcification will reflect sound back and tends to prevent adequate sonographic evaluation of a mass.

Recently, attempts have been made to non-invasively characterize renal masses as benign or malignant using pulsed Doppler ultrasound.[25,26] Hypervascular carcinomas demonstrate high-frequency signals with a large systolic–diastolic gradient, which has been attributed to arterio-venous shunting. High-frequency Doppler shifts of 4 kHz or more were seen in all of the hypervascular carcinomas in one series.[25] In another study,[26] 83% of patients with renal-cell carcinoma exhibited higher Doppler-shift frequencies in the carcinoma relative to the frequency in the main renal artery. All of the benign lesions demonstrated

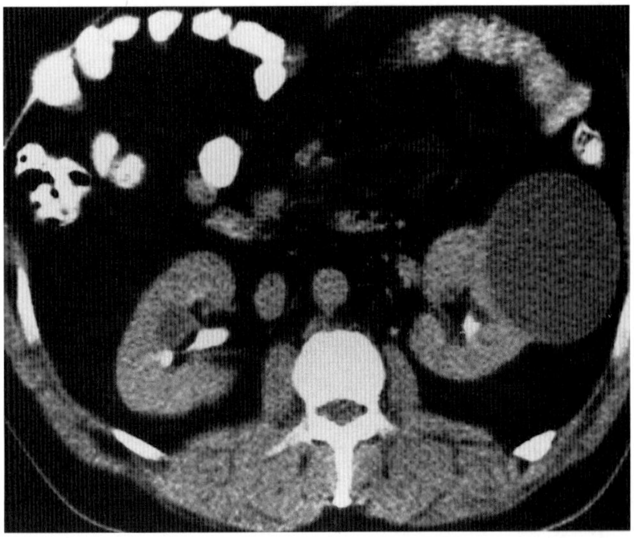

A

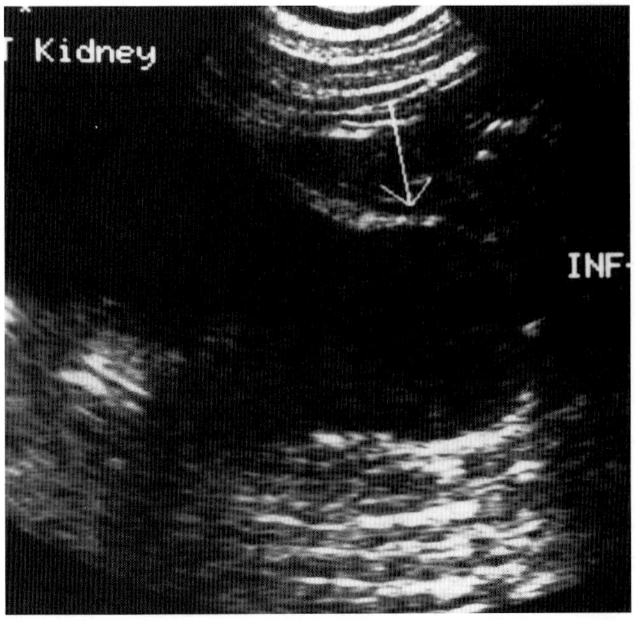

B

Figure 10.5

Papillary cystadenocarcinoma.

A CT of the left kidney demonstrates a large lesion which could be mistaken for a cyst. However, there is a suggestion of a wall, which should raise the suspicion that this is not a simple cyst.

B Sonography clearly demonstrates echogenic material within the lesion. The arrow points to a septum that was not appreciated on CT.

Doppler-shift frequencies lower than those in the control renal arteries. One potential application of this technology is to determine which renal lesions can be safely biopsied without fear of bleeding.

A major drawback of both conventional and Doppler ultrasound is that the techniques are extremely operator-dependent and only as good as the radiologists performing them. Doppler ultrasound, especially with color capability, also requires specialized, expensive equipment, the technology of which is still evolving.

Staging

The principal features to be sought in the preoperative staging of a renal neoplasm are:

- perinephric extension;
- lymph node involvement;
- extension into the renal vein and inferior vena cava;
- invasion of adjacent viscera (e.g. bowel);
- invasion of posterior abdominal musculature (e.g. psoas muscle);
- distant metastases (e.g. liver).

Two different staging systems are currently in use. Robson's staging scheme groups renal neoplasms into four stages (Table 10.1).[27]

Table 10.1 Robson's staging of renal-cell carcinoma.[27]

Stage I	Tumors are confined to the kidney
Stage II	Tumors may extend to the perinephric fat but are confined within Gerota's fascia
Stage III	Tumors have renal vein and/or caval involvement or lymph node involvement
Stage IV	Tumors have either spread to contiguous organs or have distant metastases

Robson's staging scheme has been criticized for grouping venous extension into the renal vein or inferior vena cava together with regional lymph node involvement in the same stage (stage III). The more recent TNM classification, devised by the American Joint Committee for Tumor Staging (Table 10.2),[28] attempts to rectify this shortcoming by making separate assessments of the extent of

Table 10.2 TNM staging of renal-cell carcinoma.

TNM stage		*Robson scheme*
Primary tumor		
T0	No evidence of primary tumor	–
T1	Small intrarenal tumor with minimal renal and calyceal deformity	I
T2	Large intrarenal tumor deforming and/or enlarging kidney and/or collecting system	
T3a	Tumor spread to perinephric tissues but within Gerota's fascia	II
T3b	Tumor spread to renal vein	IIIa
T3c	Tumor spread to renal vein and infradiaphragmatic cava	
T3d	Tumor spread to renal vein and infra- and supradiaphragmatic cava	
T4a	Local tumor extension into adjacent organs and abdominal wall	IVa
T4b	Intracardiac tumor	IIIa
Nodal involvement		
N0	No nodal involvement	IIIb
N1	Single ipsilateral, bilateral or contralateral nodes	
N2	Multiple ipsilateral, bilateral or contralateral nodes	
N3	Fixed surgical nodes (at surgery)	
Distant metastases		
M0	No distant metastases	IVb
M1	Distant metastases present	

the primary tumor (T), status of regional lymph nodes (N) and the presence of metastases (M). However, the TNM classification is unwieldy and the Robson staging remains popular in clinical use.

Accurate pre-operative tumor staging is important in planning appropriate management and in determining long-term prognosis. Analysis of survival by tumor stage at 5 years and 10 years (the latter in parentheses) has shown survival rates of 67% (56%), 51% (28%), 33.5% (20%) and 13.5% (3%) in stages I, II, III and IV disease, respectively.[29]

Ultrasound, CT and MR are all in use for the pre-operative staging of renal-cell carcinoma. The strengths and drawbacks of these modalities are discussed below.

Ultrasonography

Sonography is inaccurate in staging renal neoplasms. Stage I and II disease cannot be separated as the perinephric fat and renal fascia cannot be discriminated as separate structures in most patients.[30] In stage III disease, retroperitoneal adenopathy may be difficult to evaluate due to masking by overlying bowel gas. The renal vein and the infrahepatic inferior vena cava can be visualized well in only 50% of patients, although color-coded Doppler ultrasound may improve this figure in the future.

CT and MR have supplanted ultrasound in the pre-operative staging of renal neoplasms. Sonography is still occasionally useful in determining the origin of a large abdominal mass and in determining the true relationship of such masses to the kidneys.

Computed tomography

CT has proven to be accurate in staging renal-cell carcinoma, with an overall accuracy of 91%,[31] in comparison with surgical and pathologic staging. It remains the modality of choice for pre-operative staging of renal-cell carcinoma as it accurately and consistently demonstrates the tumor mass and local extension (Figure 10.6). In the following summary of the expected findings in the different stages, Robson's classification is used.

Stage I and Stage II tumors

In most patients with adequate retroperitoneal fat, normal perinephric fat and renal fascia are seen clearly in stage I tumors. With stage II tumors, tumor infiltration in the perinephric fat occurs and soft tissue masses will be seen encroaching on this area.

Perinephric extension is the most difficult finding to evaluate and accounts for more than half of the staging errors with CT: in one series,[31] perinephric soft tissue masses were seen only in 46% of patients with proven tumor. Perinephric stranding, since it can be attributable to collateral vessels as well as tumor, is a non-specific sign and was present in half the patients who had stage I tumors.

Stage III tumors

Dynamic, thin-section CT scanning with bolus administration of contrast will demonstrate the renal veins in 99% of patients.[16] Normal variations in the number and position of the renal veins can be recognized. Renal vein enlargement per se is not indicative of tumor extension into the renal veins; 30/80 patients had ipsilateral renal vein enlargement with no tumor thrombus.[16] The increase in size of the renal vein in such cases is probably related to the increased flow from a hypervascular tumor. Since spread to the inferior vena cava is by way of the renal vein, it is highly unlikely that caval tumor thrombus is present if the renal vein is tumor-free.

Tumor thrombus is seen as a filling defect in the opacified renal vein and inferior vena cava (Figure 10.7). Assessment of tumor thrombus vascularity has been found to be inconsistent and of little help in trying to distinguish tumor thrombus from bland thrombus.

Renal-cell carcinoma metastasizes to retroperitoneal and retrocrural lymph nodes (stage IIIb). Nodes less than 1 cm in diameter are considered normal, those of 1–2 cm are indeterminate or suspicious and nodes greater than 2 cm are definitely abnormal. CT scanning cannot separate nodal enlargement due to reactive hyperplasia from that due to metastatic disease – enhancement after contrast administration can be identical with both pathologies, and CT-guided biopsies are often required to make this distinction.

Stage IV

Direct extension into adjacent muscles, diaphragm and adjacent organs is depicted well by CT. With

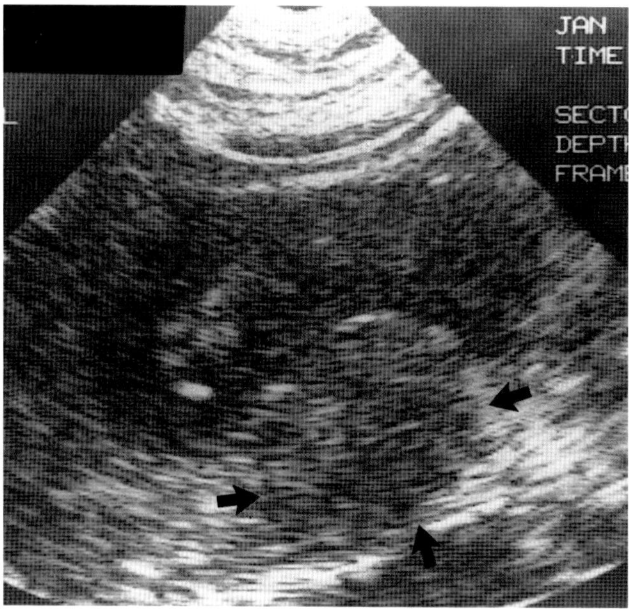

A

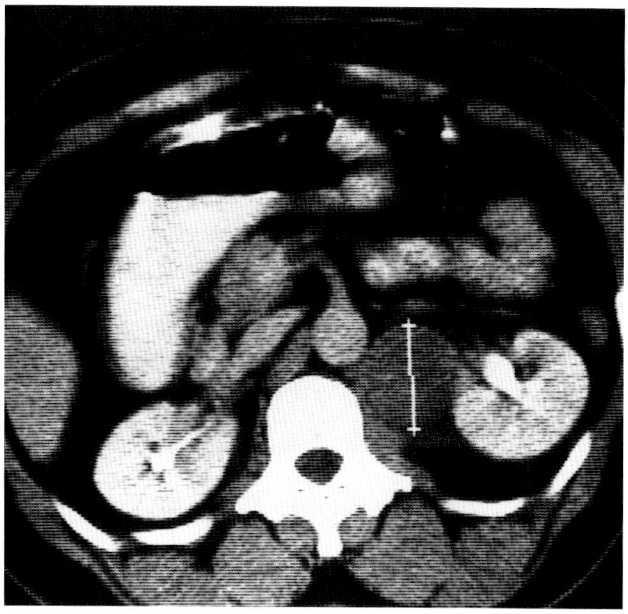

C

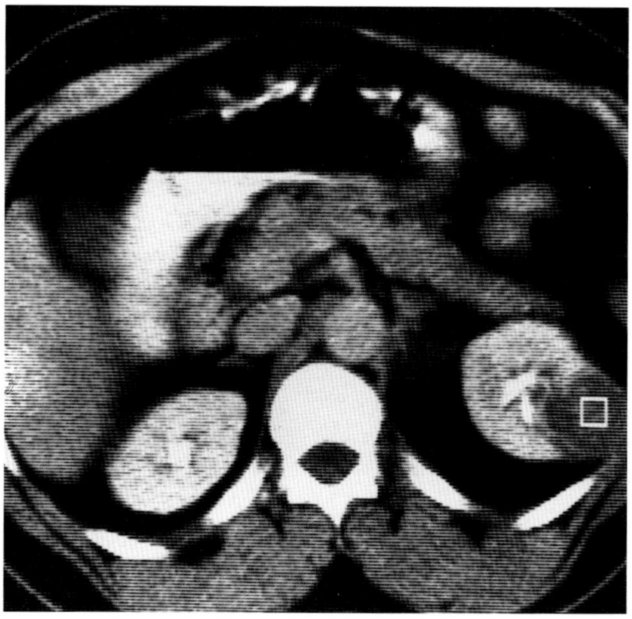

B

Figure 10.6

Renal-cell carcinoma with hilar metastasis.

A 47-year-old man with hematuria, found to have a left renal mass on excretory urography. Ultrasonography showed the renal mass to be solid (not illustrated) but also demonstrated an unexpected left renal hilar mass (arrows).

B Post-contrast CT demonstrates the renal mass to be of soft-tissue attenuation. Note the extension to the posterior abdominal wall.

C A large hilar mass seen well with CT. The left renal vein was free of tumor. Percutaneous CT-guided biopsy established that the mass was a metastasis from the left renal carcinoma.

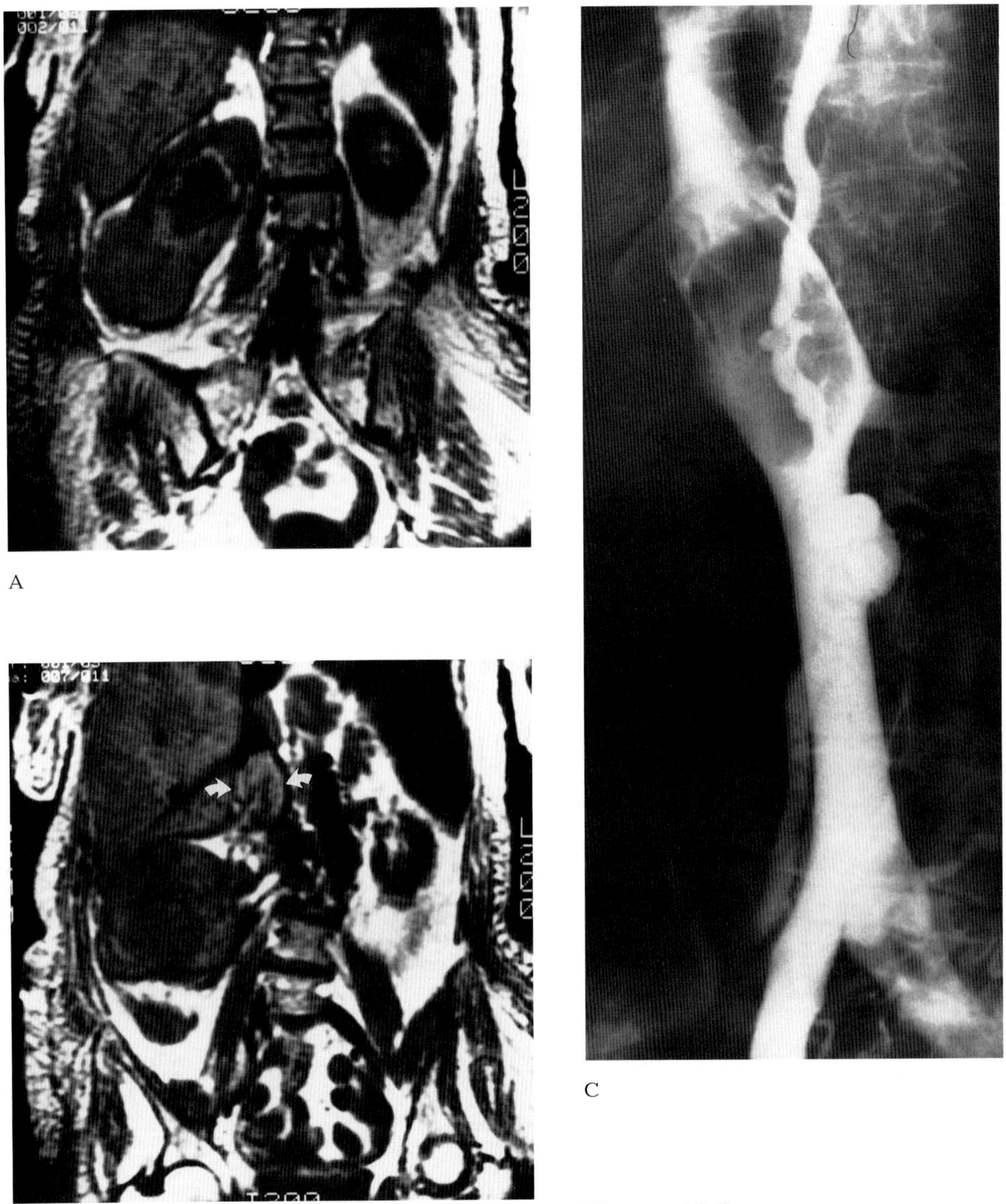

A

B

C

Figure 10.7

Caval extension of renal-cell carcinoma.

A,B Coronal MR (TR 600/TE 20) show a large lower pole renal mass with extension into the inferior vena cava (arrows).

C Inferior vena cavagram demonstrates the large thrombus in the cava.

axial images alone (the norm in CT) it is often difficult to distinguish whether the tumor is in close proximity to an adjacent organ or has actually invaded it.

Hematogenous metastases to liver, adrenals, opposite kidney, vertebrae and lungs are all easily and accurately demonstrated by CT. The metastases tend to mimic the vascularity of the primary tumor. Pre-contrast scans are important when assessing the liver as the metastases may become isodense once contrast is given.

Magnetic resonance imaging

In staging a known renal carcinoma, the accuracy of MR is comparable to or even slightly better than that of CT.[32] The capability of multiplanar imaging without loss of resolution (as occurs with reformatting in CT) is of great advantage in evaluating the great vessels and distinguishing extrinsic displacement from intraluminal tumor.[33] Collateral vessels in the renal hilus can be clearly separated from nodal enlargement due to the lack of signal in blood vessels with normal velocity of flow.

Gradient images with fast scan MR are particularly helpful in demonstrating intravascular tumor and also actual invasion of the caval wall,[34] whilst sagittal and coronal planes are a distinct aid in depicting the superior extent of the thrombus and also the relationship of a large renal mass to other abdominal organs.

Both slow flow and thrombus will give an abnormal signal in the cava. Bland thrombus has high signal intensity in both first and second echo images.[35] Tumor thrombus behavior is similar to that of the primary tumor mass, with different pulse sequences. Slow flow causes either a signal void or medium-intensity signal on first echo and absolute increase in signal intensity in the second image. It may be difficult at times to distinguish whether an intravascular signal is from slow flow or intraluminal thrombus, but gadolinium-enhanced studies can be very helpful here because the tumor thrombus usually enhances. However, MR cannot reliably predict tumor spread through the renal capsule and this is also a shortcoming of CT. Thus, the two technologies are comparable in their accuracy in depicting perinephric extension. Lymph-node size is also the main criterion for predicting nodal extension of disease by MR. Signal intensities have proved unreliable so far in determining the presence of tumor within regional lymph nodes.

Summary

To summarize, dynamic, thin-section CT remains the modality of choice in staging renal-cell carcinoma. However, MR is an equally attractive alternative, both as the primary modality for staging and as an adjunct in patients with equivocal CT findings with respect to renal veins or inferior cava, or in patients who should not receive iodinated contrast media.[32] MR is also useful in determining the origin of a large mass and in differentiating tumor invasion from tumor compression.

Diagram 10.1 is a suggested algorithm for the current work up of a renal mass.

Angiography, venography and phlebography

Angiography is seldom used nowadays for either the diagnosis or the staging of renal-cell carcinoma. The current indications for tumor angiography are as follows:

- Work up of an equivocal renal mass, in the hope of demonstrating tumor neovascularity and establishing that the mass is indeed neoplastic: papillary neoplasms are typically hypovascular and the arteriogram may be as unhelpful in establishing a diagnosis as the other imaging modalities.
- Prior to embolization in large, hypervascular neoplasms to demonstrate renal arterial anatomy and the vessels feeding the tumor: pre-operative embolization (with absolute alcohol or gelfoam) usually is performed immediately before surgery to minimize perioperative blood loss. Delayed nephrectomy, several days after renal infarction, has not been found to be an effective modality in the treatment of metastatic renal-cell carcinoma.[36]
- Vascular mapping in patients with solitary kidneys who are being considered for partial nephrectomies.

Inferior vena cavography and renal phlebography in the management of renal carcinoma are of historical interest only. The vascular structures can be adequately evaluated by noninvasive techniques such as CT, MR or ultrasonography.[35]

Percutaneous aspiration biopsy

Routine biopsy of renal-cell carcinoma is probably not justified if the lesion meets the imaging criteria for a carcinoma. The risk of possible complications, such as bleeding and the rare seeding of needle track with tumor cells, makes the risk:benefit ratio too high.

In selected situations, aspiration biopsy is a valuable adjunct in the management of renal-cell carcinoma. In patients with renal masses in association with a primary neoplasm elsewhere or in patients with known lymphoma, aspiration biopsy may help to histologically diagnose the renal mass. It is also useful in the work up of indeterminate renal masses when imaging modalities fail to establish a diagnosis. Although a positive biopsy is helpful in this circumstance, a negative biopsy may simply represent sampling error rather than indicate that the lesion is benign.

Detection of metastases

Lung metastases are found at autopsy in 55% of patients who have died of renal-cell cancer and the lung is at autopsy the most common site for metastases from renal-cell carcinoma.[37] Mediastinal lymph node involvement is an associated finding in 10% of cases.[38]

A chest radiograph should be obtained for all patients. If metastases are seen, no further chest work up is required. If the radiograph is normal or demonstrates a single metastasis, chest CT should be performed. Of patients with apparently solitary metastases on chest radiography, 45% had multiple lesions on whole lung tomography in one study.[39] Chest CT is more accurate than conventional tomography at demonstrating metastates and is the preferred examination.[40]

Bone metastases are found at autopsy in 33% of patients;[37] it can involve the axial skeleton or the long bones. Bone pain is frequent and pathologic fractures may occur. Embolization of the bony metastasis prior to fracture fixation helps both in reducing perioperative blood loss and in dramatically reducing pain. The lesions are lytic and are seen as areas of increased radionuclide uptake on bone scans.[41]

Post-operative follow up

Radical nephrectomy is the usual surgical procedure for renal-cell carcinoma unless the patient has a compromised contralateral kidney, in which case kidney-sparing surgery is performed.

CT scanning is the modality of choice in following for recurrence in the operative bed, evaluation of the contralateral kidney and in the search for distant metastases; 2–3% of patients have or will develop tumors in the other kidney. Ultrasonography is insensitive in detecting tumors in the operative bed or small tumors in the opposite kidney. MR has been unreliable in consistently depicting renal masses. However, tumor-bed recurrence is easier to image with MR as surgical clip artifact does not degrade the whole MR image, as it would the CT scan.

Other malignant renal parenchymal neoplasms

Renal metastasis

Renal metastasis is the most common malignant neoplasm of the kidney, probably because of the rich vascular supply of the kidneys. The common primaries are lung, breast, gastrointestinal tract and melanoma.

Most renal metastases are asymptomatic and occur when there is widespread disease. If large enough, they will be seen on excretory urography (hematuria is a frequent abnormality in these patients). The ultrasound appearance is nonspecific, and metastatic lesions appear as solid masses.

CT is the most sensitive imaging modality for detecting metastases. The lesions are usually hypovascular and appear as low-attenuation lesions in the enhanced renal parenchyma. Central necrosis and calcification is rare.

Differentiating a metastasis from a primary renal carcinoma on the basis of imaging characteristics alone is difficult. Aspiration biopsy will help to establish a diagnosis if this is of clinical importance.

Renal lymphoma

Renal involvement can be due to hematogenous spread or contiguous invasion from adjacent retroperitoneal adenopathy. It occurs more commonly with non-Hodgkin's lymphoma, usually late in the disease.

CT is the most sensitive imaging technique for detecting renal lymphomatous involvement. The appearance is non-specific and either percutaneous aspiration biopsy or open surgical biopsy is required to establish the diagnosis.[42,43]

Renal sarcoma

Renal sarcoma is a very unusual tumor which probably originates from the renal capsule. Abdominal pain and a palpable mass are the presenting symptoms in a third of patients. Prognosis is poor, with 10% survival beyond 8 years. The tumors can propagate into the renal vein and inferior vena cava. Distinguishing a renal sarcoma from a renal-cell carcinoma is difficult.[44]

Adult Wilm's tumor

In adults, Wilm's tumor is an uncommon lesion. The pathology is identical to the tumors of childhood, but the response to therapy and prognosis is poorer. There are no specific identifying imaging criteria to distinguish it from a renal-cell carcinoma.[44]

Renal oncocytoma

Oncocytomas are somewhat controversial lesions, since recent claims have been made that they are not always benign, as was thought previously.[45] In 1975, enthusiasm was regenerated among pathologists, radiologists and urologists about the benign nature of oncocytomas. It was shown that they consisted of clusters of uniform cells, probably of proximal tubular origin, containing granular eosinophilic cytoplasm.[46] The concept of the oncocytoma as a unique, benign renal mass led to vigorous efforts by radiologists to devise imaging criteria by which oncocytomas could be differentiated from malignant renal parenchymal lesions. While such criteria were once thought to be firmly established, it now appears that the radiological recognition of oncocytomas is problematic for two reasons.

Firstly, some lesions that appear to satisfy all the imaging requirements for oncocytomas prove to be renal-cell carcinomas, none the less. There are two main features on which the radiological suspicion of oncocytoma is based: a central scar and a 'spoke wheel' appearance. These characteristics may be recognized, at times, on CT, ultrasonography, angiography and MR. CT and ultrasonography demonstrate a smooth, relatively homogeneous mass with a stellate central scar (identified by CT in a third of cases and by ultrasound in a quarter of cases).[47] When the spoke wheel pattern is unusually prominent, it can be appreciated on CT and ultrasonography. On angiography, a spoke wheel pattern with a peripheral rim vessel may be seen more often.[48] MR demonstrates a well-defined low-intensity capsule on T2-weighted spin-echo images; the central scar may be seen as an area of low intensity.[49]

Secondly, there is evidence suggesting that not all oncocytomas are benign. Oncocytic tumors have been graded on the basis of their nuclear features into two grades – I and II. Grade I tumors have small, regular nuclei with no necrosis, nuclear anaplasia or mitotic activity. These tumors behave in a benign fashion and can be termed benign oncocytomas.[50] Oncocytic tumors that are grade II or higher demonstrate moderate to marked anaplasia and should not be considered benign.[45] In one series,[45] 4 of 28 patients with grade II tumors died of metastatic disease, whilst 62 patients with grade I tumors demonstrated no metastases.

Percutaneous needle biopsy may be unreliable in distinguishing renal-cell carcinoma from oncocytomas as the former may contain clusters of benign appearing oncocytic cells and sampling errors can thus occur. Open surgical biopsy may be indicated to establish the diagnosis if there is a high pre-operative suspicion of an oncocytoma.

References

1. Sufrin G, Murphy GP, Renal adenocarcinoma, *Urol Surv* (1980) **30**:129–44.
2. Skinner DG, Colvin RB, Vermillion CD, et al, Diagnosis and management of renal cell carcinoma. A clinical and pathological study of 309 cases, *Cancer* (1971) **28**:1165.
3. Murphy GP, Schirmer HKA, The diagnosis and treatment of hypernephroma, *Geriatrics* (1963) **18**:354.

4. Lieber MM, Renal cell carcinoma: new developments, *Mayo Clin Proc* (1985) **60**:715.
5. Provet J, Tessler A, Brown J, et al, Partial nephrectomy for renal cell carcinoma: indications, results and implications, *J Urol* (1991) **145**:472–6.
6. Smith SJ, Bosniak MA, Megibow J, et al, Renal cell carcinoma: earlier discovery and increased detection, *Radiology* (1989) **170**:699–703.
7. Amendola MA, Bree RL, Pollack HM, et al, Small renal cell carcinomas: resolving a diagnostic dilemma, *Radiology* (1988) **166**:637–41.
8. Mydlo JH, Bard RH, Analysis of papillary renal adenocarcinoma, *Urology* (1987) **30**:529–34.
9. Daniel WW, Hartman GW, Witten DM, et al, Calcified renal masses: a review of ten years experience at the Mayo Clinic, *Radiology* (1972) **103**:503.
10. Sniderman KW, Kreiger JN, Seligson GR, et al, The radiologic and clinical aspects of calcified hypernephroma, *Radiology* (1979) **131**:13.
11. Warshauer DM, McCarthy SM, Street L, et al, Detection of renal masses: sensitivities and specificities of excretory urography/linear tomography, US and CT, *Radiology* (1988) **169**:363–5.
12. Demos TC, Schiffer M, Love L, et al, Normal excretory urography in patients with primary kidney neoplasms, *Urol Radiol* (1985) **7**:75–9.
13. Curry NS, Schabel SI, Betsill WL Jr, Small renal neoplasms: diagnostic imaging, pathologic features and clinical course, *Radiology* (1986) **158**:113–17.
14. Weyman PJ, McClennan BL, Lee JKT, et al, CT of calcified renal masses, *AJR* (1982) **138**:1095.
15. Levine E, Huntrakoon M, Wetzel LH, Small renal neoplasms: clinical, pathologic and imaging features, *AJR* (1989) **153**:69–73.
16. Zeman RK, Cronan JJ, Rosenfield AT, et al, Renal cell carcinoma: dynamic thin-section CT assessment of vascular invasion and tumor vascularity, *Radiology* (1988) **167**:393–6.
17. Zirinsky K, Auh YH, Rubenstein WA, et al, CT of the hyperdense renal cyst: sonographic correlation, *AJR* (1984) **143**:151–6.
18. Quint LE, Glazer GM, Chenevert TL, et al, In vivo and in vitro MR imaging of renal tumors: histopathologic correlation and pulse sequence optimization, *Radiology* (1988) **169**:359–62.
19. Glazer GM, MR imaging of the liver, kidneys and adrenal glands, *Radiology* (1988) **166**:303–12.
20. Fein AB, Lee JKT, Balfe DM et al, Diagnosis and staging of renal cell carcinoma: a comparison of MR imaging and CT, *AJR* (1987) **148**:749–53.
21. Semelka RC, Hricak H, Stevens SK, et al, Combined gadolinium-enhanced and fat saturation MR imaging of renal masses, *Radiology* (1991) **178**:803.
22. Marotti M, Hricak H, Fritzsche P, et al, Complex and simple renal cysts: comparative evaluation with MR imaging, *Radiology* (1987) **162**:679–84.
23. Coleman BG, Arger PH, Mulhern CB, et al, Gray scale sonographic spectrum of hypernephromas, *Radiology* (1980) **137**:757–65.
24. Charboneau JW, Hattery RR, Ernst CC, et al, Spectrum of sonographic findings in 125 renal masses other than benign simple cysts, *AJR* (1983) **140**:87.
25. Kiujpers D, Jaspers, R, Renal masses: differential diagnosis with pulsed doppler ultrasound, *Radiology* (1989) **170**:59–60.
26. Ramos IM, Taylor KJW, Kier Ruben, et al, Tumor vascular signals in renal masses: detection with doppler ultrasound, *Radiology* (1988) **168**:633–7.
27. Robson CJ, Churchill BM, Anderson W, The results of radical nephrectomy for renal cell carcinoma, *J Urol* (1969) **101**:297.
28. Beahrs OH, Myers MH (eds), *Manual for staging of cancer* 2nd edn (JB Lippincott: Philadelphia 1983) 177.
29. McNichols DW, Segura JW, Deweerd JH, Renal cell carcinoma: long term survival and late recurrence, *J Urol* (1981) **126**:17.
30. Levine E, Maklad NF, Rosenthal SJ, et al, Comparison of computed tomography and ultrasound in abdominal staging of renal cancer, *Urology* (1980) **16**:317.
31. Johnson CD, Dunnick NR, Cohan RH, et al, Renal adenocarcinoma: CT staging of 100 tumors, *AJR* (1987) **148**:59–63.
32. Amendola MA, King LR, Pollack HM, et al, Staging of renal carcinoma using magnetic resonance imaging at 1.5 Tesla, *Cancer* (1990) **66**:40–4.
33. Ramchandani P, Soulen RL, Schnall RI, et al, Impact of magnetic resonance on staging of renal carcinoma, *Urology* (1986) **27**:564–8.
34. Levine E, Malignant renal parenchymal tumors in adults. In: Pollack HM, ed, *Clinical urography* (WB Saunders: Philadelphia 1990) 1254–5.
35. Hricak H, Thoeni RF, Carroll PR, et al, Detection and staging of renal neoplasms; a reassessment of MR imaging, *Radiology* (1988) **166**:643–9.
36. Gottesman JE, Crawford ED, Grossman HB, et al, Infarction nephrectomy for metastatic renal carcinoma, Southwest Oncology Group Study, *Urology* (1985) **25**:248–50.
37. Bennington JL, Beckwith JB, *Atlas of tumor pathology*, series 2, fascicle 12, *Tumors of the kidney, pelvis and ureter* (Armed Forces Institute of Pathology: Washington DC 1975) 93.
38. Lang, EK, Renal cell carcinoma presenting with metastases to pulmonary hilar nodes, *J Urol* (1977) **118**:543.
39. Bergman SM, Lippert M, Javadpour N, The value of whole lung tomography in the early detection of metastatic disease in patients with renal cell carcinoma and testicular tumors, *J Urol* (1980) **124**:860.
40. Muhm JR, Brown LR, Crowe JK, et al, Comparison of whole lung tomography and computed tomography for detecting pulmonary nodules, *AJR* (1975) **131**:981.
41. Forbes GS, McLeod RA, Hattery RR, Radiologic manifestations of bone metastases from renal carcinoma, *AJR* (1977) **129**:61.
42. Cohan RH, Dunnick NR, Leder RA, Baker ME, Computed tomography of renal lymphoma, *J Comput Assist Tomogr* (1990) **14**:933–8.

43. Reznek RH, Mootoosamy I, Webb JAW, et al, CT in renal and perirenal lymphoma: a further look, *Clin Radiol* (1990) **41**:233–8.
44. Pollack HM, Banner MP, Amendola MA, Other malignant neoplasms of the renal parenchyma, *Semin Roentgenol* (1987) **22**:260–74.
45. Lieber MM, Tomera KM, Farrow GM, Renal oncocytoma, *J Urol* (1981) **125**:481.
46. Klein MJ, Valensi QJ, Proximal tubular adenomas of the kidney with so called oncocytic features: a clinicopathological study of 13 cases of a rarely reported neoplasm, *Cancer* (1976) **38**:906.
47. Quinn MJ, Hartman DS, Friedman AC, et al, Renal oncocytoma: new observations, *Radiology* (1984) **153**:49.
48. Bonavita JA, Pollack HM, Banner MP, Renal oncocytomas: further observations and literature review, *Urol Radiol* (1981) **2**:229.
49. Remark RR, Berquist TH, Lieber MM, et al, Case report: magnetic resonance imaging of renal oncocytoma, *Urology* (1988), **31**:176.
50. Farrow GM, Diseases of the kidney. In: Murphy WM, ed, *Urological pathology* (WB Saunders: Philadelphia 1989) 445–51.

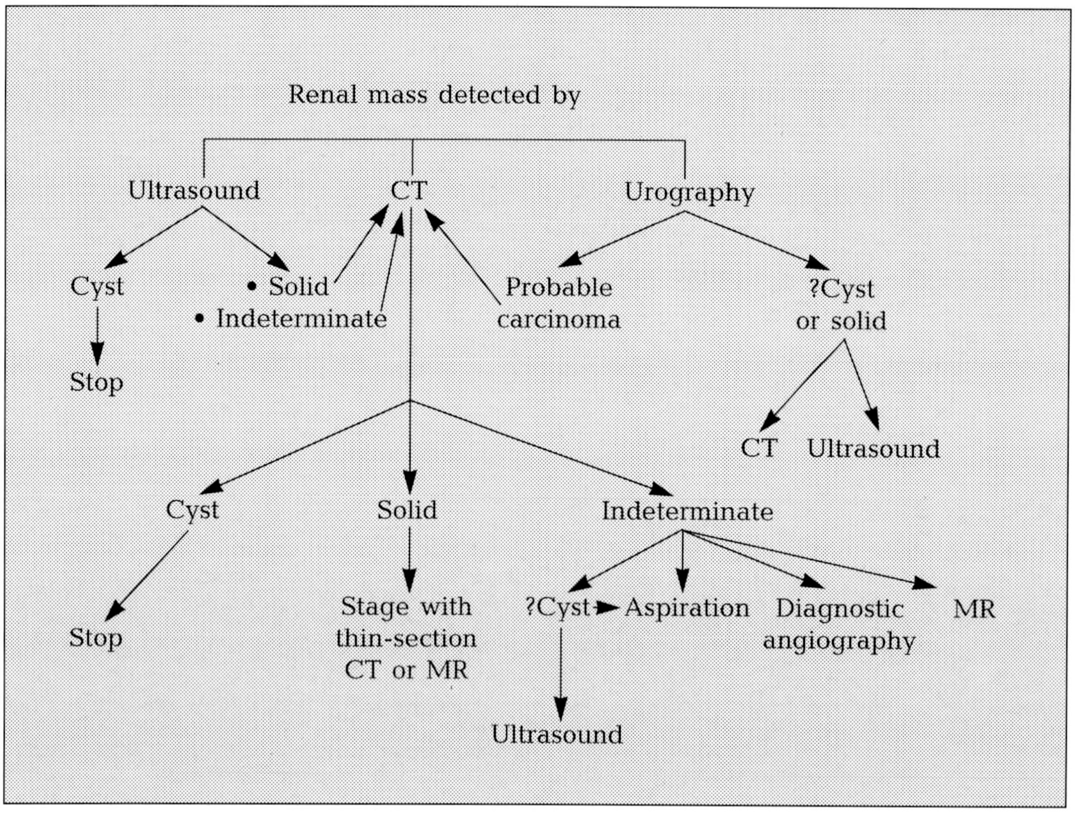

Diagram 10.1

Evaluation of a renal mass.

11

The renal collecting system

Peter McCarthy, Parvati Ramchandani and Howard Pollack

Introduction

The renal collecting systems and ureters are derived from the fetal mesonephros while the renal parenchyma originates from the metanephric blastema. Hence, there is an embryologic basis for the histologically distinct neoplasms that affect the renal calyces, pelvis and ureters.

Both epithelial and mesodermal tumors can occur in the collecting system, the former being much more common. The epithelial neoplasm most frequently encountered is transitional-cell carcinoma (TCC), which accounts for 7–10% of all malignant renal tumors and over 80% of renal pelvic tumors. Other epithelial tumors are squamous-cell carcinomas, which account for 6% of renal pelvic tumors and 0.5% of all renal neoplasms.[1] Adenocarcinoma and carcinosarcoma are other, rarer epithelial neoplasms. Both squamous-cell carcinoma and adenocarcinoma occur most often in association with chronic urinary tract infection, and a renal calculus is present in two-thirds of cases. Carcinosarcomas have a very poor prognosis. Non-function of the affected kidney is a common finding with non-transitional cell neoplasms, as these tumors usually present late in the course of the disease.[2]

Malignant mesodermal tumors (sarcomas) are extremely rare. The lesions are very aggressive and far advanced at diagnosis, generally presenting as large abdominal masses. Sarcomas arising in the renal pelvis are generally indistinguishable from those arising in the renal capsule or retroperitoneum, both radiologically and pathologically.

Secondary tumors of the renal pelvis and ureter can occur by direct extension of an adjacent neoplasm, or by lymphatic or hematogenous spread from a variety of primary neoplasms.

Diagnosis of transitional-cell carcinoma

TCCs of the renal collecting system and ureters occurs most frequently in the fifth to seventh decades, with males more commonly affected. Hematuria, whether gross or microscopic, is the most common symptom and affects 70–80% of patients who have renal pelvic involvement and 55–75% of patients who have ureteral involvement. Dysuria and pain is more frequent with ureteral tumors. The pain can be either colicky due to obstruction, or constant due to local tumor extension.

A variety of carcinogens and drugs, as well as chronic irritation, have been implicated in the development of TCC.[1,3] Aniline dyes and aromatic amines used in the manufacture of rubber, cable, dyes and plastics have been found to be carcinogenic, as are also smoking, phenacetin abuse and chronic urinary infection with or without calculi. All of these stimuli cause hyperplastic and metaplastic changes in the urothelium, with eventual progression to TCC. Thorotrast(thorium dioxide)-induced renal neoplasms are occasionally still encountered, with squamous-cell carcinoma being most frequent, followed by TCC. Multicentricity and multiplicity is an important, well-recognized feature of TCC of the urinary tract. A recent study[4] reported that in patients with renal TCC, synchronous lesions were present in 24% of the patients – in the ureter in 11%, in the bladder in 10%, and in the contralateral kidney in 3%. With ureteral TCC, synchronous lesions were identified in 39–21% of patients in the bladder and in 18% in the kidney. Other studies have reported similar results.[5] Thus, imaging studies have to be directed towards precise delineation of the entire collecting system so that all coexisting lesions can be identified.

Primary renal TCC is two to three times more common than ureteric TCC (bladder carcinomas are 50 times more frequent than renal TCC). Overall, primary ureteral neoplasms constitute 1% of all cancers of the upper genitourinary tract.

TCCs have an unusually high incidence in Balkan countries and are a part of the syndrome of Balkan nephropathy. Men and women are equally affected.

Histologic grading and staging

There is no universally accepted staging system for TCC of the renal pelvis or ureter. As with tumors of other organs, the stages are determined by the depth of invasion of the underlying submucosa and muscular layers. Tumors at a lower stage (limited to mucosa or superficially invasive into the lamina propria) tend to have a better prognosis. Invasion may be difficult to recognize in early lesions as it can occur in a tentacular fashion, rather than en bloc, and thus can be missed even on histologic examination.

The prognosis of renal and ureteral TCC is much poorer than that of urinary bladder TCC because the renal pelvis and ureter are thin-walled and lack a protective muscle coat to act as a barrier for tumor extension. An extensive lymphatic drainage system in the renal pelvis and ureter makes the lymphatic route the common mode of spread early in the course of the disease. Metastases occur to the retroperitoneal lymph nodes, lungs, liver and bones. Direct extension into the retroperitoneum is also common.

TCC of the renal pelvis is papillary in 80% of cases. The tumors tend to be large and are usually sessile but can be pedunculated. Papillary TCC of the ureter tends to be infiltrative much less frequently than in the renal pelvis, only 40% being infiltrating at the time of diagnosis.

Non-papillary tumors constitute 20% of renal TCC and 40% of ureteral TCC. Early invasion is common with early metastases.

TCCs are cytologically graded from I (slight anaplasia) to IV (marked anaplasia).[1,6] Some pathologists use five or even seven grades. Renal pelvic papillomas are a diagnostic dilemma because their significance is uncertain. Some pathologists believe that they represent low-grade tumors and label them as grade I papillary carcinomas;[1] others believe that they are non-malignant proliferations of transitional epithelial cells which are merely associated with TCC. Of patients with a renal pelvic papilloma, 25% ultimately develop TCC, whilst of patients with multiple papillomas, 50% develop TCC.

Cytologic analysis of urine

Cytologic analysis of the urine is inaccurate in the diagnosis of early, low-grade tumors, with a high rate of false-negative results.[7,8] The overall accuracy is reported as 10–20% for grade I lesions, increasing to 77–83% for grade IV tumors. Clearly, the skill of the pathologists will affect the rate of accurate detection at different institutions. Despite this, urine cytology remains an important step in the initial screening and subsequent follow up of patients with TCC.

Chemical tests have proved to be of little value in diagnosing TCC. An elevated urine lactate dehydrogenase level has been reported in some patients, but this is a non-specific finding.

Radiologic imaging

Plain radiography

The primary use of plain radiography is in the demonstration of renal or ureteric calculi, seen most often in association with squamous-cell carcinoma or adenocarcinoma. Tumor calcification is rarely seen in TCC of the renal pelvis or ureter. When it has been present, no pathognomonic pattern of calcification has been seen.[9] The calcifications generally have an indistinct border coupled with a mucosal lesion as seen on retrograde or excretory urography.

Bony metastases are occasionally seen and these can be both osteoblastic and osteoclastic.

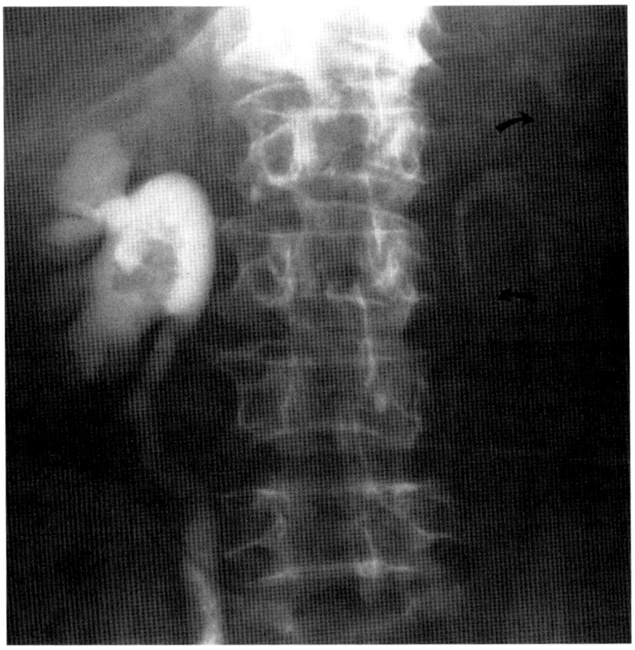

A

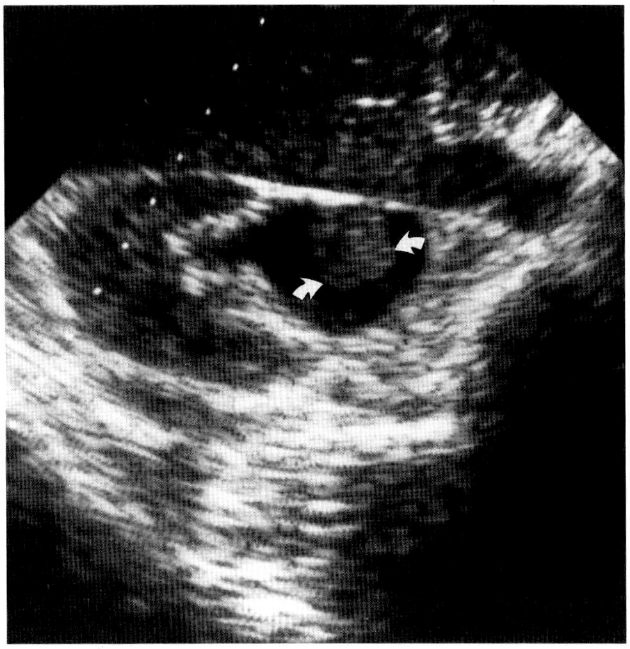

B

Figure 11.1

Bilateral transitional-cell carcinoma (TCC).

A Excretory urography demonstrates a large filling defect in the right renal pelvis. Lesions in the left upper pole infundibulum and proximal left ureter (arrows) were also TCC.

B Sonogram of the right kidney demonstrates the solid tumor mass projecting into the renal pelvis (arrows).

Excretory urography

Excretory urography (EU) is the initial imaging modality for the evaluation of the collecting system (see Diagram 11.1). Adequate distension of the pyelocalyceal systems and the ureters is essential for the detection of subtle lesions, and a high degree of suspicion is needed to appreciate and diagnose early disease.

Five urographic patterns have been described in TCC of the kidney:[10]

- Discrete filling defects, either single or multiple (Figures 11.1 and 11.2): this is the most common urographic finding and is seen in 35% of cases. The surface of the mass/defect may be smooth or irregular. In non-papillary carcinoma, the mass may be flat with little intraluminal intrusion. A pedicle of varying length is seen in the papillary types. A 'stipple sign' has also been described in papillary carcinoma;[11] it is due to the trapping of contrast between the fronds of the tumor, which then appears stippled when viewed en face.

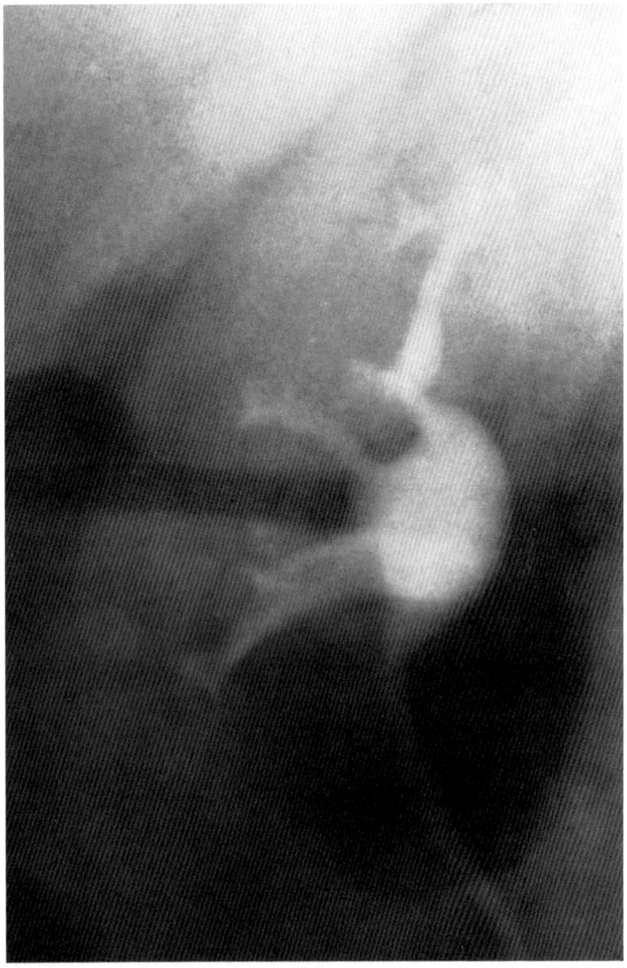

A

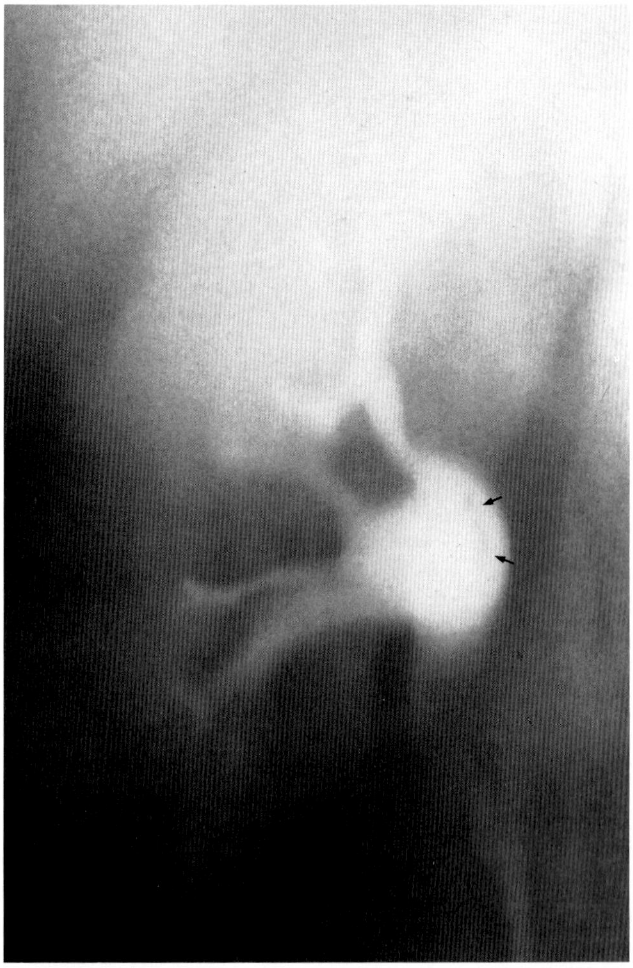

B

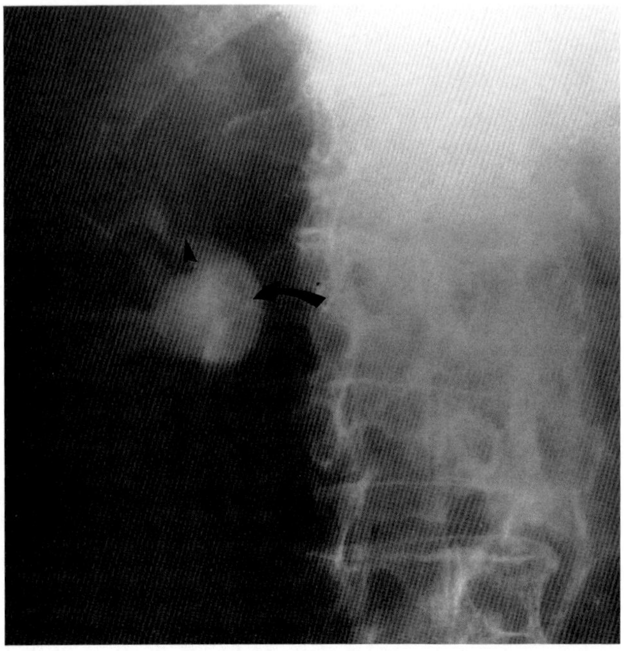

C

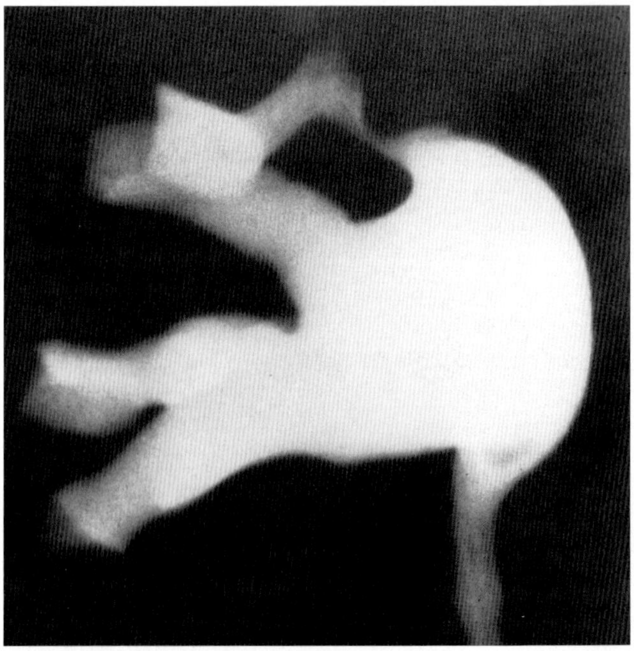

D

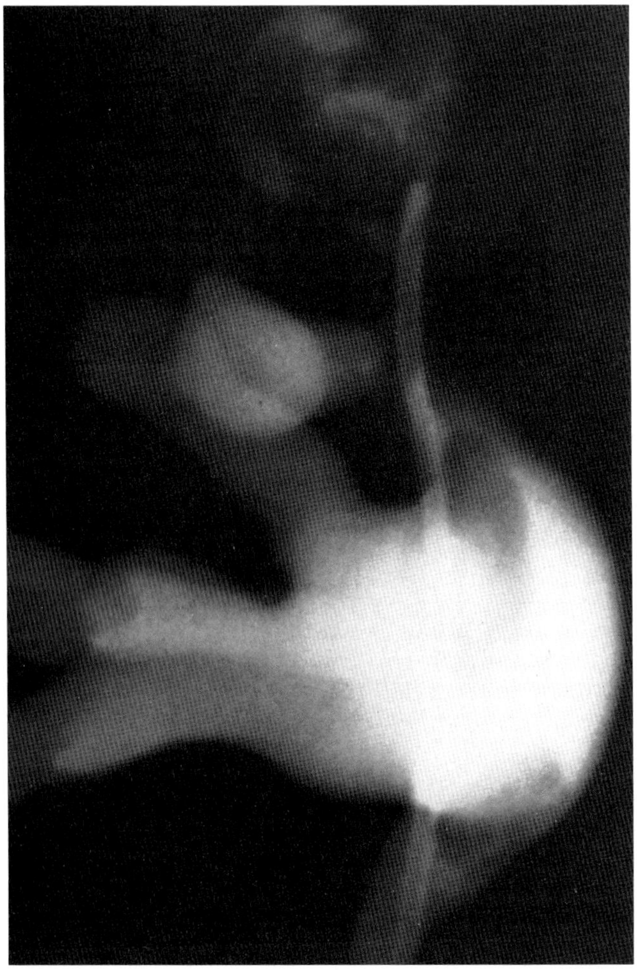

E

Figure 11.2

Evolution of transitional-cell carcinoma.

A Frontal film from excretory urography demonstrates normal pelvicalyceal system and ureter.

B Tomography at the same time as (**A**) shows a small filling defect in the renal pelvis (arrows) which was overlooked.

C Excretory urography 2 years later demonstrates no filling of upper pole infundibulum (arrowhead) or calyces ('phantom' calyx). A filling defect in the renal pelvis is now obvious (arrow).

D Retrograde pyelography at same time as (**C**): contrast injection through a catheter placed in the renal pelvis fails to opacify the tumor-laden upper pole infundibulum and calyces.

E Retrograde brush biopsy of the tumor-filled upper pole calyces: note the irregular filling defects within the upper pole calyces.

F CT shows obliteration of the sinus fat in the upper pole of the right kidney due to tumor infiltration. Note the normal sinus fat in left kidney.

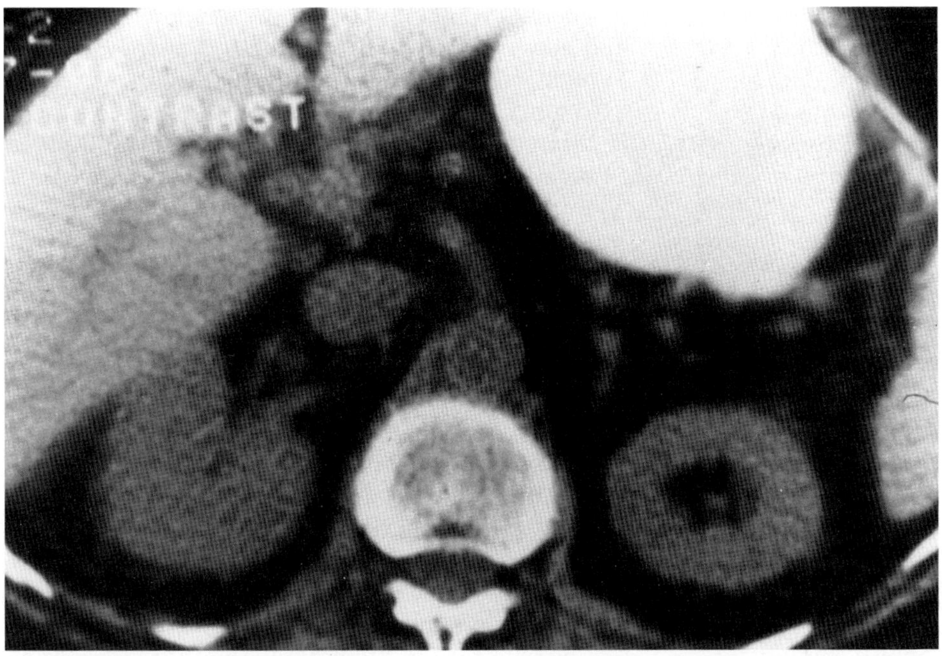

F

- Filling defects within distended calyces: these are seen in 26% of cases. If a calyceal infundibulum is involved with tumor and there is partial obstruction, the calyx will be dilated (focal hydrocalycosis). If there is complete infundibular obstruction, the calyx may not be opaque at all ('phantom' calyx) (Figure 11.2). The nephrogram may show a defect in such cases, with focal increase in density on delayed films, referred to as a focal intensifying nephrogram.[12] A tumor-filled, ballooned calyx will also appear as a defect on the nephrogram.
- Calyceal obliteration: this is seen in 19% of cases. If the cut-off is smooth, inflammatory narrowing would be difficult to separate from tumor. A retrograde pyelogram helps to define better the anatomy in such cases.
- Hydronephrosis with renal enlargement: this is seen in 6% of cases and is due to partial obstruction at the ureteropelvic junction. A notable feature of both TCC and squamous-cell carcinoma is that the reniform outline of the kidney is preserved.
- Reduced function/non-function without renal enlargement: complete obstruction at the ureteropelvic junction will cause global nonfunction and is seen in 13% of patients. A retrograde pyelogram is then required to evaluate the collecting system.

In ureteral TCC, decreased or absent renal function is more common and is seen in a quarter to a third of all cases. Filling defects in the ureter and hydronephrosis have been reported in 33 and 25% of cases, respectively[13] (Figure 11.3). Papillary tumors tend to be multicentric while non-papillary lesions are frequently solitary. Papillary ureteral neoplasms often cause dilatation of the ureter immediately below as well as above the tumor site (Bergman's sign or 'goblet sign') (Figure 11.4). This dilatation is attributed to repeated prolapse of the tumor, with ureteral peristalsis causing ureteral dilatation. The sign, if present, is useful in separating obstruction due to a calculus (the ureter below the calculus will be smaller in caliber than the obstructed ureter above it) from tumor obstruction. The goblet sign refers to the meniscus-like appearance of the inferior edge of the tumor when it is outlined by contrast.

Retrograde pyelography

Ideally, retrograde pyelography should be performed with fluoroscopic monitoring during contrast injection so that optimal projections can be obtained during adequate distension of the collecting system. It is the mainstay for the evaluation of the ureters. It is invaluable in patients in whom the excretory urogram fails to visualize the collecting system due to non-function. It is also indicated in patients in whom the entire collecting system cannot be satisfactorily distended and evaluated on the urogram.

The radiographic findings are similar to those seen on excretory urography. The mucosal surface will usually be better demonstrated (see Figures 11.2, 11.4 and 11.5). Underfilled or unopacified segments can also be better evaluated by advancing the retrograde catheter and injecting in close proximity to the affected calyx or infundibulum. In addition to the findings of filling defects and hydronephrosis, ureteral TCC will sometimes appear as areas of long or short segment-narrowing due to desmoplastic reaction. Unexplained strictures in the elderly are worrisome, and an effort should be made to exclude TCC in such cases.

As mentioned before, the frequent multiplicity of these tumors makes it important to carefully examine the entire urinary tract for other, synchronous tumors.

If an abnormality is seen on the retrograde pyelogram or excretory urogram, a brush biopsy can be performed through the retrograde route to confirm the malignant nature of the defect (see Figure 11.2). Fluoroscopic monitoring is again preferable, so that precise sampling of the questioned areas can be performed. The reported sensitivity and specificity is 92%, with positive predictive value of 100% in cytologic grades III and above.[6] The predictive value of a class I biopsy is 86%. Thus, although a positive biopsy is extremely accurate and reliable, a negative biopsy is less reliable because malignancy could have been missed.

Antegrade pyelography

Percutaneous needle pyelography may be performed in the non-functioning, hydronephrotic kidney if the presence of a TCC has not been recognized (see Figure 11.3). The upper margins of the obstructing tumor could be outlined with contrast, but the inferior extension can be outlined only by a retrograde injection. Antegrade pyelography (as well as antegrade brush biopsy) is frowned upon by most urologists due to the real risk of seeding the biopsy track with tumor, which is estimated to be as high as 10%.[14]

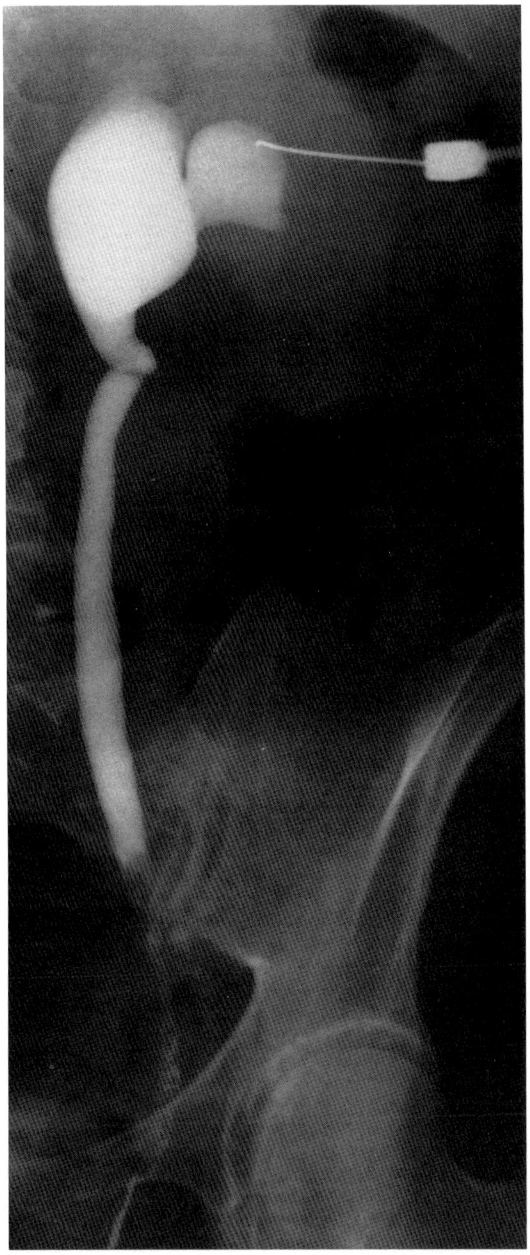

A

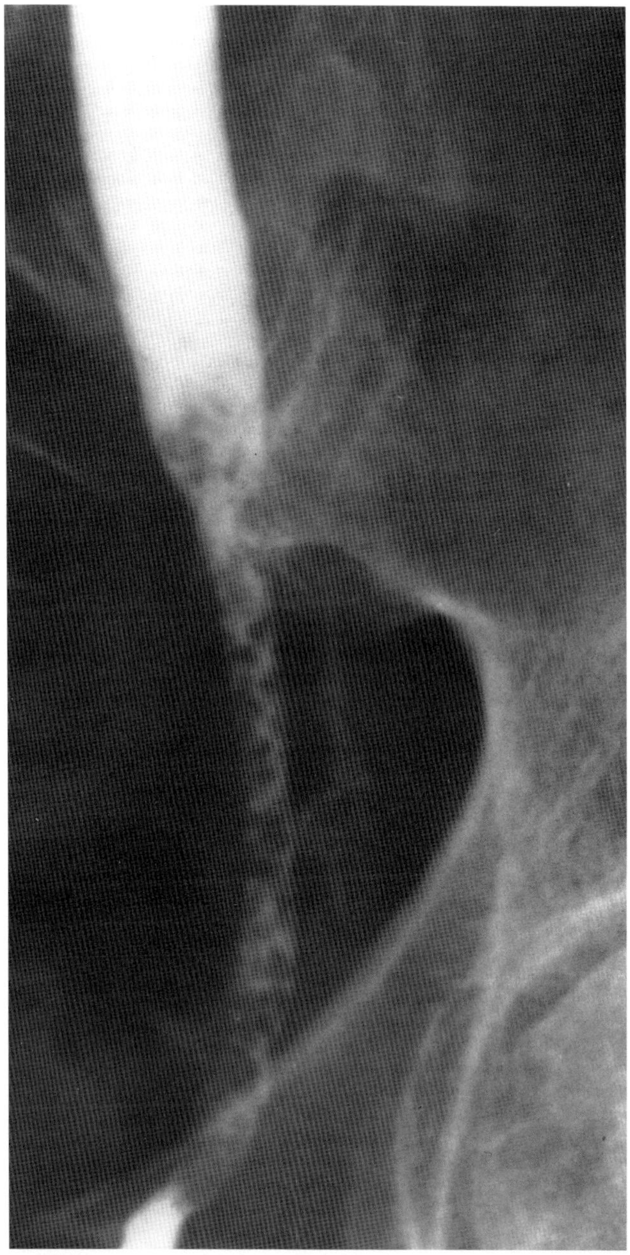

B

Figure 11.3

Antegrade pyelography of transitional-cell carcinoma (TCC) of the distal ureter.

A Excretory urography (not shown) of patient with bladder TCC resected 2 years previously demonstrated poor function, and the left ureter could not be catheterized in a retrograde fashion. Antegrade pyelography demonstrates left hydronephrosis, with multiple filling defects in the distal ureter.

B A close-up view demonstrates the long ureteral lesion and the cobblestone appearance of the mucosa. Note the irregular distal margin which helps to distinguish tumor from a benign condition such as ureteritis cystica.

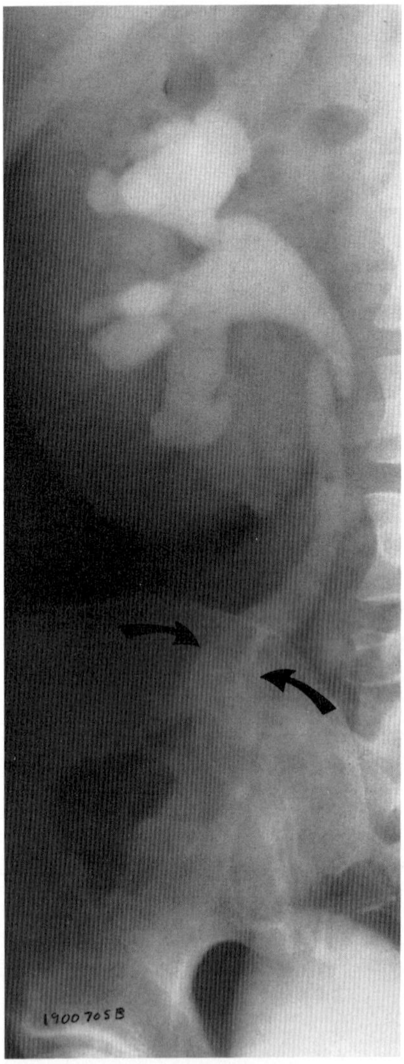

A

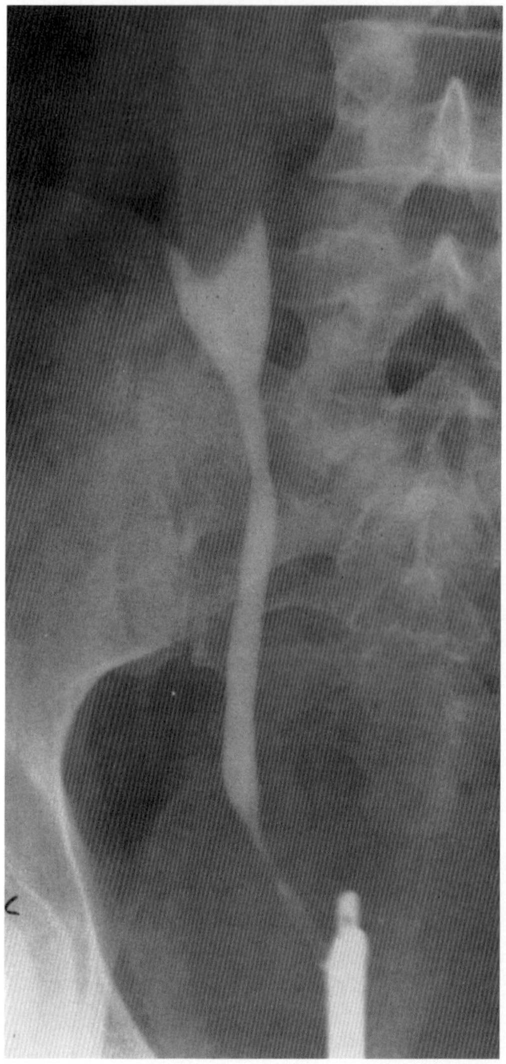

B

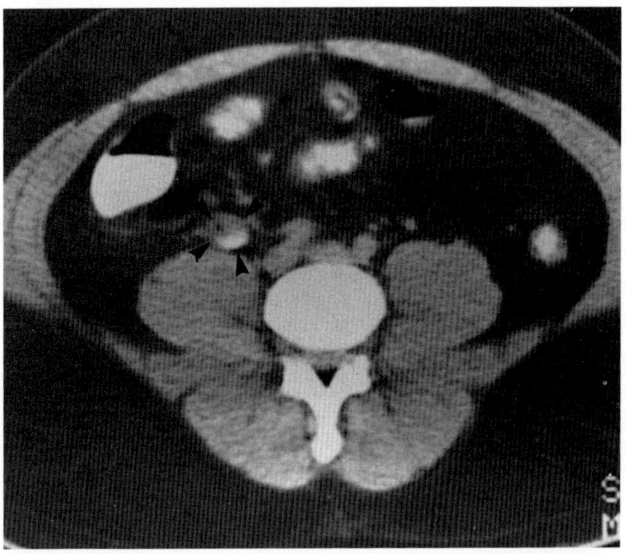

C

Figure 11.4

Ureteral transitional-cell carcinoma.

A Excretory urography demonstrates right hydronephrosis with a filling defect in the right mid ureter (arrows).

B Retrograde pyelography demonstrates the irregular inferior margin of the ureteral mass. Note the dilation of the ureter distal to the tumor (Bergman's sign, 'goblet' sign).

C CT demonstrates the soft tissue mass in the dilated right ureter (arrowheads).

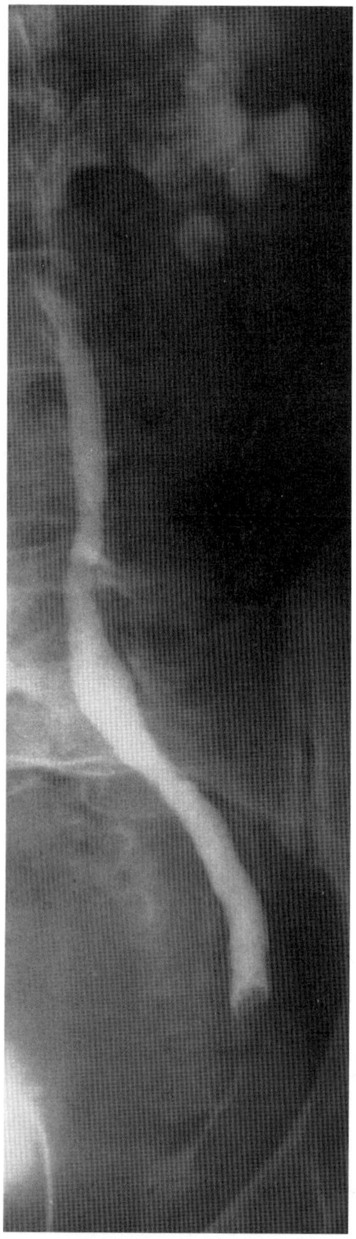

Figure 11.5

Renal and ureteral transitional-cell carcinoma (TCC). Retrograde pyelogram of a 47-year-old female with a 20-year history of recurrent TCC of bladder.

Computed tomography

The primary role of CT is in demonstrating local extension of the tumors. Renal TCC tends to spread medially through the hilus and invade adjacent retroperitoneal structures such as the psoas muscle. Renal hilar and retroperitoneal adenopathy will also be demonstrated well by CT. CT should be a routine part of the work up of all patients with renal TCC. In general, even with large tumors, the reniform outline of the kidney is preserved so that the appearance is that of an infiltrating, rather than an exophytic, process.

CT scans should be performed both before and after contrast administration. Minimal contrast enhancement is seen as these tumors are hypovascular (Figure 11.6). The tumors appear as filling defects in the renal pelvis, calyces or ureters (see Figures 11.2 and 11.4). Hydronephrosis and hydroureter will also be demonstrated, proximal to the tumor. Thus CT is of value in diagnosing the presence of TCC in the non-functioning kidney. It is also of value in excluding calculi as the cause of ureteral obstruction. An accuracy of 94% has been reported in determining which tumors are confined to the pelvis.[15] In tumors limited to a calyx, a focal obstructive nephrogram may be observed.

As with renal-cell carcinoma, renal TCC can also invade the renal vein and inferior vena cava and is estimated to do so in 5% of patients. CT scanning with bolus contrast technique is usually adequate to detect this.[16]

Ultrasonography

The primary role of ultrasonography is in establishing the nature of a renal pelvic defect and distinguishing renal calculi from tumor (see Figure 11.1). The former are echogenic and will shadow. Blood clots can mimic tumors on both urography and ultrasound. However, they are usually mobile and should decrease in size or disappear on subsequent scans.

Separation of the high-intensity central echo complex by low-intensity echoes from a renal pelvic TCC may be seen. Invasive, infiltrating tumors will cause loss of the normal parenchymal architecture.

Magnetic resonance imaging

At present, MR has no definite role in the diagnosis or management of renal TCC. Small lesions are

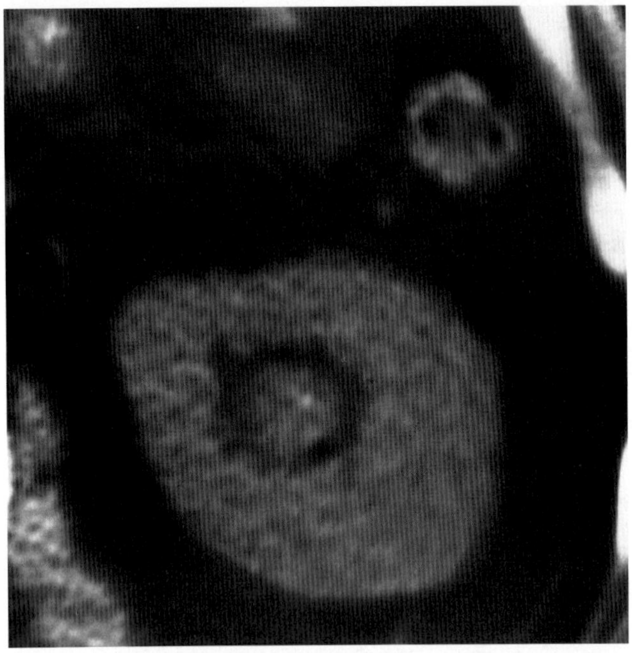

A

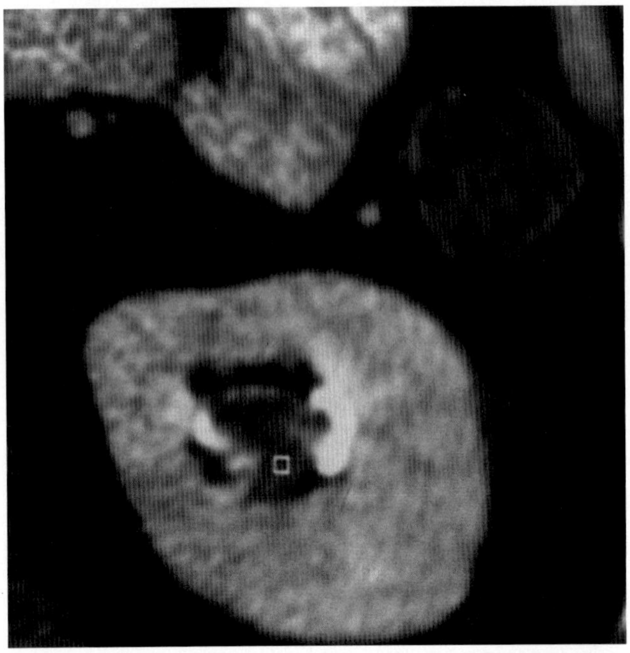

B

Figure 11.6

Transitional-cell carcinoma in renal pelvis.

A CT prior to contrast administration shows a solid mass occupying the left renal sinus.

B Post-contrast, the tumor mass does not enhance.

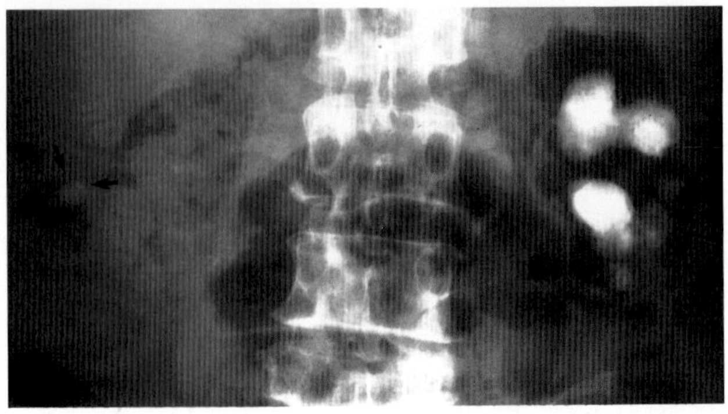

A

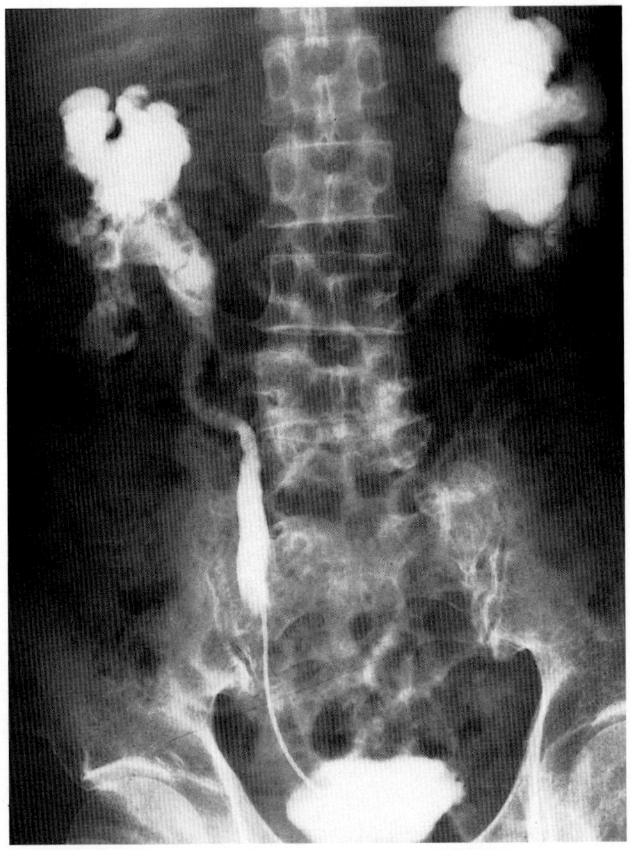

B

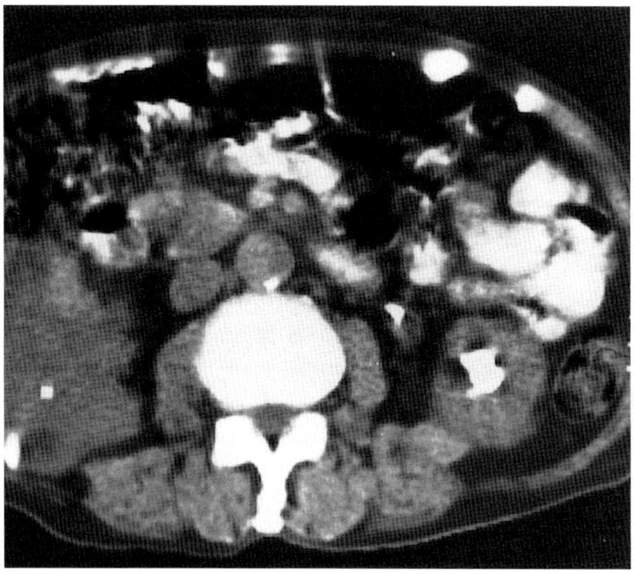

C

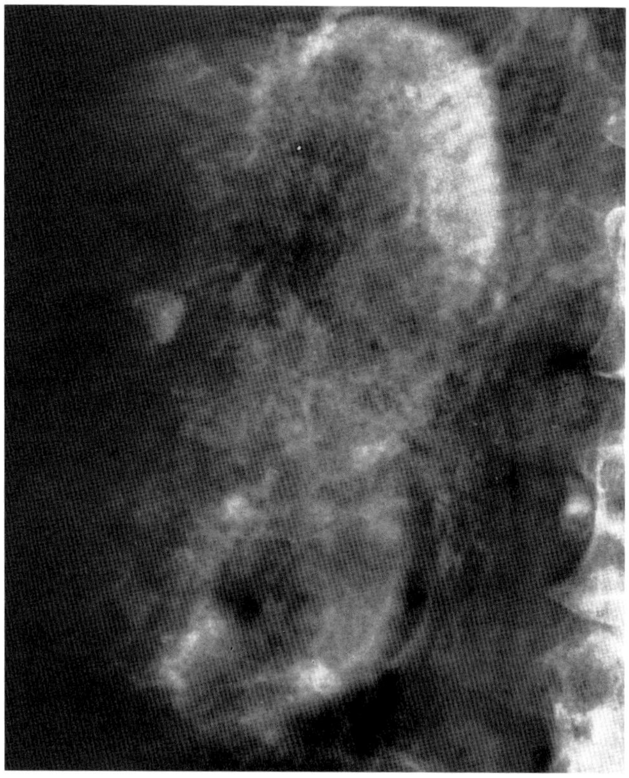

E

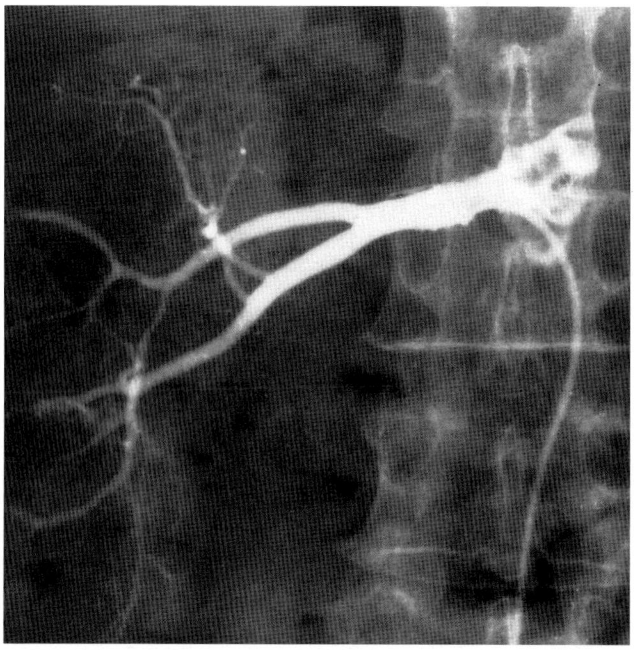

D

Figure 11.7

Squamous-cell carcinoma in a 74-year-old male who had hematuria and a history of surgical removal of right renal calculi 10 years previously.

A Abdominal film shows a small right renal calculus (arrows) and a large left renal staghorn calculus.

B Retrograde pyelography shows infiltration of the entire right pelvicalyceal system and proximal ureter by an irregular mass.

C CT demonstrates a large mass replacing the right kidney. Note how the reniform shape of the kidney is preserved. Calculi in both kidneys are well demonstrated.

D Right renal arteriography, early arterial phase: note the encasement of the intrarenal arterial branches.

E Right renal arteriography, capillary phase: tumor neovascularity involves the entire right kidney and extends into the hilus.

likely to be missed by MR, due to motion artifact. When identified, the tumors are similar in intensity to normal renal parenchyma on T1-weighted images and are slightly increased in signal intensity on T2-weighted images.

MR is excellent at depicting vascular invasion if the CT is equivocal or if iodine-containing contrast media cannot be used. Parenchymal and perinephric invasion can also be identified.

Angiography

At present, angiography has no clear role in the diagnosis or work up of urothelial neoplasms. TCCs are hypovascular to avascular and may be difficult to identify with certainty, even with selective angiography. In equivocal cases where inflammatory strictures cannot be separated from tumor, angiography is unlikely to be helpful because tumor vascularity and inflammatory neovascularity may be indistinguishable.

Phlebography and cavography

With MR and rapid CT scanning available, renal phlebography and cavography are rarely needed.

Squamous-cell carcinomas

Squamous-cell carcinomas constitute 6.2% of renal pelvic tumors. They are non-papillary and are obviously invasive at presentation (Figure 11.7). These tumors are aggressive and have a poor prognosis. There is a strong association between squamous-cell carcinoma and chronic infection. Thus, the onset of symptoms due to the tumor is hard to distinguish from symptoms due to the underlying infection.

Squamous-cell carcinoma may mimic xanthogranulomatous pyelonephritis both clinically and radiographically. In both conditions imaging studies show that the kidney is often non-functional and has stones within it. However, the perinephric space is usually invaded at presentation in patients with squamous-cell carcinoma. An irregular cobblestone appearance to the mucosa is sometimes seen.

Metastases to the urothelium

The renal pelvis and ureter can be involved either by direct spread or spread from a distant primary site. Direct extension is most frequent from retroperitoneal tumors such as lymphoma and pancreatic carcinoma and can rarely occur also in colon carcinoma and hypernephromas. Direct extension from cervical carcinoma, prostate and other malignancies of the reproductive system can cause ureteral obstruction.

Metastases to the urothelium usually occur when widespread metastatic disease is already present. Melanoma can cause multiple mucosal nodules that mimic TCC. Almost any primary tumor can metastasize to the renal pelvis or ureter.

Post-operative follow up

The high incidence of recurrent TCC makes post-operative screening problematic. Two recent publications address this issue with clarity.[4,17] One of these recommends annual intravenous or retrograde urography or both in addition to urine cytology in patients who have undergone surgery.[4] Special vigilance is required in the first 2 years following initial diagnosis, when the rate of recurrence is highest.

References

1. Bennington JL, Beckwith JB (eds), *Atlas of tumor pathology*, series 2, fascicle 12, *Tumors of the kidney, renal pelvis and ureter* (Armed Forces Institute of Pathology: Washington DC 1975) 243–311.
2. Goldman SM, Gatewood OMB, Neoplasms of the renal collecting system, pelvis and ureters. In: Pollack HM, ed, *Clinical urography* (WB Saunders: Philadelphia 1990) 1292–1352.
3. Werth DD, Weigel JW, Mebust WR, Primary neoplasms of the ureter, *J Urol* (1981) **125**:628.
4. Yousem DM, Gatewood OMB, Goldman SM, et al, Synchronous and metachronous transitional cell carcinoma of the urinary tract: prevalence, incidence and radiographic detection, *Radiology* (1988) **167**:613–18.

5. Johansson S, Angervall L, Bengtsson U, et al, A clinicopathologic and prognostic study of epithelial tumors of the renal pelvis, *Cancer* (1976) **3**:1376.
6. Sheline M, Amendola MA, Pollack HM, et al, Fluoroscopically guided retrograde brush biopsy in the diagnosis of transitional cell carcinoma of the upper urinary tract: results in 45 patients, *AJR* (1989) **153**:313–16.
7. Zincke H, Aguilo JJ, Farrow GM, et al, Significance of urinary cytology in the early detection of transitional cell cancer of the upper urinary tract, *J Urol* (1976) **116**:781–3.
8. Sarnacki CT, McCormack LJ, Kiser WS, et al, Urinary cytology and the clinical diagnosis of urinary tract malignancy: a clinicopathologic study of 1400 patients, *J Urol* (1971) **106**:761–4.
9. Dinsmore BJ, Pollack HM, Banner MP, Calcified transitional cell carcinoma of the renal pelvis, *Radiology* (1988) **167**:401–4.
10. Lowe PP, Roylance J, Transitional cell carcinoma of the kidney, *Clin Radiol* (1976) **27**:503.
11. McLean GK, Pollack HM, Banner MP, The "Stipple sign" – urographic harbinger of transitional cell neoplasms, *Urol Radiol* (1979) **1**:77.
12. Brennan RE, Pollack HM, Non visualized ("phantom") renal calyx: causes and radiological approach to diagnosis, *Urol Radiol* (1979) **1**:17.
13. Ghazi MR, Morales PA, Al-Askari S, Primary carcinoma of ureter. Report of 27 new cases. *Urology* (1979) **14**:18.
14. Mcdonald MW, Zincke H, Urothelial tumors of the upper urinary tract. In: de Kernion JB, Paulson DF, eds, *Genitourinary cancer management* (Lea and Febiger: Philadelphia 1987) 12.
15. Baron RL, McClennan BL, Lee JKT, et al, Computed tomography of transitional-cell carcinoma of the renal pelvis and ureter, *Radiology* (1982) **144**:125.
16. Jitsukawa S, Nakamura K, Nakayama M, et al, Transitional cell carcinoma of the kidney extending into renal vein and inferior vena cava, *Urology* (1985) **25**:310.
17. Pollack HM, Long-term follow up of the upper urinary tract for transitional cell carcinoma: how much is enough? *Radiology* (1988) **167**:871–2.

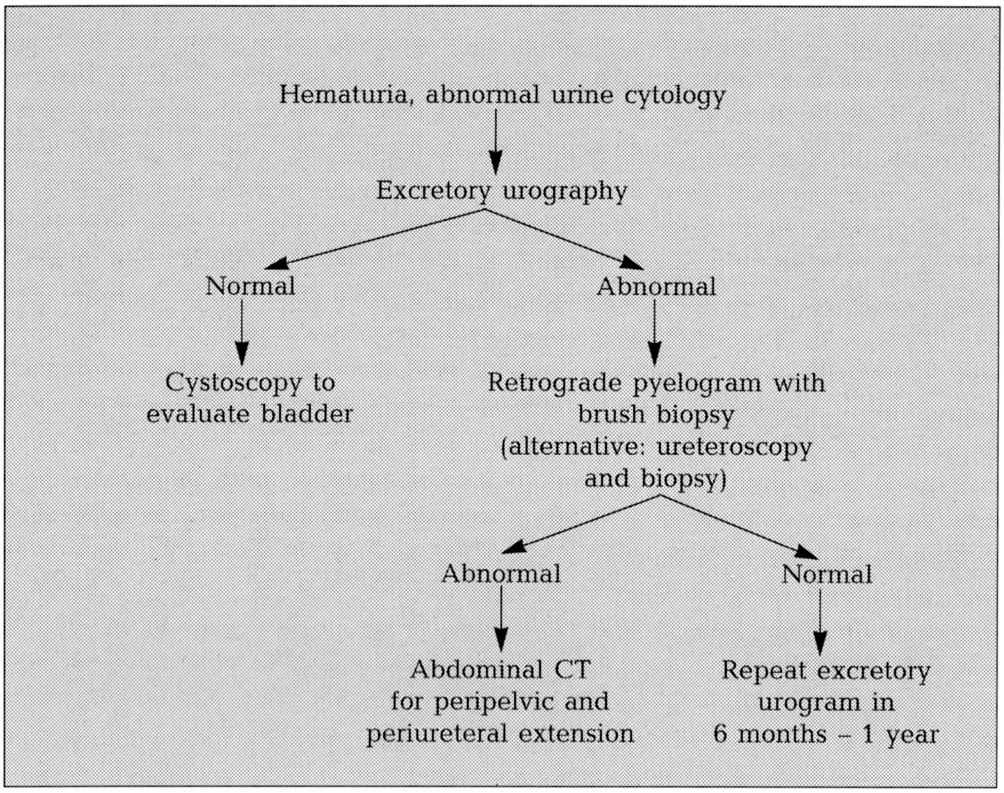

Diagram 11.1

Imaging strategy for suspected abnormalities of the collecting system.

12

The bladder and urethra

Peter McCarthy, Parvati Ramchandani and Howard Pollack

Carcinoma of the bladder

In the USA there has been a substantial rise in the number of bladder cancers diagnosed in 1989 (47 000) from the 37 000 diagnosed in 1984.[1] This has been ascribed to exposure to environmental carcinogens.[2] There are some suggestions, however, that while the number of cases has increased, the mortality has not changed, possibly because the carcinogens lead to an increase primarily in the number of less aggressive tumors. In 1988, it was estimated that in the USA 10 400 patients died of bladder cancer,[3] a number that has subsequently changed little.

Malignant bladder tumors are a varied group, but 90% are composed of a single histologic type: transitional-cell carcinomas. Squamous-cell carcinoma accounts for 5%, adenocarcinoma 2%, and others, including leiomyosarcoma, for the remaining 3%. Most bladder neoplasms arise near the trigone, presumably because this area is close to the ureteric orifices to which carcinogenic urine has been transmitted from the upper tracts.

There has been no thrust towards large-scale population screening for bladder tumors as there has been with prostate carcinoma because of the smaller number of cases, the lack of a specific screening test and the common presentation in the former, which is almost invariably with hematuria.

The staging of bladder cancer was organized according to its depth of penetration, first proposed in a classification system by Jewett and Strong in 1946 (and later revised by Marshall in 1952). While not the first to recognize that prognosis was related to the depth of mural invasion, Jewett and Strong made the important observation that survival dropped sharply with tumors which penetrated more than half-way through the bladder wall. In 1974, the American Joint Committee and Union International Contre Cancer (UICC) modified the classifications, and tumors superficially invading muscle (T2) were separated from those that invaded deep muscle (T3A) (Table 12.1).

Table 12.1 Staging of bladder carcinoma.

American Joint Committee/UICC	*Jewett–Marshall*	*Clinical stage*
To/Tis/Ta		Carcinoma in situ, noninvasive lesion
T1	A	Superficial tumor with lamina propria invasion
T2	B1	Superficial muscle invasion
T3A	B2	Deep muscle invasion
T3B	C	Invasion of perivesical fat
T4	D1	Local organ and local node involvement
T4	D2	Distant organ and distant node involvement

Techniques for staging bladder cancers

Excretory urography

Only 60% of cystoscopically proved bladder tumors can be visualized on intravenous (IVU) urography.[4] Multiple projections can be used to aid visualization of a tumor, for example oblique views, but in a study by Hillman et al[4] were not found to improve detection significantly. Hillman et al concluded that the single most useful view was the post-void film. From a prognostic point of view, patients with carcinoma of the bladder are more likely to have a lower grade of tumor and a lower mortality rate if their bladder tumors cannot be visualized on the excretory urography (EU), presumably because larger tumors are more easily visualized.

The IVU is still a useful investigation in bladder cancer and the commonest way in which radiologic diagnosis is made. In practice, however, the diagnosis of carcinoma of bladder is most often made at cystoscopy. The urogram is helpful in assessing the upper tracts for two reasons: (1) for the identification of further tumors (found in approximately 4%),[5] and (2) because the ureteric orifice is at particular risk of obstruction, due to the high frequency of trigonal tumor.

The appearance of bladder tumor on EU is usually of a filling defect, which may be very large. Frequently, contrast can be seen to track into the crevices of the tumor. Filling defects have no specific feature correlated with histologic type, though calcifications on the plain film (Figure 12.1) in conjunction with a filling defect on the IVU is suggestive of transitional-cell tumor.

The IVU is not an appropriate method for staging bladder carcinoma because structures in the pelvis are not visualized and are most appropriately studied by a cross-sectional imaging technique (e.g. CT or MRI). Lymphadenopathy is not directly visualized but may be appreciated as an extravesical mass. Bone destruction due to metastatic lesions on the pelvis or lumbar region may also be identified.

The follow up by EU of bladder carcinoma has generated some controversy. Further tumors may be found in the upper tracts at a later stage. In a study of 645 patients,[5,6] 3.9% later developed tumors in the ureter or renal collecting system. However, two-thirds of these were found in the first 2 years, so routine surveillance should be performed later than this only if the patient is at high risk for development of another lesion (for example, if they have developed a second bladder tumor during the period of surveillance).

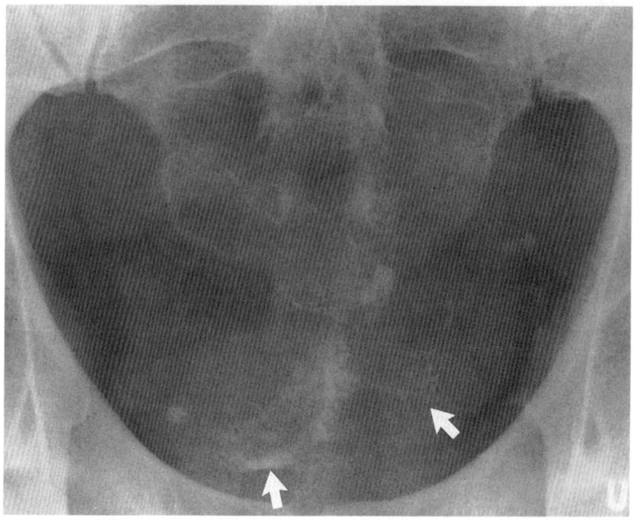

Figure 12.1

Transitional-cell carcinoma. Plain view of the pelvis showing amorphous calcification projected over the region of the bladder (arrow), due to calcification of a transitional-cell carcinoma.

Cystography

Cystography has never really enjoyed a prominent role in the diagnosis and staging of bladder carcinoma. MR and CT have largely replaced its use, though CT is occasionally used with single- or double-contrast cystography.

Lymphography

Lymph node involvement in patients with bladder cancer is a serious finding. In a study by Smith and Whitmore[7] 82% of patients with nodal involvement from bladder carcinoma at radical cystectomy died in 5 years. This study also suggested that extrapelvic disease was the major determinant of survival, though there was still a substantial mortality from pelvic node disease alone. Lymphography alone has proved disappointing in staging bladder carcinoma, various studies showing rates of 15–40% false negatives and 5–10% false positives.

Attempts to upgrade the accuracy of Smith's and Whitmore's study were made by combining lymphography with fine-needle aspiration biopsy of suspicious nodes under fluoroscopic guidance. Several groups reported significant advantages with this technique, but negative biopsy was found not to exclude node disease and such patients needed staging lymphadenectomy.[8] However, patients with positive cystological aspirates were spared the morbidity of this procedure.

Lymphography is the only technique that will demonstrate abnormality in normal-sized nodes.[9] Despite this, it has largely been abandoned in favor of cross-sectional studies.

Other staging techniques

No imaging technique is sensitive enough to detect microscopic invasion either perivesically or into lymph nodes. Therefore, all imaging is beset with the problem of inaccuracy, and this has been a significant problem with carcinoma of the bladder. With superficial tumors, pathologic assessment has revealed clinical understaging in 25% of cases. With more deeply invasive lesions, errors are even more frequent. Consequently, the development of high-quality cross-sectional imaging has had an impact. One of the most critical distinctions has been how to distinguish B1 from B2 disease (superficial vs. deep muscle invasion). Allied to this is the question of how to predict which superficial lesion will progress to deeper invasion at a later stage.

Magnetic resonance imaging

Initial MR images are obtained with the standard body coil and are if possible then supplemented with the use of an endorectal surface coil, which is part of a multicoil array. This technique renders all surfaces and parts of the bladder accessible to high-resolution imaging with MR. Images are obtained both with and without gadolinium enhancement. MR has superior contrast resolution

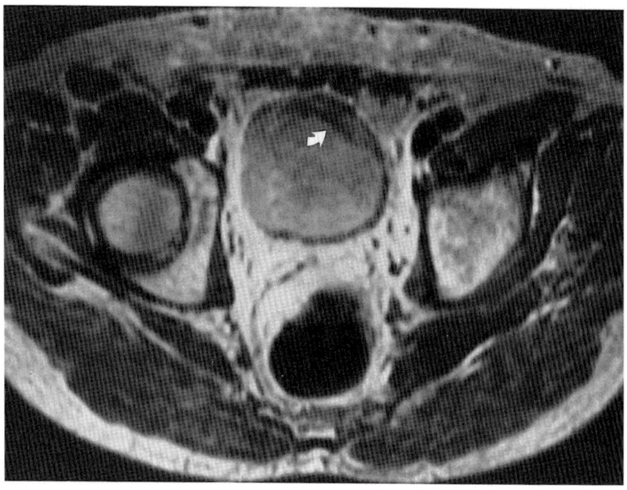

A

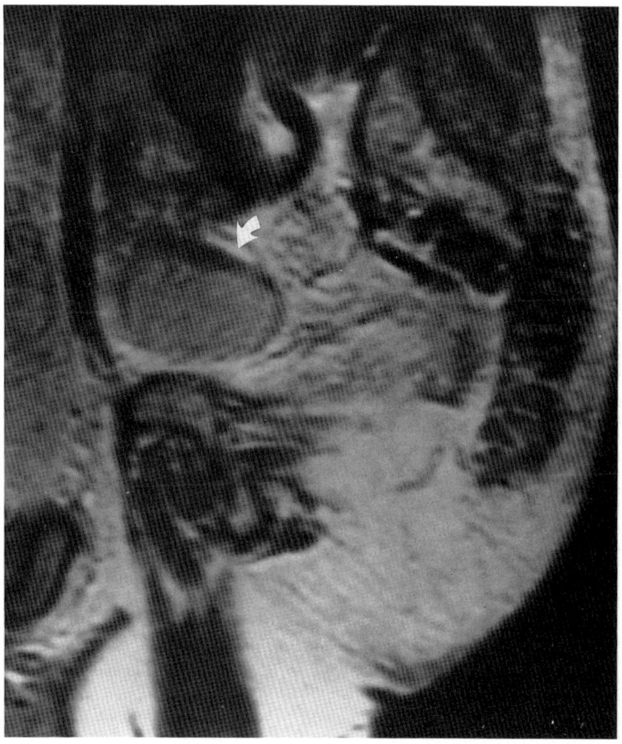

B

Figure 12.2

Stage B carcinoma. Axial (**A**) and sagittal (**B**) (TR 2500/TE 40) MR scans with a body coil, showing a plaque like lesion (arrow) in the superolateral aspect of the bladder.

to CT and it has multiplanar capability, giving it major advantages. However, carcinoma in situ is not detectable by current imaging methods. MR cannot distinguish between mucosal, submucosal and superficial muscle invasion.

When the tumor is confined to the bladder (i.e. A or B1), on MR the bladder wall (or at least its outer rim) will be intact. This is represented by a low-signal rim and visualized best on T2-weighted or T1-weighted, gadolinium-enhanced sequences. In stage B2 lesions, the tumor is seen to extend to involve the low-signal rim of the outer bladder wall. In tumors of this grade, the perivesical fat (high signal) is intact, best seen on T1-weighted sequences (Figure 12.2). In stage C lesions, the tumor is seen to invade the perivesical fat (Figure 12.3). If the tumor extends into adjacent pelvic organs (for example the rectum or uterus), then stage D1 disease is present.

Some early reports showed variable levels of accuracy which did not lead to widespread acceptance of the value of MR in staging bladder tumors. One study showed an accuracy of 73% (using Jewett–Strong–Marshall Staging) and 64% (using TNM staging).[10] More recently, a large study showed high specificity levels for invasion of deep muscle, fat and adjacent organs. Sensitivity was variable, however, with the highest levels (95%) for deep muscle invasion. Overall, however, using TNM staging, an accuracy of 60% only could be achieved with MR. A third of patients were understaged by MR.[11] Most studies point to the failure to adequately visualize lymphatic metastases. Also the difficulty of distinguishing between tumor recurrence and radiotherapy or postoperative fibrosis has been a problem.

In general, the difficulty of distinguishing between B1 and B2 lesions has been resolved by some groups by combining B1 and early B2 lesions (in which the outer bladder wall is intact) and separating these from advanced B2 lesions.[12] Early invasion of the deep muscle layer does not preclude endoscopic resection by the urologist. Endoscopic resection poses staging problems for the radiologist because of post-operative edema which can not only cause bladder wall thickening, but also hemorrhage and edema obscuring the MR signal derived from the bladder wall. The same masking effect can result from inflammation, which often accompanies bladder tumors.

The accuracy of detection of lymphadenopathy by MR, using 1 cm as the upper limit of normal for diameter of pelvic nodes, was approximately 80% in one study, the specificity being 100%.[13] In another study, all patients deemed either positive or negative at pre-operative MR were found to have been correctly assessed[12] (in this study, sensitivity or specificity could not be calculated, since not all of the nodes were sampled).

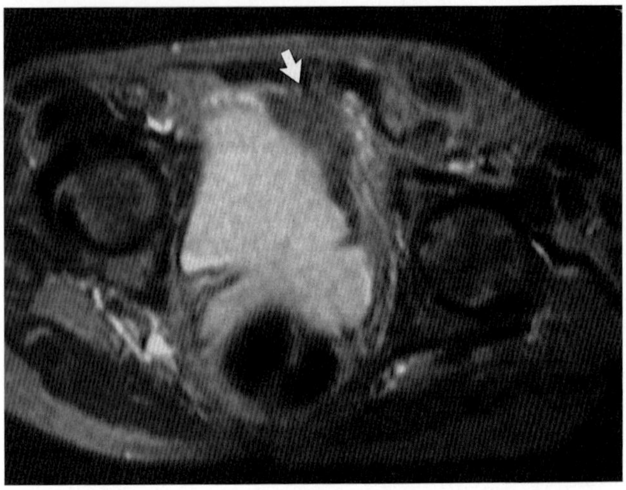

A

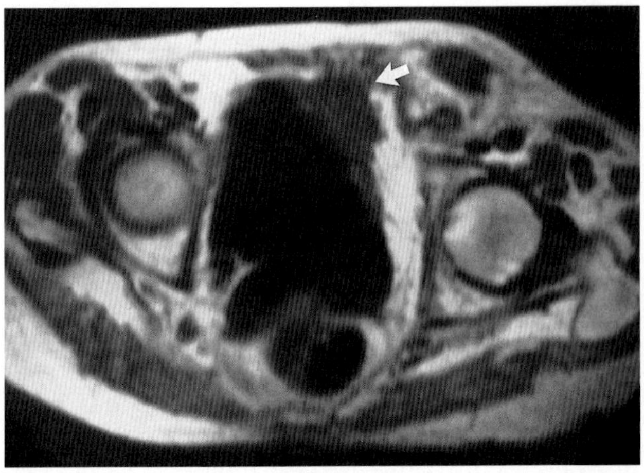

B

Figure 12.3

Stage C carcinoma of the bladder. Axial TR 2000/TE 100 (**A**) and TR 400/TE 20 (**B**) MR sequences show a left-sided bladder mass of intermediate signal clearly extending outside the bladder and into the perivesical fat (anterior, arrow).

The post-treatment follow up by MR of patients with carcinoma of the bladder is fraught with difficulty. Radiotherapy causes bladder-wall thickening, and some patients can develop signal change on T2-weighted sequences which may not be distinguishable from recurrence of tumor. Radiation fibrosis can typically be identified showing low-signal on the T2-weighted sequence, but unfortunately many bladder tumors also impart a low signal. Enhancement after gadolinium, however, is a property much more likely to be demonstrated by neoplasms than fibrotic tissue. An exception is early, developing fibrosis in which granulation tissue is prominent.

MR may find its most appropriate role in imaging locally advanced pelvic disease, in which circumstances its diagnostic value is high.[13]

Computed tomography

CT was the first cross-sectional imaging technique used, but unfortunately it has been found wanting in several respects. It is distinctly limited in identifying how deeply muscle invasion has occurred. Bladder-wall thickening due to a B2 lesion may be mistaken for muscle hypertrophy, edema or radiation change. Therefore, it is generally agreed that tumors up to and including stage B2 lesions cannot be differentiated by CT.

Overall staging accuracy using CT is between 50 and 90%.[14] Lymph-node disease detection by CT is thought to be between 70 and 90%, similar to that by MR. A possible source of error in misinterpreting enhancing nodes has been recently pointed out.[15] Again it appears that the comments applied to the most appropriate role for MR also apply to CT.

Occasionally, CT with intravenous contrast can be combined with another contrast medium (for example air) to better delineate a particular lesion in the bladder. In addition, decubitus views may be useful.

Ultrasonography

Ultrasonography of the bladder can be performed in several different ways—transabdominal (Figure 12.4), transrectal (TRUS) and transurethral. The first of these is limited by its ability for depth penetration. Some promising results have been achieved with transurethral ultrasound. This allows good visualization of the bladder wall but is a poor discriminator of perivesical invasion and, in particular, lymphadenopathy. The test is also invasive and may require general anesthesia for adequate performance. On the other hand, TRUS is relatively noninvasive and can be performed readily. Claims have been made for high levels of accuracy in staging tumors in the main part of the bladder, excluding the neck. A major advantage of TRUS is the good visualization of the prostate and seminal vesicles.

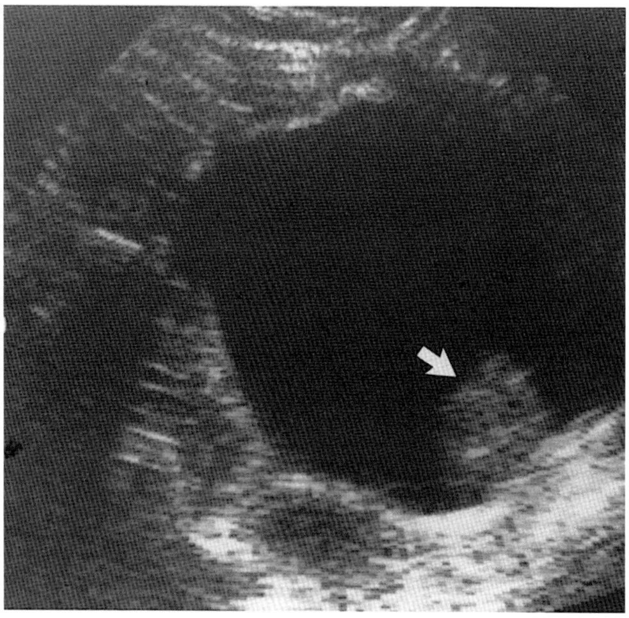

Figure 12.4

Polypoid bladder carcinoma. Longitudinal right parasagittal pelvic ultrasound scan shows a polypoid bladder carcinoma (arrow).

Radionuclide skeletal scintigraphy

The incidence of skeletal metastases in bladder carcinoma is low, apparently less than 5%, though autopsy study shows 25% have metastases. One study showed that even with this incidence, cystectomy was carried out despite the findings of metastatic disease. Therefore routine isotope bone scanning may be useful only as a baseline, and routine further evaluation in the absence of symptoms is not necessary. Occasionally an incidental finding of a photon-deficit is seen in the bladder (Figure 12.5).

Chest radiography

Plain chest films are useful in the evaluation of bladder cancer. In one study, 6% of patients had intrathoracic disease.[16] A whole range of findings were seen: nodules (which may cavitate), pleural effusion, pulmonary infiltrates and edema (Figure 12.6).

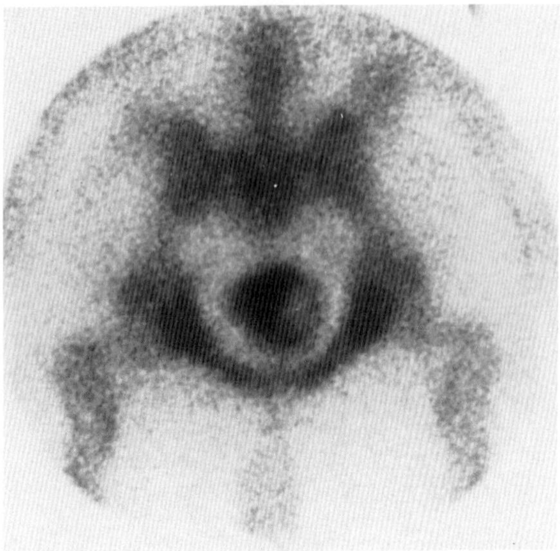

Figure 12.5

Carcinoma. Anterior view of the pelvis from a ^{99m}Tc bone scan shows a filling defect in the left side of the bladder, due to the carcinoma. This was a incidental finding.

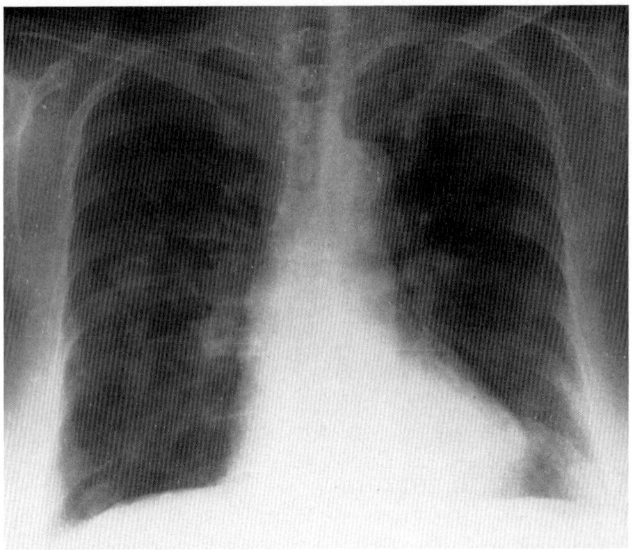

Figure 12.6

Metastasis from bladder carcinoma. This chest radiograph shows widespread cavitating metastatic lesions.

Summary of imaging strategies

- The mainstay of diagnosis of bladder carcinoma, whatever the histologic type, is cystoscopy. The IVU is a key study not because of its diagnostic accuracy in detecting bladder tumors but because of the risk of accompanying upper tract disease, or perhaps because of hematuria, which is the most common symptom of bladder neoplasia.
- A normal EU does not exclude bladder carcinoma, and cystoscopy is indicated in all patients with hematuria.
- Follow-up studies using the EU to assess the upper tracts after 2 years should be subsequently continued only in selected patients, but interval cytology should be continued in all. Neither sonography nor CT is a substitute for EU in surveying the upper urinary tract for urothelial tumors.
- Although CT and MR are reliable in determining perivesical invasion, their poor discrimination of the degree of bladder wall invasion and their modest performance in staging of lymph-node disease makes them of limited usefulness for clinical staging. Of the two, MR seems somewhat more accurate in gauging depth of mural invasion.
- Chest radiography is mandatory in the work up, but isotope bone scanning is not.
- Lymphography with fine-needle biopsy could be valuable in disclosing unsuspected stage D disease, but probably because it is an inconvenient procedure for radiologists, it is underutilized.
- An algorithm showing the prospective work up of patients is given in Diagram 12.1.

Carcinoma of the urethra

Carcinoma of the urethra is rare and is a more mixed histologic group than carcinoma of the bladder. Seventy-eight per cent are squamous-cell, 15% transitional-cell, 6% adenocarcinoma and 1% are undifferentiated. Squamous-cell carcinomas are believed to be associated with chronic irritation and urethral stricture, and are common in the bulbomembranous urethra. Transitional-cell tumors are most frequently seen in the prostatic urethra and have been reported in the remaining urethra of 7–18% of patients after total cystectomy for bladder cancer. Urethral carcinoma is the only epithelial neoplasm that is more common in females than males.

Table 12.2 Staging of carcinoma of the urethra.

Stage O	Carcinoma in situ
Stage A	Submucosal involvement only
Stage B	Extending into but not beyond either the corpus spongiosum or the prostate
Stage C	Extending beyond the corpus spongiosum or prostate
Stage D	Metastases to: inguinal nodes pelvic nodes para-aortic nodes distant

Staging

No uniform agreement regarding staging has been reached but a staging system was proposed by Ray in 1977 and modified by Levine in 1980[17] (Table 12.2).

The presenting symptom is most frequently obstructive in origin, with hematuria being much less common.

Retrograde urethrogram

Typically this will show an irregular filling defect in the urethra, often with proximal dilation. A periurethral fistula is not uncommon. None of these features is diagnostic.

Other staging techniques

Metastatic disease at presentation is uncommon but is seen in 10–14% of patients. The comments on CT and lymphangiography in the assessment of bladder carcinoma (see earlier) also apply to urethral malignancy.

An MR study of 6 patients with urethral neoplasms has been made with good results.[18] Some notable features arose. There was no difference in signal between transitional-cell and squamous-cell tumors. The signal in tumors was variable but mainly lower than in the surrounding corpus spongiosum on T1-weighted and T2-weighted sequences.

MR will not demonstrate stage O lesions, nor will it differentiate stage A from stage B lesions. A high level of correlation between MR and surgical findings has been noted.

For prognostic purposes, two groups of patients are defined.[19] Group 1 patients have distal lesions (at least in the distal bulbar urethra). These patients present earlier and have a better 5-year survival. Group 2 patients have lesions that are more proximal; they do less well, having presented later, and can develop periurethral fistulae, which are not common in group 1.

References

1. Silverberg E, Laterra JA, Cancer Statistics 1989, *CA* (1989) **39**: 3–20.
2. Droller M, Transitional cell cancer: upper tracts and bladder. In: Walsh PC, Gittes R, Perlmutter A, Stamey T, eds, *Campbell's urology* (WB Saunders: Philadelphia 1986) 1343.
3. Hahn D, Neoplasms of the urinary bladder. In: Pollack HM, ed, *Clinical urography* (WB Saunders: Philadelphia 1989) 1353.
4. Hillman BJ, Silvert M, Cook G, et al., Recognition of bladder tumors by excretory urography, *Radiology* (1981) **139**:319–23.

5. Yousem D, Gatewood O, Goldman S, et al, Synchronous and metachronous transitional cell carcinoma of the urinary tract: prevalence, incidence and radiographic detection, *Radiology* (1988) **167**:613.
6. Pollack HM, Long term follow-up of the upper urinary tract for transitional cell carcinoma: how much is enough? *Radiology* (1988) **167**:871.
7. Smith J and Whitmore W, Regional lymph node metastasis from bladder cancer, *J Urol* (1981) **126**:591.
8. Boccon-Gibod L, Katz M, Cochard B, et al, Lymphography and percutaneous fine needle aspiration biopsy in the staging of bladder carcinoma, *J Urol* (1984) **132**:24.
9. Zoretic S, Wajsman Z, Beckley S et al, Filling of the obturator nodes in pedal lymphangiography: fact or fiction, *J Urol* (1986) **129**:533.
10. Amedola N, Glazer G, Grossman H, et al, Staging of bladder carcinoma: MRI–CT–surgical correlation, *AJR* (1986) **146**:1179–83.
11. Buy J-N, Moss A, Guinet C, et al, MR staging of bladder carcinoma: correlation with pathologic findings, *Radiology* (1988) **169**:695–700.
12. Johnson R, Carrington B, Jenkins J, et al, Accuracy in staging carcinoma of the bladder by magnetic resonance imaging, *Clin Radiol* (1990) **41**:258–63.
13. Tavares N, Demas B, Hricak H, MR imaging of bladder neoplasms: correlation with pathologic staging, *Urol Radiol* (1990) **12**:27–33.
14. Singer J, McClennan B, The diagnosis staging and follow-up of carcinomas of the kidney, bladder and prostate: the role of cross sectional imaging, *Semin Ultrasound CT MR* (1989) **10**(6):481–97.
15. Husband J, Robinson L, Thomas G, Contrast enhancing lymph nodes in bladder cancer: a potential pitfall on CT, *Clin Radiol* (1992) **45**:395–8.
16. Goldman S, Fajardo A, Maraval R, et al, Metastatic transitional cell carcinoma of the bladder: radiographic manifestations, *AJR* (1979) **132**:419.
17. Hopkins S, Grabstald H, Benign and malignant neoplasms of the male and female urethra. In: Walsh P, Gittes R, Perlmutter A, Stamey TA, eds, *Campbell's urology* (WB Saunders: Philadelphia 1986) 1441–62.
18. McCallum R, Urethral neoplasms. In: Pollack HM, ed, *Clinical urography* (WB Saunders: Philadelphia 1989) 1404–12.
19. Hricak H, Mariotti M, Gilbert T, et al, Normal penile anatomy and abnormal penile conditions: evaluation with MR imaging, *Radiology* (1988) **169**:683.

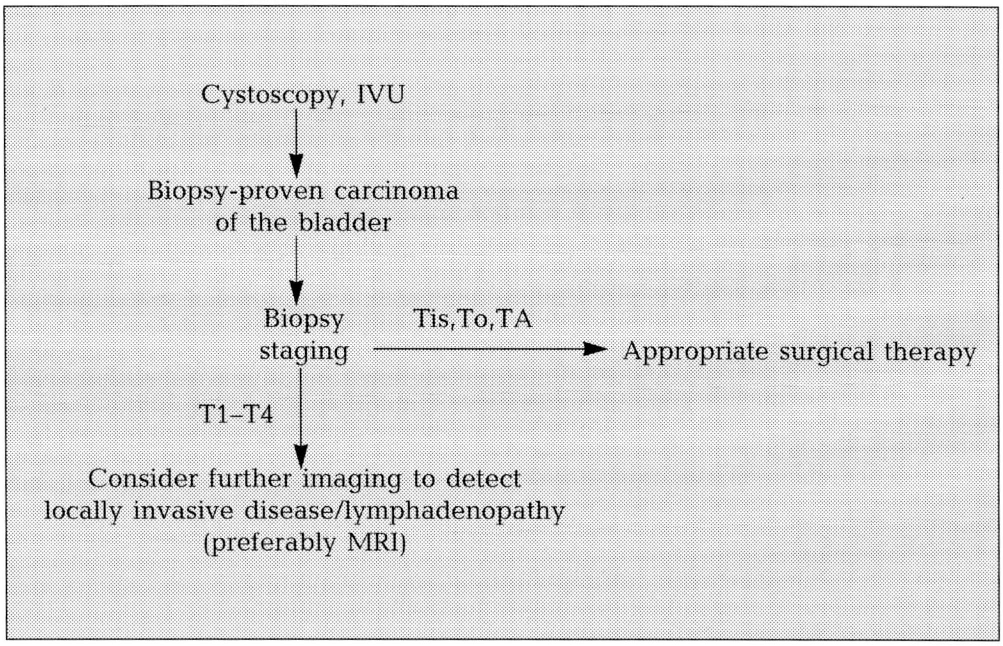

Diagram 12.1

Carcinoma of the bladder.

13

The prostate

Peter McCarthy, Parvati Ramchandani and Howard Pollack

Introduction

In 1989, it was projected that in that year there would be 103 000 new cases of adenocarcinoma of the prostate diagnosed in the USA.[1] This represented an increase from the 75 000 new cases diagnosed annually 10 years previously.[2] In 1983, 24 000 men died from this disease in the USA,[3] and it is estimated that this figure will rise to 32 000 in 1991. The incidental findings of carcinomas in 40% of autopsy and simple prostatectomy specimens in males over 50 years of age,[4] combined with the increasing number of men living into their seventies, indicates that a potentially vast drainage of health-care resources could result from attempts to care for so many patients. It is not clear yet, however, whether the increase in the prevalence of prostate cancer is real or whether the increased numbers are due to improved methods of detection. None the less, it behoves radiologists involved in the initial diagnosis, staging and follow up of prostate cancer to be *au fait* with the newer technologies: MR, CT and transrectal ultrasound (TRUS) as well as such traditional investigations as excretory urography (EU), isotope scintigraphy and plain chest radiography.

Sarcomas of the prostate are the only other malignant tumors of the prostate that need to be considered. They are exceedingly rare. These tumors are usually larger and invade locally early including into lymph nodes. Such findings in a younger patient should favor the diagnosis of sarcoma rather than adenocarcinoma. Embryonal sarcoma (rhabdomyosarcoma) of the prostate is primarily a disease of the pediatric age group.

In this chapter we will discuss the initial radiological diagnosis of prostatic carcinoma, suggest

Table 13.1 Comparison of UICC and modified Whitmore–Jewett staging for prostatic carcinoma.

Whitmore–Jewett	*UICC*	*Clinical*
A1	T0a	Impalpable tumor—focal
A2	T0b	Impalpable tumor—diffuse
B1	T1a, T1b	Lesion up to 2 cm in size within the gland
B2	T1c, T2	Lesion more than 2 cm confined within the capsule
C	T3	Extension beyond gland capsule
D0		Palpably normal gland but elevated acid phosphatase
D1	T4	Pelvic node metatases
D2		Bone or other organ metastases
D3		Unresponsive to hormone therapy

appropriate staging investigations and discuss how patients should be followed radiologically. The staging classification used most frequently is the Whitmore–Jewett system,[5,6] which is compared with the Union International Contre Cancer (UICC) system in Table 13.1.

Screening

Considerable controversy has arisen recently regarding screening to detect early carcinoma of the prostate. A substantial proportion of men with carcinoma of the prostate do not die of the disease. The American College of Surgeons Survey in 1982 found that 55% of patients had stage A or B carcinoma (20% had stage A disease) at presentation.[7] Stage A1 carcinoma was once considered a relatively benign disorder,[8] but more prolonged follow-up studies have suggested this may not be the case[9] and that some patients with stage A1 tumors may benefit from radical prostatectomy, particularly the younger age group. This is the rationale for screening, i.e. diagnosing early disease and treating it aggressively. However, some are not in complete agreement with this strategy and favor a less radical approach, reserving such surgery for highly selected cases.[10]

Can ultrasound be used for screening impalpable cancers? Two studies showed promising results,[11,12] noting that detection of cancers by transrectal ultrasonography (TRUS) was greater than that of digital rectal examination; nevertheless the specificity was found to be only 20% in one of these studies.[11] In another study the contralateral (clinically normal) lobes of patients with proven carcinoma in the other lobe were preoperatively assessed.[13] Ultrasound detected only 13 of 25 previously unsuspected cancers, with a positive predictive value of 54%. It was concluded that such a high level of false-negative results made it difficult to recommend TRUS to screen for impalpable cancers. Besides, the cost of implementing such a program would seem to be prohibitive.[14] In contrast, a recent Swedish report has concluded that screening by digital rectal examination and biopsy as indicated is a cost-effective method, but doubted if such a program had any impact on survival.[15] Of note is a study that found that a combination of digital rectal examination and serum prostatic-specific antigen (PSA) detected as many cancers as did TRUS.[14]

At present, there is no general consensus regarding even the need for screening, quite apart from how it should be done or what the cost would be. However, as the Stanford group suggest,[16] if screening is to be attempted it makes more sense to do this by screening for palpable abnormalities on digital rectal examination, knowing that 66% will show cancer on ultrasound-guided biopsy, whereas in those with palpably benign prostates only 5% have cancer. The prevalent mood is away from the use of TRUS as a routine screening tool.

Techniques

Magnetic resonance imaging

The evolution of high-quality MR has changed the imaging approach to prostatic carcinoma. Its main advantages are its multiplanar capability, high contrast resolution and the lack of associated ionizing radiation. Examination of the prostate includes T1-weighted (short TR/TE) and T2-weighted (long TR/TE) spin-echo sequence. Axial images are best, but coronal and sagittal imaging is also used as required. These images are best performed at 1.5 T and generated in the body coil at a slice thickness of 5 or 10 mm and a field of view of 30–36 cm.[17,18] When staging examinations are performed, the region from the renal hila to the symphysis pubis is imaged in 10 slices. The study can be terminated at the aortic bifurcation, if the pelvic nodes are negative because para-aortic node disease is rare in the absence of pelvic node disease.[19]

Though not yet generally available, the recent development of a balloon-mounted endorectal surface coil (Figure 13.1) seems certain to have a major impact on the assessment of prostate cancer,[20] especially in relation to some recent reports which suggest that body-coil imaging alone is not accurate for detection of stage C disease.[21] These images are generated with a 10–12 cm field of view at a slice thickness of 3–4 mm, though slice thickness of 1.5 mm can be achieved using spoiled gradient-echo sequences.[22] The addition of a multicoil array has further improved imaging by preventing the far-field fall-off so prevalent with surface monocoil imaging.

Carcinoma of the prostate arises mainly in the peripheral zone (68%) and to a lesser extent in the transition zone (24%) and central zone (8%).[23] As many as 50% of all prostate cancers involve the anterior half of the gland, which has important implications for the use of both MR and TRUS.

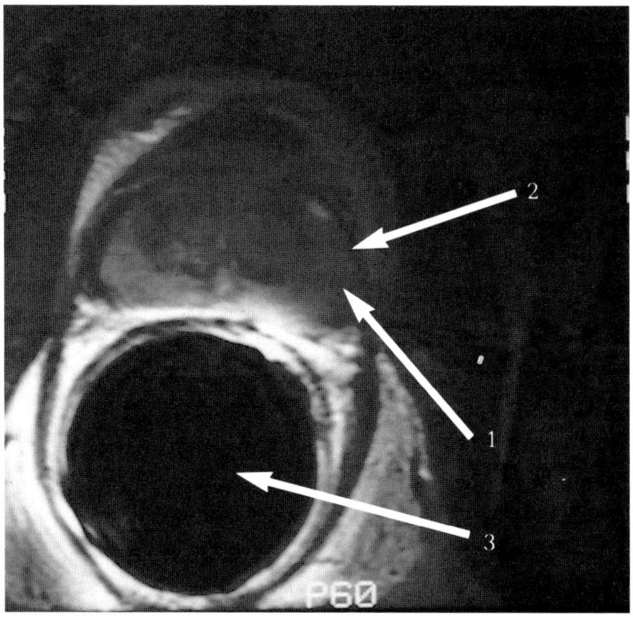

Figure 13.1

Axial image (TR 2500/TE 40) from an endorectal surface-coil MR scan. This is a T2-weighted image: it shows a low signal intensity focus in the left peripheral zone (arrow 1), consistent with a carcinoma. This extends up to but does not involve the prostatic venous plexus (arrow 2). The diagnosis was stage B carcinoma of the prostate. The inflated balloon coil is seen in the rectum (arrow 3).

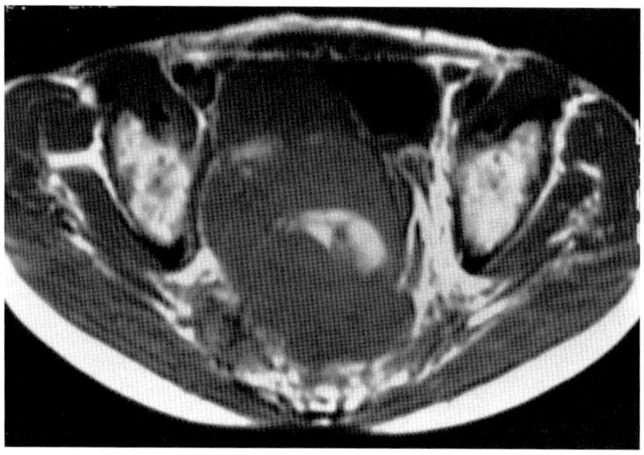

A

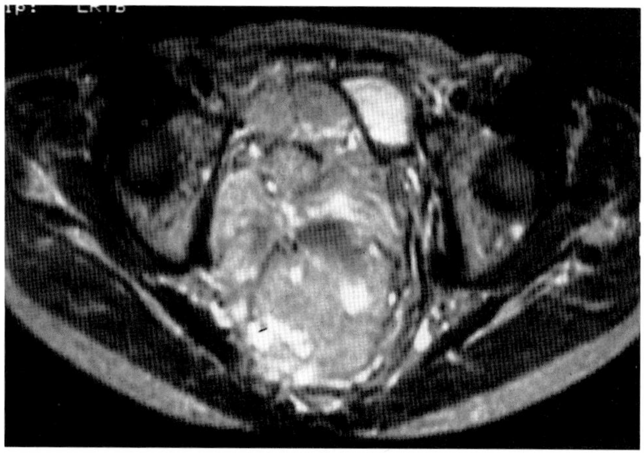

B

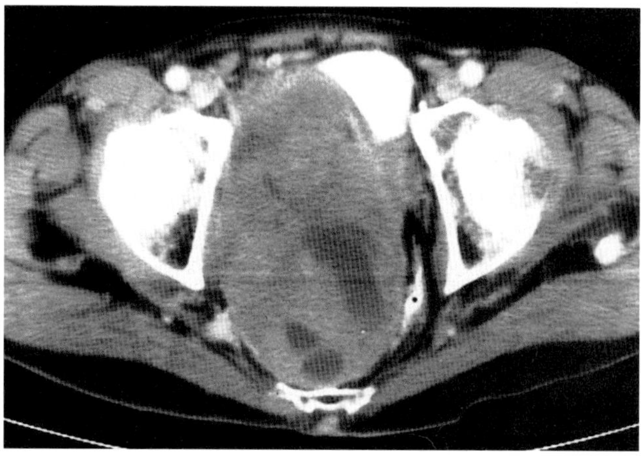

C

Figure 13.2

MR scans—TR 600/TE 25 (**A**) and TR 2500/TE 80 (**B**)—and a corresponding axial CT slice (**C**) through the prostate show an unusually large prostate mass, compressing the bladder to the left. Areas of high signal on both MR sequences are due to hemorrhage.

The anatomic detail displayed by MR is excellent. T1-weighted images are best used to display the periprostatic fat and venous plexus, the perivesicular tissues and lymph nodes, whereas T2-weighted sequences show the internal prostatic architecture to best effect.[18] The balloon-mounted endorectal surface coil shows very clearly the neurovascular bundle and prostatic capsule. Carcinoma of the prostate is usually denoted by low-signal areas in the peripheral zone, the conspicuousness of which increases with age, making the low-signal tumor stand out more clearly (Figure 13.2). High signal can occasionally be seen with mucinous cystadenocarcinoma.

There are certain pitfalls in using MR to make the diagnosis of prostate carcinoma. The low-signal foci seen in carcinoma can be identified in other conditions, for example chronic prostatitis. This precludes the use of MR as a screening tool.

Furthermore, since carcinomas may involve central structures, they can be missed as the low-signal areas blend with the low signal of benign nodular hyperplasia in the transitional zone. Many scans are performed after biopsy, and one must recognize the appearance of post-biopsy hemorrhage and not confuse it with other abnormality. The giveaway is that hemorrhage is of high signal on both T1- and T2-weighted sequences 1–3 weeks after biopsy. Tumors are invariably of low signal on such sequences.

The volume of tumor itself in the prostate has been shown to be the single most important prognostic indicator of disease.[24] MR has been used to assess volume, a study in our department noting that tumors of less than 1.9 cm^3 were likely to be stage B lesions; if they were greater than 6 cm^3 then stage D disease was likely. There was little correlation between disease and volume at volumes of 2–6 cm^3.[25]

The most important role for MR is its ability to differentiate stages A and B from stages C and D disease. Particularly it is known that body-coil MR has an overall accuracy in this respect of 78%, with 84% specificity.[25] Surface coil MR, however, promises to exceed this value, with initial reports suggesting accuracies of up to 90%.[20] MR is also particularly useful in assessing involvement of the seminal vesicles, either by direct tumor invasion or by invading around the ejaculatory ducts and ductus deferens and then around and into the seminal vesicles.[26] The finding of low signal in the seminal vesicles on T2-weighted sequences is highly suggestive of invasion.[27]

Regarding nodal disease, detection by MR, like CT, depends on the involved nodes being enlarged: nodes of greater than 1.5 cm are considered to be definitely abnormal, those of less than 1 cm considered normal and those between 1.0 and 1.5 cm suspicious. MR has a 69% sensitivity in detecting node disease on this basis, with an accuracy of 88%. These figures are very similar to those of CT in assessing node status. Overall, however, MR is significantly more accurate for staging (83%) than CT (65%) or clinical examination (61%).

Other visceral metastases in prostate carcinoma are not unknown. In one autopsy study of 1885 patients liver lesions were found in 35%, 17% had adrenal metastases and 10% each had disease in the kidney and retroperitoneum. As most of this disease is clinically silent during life, routine MR above the renal hila is not indicated, bearing in mind the proviso for scanning to this level as mentioned earlier. If the primary tumor is poorly differentiated and nodes are enlarged more than 3 cm, especially if the patient is symptomatic from possible renal or hepatic metastases, then further scanning should be performed. MR and CT are probably of equal usefulness in this respect.

Using MR to follow patients after therapy for prostate carcinoma is dependent on the type of therapy and the extent of the disease prior to therapy. MR has a distinct advantage over CT and ultrasonography as it can in some cases distinguish post-operative scar tissue from recurrent or residual tumor.[28] However, a disadvantage of MR is that the zonal anatomic differentiation is distorted after radiation therapy, which may make interpretation difficult. Imaging takes a back seat to monitoring PSA levels after hormonal therapy.

Follow up should include an attempt to assess the tumor volume and extent of primary disease as well as lymph nodes and distant metastases. In patients who have had localized disease there seems little point in re-assessing lymph-node status, but the primary (i.e. prostatic) lesion should be evaluated every 6 months for a year and then yearly or on the basis of clinical condition subsequently. With more advanced disease, lymph-node status should be assessed at intervals of 1 and 3 years if the initial study is negative, but more frequently (even up to 3 month intervals) if positive.

Computed tomography

Pelvic CT scans for staging prostatic carcinoma are performed with the patient supine, using intravenous contrast to opacify the bladder and ureters and oral contrast to opacify bowel loops. Usually patients are examined with 8 mm contiguous slices but slice thickness of 1.5 mm can be used for greater detail. The greatest deficiency of CT is its inability to assess the internal architecture of the prostate. It is thus unsuitable for screening for cancer.

If CT is not useful for intracapsular carcinoma, can it be reliably used to differentiate stage B from C? Unfortunately, the results have been disappointing, with accuracy of 58% for seminal vesicle involvement and 64% for periprostatic fat invasion[29] (Figure 13.3). Some features are worth looking for on CT:

- Is the periprostatic fat/seminal vesicle angle obliterated? Unfortunately contour deformity due to a very enlarged prostate can obliterate the fat plane between the gland and the bladder wall and lead to false-positive diagnosis.

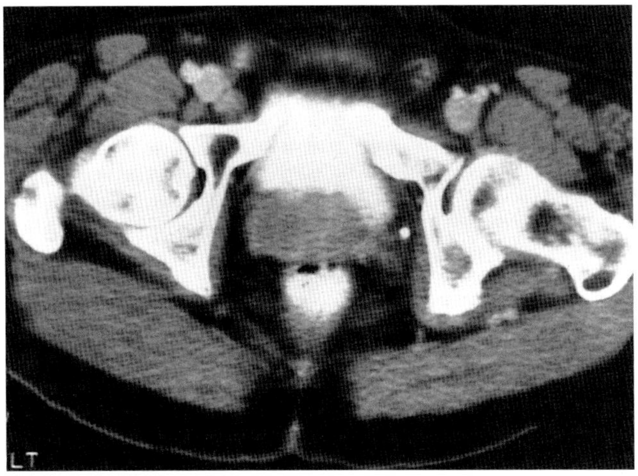

Figure 13.3

Stage C carcinoma of the prostate. This axial CT scan of the prostate shows irregularity of gland contours and extension of soft tissue thickening into the left perirectal region.

- Is the seminal vesicle involved? The signal change detected on MR (on T2-weighted images), even if the gland is not enlarged, is a much more reliable sign of invasion than anything detected by CT.
- Is the bladder wall involved?
- Are the pelvic nodes involved? An accuracy of 81% for the assessment of nodal metastasis has been achieved (somewhat similar to MR).[29] As with MR, the node must be enlarged to visualize abnormality by CT.

Other deficiencies of CT include inability to visualize the prostatic capsule and neurovascular bundles.

For distant lesions (i.e. liver, adrenal, etc.), CT and MR are probably equally useful. CT is less expensive than MR, the latter does however have the ability to provide all answers from just a single study, while CT cannot easily visualize the primary malignancy.

Why use CT at all? It is in fact a reliable method for assessing the prostatic volume (not the actual tumor volume); for determining the correct dosage of iodine-125 seeds, and for the determination of spatial localization of the seeds, within the gland.[30]

For the follow up of prostate carcinoma after treatment CT has a proven role. Issues related to the timing of the repeat scans are the same as those mentioned earlier for MR. However, when assessing pelvic recurrence with CT it should be remembered that surgical clips in patients who have had radical prostatectomy cause significant metallic artifacts which may invalidate the study. MR is an evolving technology and a definitive role for this technique in following such patients has yet not been firmly established.

Transrectal ultrasonography

Nothing is guaranteed to cause more controversy than this technique and its role in the imaging of prostatic carcinoma. Aside from philosophical discussions as to who should perform it (radiologists or urologists), several other bones of contention exist.

The spatial resolution of the transabdominal approach to scanning the prostate cannot reliably detect small carcinomas of the prostate. The development of 5.0 and 7.5 MHz rectal transducers has thus had a major impact.

Carcinoma of the prostate is generally thought to appear as a hypoechoic focus in the peripheral zone (Figure 13.4). However, an incidence of 24% isoechoic tumors has been noted, thus making them effectively invisible with TRUS.[31] Even worse, it has been noted that up to 40% of cancers greater than 5 mm in diameter will be missed by TRUS.[32]

Ultrasonography has diagnosed twice as many cancers as has digital rectal examination.[11] However, if a hypoechoic area is seen on TRUS, the chance that a biopsy of this area would show cancer depends heavily on the PSA level and the digital rectal examination. Thus, the positive predictive value of a hypoechoic lesion on TRUS is 62% if both of the latter evaluations are abnormal. If both are normal, however, the probability of a hypoechoic area showing cancer on biopsy is low (only 16%), and this finding has been particularly notable in patients aged 50–64. An even lower likelihood of cancer being present if DRE and PSA are normal has been found.[14] These findings strongly militate against use of TRUS alone as a screening technique.

Some controversy also exists regarding whether TRUS is necessary to biopsy the prostate. In one study, no added benefit in using TRUS to guide biopsy of palpable nodules was found, but this is

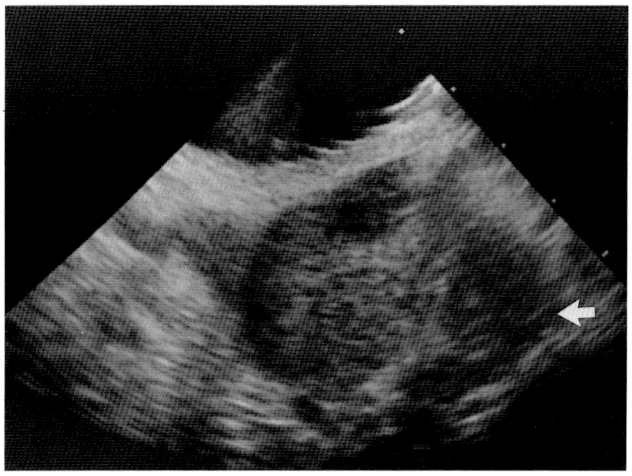

Figure 13.4

Pathologically confirmed stage B2 carcinoma. A transrectal ultrasound scan of the prostate shows a hypoechoic lesion in the peripheral zone on the left side (arrow), bulging the capsule but not clearly extending outside.

a view not universally shared. The Stanford group[16] found that 90% of abnormally firm prostates on palpation were accompanied by a hypoechoic defect on TRUS. This group suggested that in the presence of a negative biopsy of a palpable abnormality without TRUS, biopsy should be repeated using TRUS. In another study, this same group found that random biopsies, including biopsies of the opposite lobe, in patients with palpable nodules yielded as high a rate for cancer as did biopsy of the nodules themselves.[32] However, there appears to be a trend toward progressively greater use of TRUS, in conjunction with automated spring-loaded biopsy needles, in carrying out prostatic biopsy.[34]

In the assessment of actual tumor volume, the value of TRUS is dubious. Since carcinoma of the prostate can be multifocal or an infiltrative disorder, it is felt that 50% or more tumors may have the volume incorrectly estimated by TRUS.[32]

There are some claims for TRUS in staging prostate carcinoma that suggest very high levels of accuracy. However, these have not been generally corroborated and a recent multi-institutional study suggested that 58% accuracy is a more realistic figure for TRUS,[32] while the accuracy of body coil MR is somewhat higher, at 68%. Some features suggested to be sonographically indicative of periprostatic local extension are: hypoechogenicity in the peripheral zone with irregular echoes in the periprostatic fat, a focal bulge extending outside the prostate and irregularity of the capsular or pericapsular region. The most significant drawback of TRUS is its inability to visualize pelvic lymph nodes, because the high frequency probes have only a limited range of view. TRUS compares even less favorably with the alleged higher accuracy of endorectal multiarray surface coil MR.

Lymphography

This technique has been largely supplanted by more recently developed ones (MR, CT). Since pedal lymphatic channels are cannulated, only the external iliac nodes are filled in the pelvis (this includes the obturator group). However presacral and internal iliac nodes are not filled, and lesions in these areas will be missed.

The best staging accuracy claimed for lymphography is 75%,[35] comparable with MR and CT. However, unlike MR and CT, lymphography is uncomfortable, time-consuming and tedious for the physician and patient. Aside from the earlier mentioned disadvantage, there are several contraindications, including recent radiotherapy to the chest and past contrast reactions.

There are some advantages to lymphography, however. It is the only imaging technique that will detect disease in nodes of normal size. This is because invasion will be associated with a filling defect in the node. The technique is also ideal for fluoroscopic guidance of needles for biopsy of both suspicious and normal appearing nodes. Using this combined technique, which can be performed on outpatients, many patients will be found to have unsuspected metastatic disease and can be spared the morbidity and expense of needless surgery. Lymphography can therefore be very cost-effective in the management of patients with cancer of the prostate. The oily contrast material can stay in lymph nodes and be visualized for up to a year on radiographs. Thus patients can be followed simply by taking plain abdominal films at suitable intervals. However, because contrast is lost from the nodes in patchy fashion, one cannot infer disease progression on the appearance of the internal nodal architecture. Disease progression can only be confidently diagnosed by an increase in size of the nodes.

At present, lymphography has only a limited role in staging prostate carcinoma. It is usually reserved for situations in which CT or MR assessment of nodal status is equivocal, when it could save the patient from pelvic lymphadenectomy if positive. It seems a shame, however, that there is not more widespread enthusiasm for performance of this informative study which has the potential to spare many patients the hazards of inopportune radical surgery.

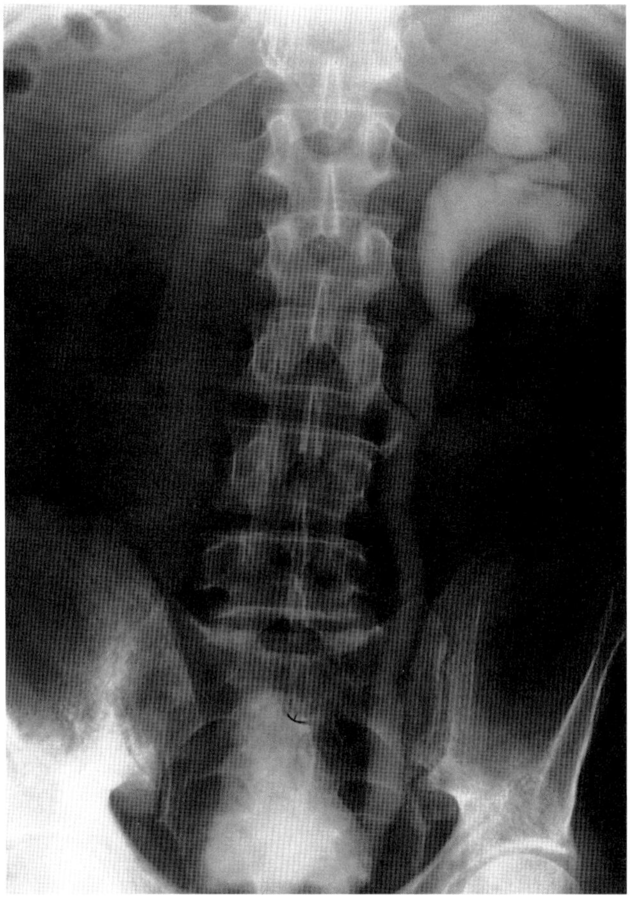

Figure 13.5

Carcinoma of the prostate invading the bladder base. This excretory urogram shows dilation of both ureters and excreting systems, more severe on the right due to invasion of the bladder base.

Excretory urography

This technique can only indirectly visualize the prostate gland and detect disease by its impact on surrounding structures (e.g. the bladder). Hence its routine use in the evaluation and staging of prostatic carcinoma is not warranted.

Most clinicians will, quite properly, wish to evaluate the upper urinary tracts prior to initiating treatment, as the ureters are frequently obstructed (Figure 13.5). In this respect, the use of EU has diminished as other techniques (MR, CT, abdominal ultrasonography) can now visualize hydronephrosis with high degrees of accuracy. Nevertheless there remain some primary indications for EU in patients with prostatic carcinoma, for example hematuria and pyuria, and these patients should be evaluated accordingly. Follow up of patients with upper tracts that are initially normal on CT or ultrasonography should be repeated periodically. If the initial study is positive, studies should be repeated at 3-month intervals until the hydronephrosis resolves or is stable, at which point yearly studies are adequate. If hydronephrosis persists, then more frequent studies may be necessary.

Radionuclide skeletal scintigraphy and skeletal radiography

Bone metastases are very common in carcinoma of the prostate, with an incidence of 7% in patients thought to have stage A or B disease, 18% in stage C and even higher in stage D.[36] Because bone pain is often the most distressing complaint in advanced prostate carcinoma, accurate documentation of skeletal disease is essential.

The commonest isotope in current use is technetium-99m linked to methyl diphosphonate (MDP). Isotope scintigraphy is known to be significantly more accurate in assessing bone metastases than plain radiography. Nearly a quarter of patients judged to be skeletally normal on plain film, require upstaging after scintigraphy. Therefore the routine use of skeletal radiological survey is time-consuming, wasteful and scientifically unsound. The use of plain films should be tailored to the indications from scan, with equivocal areas being radiographed and highly suspicious areas being confirmed. Recourse to bone biopsy may even be necessary occasionally. MR is also useful in the assessment of bone marrow involvement (no signal is returned from cortical bone), but its expense precludes its routine use. However, in the future it may be that routine sagittal T1-weighted sequences of the spine will be performed.

In patients with prostate carcinoma the skeletal scintigram typically shows multple areas of high photon activity. False-negative scans are thought to occur in approximately 8% of patients.[30]

Because of its renal excretion pathway, isotope scintigraphy has a further advantage in addition to its use in skeletal survey. The kidneys can be visualized and this is particularly useful if they are abnormal: unsuspected hydronephrosis and other disorders can be identified.

For follow up of bone metastases, skeletal scintigraphy is inexpensive and is the method of choice. Because there is a high likelihood of developing bone metastases early, a repeat scan should be obtained at 6 and 12 months after the initial study, and then yearly if the initial evaluation was normal. However, 3–6 month intervals are appropriate if metastases are detected initially: 80% of these patients will have died of their disease in 5 years.

It is worth noting that the 'flare' reaction has been found in one study to occur in 28% of patients.[37] It occurs due to increased isotope uptake secondary to healing and can be a source of confusion.

Prostatic metastases are almost always sclerotic (Figure 13.6) but there is a small but definite incidence of purely lytic and mixed lytic/sclerotic lesions. Typically the sclerotic lesions are small and dense involving the axial skeleton and skull. Paget's disease of bone and metastases from carcinoma of the prostate are usually recognized readily but they can be confused when the two coexist. It is thought by some that the incidence of metastases in pagetic bone possibly increases due to increased blood flow.

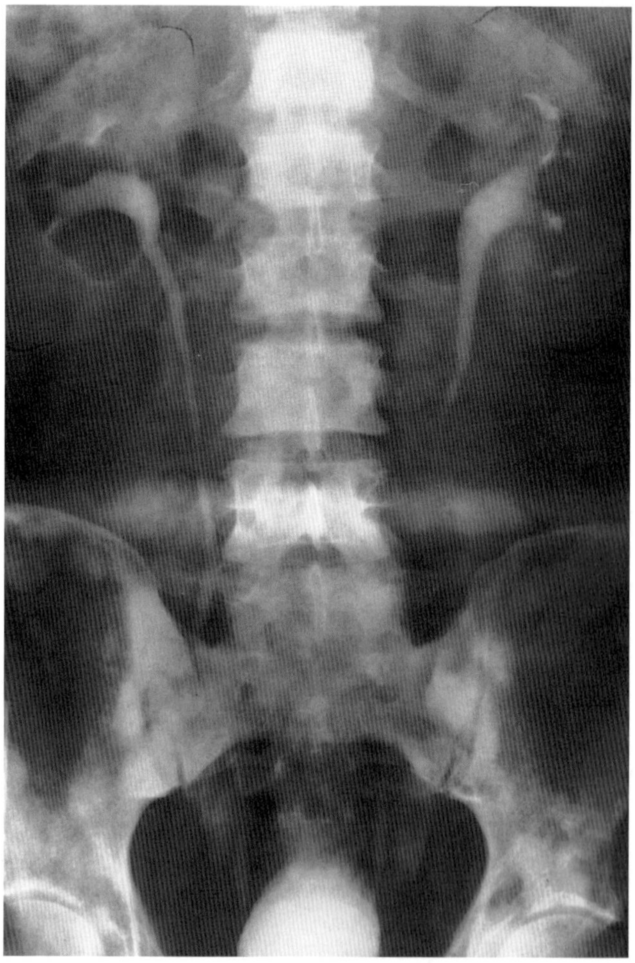

Figure 13.6

Metastases from carcinoma of the prostate. Excretory urography shows extensive sclerotic, bony deposits due to metastases.

Chest radiography

Metastases to the chest, including the thoracic cage, from prostate carcinoma are relatively common, especially in advanced disease, in which the incidence is 25%.[38] The typical finding is lymphangitic spread with coarse reticular shadowing peripherally and basally. Discrete nodular opacities are less common but have been described (Figure 13.7). Mediastinal lymphadenopathy is also a feature. However, the commonest manifestation is probably pleural effusion, though one study showed that this was as likely to be due to other causes as to prostate malignancy.[39]

Plain radiography is the cheapest and most effective way of detecting intrathoracic metastases. Routine chest CT or plain whole lung tomography has no role. A chest radiograph should be part of the initial evaluation in patients with prostatic carcinoma and should then be performed as clinically indicated on follow up.

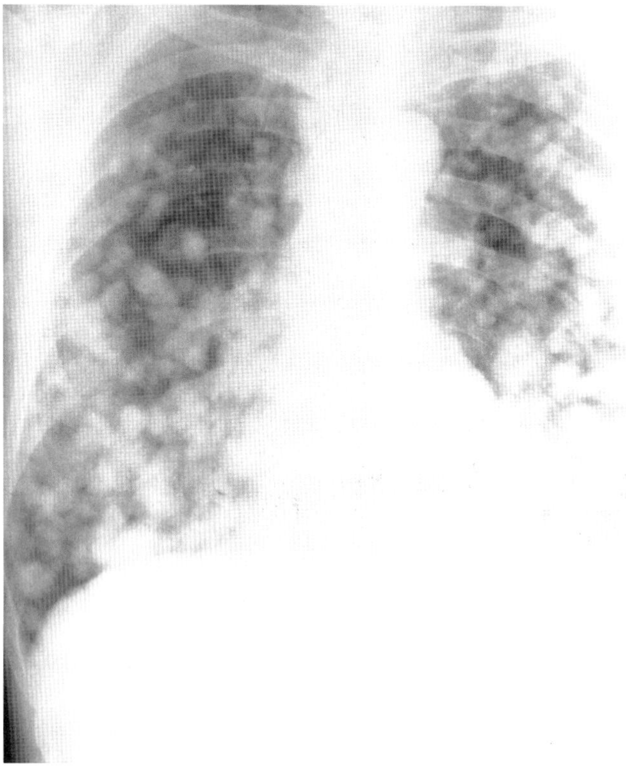

Figure 13.7

Metastases from carcinoma of the prostate. The chest radiograph showing extensive nodular deposits due to metastases.

Summary of imaging strategies

- The only technique which has been shown to be effective in imaging the primary lesion and pelvic abdominal spread is MR, ideally by combining standard body coil images with an endorectal surface coil, which will, we feel, soon be standard practice. This is the method of choice.
- The role of CT has diminished since the advent of MR and there are now few primary indications for CT which cannot be better evaluated by other techniques (especially MR). A possible exception is the placement of radioactive seeds in the prostate.
- The role of TRUS has yet to be defined; however, it appears to have no role in assessing tumor volume or in staging extraprostatic spread. It is valuable for biopsy guidance and may be useful in preference to MR for follow up of patients who have had radiation therapy and also of patients with elevated PSA levels and a normal rectal examination. Its use as a screening tool for carcinoma of the prostate is, at present, controversial.
- Radionuclide scintigraphy is the primary method of investigating and following bone metastases. Suspected spinal metastases are best studied by MR.
- An algorithm of the work up of prostate cancer is shown in Diagram 13.1.

Myelography and spinal magnetic resonance imaging

These techniques are not routine but are considered here because spinal disease is common. Metastatic disease to the vertebral column can lead to extradural compression of nerve roots or the spinal cord. Economics may dictate local practices, but myelography is a very effective investigation in this disorder. MR is the investigation of choice, however, especially when there are multiple lesions as there may be an extradural block beyond which the myelographic contrast cannot be run. MR is also superior to myelography in demonstrating soft-tissue masses. CT combined with myelography is helpful in such circumstances, but again MR is the investigation of choice for imaging the whole spine.

References

1. Silverberg E, Lubera JA, Cancer statistics 1989, *CA* (1989) **39** (1):3–20.
2. de Vere White R, Surgery in the treatment of prostate cancer. In: Wein AJ, Malkowicz SB, eds, *Cancer of the prostate: current practice/future directions* (Philadelphia Co. Med. Communications: Philadelphia 1989) **1**:4–11.
3. Silverberg E, Lubera JA, A review of American Cancer Society estimates of cancer cases and deaths, *CA* (1983) **33**:2.
4. Catolona W, Scott W, Carcinoma of the prostate. In: Walsh Gittes R, Perlmutter A, Stamey T, eds, *Campbell's urology* (WB Saunders: Philadelphia 1986) 1463–534.
5. Jewett HJ, The present status of radical prostatectomy for stages A and B prostatic cancer, *Urol Clin N Am* (1975) **2**:105.
6. Whitmore W Jr, Hormone therapy in prostate cancer, *Am J Med* (1956) **21**:697.

7. Murphy GP, Nararajan N, Pontes J, et al, The national survey of prostate cancer in the United States by the American College of Surgeons, *J Urol* (1982) **127**:928–34.
8. Oesterling JE, The rationale for radical prostatectomy in selected patients with stage A1 prostate cancer. In: Wein AJ, Malkowicz SB, eds, *Controversies in the management of prostate cancer* (Philadelphia Co. Med. Communications: Philadelphia 1990) 8–13.
9. Brawn PN, The differentiation of prostate carcinoma, *Cancer* (1983) **52**:246.
10. Smith JA, Management of patients with stage A1 adenocarcinoma of the prostate. In: Wein AJ, Malkowicz SB, eds, *Controversies in the management of prostate cancer* (Philadelphia Co. Med. Communications: Philadelphia 1990) 4–8.
11. Lee F, Littrup P, Torp-Pedersen S, et al, Prostate cancer: comparison of transrectal US and digital rectal examination for screening, *Radiology* (1988) **168**:389.
12. Cooner WH, Mosley BR, Rutherford CL, et al, Clinical application of transrectal ultrasonography and prostate specific antigen in the search for prostate cancer, *J Urol* (1988) **139**:758.
13. Carter HB, Hamper UM, Sheth S, et al, Evaluation of transrectal ultrasound in the early detection of prostate cancer, *J Urol* (1987) **162**:331–6.
14. Cooner W, Mosley B, Rutherford C, et al, Prostate cancer detection in clinical urological practice by ultrasonography, digital rectal examination and prostate specific antigen, *J Urol* (1990) **143**:1146–54.
15. Pedersen K, Carlsson P, Varenhorst E, et al, Screening for carcinoma of the prostate by digital rectal examination in a randomly selected population, *Br Med J* (1990) **300**:1041–4.
16. Hodge K, McNeal JE, Terris MK et al, Random systematic versus directed ultrasound guided transrectal core biopsies of the prostate, *J Urol* (1989) **142**:71–5.
17. McCarthy P, Pollack HM, Imaging of patients with stage D prostatic carcinoma, *Urol Clin N Am* (1991) **18**:35–53.
18. Phillips ME, Kressel HY, Spritzer CE, et al, Normal prostate and adjacent structures: MR imaging at 1.5T, *Radiology* (1987) **164**:381.
19. Styles RA, Seltzer R, CT staging of prostate cancer, *Radiology* (1985) **157**:838.
20. Schnall M, Imai Y, Tomaszewski J, et al, Prostate cancer: local staging with endorectal surface coil MR Imaging, *Radiology* (1991) **178**:797–802.
21. Scheibler M, Yankaskas B, Tempany C et al, MR imaging in adenocarcinoma of the prostate: interobserver variation and efficacy for detecting stage C disease, *AJR* (1992) **158**:559–62.
22. Schnall M, Bezzi M, Pollack HM, et al, Magnetic resonance imaging of the prostate, *Magn Reson Q* (1990) **6**:1–16.
23. McNeal JE, Redwine EA, Freiha FS, et al, Zonal distribution of prostatic adenocarcinoma: correlation with histologic patterns and direction of spread, *Am J Surg Pathol* (1988) **12**:897.
24. McNeal J, Kindrachuck R, Freiha F, et al, Patterns of progression of prostatic cancer, *Lancet* (1986) **1**:60.
25. Bezzie M, Kressel HY, Allen KS, et al, Prostatic carcinoma: staging with MR imaging at 1.5T, *Radiology* (1988) **169**:339–46.
26. Wheeler T, Anatomic considerations in carcinoma of the prostate, *Urol Clin N Am* (1989) **16**:623–34.
27. Hricak H, Dooms G, Jeffery RB, et al, Prostatic carcinoma: staging by clinical assessment, CT and MR imaging, *Radiology* (1987) **162**:331–6.
28. Ebner F, Kressel HY, Mintz M, et al, Tumor recurrence versus fibrosis in the female pelvis: differentiation with MR imaging at 1.5T, *Radiology* (1988) **166**:333–40.
29. Platt J, Bree R, Seltzer R. The accuracy of CT in staging carcinoma of the prostate, *AJR* (1987) **149**:315–18.
30. Hricak H, Theoni RF, Neoplasms of the prostate gland. In: Pollack HM, ed, *Clinical urography* (WB Saunders: Philadelphia 1989) 1394.
31. Danhert WF, Hamper UM, Walsh PC, et al, The echogenic focus in prostatic sonograms with xeroradiographic, and histopathologic correlation, *Radiology* (1986) **159**:95–100.
32. Rifkin MD, Dahnert W, Kurtz AB, State of the art: endorectal sonography of the prostate gland, *AJR* (1990) **154**:691–700.
33. Hodge K, McNeal JE, Stamey TA, Ultrasound guided transrectal core biopsies of the palpably abnormal prostate, *J Urol* (1989) **142**:66–70.
34. Rifkin M, Alexander A, Pisarchick J, et al, Palpable masses in the prostate: superior accuracy of US-guided biopsy compared with digitally guided biopsy, *Radiology* (1991) **179**:41–2.
35. Castellino R, Lymphography. In: Pollack HM, ed, *Clinical urography* (WB Saunders: Philadelphia 1989) 513.
36. McNeil BJ, Rationale for the use of bone scan in selected metastatic and primary bone tumors, *Semin Nucl Med* (1978) **8**:336.
37. Grinis G, Guinan P, Lopez-Majano V, et al, Prostate cancer: monitoring response to therapy—the bone scan. In: Resnick M, Watanabe H, Karr J, eds, *Diagnostic ultrasound of the prostate (Proceedings of the first international workshop, 1988)* (Elsevier: Amsterdam 1989) 168–70.
38. Lindell M, Doubleday L, von Eschenbach A, et al, Mediastinal metastasis from prostatic carcinoma, *J Urol* (1982) **128**:331.
39. Apple J, Paulson D, Baber C, et al, Advanced prostatic carcinoma: pulmonary manifestations, *Radiology* (1985) **154**:601–4.

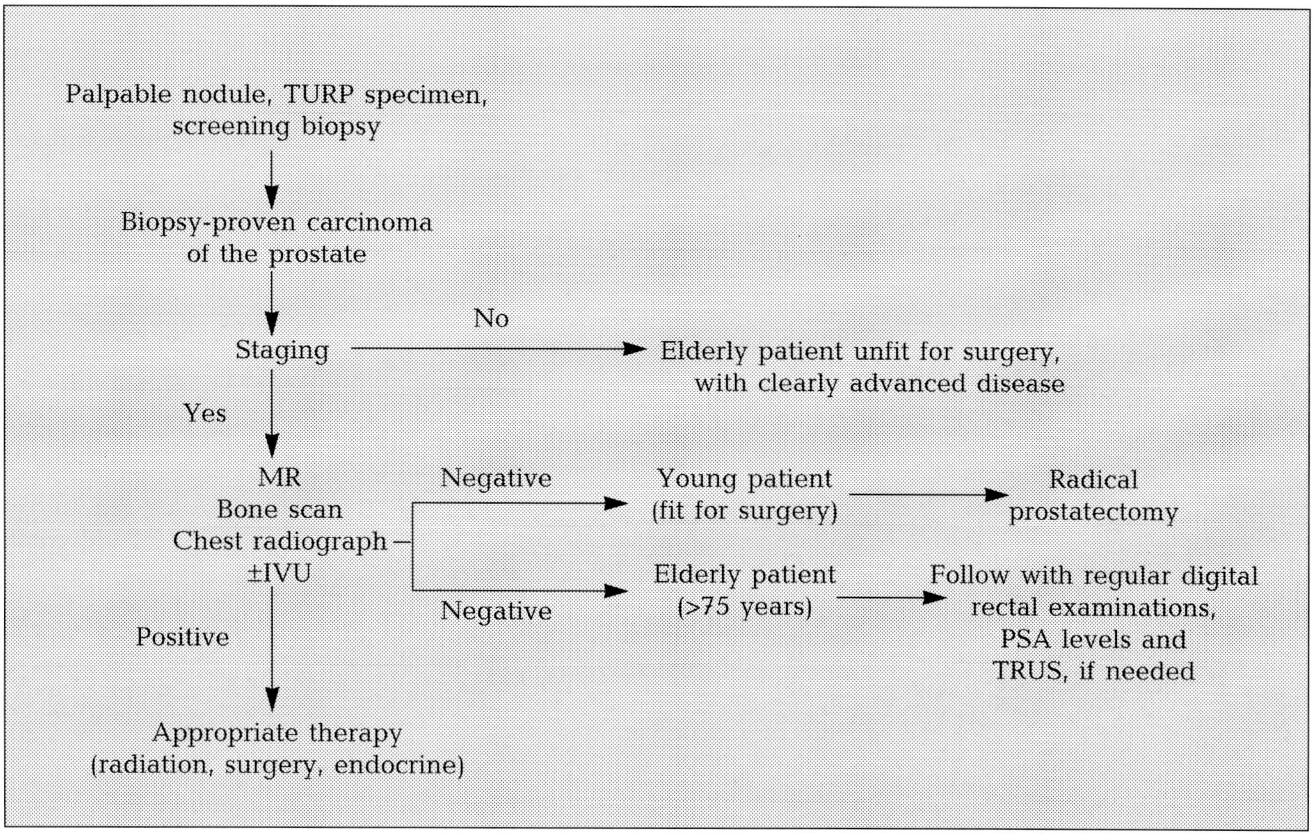

Diagram 13.1

Imaging strategy in carcinoma of the prostate. TURP = transurethral resection of the prostate.

14

The testes

Peter McCarthy, Parvati Ramchandani and Howard Pollack

Introduction

Testicular tumors are uncommon but have in recent times generated much interest in view of the dramatic change in their prognosis. Before 1970, survival was approximately 50%, whereas today the mortality is in the region of 10%. Approximately 5000 new cases of testicular malignancy are reported annually in the USA.[1] It is mainly a disease of the younger population, with a peak incidence in the 15- to 34-year-old age-group and a second peak occurring in men over 70. Bilateral tumors are recognized, occurring in 1–3% of cases.

Cryptorchidism is a risk factor for the development of a testicular malignancy, the risk being 30–50 times that of a normal man. Approximately 5–10% of the tumors developing in the former occur in the contralateral (normal) testis. The commonest type of malignancy in cryptorchids is seminoma. The risk appears not to be mitigated by orchiopexy, which may however preserve spermatogenesis if performed before the age 2 or 3 years. If this is done later, the organ is nearly useless in terms of fertility, so most urologists remove undescended testes if found in young or older men. What course of action to take in teenagers however is controversial.

There are two main types of testicular tumor: (1) about 90% are germ cell tumors and are, with the exception of the occasional 'pure' teratoma, invariably malignant, and (2) non-germ cell tumors (e.g. Leydig cell and Sertoli cell tumors) which are invariably benign and are not discussed further in this chapter. Lymphoma of the testis is a rare tumor but is of interest as it is the most common neoplasm found in the testis of men over 60 years of age. Tumorous metastases to the testis are rare, with the exception of acute leukemia which not infrequently involves the testis of boys.

The germ cell tumors are further subdivided into (a) seminomas and (b) non-seminomatous germ cell tumors (NSGCT). The latter group comprises embryonal carcinoma, choriocarcinoma, teratoma and yolk-sac tumor. A testicular tumor is considered to be NSGCT even when it is comprised mainly of seminoma. Forty per cent of NSGCT are of mixed pattern. The distinction between these two groups is made because seminoma is treated primarily by orchiectomy and radiotherapy, whilst NSGCT are treated by a combination of orchiectomy, surgery, chemotherapy and, in many cases, retroperitoneal lymphadenectomy. The incidence of seminoma peaks in the fourth decade and has an excellent survival rate—approximately 90% in 5 years. Embryonal cell carcinomas and teratoma incidences peak at an earlier age, whilst yolk-sac tumors usually present in infancy and early childhood. The long-term outlook in NSGCT is variable but is best in embryonal cell tumors and teratoma, while choriocarcinoma patients have an extremely poor prognosis.

Staging

No single method of staging testicular malignancy has achieved uniform acceptance. Most departments use the basic framework outlined by Boden and Gibb in 1951 and revised by Maier's group in 1968[3,4] (Table 14.1).

Table 14.1 Staging systems for testicular malignancy.

Boden and Gibb[3]		*Maier et al*[4]	
Stage A	Tumor confined to the testis	IA	Tumor confined to testis
Stage B	Retroperitoneal metastasis	IB	Histologic evidence of spread to iliac or para-aortic nodes at surgery
		II	Clinical or radiographic evidence of metastasis to femoral, inguinal iliac or para-aortic nodes
Stage C	Distant metastases	III	Clinical or radiographic signs of metastases above the diaphragm or distant metastases to other organs

Radiologic assessment

Unfortunately delay in presentation and delay in diagnosis still occur in testicular carcinoma: up to 15% of patients present with metastatic disease. We will here discuss the imaging modalities used and their relative usefulness.

Ultrasonography

This technique is inexpensive, non-invasive and excellently visualizes the primary tumor in the testis. The development of high-frequency probes (of the order of 7.5 MHz) has been the main reason that sonography has become the major imaging method used for studying the testis. Even higher frequency probes (10 MHz) are also now in routine use and provide high resolution images.

Prior to the emergence of ultrasonography (US), the mainstay of the diagnosis of testicular tumors was clinical examination and laboratory studies (serum tumor markers). An advantage of US is that it can detect clinically impalpable lesions; in fact, its spatial resolution allows detection of lesions of 3–4 mm in diameter.

The characteristic features of tumor on US are the finding of a mass, a diffuse textural change in the echotexture of the testis and echogenic foci related to either (Figure 14.1).[5] The mass can be either well- or ill-defined. Tumor masses are of low echogenicity in 81% of cases, while mixed echo patterns are seen in 19%.[6]

A diffuse hypoechoic area is a relatively frequent finding. The finding of small echogenic foci, with or without acoustic shadowing, associated with the edges of a mass or at the periphery of a diffuse textural change is thought to be highly suggestive of neoplasm. It has been found by careful biopsy that not all of these foci are due to calcification.[5] Calcification within a testicular neoplasm often indicates that the lesion is teratomatous.

Many of the findings outlined above are non-specific. Attempts have been made to differentiate benign from malignant processes and specifically to differentiate neoplasms from inflammatory processes, but usually without success. In malignancy, the testis is more likely to be enlarged and to have a globular shape, with a lobulated contour and heterogeneity of texture.[6] In inflammatory processes, the testicular enlargement is less prominent and more dramatic features are the finding of epididymal enlargement and thickening of the scrotal skin, which are not found in malignancy. Rifkin et al[7] have suggested that if the acoustic reflectively is increased, a benign process is more likely. The same authors suggested that the finding of small hydroceles is not helpful in confirming malignancy in that although they are said to be found in inflammatory and neoplastic conditions, another study indicated that a large amount of fluid was more likely indicative of benign pathology.[8]

It is worth stressing the almost 100% accuracy of US in distinguishing testicular from extratesticular pathology, the latter being a problem which may arise on clinical examination, especially when a very large mass or fluid is present.[7]

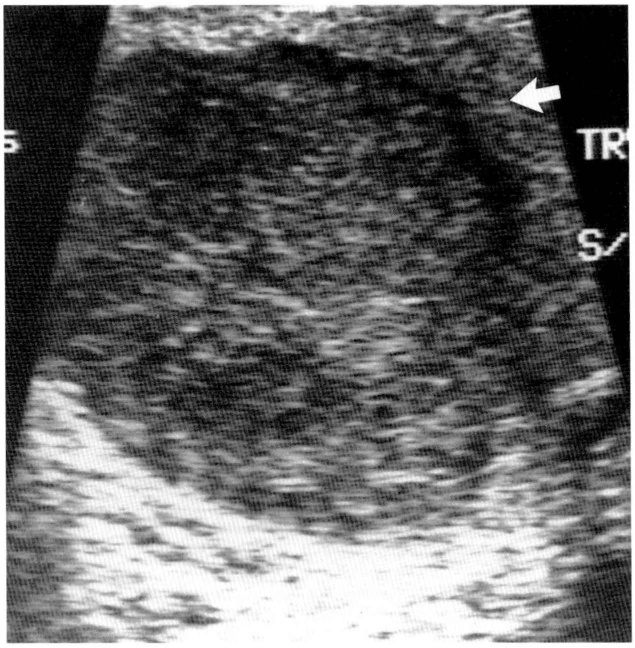

A

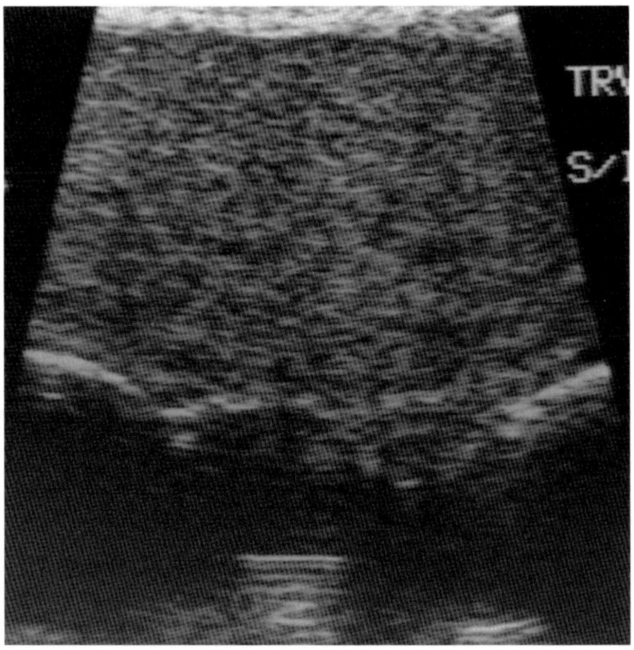

B

Figure 14.1

Seminoma. (**A**) Testicular ultrasound shows a large testicular lesion of mixed echogenicity with a surrounding capsule of low echogenicity. Some normal testicular tissue is seen peripherally (arrow). (**B**) An example of a normal testicular ultrasound is shown (opposite testis).

Regarding staging, US is occasionally but not always reliably used to image pelvic and retroperitoneal nodal disease. However, it pales by comparison with other cross-sectional imaging techniques. In following up testicular neoplasms, US can also be used to image the contralateral testis in patients who have had orchiectomy, or in assessing tumor progression/regression in patients who have not had such surgery.

Magnetic resonance imaging

MR is useful for imaging primary lesions and also in staging. Use of thin slices with a high-resolution surface coil for directly imaging the testis and standard body-coil imaging for the pelvis and abdomen is a good way of staging the disease.

On T1-weighted MR images, testicular tumors are generally isointense with the surrounding testis, but some tumors are found to be hyperintense (Figure 14.2). On T2-weighted sequences, most will to a variable degree demonstrate low signal in comparison with the surrounding testis. Hemorrhage may be present, complicating the picture. MR may also show that the entire testis has been infiltrated, though more commonly some residual normal testis will be identified. Some recent work has suggested that it may be possible by MR to distinguish seminomas from NSGCT.[9] In this study, the seminomas appeared on MR as hypointense, homogeneous masses on T2-weighted sequences, while the NSGCT appeared much more heterogeneous than normal testis tissue on proton density and T2-weighted sequences. A capsule was identified around these tumors, which was absent from seminomas. The sample in this study included only a small number of cases and it is too early yet to say if the findings will have an impact on diagnoses.

One study compared ultrasound and MR and found the major limitation of both to be their inability to differentiate benign and malignant processes.[10] Both yielded poor figures for accuracy of local staging (US 45%, MR 63%). Thus it was suggested that MR had no significant advantages over US and that US should remain the primary method of studying the testicular lesion, MR being reserved for selected cases.

The question of the use of MR in the assessment of retroperitoneal nodal spread is one about which little has been written with reference to testicular cancer, but it is discussed more fully in the following sections on lymphography and CT.

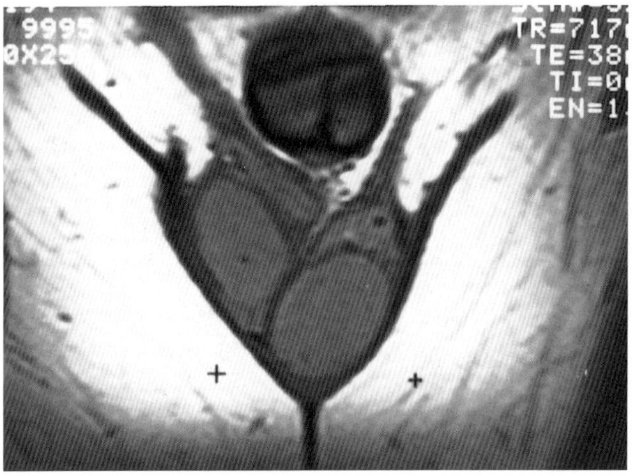

A

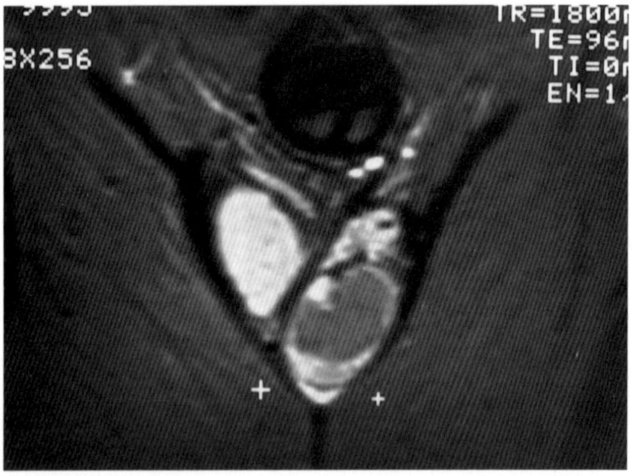

B

Figure 14.2

Coronal MR of the testis (spin-echo scans: **A**, TR 717/TE 38; **B**, TR 1800/TE 96) shows isointensity signal on the T1-weighted scan (**A**), but on the T2-weighted scan (**B**), the lesion stands out clearly as a low-signal area. The lesion was a seminoma; the epididymis was also involved.

Lymphography

Debate has raged in the radiologic literature over which study is more appropriate in the node staging of testicular cancers, lymphography or CT, the consensus now being that cross-sectional imaging has superseded lymphography.[11]

Lymphatic spread is typically the primary method of spread of testis cancer. The drainage is initially to the nodes along the testicular artery in the paralumbar region and from there to para-aortic nodes. Spread to mediastinal nodes along the thoracic duct can also occur. The detection of lymphatic spread is the key determinant of treatment. In the past, however, many stage I patients were treated as if they had stage II disease, i.e. patients with seminoma were given radiotherapy and NSGCT patients underwent retroperitoneal node dissections. More recently, however, this has been challenged and orchiectomy used alone in stage I seminoma, without radiotherapy, with good result.[12] However, were imaging to detect nodal disease, radiotherapy would undoubtedly be given. It is now clear that radiology will be placed under even greater pressure to exclude nodal invasion. In order to predict the likelihood of occult retroperitoneal metastasis in stage I disease, four factors are suggested to have an effect: lymphatic and vascular invasion, primary tumor stage and histological status.[13]

Lymphographic abnormalities which indicate disease are filling defects within nodes (even those which are normal in size), change in flow patterns of the lymphatics and nodal enlargement. Follow-up chest films 24 h after injection are probably useful in the assessment of the presence of mediastinal and supraclavicular lymphadenopathy.

Computed tomography

This technique has revolutionized the assessment of intrathoracic and intra-abdominal disease since its introduction in the 1970s. CT is, however, of little or no value in assessing the primary testicular lesion. Its main disadvantage is its inability to detect disease in normal sized nodes. Normal-sized adenopathies are nevertheless very rare in testicular tumors. However CT gives an overview of the abdomen and chest not afforded by lymphography and reveals areas not well imaged by lymphography, such as renal perihilar nodes. It can also visualize the hydronephrosis that may be due to large retroperitoneal masses.[14]

On retroperitoneal CT scans, nodes can be discrete and nodular or they may coalesce and form confluent masses, which may reach very large proportions (Figures 14.3 and 14.4). Any node of greater than 1 cm is considered abnormal. Central necrosis of the nodes prior to treatment is

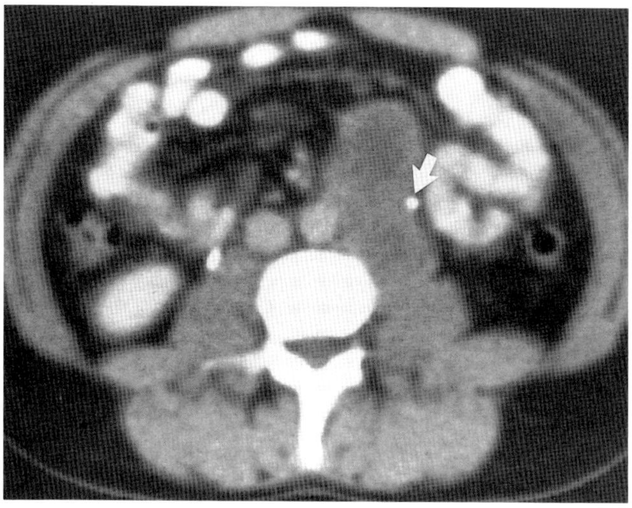

Figure 14.3

Teratoma, prior to therapy. Abdominal CT scan below the kidneys shows a large low-attenuation mass adjacent to the aorta, involving the anterior surface of the left psoas muscle and displacing the high attenuation ureter to the left (arrow).

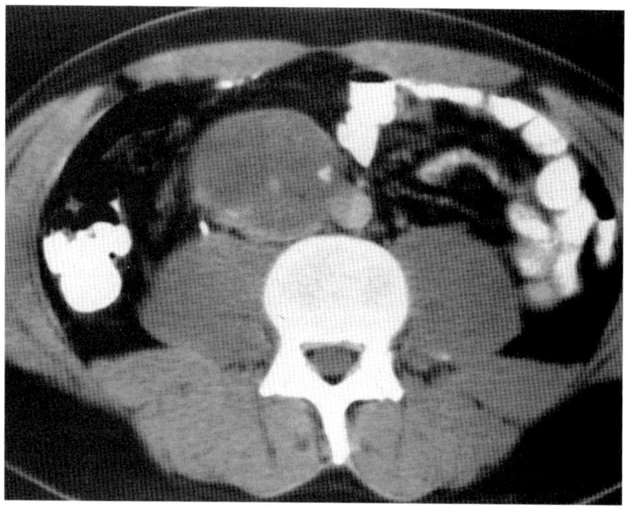

A

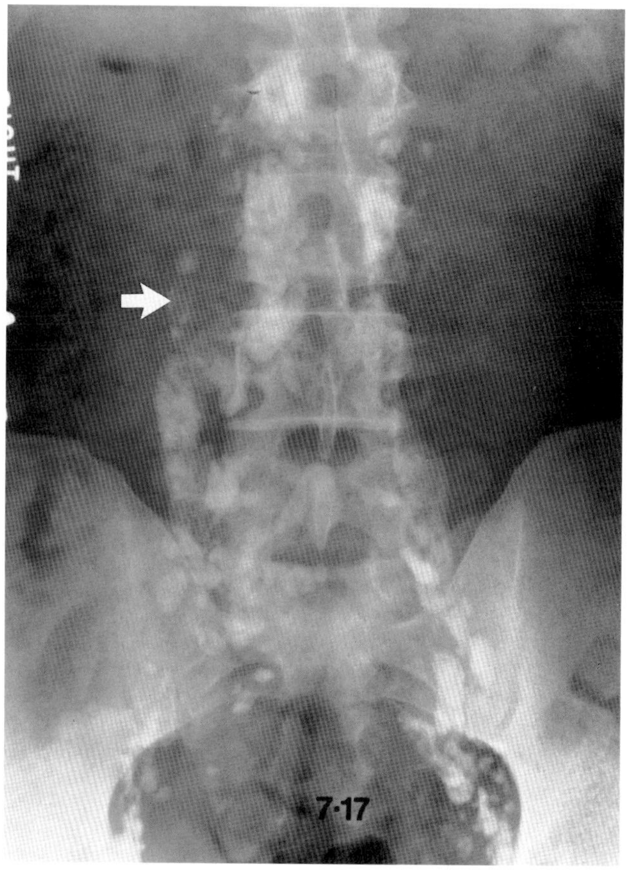

B

Figure 14.4

Seminoma, prior to therapy. (**A**) Abdominal CT scan shows a large mass with central necrosis and a focus of calcification which obliterates the inferior vena cava. (**B**) A lymphogram of the nodes of the region depicted on the CT scan (arrow), shows corresponding filling defects.

a phenomenon seen in many testicular tumors but more commonly seen in teratomas. This central, low attenuation on CT is a finding more typically noted after radio- or chemotherapy. Some would even suggest that the absence of this finding in a post-treatment node on CT is suspicious of recurrent or residual malignancy.

In many departments, CT has completely supplanted lymphography. Rarely, CT and lymphography are still performed together, particularly for seminomas. There are some departments which use CT as the primary method, and if CT is normal or equivocal, then lymphography is performed. There seems to be little role for lymphography in any situation if CT shows clearly that there is nodal enlargement (Figure 14.5). There is also no role for lymphography if routine retroperitoneal lymphadenectomy is performed in patients with NSGCT. The accuracy of both techniques is very high, at around 90%.[14–16]

CT of the chest is also a useful diagnostic technique in evaluating parenchymal lung metastases as it may reveal nodular metastatic deposits,

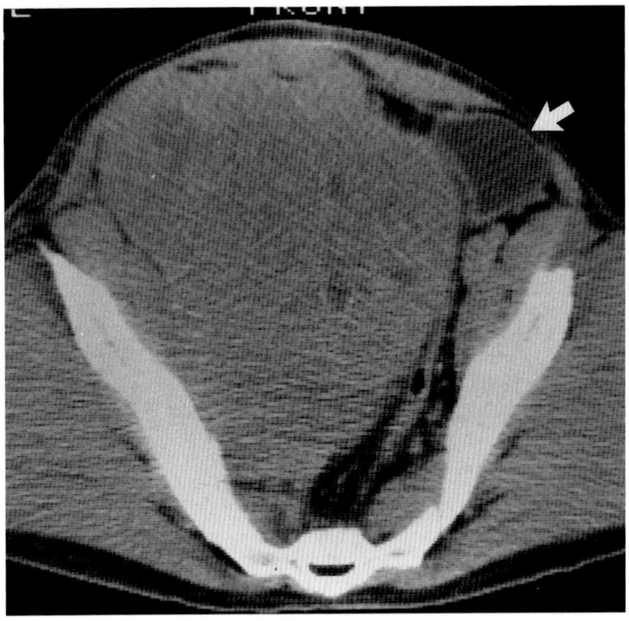

Figure 14.5

Pelvic CT scan shows a large right hemipelvic mass displacing the bladder (arrow) due to NSGCT nodal metastasis.

typically in the lung periphery. Mediastinal lymphadenopathy is also detected well on chest CT, nodes of greater than 1 cm being considered to be abnormal.

CT is the most useful method of following patients with abdominal disease. After the initial staging study, the surveillance of patients with probable stage I disease should include yearly CT scans to 36 months and retroperitoneal US at 6 and 18 months.[12] In aggressive disease, more frequent studies are appropriate and, as discussed already, many would not be satisfied with US examination of the retroperitoneum alone.

A recent study[17] noted that in a group of patients with NSGCT, enlarging masses on CT (both retroperitoneal and mediastinal) after treatment did not necessarily imply residual or recurrent malignancy. This is particularly the case in patients whose clinical signs and tumor markers suggest remission of disease. The authors suggested that such patients should have surgical removal to exclude any residual malignancy, whilst making the point that in the vast majority of cases such masses are due to maturation (but not progression) of the teratomas. Only one (6%) of their 17 patients had residual tumor. Conversely, there is no appearance on CT that guarantees that any node or group of nodes—no matter how responsive to therapy, how stable on follow up or how innocent-looking—does not in fact harbor residual malignancy.

Chest radiography

The plain chest film is a critical part of the work up, not only to assess the possibility of metastatic disease but also to assess the patient's cardiovascular status. CT of the chest is, however, more sensitive in detecting both parenchymal and mediastinal disease.

Excretory urography

Excretory urography is not routinely performed as it is a relatively insensitive method of detecting nodal disease, requiring substantial mass size to cause displacement or the ureter or kidney. Likewise, there is little or no reason any longer for cavography to assess the spread of testis tumor.

Summary

Once the initial diagnosis is made, plain chest films, CT scanning of the retroperitoneum and chest and US of both testes (if there has not previously been orchiectomy) are appropriate. If the CT findings are equivocal or if the CT is normal, and the patient is due to receive either radiotherapy, retroperitoneal dissection or chemotherapy based on the presence of known or suspected nodal metastases, then lymphography may be useful to detect nodal disease not identified on CT. This is more likely to be the case in seminomatous tumors, in which node dissection is rarely performed and tissue therefore is not usually available.

The role of MR in the accurate staging of retroperitoneal node disease is as yet unproved.

References

1. Silverberg E, Cancer statistics *CA* (1983) **33**:9.
2. Morse M, Whitmore W, Neoplasms of the testis. In: Walsh P, Gittes R, Perlmutter A, Stamey T, eds, *Campbell's urology* (WB Saunders: Philadelphia 1986) 1535–82.
3. Boden G, Gibb R, Radiotherapy and testicular neoplasms, *Lancet* (1951) **2**:1195.
4. Maier J, Mittemeyer B, Sulak M, Treatment and prognosis in seminoma of the testis, *J Urol* (1968) **99**:72.
5. Grantham J, Charbonneau W, James E, et al, Testicular neoplasms: 29 tumors studied by high resolution US, *Radiology* (1985) **157**:775–80.
6. Subramanyam B, Horii S, Hilton S, Diffuse testicular disease: sonographic features and significance, *AJR* (1985) **145**:1221.
7. Rifkin M, Kurtz A, Pasto M, et al, The sonographic diagnosis of focal and diffuse infiltrating scrotal lesions, *Urol Radiol* (1984) **6**:20–6.
8. Arger P, Mulhern C, Coleman B, et al, Prospective analysis of the value of scrotal ultrasound, *Radiology* (1981) **141**:763–5.
9. Johnson J, Mattrey R, Phillipson J, Differentiation of seminomatous from non-seminomatous testicular tumors with MR, *AJR* (1990) **154**:539–43.
10. Thurnher S, Hricak H, Carroll P, et al, Imaging the testis: comparison between MR Imaging and US, *Radiology* (1988) **167**:631–6.
11. North J, Lindell M, Jing B-S et al, Current use of lymphography for staging lymphomas and genital tumors, *AJR* (1992) **158**:725–8.
12. Duchesne G, Horwich A, Dearnaley D, et al, Orchiectomy alone for staging 1 seminoma of the testis, *Cancer* (1990) **65**:1115.
13. Hesketh P, Krane R, Prognostic assessment in nonseminomatous cancer: implications for therapy, *J Urol* (1990) **144**:1–9.
14. Epstein B, Order S, Zinreich E, Staging treatment and results in testicular seminoma, *Cancer* (1990) **65**:405.
15. Jing B, Wallace S, Zornoza J, Metastases to retroperitoneal and pelvic lymph nodes: computed tomography and lymphangiography, *Radiol Clin N Am* (1986) **20**:511.
16. Taylor R, Duncan W, Best J, Influence of computed tomography scanning and lymphangiography on management of testicular germ cell tumors, *Clin Radiol* (1986) **37**:539–42.
17. Panicek D, Toner C, Heelan R, et al, Non seminomatous germ cell tumors: enlarging masses despite chemotherapy, *Radiology* (1990) **175**:499–502.

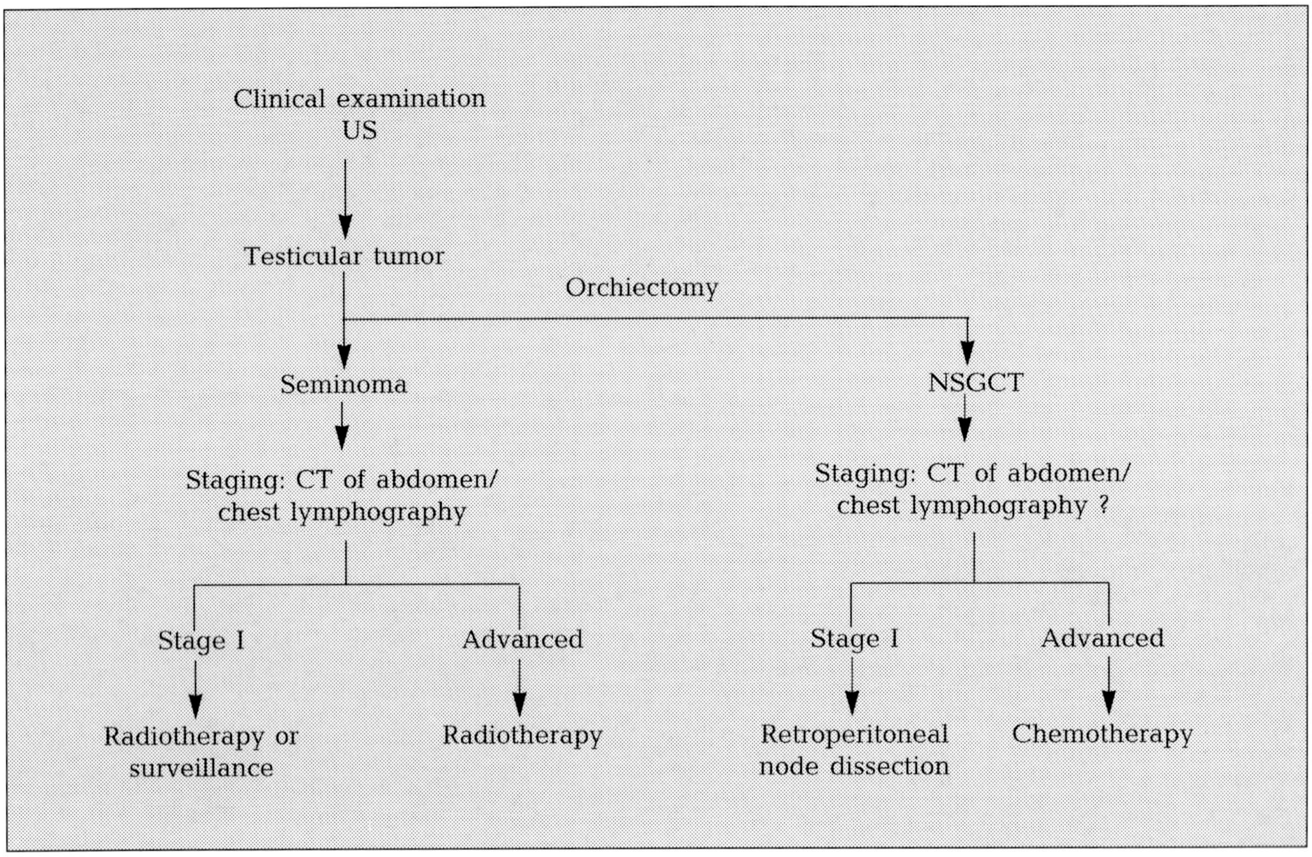

Diagram 14.1

Strategy for carcinoma of the testis.

15

The adrenal gland

Peter McCarthy, Parvati Ramchandani and Howard Pollack

Introduction

The most common malignancy affecting the adrenal gland is metastatic disease, thus the detection of metastases is the most frequent indication for adrenal imaging. Primary neoplasms of the adrenal cortex and medulla, such as primary adrenocortical carcinoma, pheochromocytoma and neuroblastoma, are much rarer.

Despite its small size, the adrenal gland is the fourth most common site for metastatic disease, after the lungs, liver and bone.[1] This may be related to its abundant arterial supply. The most common primaries metastasizing to the adrenal are lung (35–38% of cases in autopsy series), breast (50%), renal (18–25%)[2] and malignant melanoma (50% of cases in autopsy series).[3] However, almost any neoplasm can metastasize to the adrenal gland.

Most metastases begin in the medulla and remain asymptomatic until they grow large enough to cause pressure on adjacent organs or undergo hemorrhage or necrosis. Adrenal insufficiency is rare and occurs when 90% of the functioning adrenal tissue is replaced by tumor, usually with bilateral involvement.

Direct extension of contiguous malignancies can occur in patients with carcinoma of the pancreas, stomach, liver, kidney or retroperitoneum (sarcomas and lymphomas).

Lymphomatous involvement of the adrenal occurs more frequently in non-Hodgkin's lymphoma (NHL) than in Hodgkin's disease. Of patients with NHL, 4% demonstrate discrete adrenal involvement on CT at some time during the course of their disease; the involvement is bilateral in 46% of cases.[4] Adrenal involvement is most often in association with other extranodal disease in the abdomen and retroperitoneum. However, discrete involvement can occur, the only detectable disease being in the adrenal. The lesions respond to therapy in the same fashion as lymphomas elsewhere in the body.

Primary adrenal neoplasms

Cortical neoplasms

Primary adrenocortical carcinoma is an uncommon malignancy, accounting for 0.2% of all cancer deaths.[5] The peak incidence is in the 4th and 5th decades and both sexes are affected equally. The left gland is more commonly involved than the right; 10% of these tumors are bilateral.

Adrenal carcinomas can be endocrinologically active and produce excess hormones – such tumors are termed functioning carcinomas. Excess cortisol production is the most common functional abnormality, with resultant Cushing's syndrome. Next most frequent are virilization or feminization syndromes (adrenogenital syndromes). Hyperaldosteronism is rarely due to carcinomas. Functioning carcinomas occur more frequently in females, and males are more likely to have non-functioning tumors.

Most adrenal carcinomas present as large abdominal masses or with abdominal pain. Functioning tumors may present earlier, while the tumor mass is still small. Small lesions pose a diagnostic dilemma as benign adenomas are often difficult to distinguish from malignant adrenal tumors even by histology.

Neoplasms of the adrenal medulla

These fall into two main groups – the pheochromocytomas, which are usually benign but can be malignant, and the neuroblastoma series of tumors. Pheochromocytomas arise from chromaffin cells and produce, store and secrete catecholamines. They are malignant in only 10% of patients. Invasion of adjacent structures or evidence of distant metastases indicate that the tumor is malignant. Histology alone cannot differentiate benign from malignant pheochromocytomas. The tumors are functionally active and patients present with paroxysmal hypertension and associated complications. The clinical diagnosis is established by the detection of catecholamines and their metabolites in the urine. Malignant pheochromocytomas can be located in the adrenals or along the course of the sympathetic ganglia in the abdomen and pelvis. Only occasionally are they found above the diaphragm.

Neuroblastomas and ganglioneuroblastomas occur rarely in adults and hence will not be discussed in detail here. Transformation to benign ganglioneuroma can occur. CT is the imaging modality of choice to determine the full extent of the lesion, detect metastases and monitor response to therapy.

Radiological appearances and imaging strategy

Metastases

The distinction between metastases and primary adrenal tumors is very difficult to make by radiologic appearance alone. It is of prime importance to be able to separate benign non-functioning adrenal adenomas from metastases in the oncologic patient, as subsequent patient management is affected. Benign adenomas are a frequent, incidental finding in the present era of easily accessible CT. They are reported in 1.5–3.0% of autopsy series. Routine pre-operative CT staging of patients with non small cell bronchogenic carcinoma have demonstrated solid adrenal masses in 10–20% of cases in one series,[6] of which only 32% were metastases while 68% were benign adenomas. Thus, an isolated adrenal mass in non small cell lung cancer is more likely to represent a benign adenoma than a metastasis. In another series, only 46% of adrenal masses in oncologic patients with different primaries were found to be due to metastases.[7]

Computed tomography

CT is the modality of choice in searching for adrenal metastatic disease. The metastases appear as soft-tissue density masses which can be small or large and round, lobulated or irregular in shape. They can be unilateral or bilateral.

The vascularity of the metastases mimics that of the primary. Hypovascular primaries such as squamous-cell carcinoma of the lung produce metastases with relatively little contrast enhancement, whilst hypervascular primaries such as renal-cell carcinoma give rise to metastases that enhance after contrast administration. With increase in size, hemorrhage and necrosis can occur in the metastatic lesions, which then appear as low-density cystic areas within the masses.

As metastases cannot be distinguished from other adrenal masses by their appearance alone, percutaneous aspiration biopsy, generally with CT guidance, often helps in establishing the histologic diagnosis and assumes a central role in the work up of these patients. In one report, initial biopsy obtained diagnostic material in 83% of patients with a 12% incidence of minor complications in one report.[7]

The right adrenal gland is approached either transhepatically or posteriorly. The left adrenal gland is biopsied either through a left posterior approach or, rarely, an anterior approach.

Magnetic resonance imaging

MR, especially when abetted by the use of surface coils, which are well suited to adrenal imaging, provides tissue characterization unobtainable by CT or ultrasound. Characteristically, adrenal metastases are of high signal intensity on T2-weighted images and are of low intensity, similar to liver or muscle, on T1-weighted images.[8] Metastases have characteristics similar to the primary tumor. Non-functioning adenomas tend to behave similarly to liver and remain relatively low intensity on both T1- and T2-weighted images.

Overlap in signal characteristics between adenomas and metastases can make it difficult to clearly separate the two. This occurred in 21% of patients in one series.[8]

At present, the superior spatial resolution of CT compared with MR makes it the screening procedure of choice. MR is indicated in those patients who have indeterminate adrenal masses, in an attempt to further characterize the solid mass, and it is very helpful in identifying benign adenomas. If MR is equivocal, CT-guided aspiration biopsy helps to obtain the confirmatory histology. Percutaneous biopsy is indicated in any patient in whom the presence of metastatic disease would affect subsequent therapy.

Ultrasonography

Ultrasonography (US) has a limited role in both the screening and characterization of adrenal masses. The normal adrenal gland is difficult to identify ultrasonographically on a consistent basis; furthermore, subtle enlargement may be difficult to detect.[9] Moderate sized masses (4–5 cm in diameter) may be seen as solid masses anteromedial to the upper pole of the kidney. The metastases usually appear as homogeneous, hypoechoic masses but there are no specific sonographic criteria to distinguish metastases from other solid adrenal masses. Necrosis and hemorrhage can cause inhomogeneity and increased echoes within the mass. US does play an important role, however, in the case of adrenal cysts (or pseudocysts), and in children when the differential diagnoses are neuroblastoma and adrenal hemorrhage.

Plain films and intravenous urography

Intravenous urography (IVU), especially with tomography, may detect large metastases as an incidental finding. However, plain films and IVU have no role in the screening or diagnosis of adrenal masses nowadays.

Primary adrenocortical carcinoma

CT remains the mainstay for the initial detection of the adrenal mass. Most patients present with large abdominal masses (Figures 15.1 and 15.2). CT characteristics – such as size greater than 5 cm, irregular walls with calcification, central necrosis, invasion of adjacent structures or distant metastases – indicate the malignant nature of the mass. But size alone cannot be relied on as a criterion of benignancy. Small, primary carcinomas that are indistinguishable from benign adenomas do occur and are a diagnostic dilemma. In one study, 27% of patients were reported to have carcinomas of less than 6 cm in diameter, with some as small as 3 cm.[10] All of these lesions were well-defined, sharply outlined and not adherent to adjacent tissues. Large tumor size does not always indicate malignancy, however, as there are reports of benign adenomas of 13–14 cm in diameter. Nevertheless, in spite of such exceptions, the rule of thumb that tumors greater than 5 cm are malignant works rather well in practice.

The usefulness of percutaneous adrenal biopsy is limited in attempting to distinguish benign adenomas from carcinomas. This distinction is very difficult to make even histologically, and percutaneous aspiration is unlikely to yield sufficient tissue to be of any diagnostic value.

CT is also crucial in identifying the uncommon adrenal myelolipoma. This lesion, a hamartoma, is readily recognizable by the presence of fat within it. Accordingly, it can also be diagnosed by MR.

Magnetic resonance imaging

Primary adrenal carcinomas display a high signal intensity on T2-weighted images, similar to adrenal metastases. Benign adenomas, on the other hand, behave like the adrenal cortex and remain low in signal intensity on T2-weighting. However, overlap in signal characteristics can occur, and in an occasional patient the MR will be equivocal and will not allow distinction of benign adenoma from carcinoma. Close follow-up examination or removal of the mass are the only alternatives in such a case.

Another very helpful aspect of MR is its multiplanar capability. When adrenal tumors are large, as many cortical carcinomas are wont to be, axial CT images do not readily pinpoint their origin to the adrenal gland, and they can be easily misrepresented as primary renal pancreatic, retroperitoneal and other neoplasms. It becomes much easier to recognize the true nature of the tumor on sagittal or coronal images however (Figures 15.1 and 15.3).

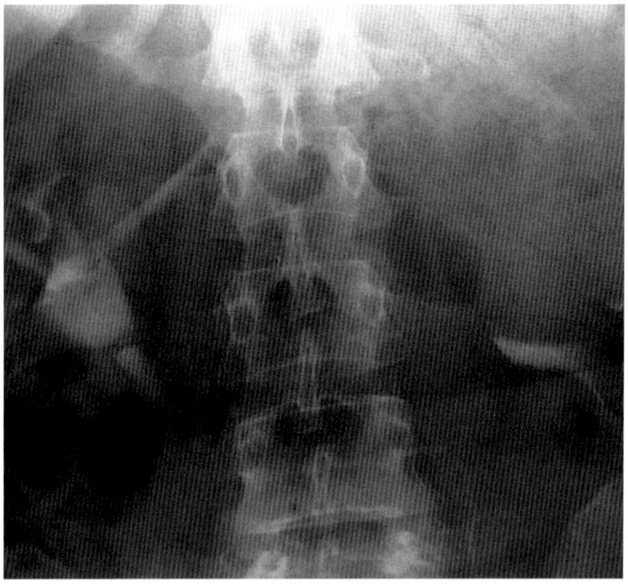

A

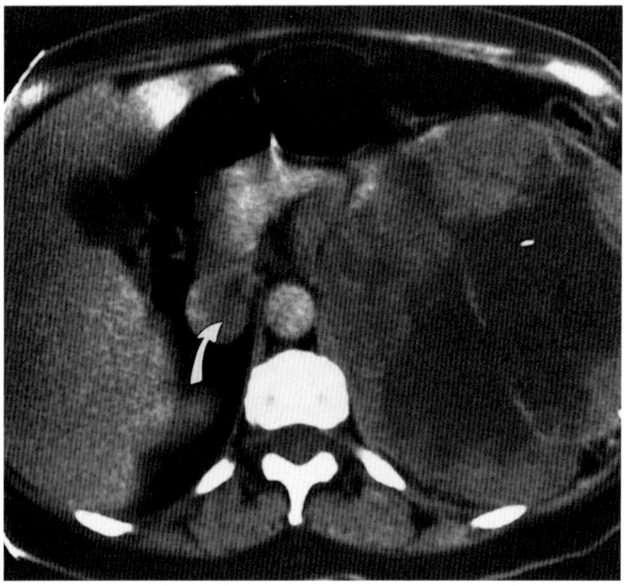

B

Figure 15.1

Primary adrenocortical carcinoma.

A Excretory urography shows caudal displacement and distortion of the left renal collecting system by the left adrenal carcinoma.

B CT scan shows a large mass with central necrosis and calcifications. With large masses, axial images may not indicate the origin of the mass, and imaging in other planes (such as with MR) is often required. Note the tumor thrombus in the inferior vena cava (arrow).

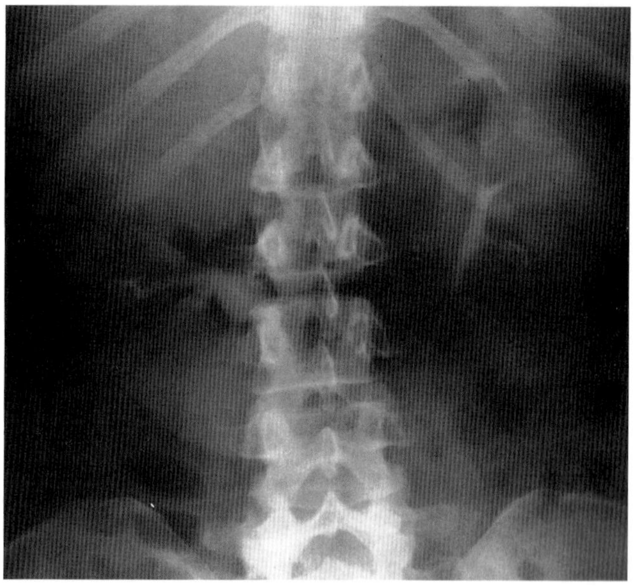

A

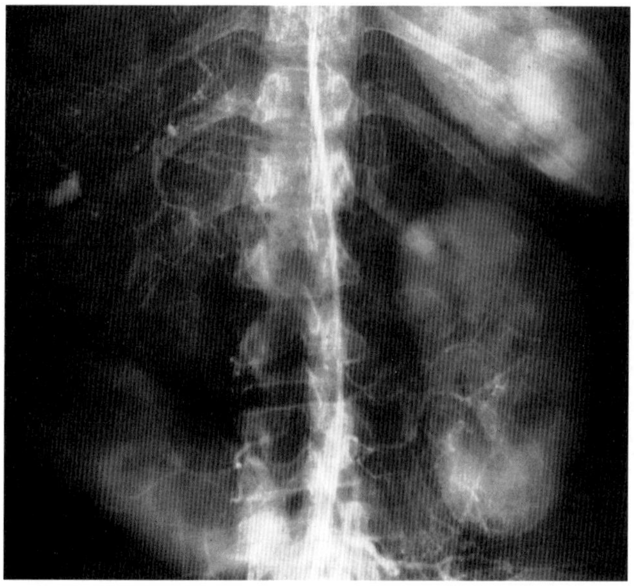

B

Figure 15.2

Primary adrenocortical carcinoma.

A Excretory urography shows caudal and lateral displacement of the right kidney.

B The late phase of an abdominal aortogram demonstrates neovascularity and contrast puddling in the right suprarenal area. Adrenal carcinomas are characteristically hypervascular.

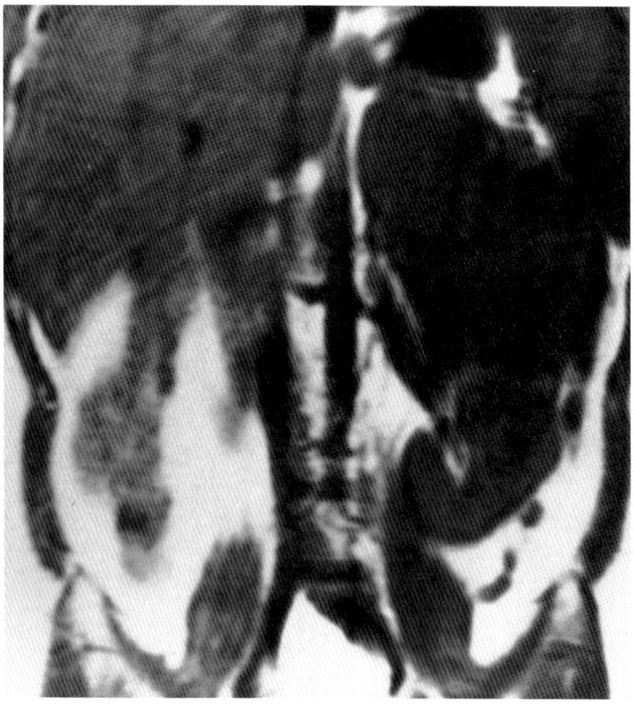

A

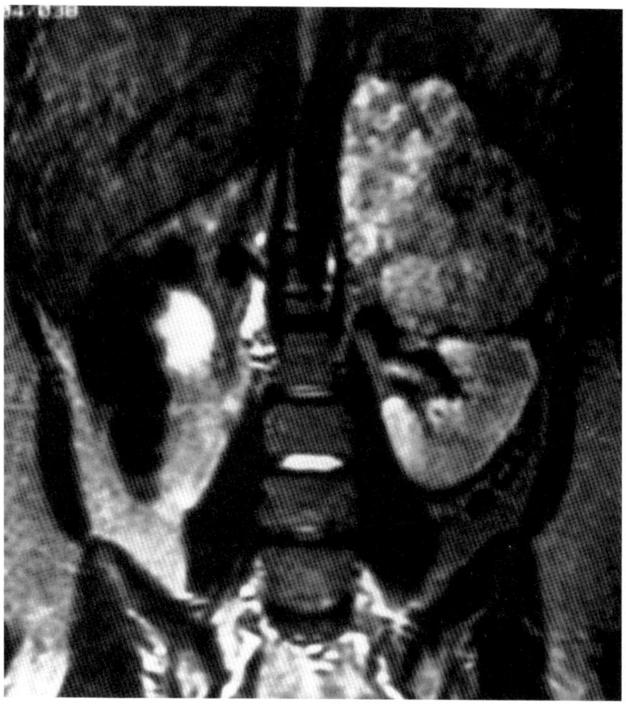

B

Figure 15.3

Primary adrenocortical carcinoma. Coronal MR scans show a large left adrenal mass displacing the left kidney (**A**, TR 600/TE 20; **B**, TR 2500/TE 80). The upper pole of the left kidney is clearly separable from the mass on these coronal images – this distinction was not possible on the axial scans.

Isotope scanning

This is performed with a cortical labelling agent, [^{131}I]6,ß-iodomethyl-19-norcholesterol (NP-59), which is administered intravenously and scans obtained 2–5 days later.[5,11] The normal adrenals visualize on or after the 5th day. Abnormally increased uptake is seen in hyperfunctioning benign adenomas. Endocrinologically active carcinomas do not accumulate the tracer but suppress pituitary adrenocorticotrophin (ACTH) and contralateral cortical function. Thus, the detection of an enlarged adrenal on CT or MR coupled with no NP-59 uptake on scintigraphy is highly suggestive of primary or secondary adrenal malignancy. Unfortunately, NP-59 is, at the time of writing, an investigational drug which is not commercially available. With small masses (2 cm in diameter) results are less reliable, further limiting its usefulness.

Neoplasms of adrenal medulla

Malignant pheochromocytomas constitute only about 10% of pheochromocytomas. The clinical presentation is that of paroxysmal or sustained hypertension and diagnosis is based on clinical and biochemical features. Histologic examination cannot differentiate benign from malignant pheochromocytomas.

Computed tomography

As for all adrenal pathology, CT is a highly accurate method to detect pheochromocytomas, both in the adrenals and in ectopic locations in the abdomen, pelvis and chest. The presence of metastases and/or local invasion would indicate malignancy. The appearance is similar to that of any other solid adrenal mass, and the CT appearance is entirely non-specific. Unenhanced CT should be performed, as contrast administration may precipitate a hypertensive crisis.

Magnetic resonance imaging

The relaxation times of pheochromocytomas are extremely long and so these tumors are dark on T1-weighted images and very bright on T2-weighted images. The unusually strong signal on T2-weighting facilitates the specific diagnosis of pheochromocytoma in most patients.[8]

Radionuclide scintigraphy

This is performed with [^{131}I]*m*-iodobenzyl guanidine (MIBG), which is a physiological analog of norepinephrine and guanethidine and is taken up by chromaffin tissue.[12] This agent has 95% specificity and 90% sensitivity in detecting pheochromocytomas. Its main use is in patients in whom the clinical suspicion of pheochromocytoma is strong but no adrenal mass is demonstrable on CT. It is also useful in ruling out multiple pheochromocytomas and in patients suspected of having metastatic tumors, as the whole body can be scanned. In post-operative patients in whom CT scans are limited due to clip artifact, [^{131}I]MIBG scanning is an alternative for detecting recurrent disease.

Angiography and venous sampling

These techniques are rarely needed today. Angiography demonstrates hypervascular lesions and can detect 85–100% of pheochromocytomas. Venous sampling at various sites is occasionally needed to localize lesions that have not been precisely defined by other imaging modalities.

References

1. Bosniak MA, Siegelman SS, Evans JA, *The adrenal, retroperitoneum and lower urinary tract* (Yearbook Medical Publishers: Chicago 1976) 29.
2. Abrams HL, Spiro R, Goldstein N, Metastases in carcinoma, *Cancer* (1950) **3**:74–85.
3. DasGupta T, Brasfield R, Metastatic melanoma, *Cancer* (1964) **17**:1323–39.
4. Pauling MR, Williamson BRJ, Adrenal involvement in non-Hodgkin's lymphoma, *AJR* (1983) **141**:303–5.
5. Dunnick NR, Adrenal imaging: current status, *AJR* (1990) **154**:927–36.
6. Oliver TW Jr, Bernardino ME, Miller JI, et al, Isolated adrenal masses in non small cell bronchogenic carcinoma, *Radiology* (1984) **153**:217–18.
7. Bernardino ME, Walther MM, Phillips VM, et al, CT guided adrenal biopsy: accuracy, safety and indications, *AJR* (1985) **144**:67–9.
8. Reinig JW, Doppman JL, Dwyer AJ, et al, MRI of indeterminate adrenal masses, *AJR* (1986) **147**:493–6.
9. Mittelstaedt CA, *Abdominal ultrasound* (Churchill Livingstone: Edinburgh 1987) 410–11.
10. Fishman EK, Deutch BM, Hartman DS, et al, Primary adenocortical carcinoma: CT evaluation with clinical correlation, *AJR* (1987) **148**:531–5.
11. Gross MD, Thompson NW, Beierwaltes WH, Scintigraphic approach to the localization of adrenal lesions causing hypertension, *Urol Radiol* (1982) **3**:241–4.
12. Quint LE, Glazer GM, Francis IR, et al, Pheochromocytoma and paraganglioma: comparison of MR imaging with CT and I-131 MIBG scintigraphy, *Radiology* (1987) **165**:89.

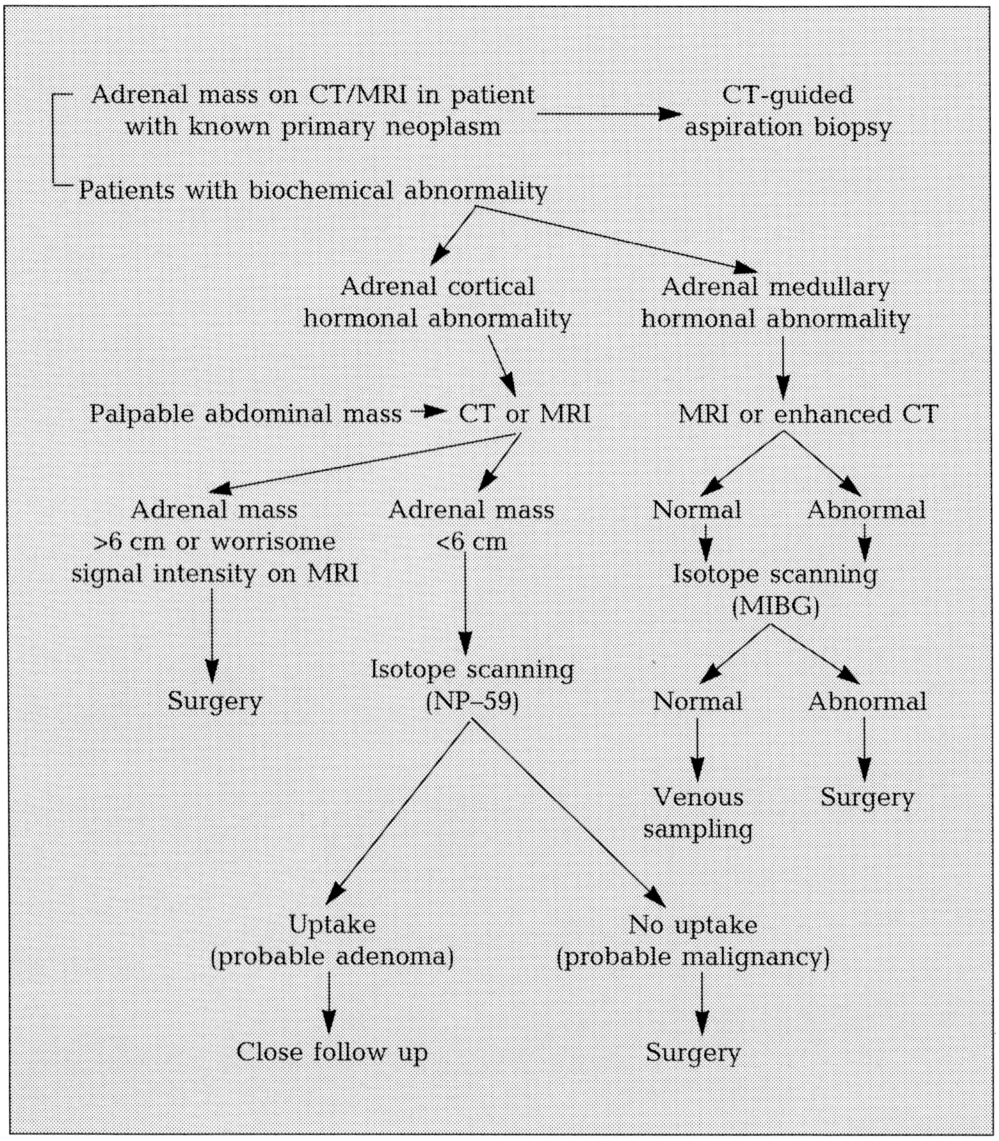

Diagram 15.1

Imaging strategy for abnormalities of the adrenal gland.

16

The retroperitoneum

Peter McCarthy, Parvati Ramchandani and Howard Pollack

Introduction

The retroperitoneum is a space occupied by fatty connective tissue. Its limits are:

- superiorly, the reflections of the diaphragm;
- inferiorly, the pelvic diaphragm (although this limit is not well defined within the pelvis and one may consider the retroperitoneal connective tissue to extend down to the most inferior reflection of the peritoneum);
- laterally, a line drawn between the tip of the 11th rib and the iliac crest;
- anteriorly, the posterior layer of the parietal peritoneum and the non-peritonealized aspects of the liver, duodenum, colon and rectosigmoid;
- posteriorly, the muscles of the body wall (psoas, iliacus, quadratus lumborum and transversalis muscle).[1]

Within the retroperitoneum reside numerous organs, such as the kidneys, ureters, adrenals, pancreas and the extraperitoneal portions of the duodenum and large bowel. Neural, lymphatic and vascular tissues abound within the retroperitoneum. Neoplasms originating within it and not arising from a specific organ are classified as primary retroperitoneal tumors.

Incidence and classification

Primary tumors of the retroperitoneum are uncommon, constituting only about 0.2% of all tumors.[2] A histologically diverse group, these lesions arise from the connective tissue that makes up the substance of the retroperitoneum. They have been divided into six major groups:[3] benign lesions (14%), germ-cell tumors (3%), lymphomas (22%), sarcomas (46%), carcinomas (7%) and undifferentiated malignancies (8%).

Regardless of their histology, retroperitoneal tumors tend to have similar presentations, usually late in their course and with few symptoms. Essentially they occur equally in men and women, primarily in the 5th to 7th decades of life, though it has been reported[2] that approximately 40% of patients are under the age of 40 and 15% less than 10 years of age.

The most characteristic feature of these lesions is their size. The average diameter of resected lesions has been reported to be 14 cm and unresectable lesions 28 cm.[4] An average weight of 1200 g has been reported, and many tumors weighing over 25 kg have been resected.[3]

Clinical features

There are no signs or symptoms specific to retroperitoneal neoplasms. At presentation, one-half to two-thirds of patients will have abdominal pain, a majority will have a palpable mass, and a smaller number will have backache or leg pain. A variety of gastrointestinal (GI) symptoms are seen, depending on the location of the mass. Urologic symptoms are uncommon. Fever may be found with lymphomas, but rarely with other tumors.

Weight loss is an inconsistent finding, reported in over 50% of patients in one series[3,5] but in less than 10% in two others.[2,6] Although hypoglycemia has been reported in association with retroperitoneal sarcomas, it is not characteristic and was not seen in any of these series. Elevated α-fetoprotein and/or β-human chorionic gonadotrophin are found in some germ-cell tumors.

Most patients will have a palpable tumor in either the abdomen, flank or pelvis. An enlarged liver and ascites have been noted in up to 20% of patients, lower extremity edema in approximately 10% and other findings even less often.

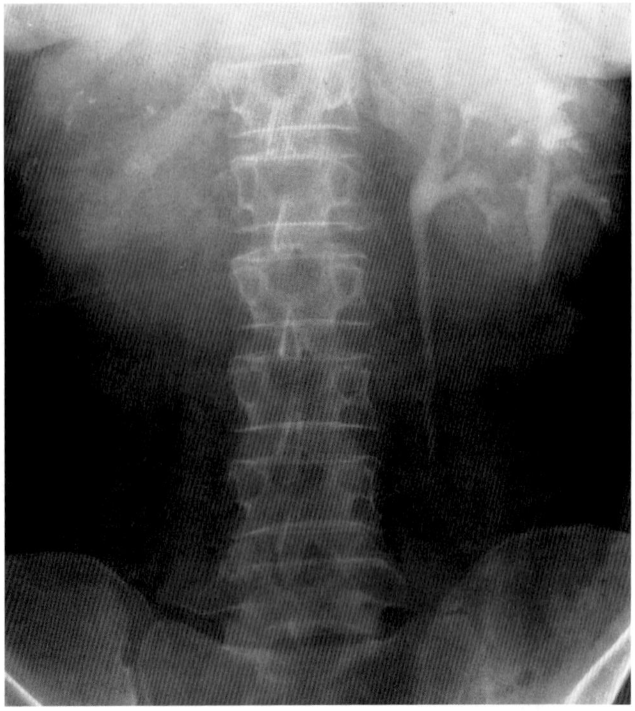

Figure 16.1

Retroperitoneal liposarcoma. Intravenous urography reveals a large right-sided abdominal mass which displaces the right kidney across the midline. Tumoral calcification is noted in the right upper quadrant.

Imaging strategy

Before the development of cross-sectional imaging the diagnosis of retroperitoneal tumors was difficult to make prior to exploration; only a third were correctly diagnosed pre-operatively.[3,5,6] Now, however, the tumors are demonstrable in nearly every case. In the past, the most useful diagnostic tools were intravenous urography (Figure 16.1), retrograde pyelography, and barium studies of the GI tract (Figure 16.2). Sensitivities ranged from 60 to 85% for urographic studies, in which the most common finding was medial deviation of a ureter, to 30–66% for gastrointestinal studies in which displacement was also the usual observation.[3,5,6] Today these studies are not used much, although the functional status of each kidney must still be known prior to surgery, since nephrectomy often accompanies the surgical extirpation of large retroperitoneal lesions.

Radiography

Plain films of the abdomen can also be helpful by suggesting a mass, a fatty tumor (unusually lucent areas) or a teratoma (teeth) (Figure 16.3). While neither aortography, selective arteriography, or venocavography have made a major impact on diagnosis, some surgeons feel that vascular studies are critically important in pre-operatively evaluating the variable, unpredictable blood supply of these tumors.[6,7] Invasion into contiguous organs such as the liver can also be detected in this way, as can tumors potentially requiring segmental resection of the aorta or vena cava. In one review,[8] angiographic data in 45 consecutive retroperitoneal tumors were considered. Although no findings were specific to a particular lesion, there was an 80% success rate in delineating the extent of the tumor, defining its blood supply and determining its nature (benign or malignant). Pre-operative intra-arterial chemotherapy of sarcomas is another indication for angiography.[3,9]

Computed tomography

CT and, later, MR have revolutionized the evaluation of retroperitoneal growths. CT has been accurate in the evaluation of the location, extent

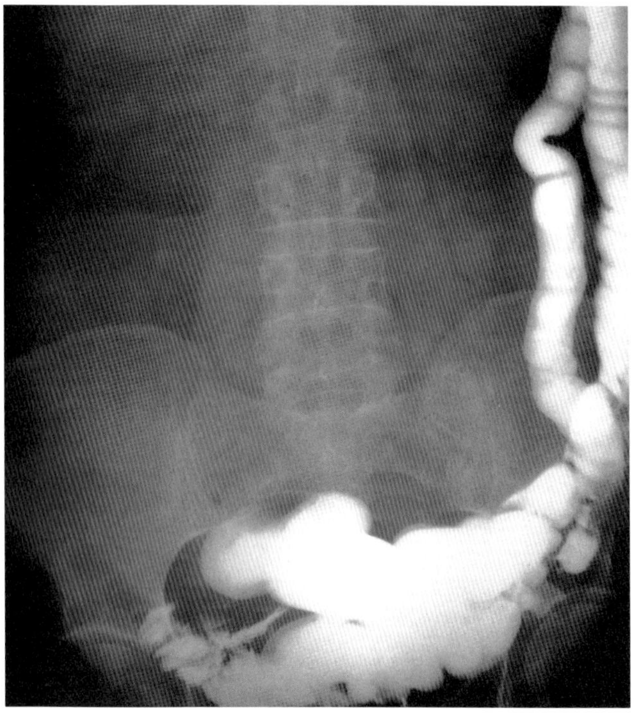

Figure 16.2

Retroperitoneal liposarcoma. Barium enema reveals marked caudal and contralateral displacement of the right-sided colon.

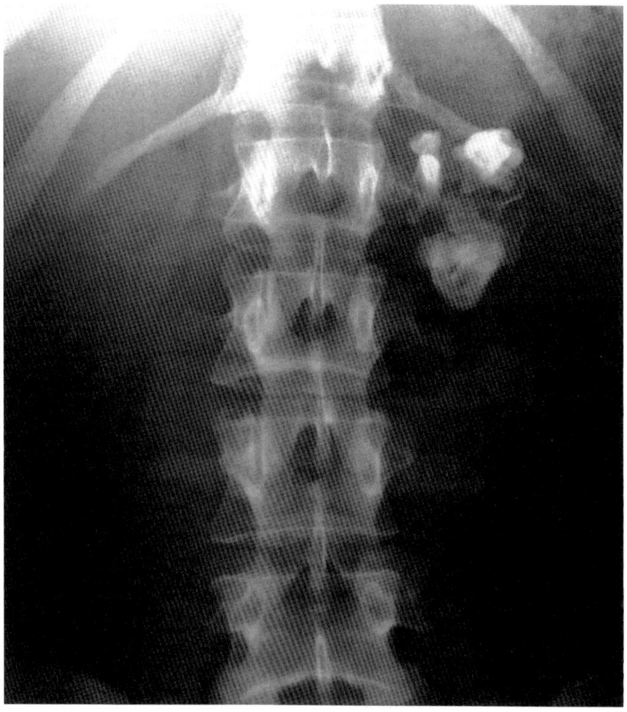

Figure 16.3

Retroperitoneal teratoma (26-year-old female). Plain abdominal radiography reveals a calcified left upper quadrant mass. The opacities proved to be teeth within a partially formed maxilla.

and make-up of a mass and can often reveal intra-abdominal metastases and involvement of adjacent structures as well.[10] One study[11] demonstrated that intraoperative assessment of the limits of a tumor is often inaccurate, while another[12] states 'often the extent of a retroperitoneal tumor is more readily apparent by CT than at surgery.' CT has good specificity for benign fatty tumors, which have a homogeneous fat density (Figure 16.4), but may fail to recognize the nature of liposarcomas (Figure 16.5), which often contain predominantly soft tissue rather than fatty components.[13,14] CT is an excellent means of following up patients receiving adjuvant therapy, identifying recurrent disease and planning radiotherapy. The sensitivity of the technique tends to be somewhat less in thin patients, in whom the contrast provided by fat planes is diminished, and following surgery, particularly if there are a large number of artifact-producing metal clips. Additionally, CT (or MR) can be used instead of myelography when intraspinal extension of a neurogenic tumor is suspected.

Ultrasonography

Ultrasonography (US) is often the first study obtained in patients – particularly children – with a retroperitoneal tumor. It has the advantages of no radiation exposure, no contrast administration and excellent accuracy in depicting the solid or cystic nature of a mass (Figure 16.6). Its sensitivity has been reported to be 84%, compared with 89%

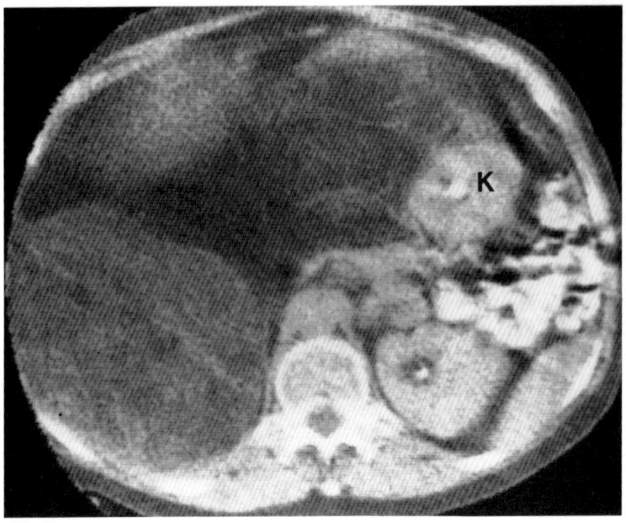

A

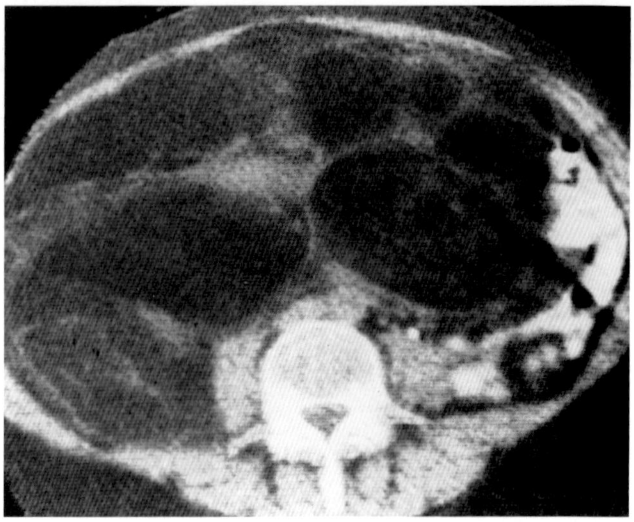

B

Figure 16.4

Retroperitoneal liposarcoma.

A CT reveals a large retroperitoneal mass of heterogeneous density. Some fat is apparent. The right kidney (K) is displaced across the midline to the left.

B CT scan at a different level now reveals the tumor to be composed primarily of fat. Liposarcomas frequently have no discernable fat on CT. The presence of an abundant non-fatty component militates against a benign lipoma.

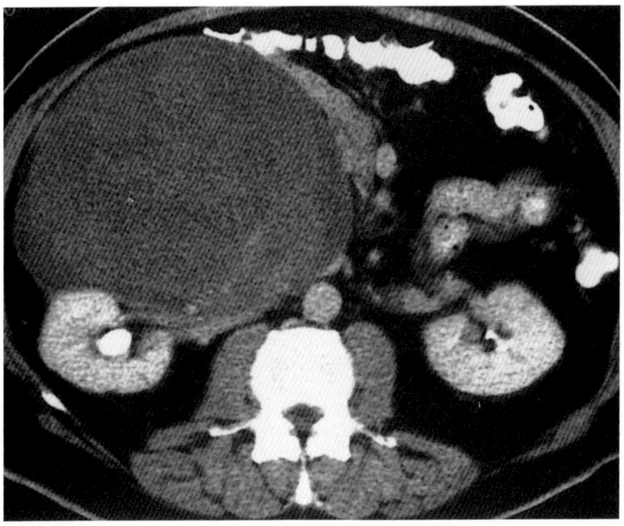

Figure 16.5

Retroperitoneal liposarcoma. There is no evidence of fat within the mass on this CT, in contrast to Figure 16.4.

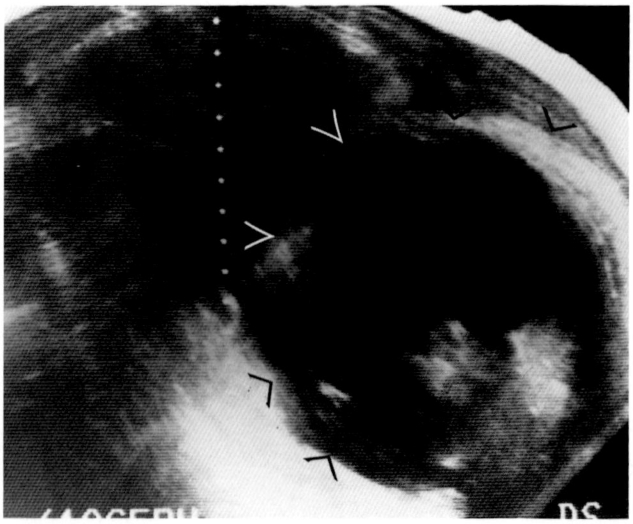

Figure 16.6

Retroperitoneal malignant mesenchymoma. Ultrasonography reveals a large complex abdominal mass (arrowheads); extensive cystic degeneration was present, accounting for the complex nature of the tumor.

for CT.[3] US can often provide adequate anatomic detail, but it is limited by bowel gas in 15–30% of patients.[15] When a mass can be clearly delineated by US, it is the most convenient way to provide guidance for percutaneous biopsy if one is to be carried out.

Magnetic resonance imaging

MR similarly delivers no ionizing radiation and requires no contrast. It offers the additional advantage of imaging in multiple planes, which can be helpful when planning resection of these large tumors. Sagittal or coronal views can sometimes establish the origin of a lesion that is unclear on CT.[16] MR is accurate in differentiating lipoma from liposarcoma (Figure 16.7).[13] It may become the diagnostic method of choice when accessibility and spatial resolution are improved, costs and imaging times are lowered, specific contrast agents are developed, and characteristics of individual tissue types are better quantified.

Benign tumors

Benign lesions constitute less than 20% of tumors in most series. The majority are stromal neoplasms and cysts (Figure 16.8, Table 16.1). Retroperitoneal cysts are classified as urogenital, lymphatic, teratomatous, mesocolic, parasitic or traumatic in origin.[17]

Urogenital cysts arise from persistent wolffian remnants and are more common in females. They can be differentiated from mesocolic cysts by the relation of the cyst to the spermatic vessels in men; mesocolic cysts must be anterior to the vessels and urogenital cysts posterior.[2] Teratomas and dermoid cysts are most commonly seen in children, and while they usually originate in the gonads or anterior mediastinum, 5% have been reported to be retroperitoneal (Figure 16.3). Ten to twenty-five per cent are malignant. It is often difficult to determine which tumors are benign and which are not.[7] The histologic evaluation of these tumors is difficult, therefore a benign report must be taken with caution. This is especially true for lipomas, which frequently harbor sarcomatous foci in the midst of an otherwise bland neoplasm.

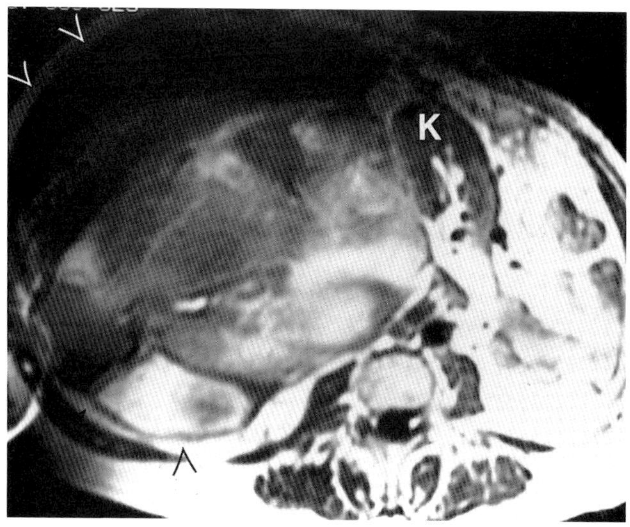

A

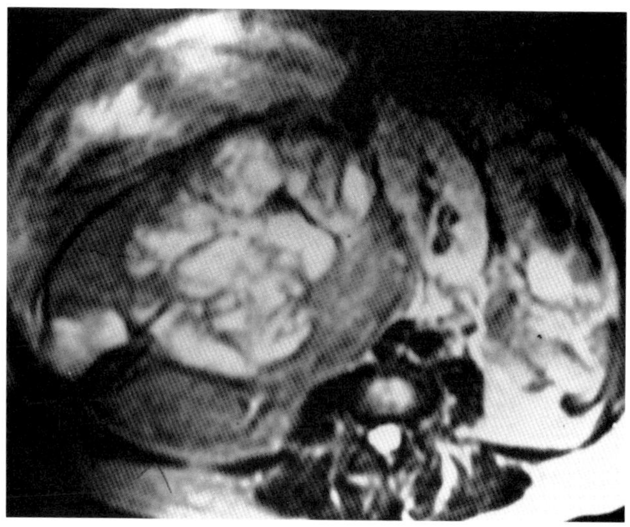

B

Figure 16.7

Retroperitoneal liposarcoma.

A T1-weighted spin-echo MR (TR 600/TE 25; 1.5 tesla). A huge retroperitoneal mass is seen (arrowheads). The signal is heterogeneous, however, and only a small dorsal portion of the lesion has the typical signal of fat. Note the transabdominal displacement of the right kidney (K).

B T2-weighted image (TR 2500/TE 80). High signal in the center of the neoplasm indicates fluid secondary to hemorrhage or cystic degeneration.

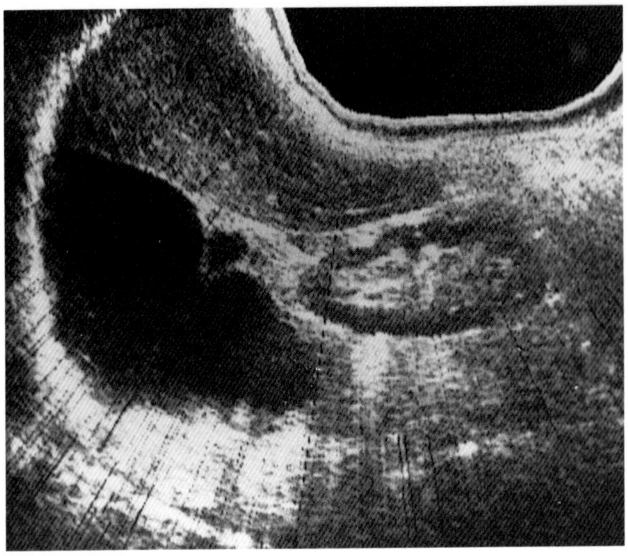

Figure 16.8

Retroperitoneal cyst. Above the right adrenal gland and behind the liver a large retroperitoneal cyst is seen by ultrasonography. The cyst was benign and lined by simple flattened epithelium.

Table 16.1 Pathology of 110 benign retroperitoneal tumors.[2,3,5–7]

Tissue type	*Total tumors*
Cystic	30
Lipoma	20
Neural	19
Fibroma	10
Leiomyoma	8
Xanthogranuloma	7
Pheochromocytoma	7
Teratoma	2
Lymphangioma	2
Hemangioma	2
Mesothelioma	2
Cystadenoma	1

Malignant tumors

About 85% of retroperitoneal tumors are malignant. Liposarcomas are the most common (Table 16.2). The sarcomas are a diverse histologic group, as malignant tumors can arise from any of the mesenchymal tissues found in the retroperitoneum (Figures 16.5 and 16.9). Only about 15% of sarcomas in the retroperitoneum are primary, the majority occurring in the extremities.[18–20] The most common retroperitoneal sarcomas are liposarcoma, leiomyosarcoma and fibrosarcoma, which comprise over half of the total. It is worth noting that the proportion of rhabdomyosarcomas in a given series is a function of the number of children in that center's referral base, since it is primarily a pediatric tumor. No other single tumor contributes a significant proportion to the total.

The neural tumors are a collection of several rare lesions including malignant schwannoma, chemodectoma, chordoma, malignant ganglioneuroma and paraganglioma. Most authors do not include extra-adrenal neuroblastomas in retroperitoneal sarcomas. Approximately one-third of neural tumors in the retroperitoneum arise from the sympathetic chain.[21] Malignant schwannomas develop in 5–15% of patients with neurofibromatosis.[22] Malignant fibrous histiocytoma comprised 21% of retroperitoneal sarcomas in a recent series in which all available pathologic specimens were reviewed,[23] and approximately 15% occur in the retroperitoneum.[24] It has been cited as the most common sarcoma overall in the elderly. The vascular tumors of the retroperitoneum include hemangiopericytomas, lymphangiosarcoma and angiosarcoma.

Table 16.2 Histology of retroperitoneal sarcomas.[2–7,9,11,23,26]

Tissue type	*Total tumors*	*(%)*
Liposarcoma	232	26.2
Leiomyosarcoma	191	21.6
Fibrosarcoma	112	12.6
Rhabdomyosarcoma	65	7.3
Neural sarcomas	65	7.3
Malignant fibrous histocytoma	38	4.3
Vascular sarcomas	20	2.2
Undifferentiated	98	11.1
All other types	64	7.2
Total	885	100.0

Malignant fibrous histocytoma is underrepresented in older series; in more recent series, it has accounted for up to 20% of retroperitoneal tumors.

Sarcomas have a diverse histopathology, ranging from well-differentiated neoplasms of which the primary question is whether the tumor is benign or malignant, to bizarre pleomorphic lesions in which even the basic cell type is uncertain. Both a grading system that subdivides lesions primarily on the presence or absence of necrosis in the specimen,[20] and a staging protocol have been proposed (Table 16.3).[18,23] Necrosis has been shown to correlate positively with time to recurrence, overall survival and survival after the first recurrence. The TMN classification classifies all T3 lesions as stage IV disease. This system also includes assessment of lymph-node status, which has rarely been reported in the literature probably because the size of these tumors makes a systematic search for nodal tissue difficult. There is a clear relationship between stage of disease and survival rates.

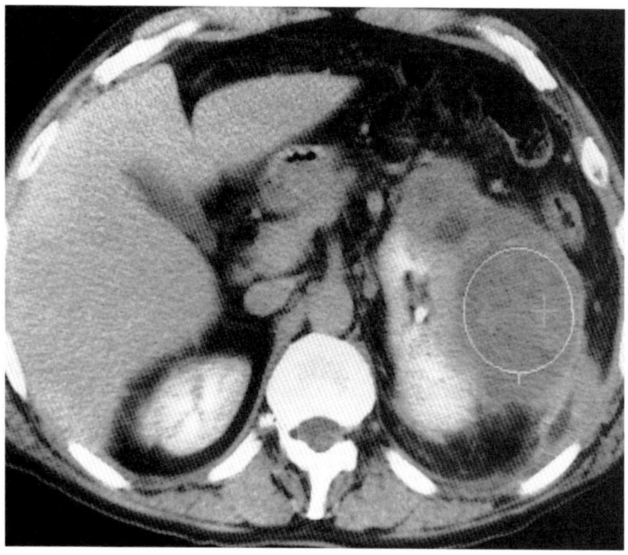

A

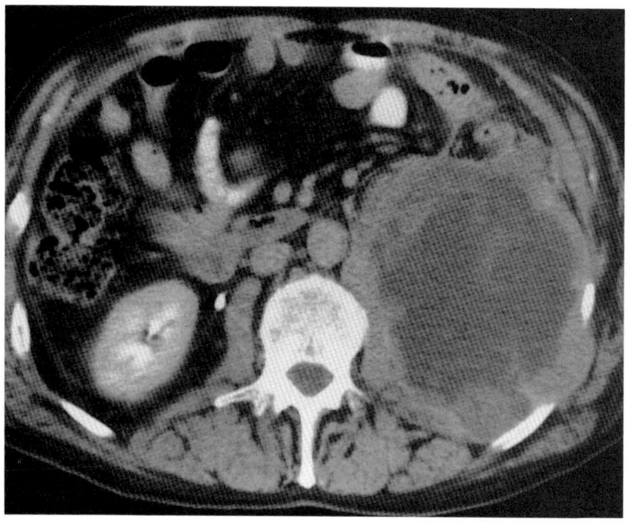

B

Figure 16.9

Retroperitoneal rhabdomyosarcoma (46-year-old male).

A On CT scan the lesion appears to involve the left kidney. At surgery, however, there was no renal involvement, although the two structures were contiguous.

B A scan at a more caudal level reveals extensive necrosis replacing most of the center of the tumor.

Table 16.3 Retroperitoneal sarcoma staging system.[18,23]

Stage	
I	G1 T1–2 N0 M0
II	G2 T1–2 N0 M0
III	G3 T1–2 N0 M0; any G, T1–2 N1 M0
IV	any G, T3, and N M0; any T, any N M1
Grade (G)	
GX	Grade cannot be assessed
G1	Lowest
G2	Intermediate
G3	Intermediate
G4	Highest
Primary tumor (T)	
TX	Primary tumor cannot be assessed
T1	Primary tumor <5 cm in greatest dimension
T2	Primary tumor ⩾5 cm in greatest dimension
T3	Primary tumor grossly invading bone, major vessels, major nerves or extensively infiltrating with fixation
Regional lymph nodes (N)	
NX	Regional lymph nodes cannot be assessed
N0	No regional node involvement
N1	Regional lymph node metastases
Metastatic disease (M)	
MX	Presence of distant metastases cannot be assessed
M0	No distant metastases
M1	Distant metastases

Treatment

Complete surgical excision offers patients with retroperitoneal sarcomas the best chance for long-term survival, but recurrent disease remains a problem. Unfortunately, complete resection of gross disease is possible in only 50–60% of patients.[11,23,25] Overall 5-year survival ranges from 25 to 40%,[4,11,23,26] with a 10-year survival of 22%.[23] However, a 54–70% 5-year survival has been reported for patients in whom complete removal of gross tumor is possible.[4,23]

Both radiation and chemotherapy have been advocated as adjuvant measures,[11,27] but conclusive evidence of their effectiveness is lacking.[23]

Other tumors

Primary germ-cell tumors

Primary retroperitoneal germ-cell tumors are rare. In fact, it can be argued that some are not primary at all but rather metastatic deposits from occult or 'burned-out' testicular primaries.[28] Any male with a retroperitoneal germ-cell tumor suspected of being primary should undergo testicular imaging (US or MR) and should undergo orchiectomy if a suspicious lesion is found. Seminoma is the most common extragonadal germ-cell tumor, and is ordinarily quite radiosensitive.

Malignant retroperitoneal fibrosis

Approximately 10% of patients with retroperitoneal fibrosis will have associated malignancy underlying the fibrotic process[29] (Figure 16.10). There are several ways in which the association may occur:

- by infiltration from lymph node metastases or lymphoma,
- by infiltration from periureteral metastases,
- by direct extension from primary retroperitoneal tumors,
- by hormonal or serotonin effect associated with appendiceal carcinoid,
- by benign idiopathic retroperitoneal fibrosis in patients with localized or metastatic tumor elsewhere in the body.[30]

At the time of clinical presentation the existence of a primary carcinoma may or may not be known. Extensive biopsies are indicated at the time of exploration and ureterolysis. Even then, biopsies may give a negative result on the first occasion, only to reveal infiltrating cancer cells on subsequent examination.

Lymphoma and lymph-node metastases

In most instances, retroperitoneal lymphomas are an expression of systemic disease and thus should be considered separately from other retroperitoneal neoplasms.[7] These tumors are also

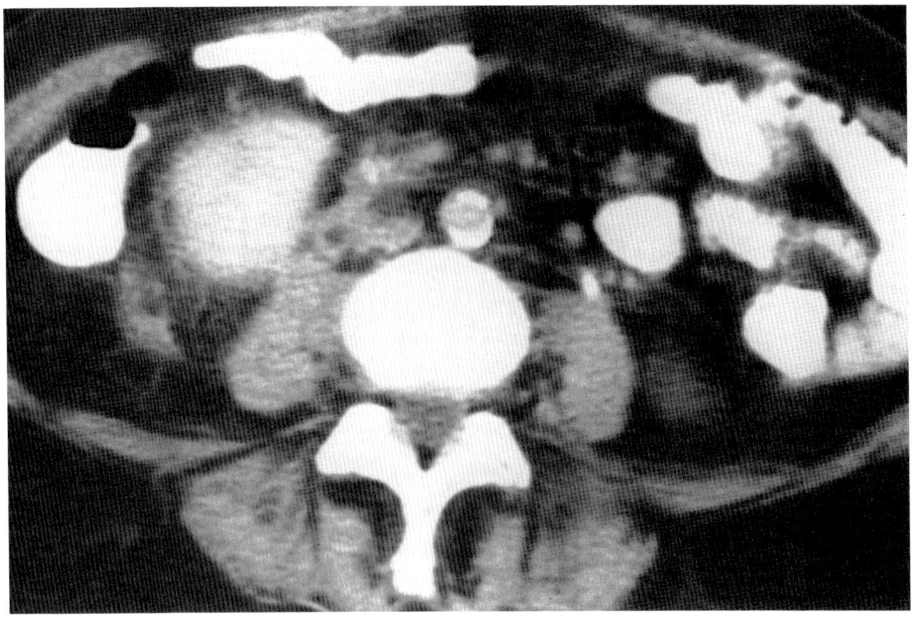

A

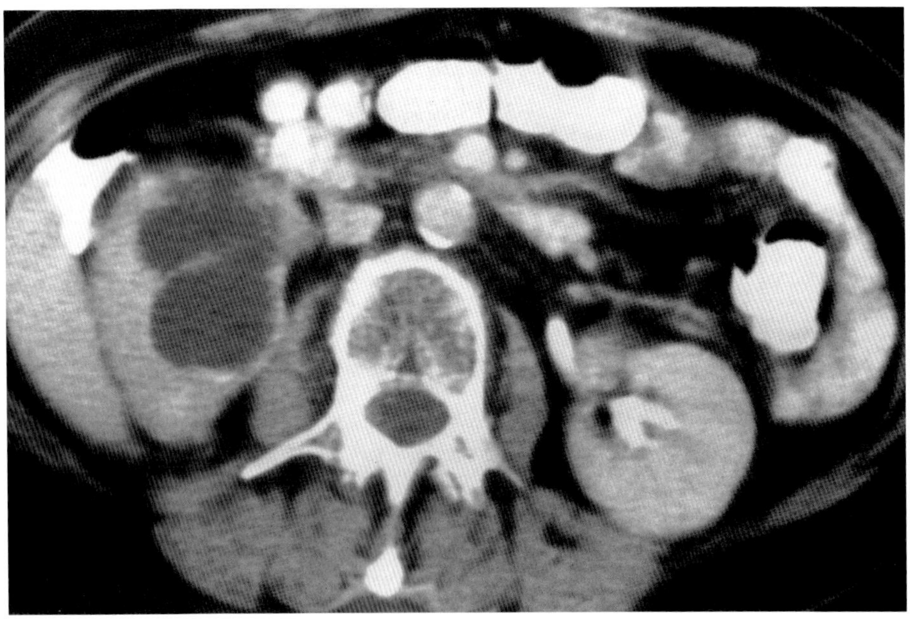

B

Figure 16.10

Malignant retroperitoneal fibrosis.

A This 46-year-old female had carcinoma of the breast. CT reveals periureteral soft tissue infiltrate entrapping right ureter. The ureter is dilated. Biopsy revealed primarily fibrous tissue with occasional foci of malignant cells.

B A scan at more cranial level reveals severe right hydronephrosis.

radio- and chemosensitive, and surgery is primarily undertaken for diagnosis and staging. Any patient with a large retroperitoneal mass should undergo careful examination for peripheral adenopathy before laparotomy is contemplated.

Rarely are isolated retroperitoneal lymph node metastases sufficiently large as to be confused with primary retroperitoneal neoplasms, but we have seen a few patients with carcinoma of the prostate in whom this was true. In these patients, the true nature of the metastases is usually evident by the distribution of the disease, especially as viewed on CT scans, but the site of the primary tumor may not be known immediately. In several of our patients, both the digital rectal examination and transrectal US were thought to be normal, but the level of prostatic specific antigen was invariably elevated.

References

1. Wheatley JK, Retroperitoneal fibrosis, tumors and cysts. In: Glen F, ed, *Urologic surgery*, 3rd edn. (JB Lippincott: Philadelphia 1983) 391–403.
2. Pack GT, Tabah EJ, Primary retroperitoneal tumors: a study of 120 cases, *Surg Gynecol Obstet* (1954) **99**:209–31, 313–14.
3. Pinson CW, Remine SG, Fletcher WS, Braasch JW, Long-term results with primary retroperitoneal tumors, *Arch Surg* (1989) **124**:1168.
4. McGrath PC, Neifeld JP, Lawrence W Jr, et al, Improved survival following complete excision of retroperitoneal sarcomas, *Ann Surg* (1984) **200**:200.
5. Braasch JW, Mon AB, Primary retroperitoneal tumors, *Surg Clin N Am* (1967) **47**:663.
6. Duncan RE, Evans AT, Diagnosis of primary retroperitoneal tumors, *J Urol* (1977) **117**:19–23.
7. Felix EL, Wood DK, DasGupta TK, Tumors of the retroperitoneum, *Curr Prob Cancer* (1981) **6**:3.
8. Damascelli B, Musumeci R, Botture M, et al, Angiography of retroperitoneal tumors: a review, *AJR* (1975) **125**:565.
9. Storm FK, Eilber FR, Mirra J, Morton DL, Retroperitoneal sarcomas: a reappraisal of treatment, *J Surg Oncol* (1981) **17**:1.
10. Stephens DH, Sheedy PF II, Hattery RR, Williamson B Jr, Diagnosis and evaluation of retroperitoneal tumors by computed tomography, *AJR* (1977) **129**:395.
11. Cody HS III, Turnbull AD, Fortner JG, Hajdu SI, The grading of soft tissue sarcomas: results of clinico-histopathologic correlation in a series of 163 cases, *Cancer* (1984) **53**:530.
12. Patel SK, Retroperitoneal tumors and cysts. In: Pollack HM, ed, *Clinical urography: an atlas and textbook of urological imaging* (WB Saunders: Philadelphia 1990).
13. Dooms GC, Hricak H, Sollitto RA, Higgins CB, Lipomatous tumors with fatty component: MR imaging potential and comparison of MR and CT results, *Radiology* (1985) **157**:479.
14. Lane RH, Stephens DH, Reiman HM, Primary retroperitoneal neoplasms: CT findings in 90 cases with clinical and pathologic correlation, *AJR* (1989) **152**:83.
15. Lindel MM Jr, Wallace S, de Santos LA, et al, Diagnostic techniques for the evaluation of soft-tissue sarcomas, *Semin Oncol* (1981) **8**:160.
16. Guz BV, Wood DP Jr, Montie JE, Pontes JE, Retroperitoneal nerve sheath tumors: the Cleveland Clinic Experience, *J Urol* (1989) **142**:1434–7.
17. Lahey FH, Eckerson EB, Retroperitoneal cysts, *Ann Surg* (1934) **100**:231.
18. Russell WO, Cohen J, Enzinger F, et al, A clinical and pathological staging system for soft tissue sarcomas, *Cancer* (1977) **40**:1562.
19. Abbas SJ, Holyoke ED, Moore R, Karakusis CP, The surgical treatment and outcome of soft-tissue sarcoma, *Arch Surg* (1981) **116**:765.
20. Costa J, Wesley RA, Glatstein E, Rosenberg SA, The grading of soft tissue sarcomas: results of clinico-histopathologic correlation in a series of 163 cases, *Cancer* (1984) **43**:530.
21. Duckett JW, Koop CE, Neuroblastoma, *Urol Clin Am* (1977) **4**:285.
22. Antoniades J, Malignant schwannoma. In: Antoniades J, ed, *Uncommon malignant tumours* (Masson: New York 1982) 245–50.
23. Dalton RR, Donohue JH, Mucha P, et al, Management of retroperitoneal sarcomas, *Surgery* (1989) **106**:725.
24. Weiss SW, Enzinger FM, Malignant fibrous histiocytoma: an analysis of 200 cases, *Cancer* (1978) **41**:2250.
25. Zhang G, Chen KK, Manivel C, Fraley EE, Sarcomas of the retroperitoneum and genitourinary tract, *J Urol* (1989) **141**:1107–10.
26. Karakousis CP, Velez AF, Emrich LJ, Management of retroperitoneal sarcomas and patient survival, *Am J Surg* (1985) **100**:376.
27. Harrison LB, Guterrez E, Fischer JJ, Retroperitoneal sarcomas: the Yale experience and a review of the literature, *J Surg Oncol* (1986) **32**:159.
28. Bohle A, Studer UE, Stonntag RW, Scheigedder JR, Primary or secondary extragonadal germ cell tumors, *J Urol* (1986) **135**:939.
29. Wagenknecht LV, Hardy JC, Value of various treatments for retroperitoneum fibrosis, *Eur Urol* (1981) **7**:193–200.
30. Lepor M, Walsh PC, Idiopathic retroperitoneal fibrosis, *J Urol* (1979) **122**:1–6.

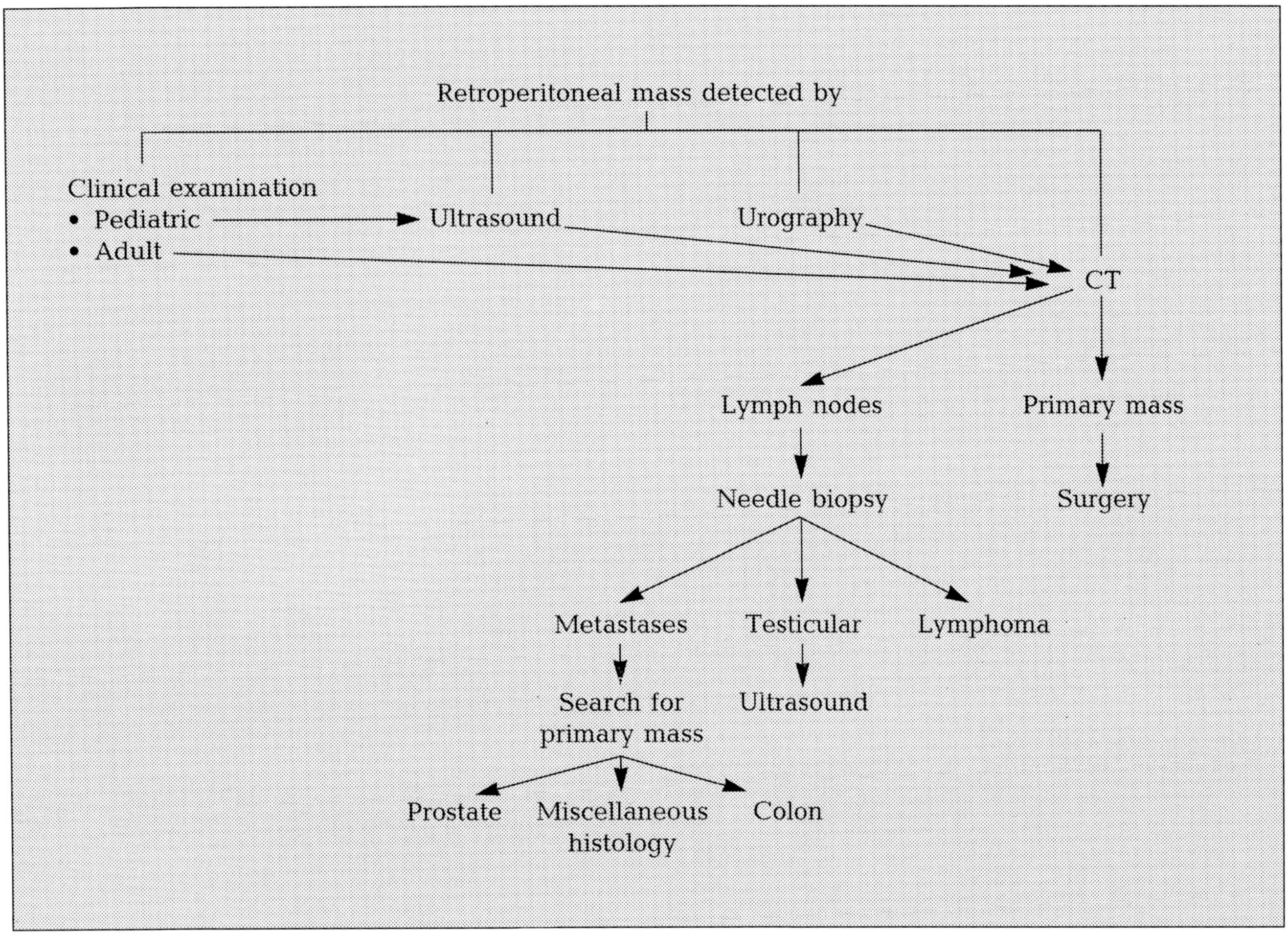

Diagram 16.1

Imaging strategy on detection of a retroperitoneal mass.

17

The female pelvis

Jacques Masselot, Philippe Soyer and Guy Michel

Introduction

A wide range of techniques in diagnostic imaging of the female pelvis is available, each having its advantages. MRI and transrectal or transvaginal ultrasound (TRUS, TVUS) raise the possibility of modifying the imaging strategies for genital tumors in the female. The purpose of this chapter is to present basic concepts in imaging strategies for the staging and follow up of genital tumors in the female.

Techniques

Hysterography

For a long time, hysterography was the sole method for the diagnosis and staging of genital tumors in females. Recent developments have improved the accuracy of tumor staging, and nowadays, hysterography is rarely indicated.

Intravenous urography

Intravenous urography (IVU) permits an appraisal of the repercussions of tumor extent on the upper urinary tract and the bladder, since obstruction of ducts in the urinary tract for the extent of the tumor worsens the prognosis. After plain abdominal radiography, a film is produced 4 min after injection. If no obvious opacification is observed at the 10th minute after IVU, we believe that the distention will be more rapidly confirmed by ultrasound.

Lymphography

Bilateral lymphography explores the para-aortic, primitive and external iliac lymph-node chains. Lymphography, which detects metastases in normal-sized lymph nodes, is the most accurate method and must be performed if the diagnosis of metastases has a therapeutic incidence. In a retrospective study,[1] the sensitivity of lymphography was 45% and the specificity 92% in the detection of lymph-node metastases of endometrial carcinoma.

Chest radiography

Chest radiography is performed to look for thoracic metastases. In the setting of suspected carcinoma, we systemically perform anteroposterior and lateral films.

Computed tomography

Patients receive oral contrast medium to outline the small bowel. A tampon can be used to outline the vagina. In some cases, an iodine enema can be useful to delineate precisely the rectosigmoid. CT slices are carried out during intravenous bolus administration of contrast medium followed by drip infusion. Contrast enhancement differentiates lymph nodes from vascular structures. CT explores both pelvis and abdomen with contiguous slices. In suspected ovarian carcinoma, the abdominal survey is performed from the iliac crests to the dome of the diaphragm in 10 mm slices. In suspected uterine carcinoma, the abdominal survey is performed from the iliac crests to the renal pedicules in 10–15 mm slices. In all cases, the pelvic survey is performed from the iliac crests to the pubic symphysis in 10 mm contiguous slices.

Ultrasonography

Ultrasonography (US) provides an evaluation of genital tumors in detection, in assessment at initial presentation and in assessing the presence of residual, recurrent or progressive disease after therapy. Real-time scanners equipped with a 3.5 or 5.0 MHz sector transducer are utilized. In some cases, TVUS is performed using a 5.0 MHz curved linear transducer which provides a better anatomical approach.[2] US explores the area of the liver, the kidneys, the retroperitoneal space, the pelvis and the pelvic lymph nodes with a fully distended urinary bladder. For ovarian neoplasms, particular attention is focused on Douglas' pouch, small bowel mesentery, the right paracolic gutter, the liver surface and the diaphragmatic domes which are frequent regions of secondary implantation. High-frequency linear transducers permit location of small subcapsular hypoechoic metastases.

Radiolabelled monoclonal antibodies

Considerable improvements have been achieved in antibody targeting, as a result of the discovery of monoclonal antibodies.[3] Radioimmunoscintigraphy allows detection and localization of metastases with an isotopically labelled tumor-specific monoclonal antibody.[4] Iodine-131 or indium-111 labelled monoclonal antibodies directed against the HMFG antigen[5] and CA 125 antigen[6] present in ovarian cancers permit imaging of tumor and metastases. This technique provides a total-body exploration but has a low sensitivity.

Magnetic resonance imaging

The examinations are carried out on patients in the supine position, with a half-full distended bladder and vaginal tampon. Rectal air insufflation and intravenous injection of glucagon can be helpful. T1- and T2-weighted images are performed with 5–10 mm thick contiguous slices. T1-weighted images are useful for searching for parametrial and vesical extension, and for identifying adenopathy. T2-weighted images are useful for analysing the uterine cervix and identifying tumoral structures. The axial plane permits the delineation of the lateral walls of the bladder, parametrium, vagina and ovary, and is of particular interest in searching for adenopathy.[7] The sagittal plane shows the uterine body and the cervix, and allows an assessment of rectal and vesical extension. The coronal plane shows the ovary and parametrium. Usually we perform T1-weighted images in the axial and T2-weighted images in the sagittal plane. The injection of gadolinium-DTPA can be helpful in differentiating tumor from intrauterine fluid retention.

Ovarian carcinoma

Epidemiology

Carcinoma of the ovary is the fifth most common cancer in females in the USA, 4% of all female cancers. It accounts for 6% of cancer deaths in females. Two-thirds of ovarian neoplasms are found in females of between 20 and 65 years of age.

Classification

Ovarian neoplasms are classified into (a) epithelial tumors accounting for 85% of ovarian cancers (serous, mucinous and clear-cell adenocarcinomas are in this category); (b) sex-cord stromal tumors; (c) lipid-cell tumors; (d) germ-cell tumors, which includes dysgerminomas, and (e) unclassified or miscellaneous tumors.

Mode of dissemination[8]

Epithelial tumors have a transcelomic spread and metastasize in the paracolic gutters, the undersurface of the diaphragm, the omentum (30%) and the surface of the peritoneal cavity. Pelvic and periaortic lymph nodes are involved in 50% of advanced stages. Germ-cell tumors have an elective lymphatic dissemination. Extensive involvement of the lymphatic channels of the diaphragm results in ascites. Dysgerminomas extend to the contralateral ovary. Blood-borne metastases are rare. At initial staging, only 1% of the patients have liver metastases.[9] At the time of death metastases are found in the liver, lung and bone in 34, 27 and 14% of patients, respectively.

Staging[10,11]

The standard staging system for ovarian neoplasms is based on surgical examination. Surgical staging consists of biopsies of the diaphragm, pelvic and periaortic lymph nodes and paracolic gutters. The usual classification is the one specified by the International Federation of Gynecology and Obstetrics (FIGO) which has been recently modified (Table 17.1).

Table 17.1 FIGO classification of ovarian carcinoma.

Stage	I	Growth limited to the ovaries
	Ia	Unilateral tumor
	Ib	Bilateral tumor; no ascites containing malignant cells
Stage	II	Growth involving one or both ovaries with pelvic extension
Stage	III	Presence of intraperitoneal metastases outside the pelvis or positive retroperitoneal node involvement; extension to small bowel or omentum
Stage	IV	Distant metastases

Prognosis

The overall 5-year survival for all stages and all histological types of ovarian neoplasms is about 30%. Stage is an important prognostic factor: for the stages I, II, III and IV, the overall 5-year survival rates are 70, 55, 14 and 4% respectively. Ascites, positive peritoneal washing and advanced age are correlated with a poor prognosis.

Imaging features

The main role of imaging techniques in ovarian malignancies is to detect an ovarian mass. Diagnosis and staging are usually confirmed by laparotomy. In ovarian malignancies, radiological examinations have a major role to play in follow up, evaluation of tumor response to therapy and assessment of recurrence.

Ultrasonography

The use of conventional US for the evaluation of pelvic masses is well established. US is a suitable examination for a first evaluation of pelvic masses. A functional solitary adnexal cyst is the most common diagnosis in pre-menopausal women with ovarian mass. These lesions are purely anechoic,

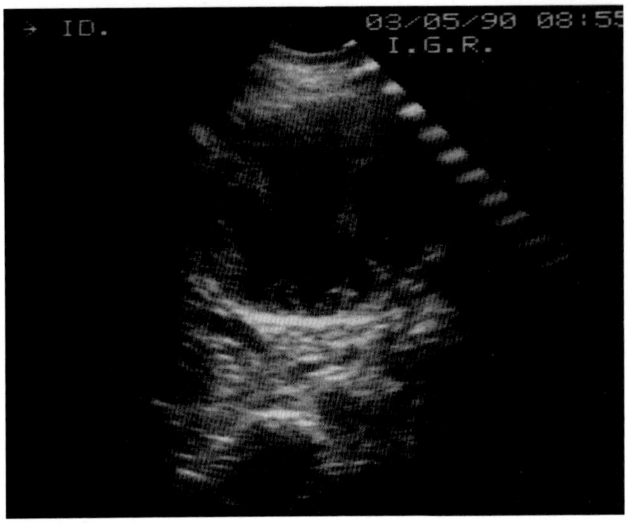

Figure 17.1

Ovarian epithelial carcinoma. US shows internal-wall thickening, solid and fluid elements.

well delineated, less than 3 cm in size and are not present on a subsequent study.

Many characteristics have been described to permit a distinction between benign and malignant tumors. This distinction is of particular interest in small tumors in young women to avoid surgical procedure for functional cysts. In a retrospective study,[12] criteria of benignity were: (a) unilaterality, found in 89% of benign tumors; (b) thin wall, in 55%; (c) purely anechoic simple cyst, in 26% and (d) calcification, in 11%. Criteria of malignancy (Figure 17.1) were (a) echogenicity, found in 94.5% of malignant tumors; (b) size more 5 cm, in 89%; (c) internal-wall thickening and solid elements, in 72.5%; (d) ascites, in 38.5% and (e) metastases, in 25%.

In many cases, US is technically difficult or uncertain (retroverted uterus, underlying obesity). TVUS is of particular interest in allowing an accurate analysis of ovarian structures,[13] in the evaluation of the unilateral enlarged ovary and diagnosis of cul-de-sac pelvic side-wall implants from ovarian carcinoma.

Computed tomography

CT findings obtained during bolus injection of contrast media are the same as those obtained during US[14] (Figure 17.2). Except for functional cysts, which are diagnosed by US, all ovarian tumors are surgically explored. The main goal of CT before surgical procedure is in planning Pfannenstiel's surgical procedure if CT can show probable benignity, instead of a large medial approach.

Magnetic resonance imaging

MR findings are similar to those obtained with CT (Figure 17.2). Because of the inherent inaccuracies of clinical staging of ovarian carcinoma, MR has been suggested as an additional method of staging. But as surgical exploration is systematically performed for each ovarian tumor, neither MR nor CT is of real interest in initial staging.

Extent

The radiologic assessment of the extent of the tumor is quite different for dysgerminomas and common epithelial carcinomas.

The diagnosis of dysgerminomas[15] is confirmed at laparotomy. Dissemination when present is

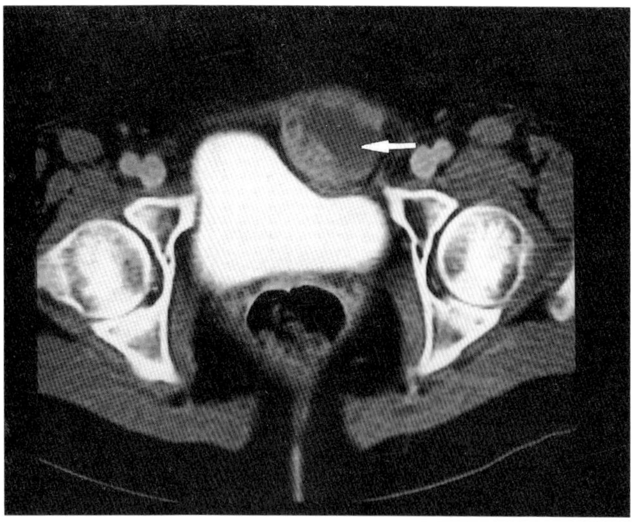

A

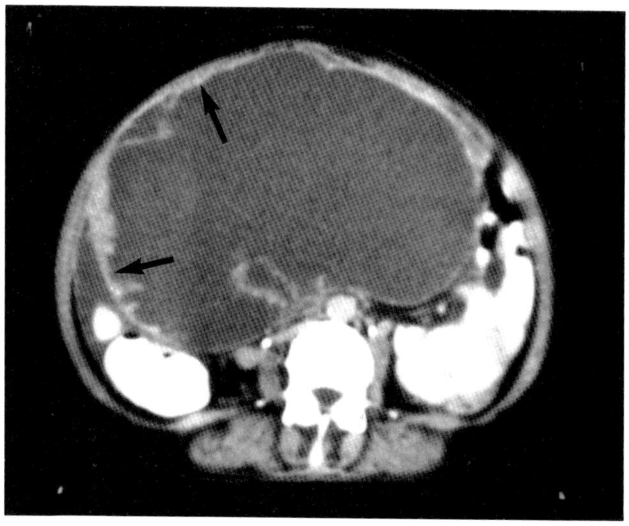

B

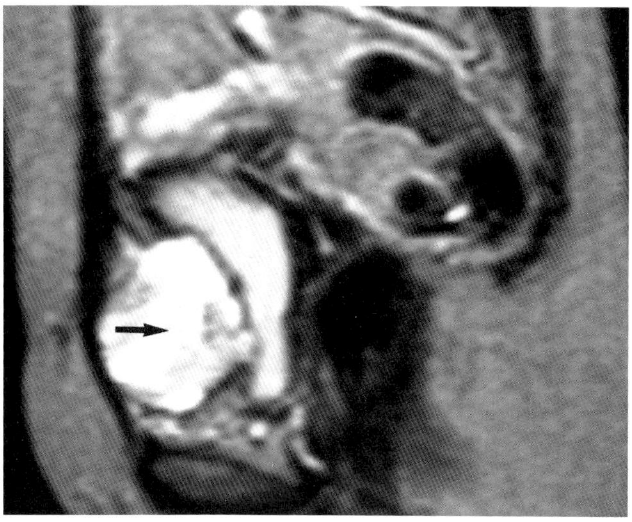

C

Figure 17.2

Ovarian epithelial carcinoma.

A CT scan during intravenous bolus injection shows mixed ovarian tumor with high and low density areas (arrow).

B CT scan during intravenous bolus injection shows extensive abdominal mass with well-defined margins. The walls of the mass are highly enhanced (arrows).

C T2-weighted MR images (SE: 2000/90) in sagittal plane shows mixed ovarian tumor with high and low signal-intensity areas (arrow). MR offers no more information than CT.

primarily via the lymphatics. Dysgerminomas are radiocurable, and therefore radiation therapy is the primary treatment modality. These tumors have a good prognosis; 75% of the patients have their tumor cured by initial treatment. A lymphography is systematically performed for planning radiation therapy.

In the diagnosis of common epithelial carcinomas, conventional radiography is still of interest, plain chest radiography reveals lung metastases and IVU assesses urinary tract distension.

Ultrasound easily depicts liver metastases, which are rare, ascites and cystic peritoneal metastases. With the use of high-frequency linear transducers, US can show peritoneal nodules on the liver surface. However, a normal examination with high-resolution transducers cannot rule out peritoneal carcinosis. It is often impossible to analyse the retroperitoneal space by US, and US is not the procedure of choice for the assessment of lymph-node involvement. US evaluates the distension of the upper urinary tract. We consider that, in comparison with US, TRUS is of no interest in the assessment of local extent.

CT can identify small foci of liver metastases and subdiaphragmatic tumor nodules.[16] The space between the abdominal wall and the lateral surface of the liver is not encroached on by small bowel loops and can be well evaluated using CT. In the presence of ascites, CT is a good useful technique and can detect peritoneal implants. Peritoneal metastases can be rounded or ill-defined masses. But carcinomatosis is the most difficult manifestation of the disease to detect by CT,[17] with a sensitivity of only 8% before a second-look operation.[16] The major drawback of CT is its incapacity to detect nodules of less than 1 cm in size,[18] except when they are calcified.

MR cannot depict peritoneal metastases and has no interest in the evaluation of ascites in a clinical setting. MR can be helpful in the evaluation of hepatic metastases.

Table 17.2 Classification of uterine carcinoma by histologic differentiation.

G1	5% or less with non-squamous or non-morular solid growth pattern
G2	6–50% with non-squamous or non-morular solid growth pattern
G3	More than 50% with non-squamous or non-morular solid growth pattern

Uterine carcinoma

Epidemiology

Carcinoma of the uterine corpus is the most common invasive cancer of the female genital tract and the third most frequent cancer in women in the USA. In France it is the second most frequent invasive cancer in women after breast cancer.

There is a causal relationship between estrogens administered exogenously and endometrial cancer. Similarly, endogenous hyperstrinism (Stein–Leventhal syndrome, obesity) increases the risk of developing endometrial cancer.

Typically, endometrial cancer occurs in postmenopausal (80% of cases) obese women, often those on estrogen therapy. Sixty per cent of these women are between 65 and 75 years old.

Classification

Endometrial carcinomas constitute 90% of carcinomas of the uterine corpus. They are classified into (a) adenocarcinomas which are the most frequent, (b) adenoacanthomas, and (c) adenosquamous carcinomas. The remaining 10% are sarcomas. Carcinomas are classified[11] according to the degree of histologic differentiation (Table 17.2).

Mode of dissemination

Endometrial carcinomas can disseminate by:

- direct extension to adjacent structures such as the myometrium, serosal surface of the uterus, peritoneal cavity, cervix, parametrium and vagina;
- through the lymphatic system from the uterus, along ovarian or uterine blood vessels to the aortic or precaval nodes and to the hypogastric lymph nodes, respectively;
- via the hematogenous route to the lung, liver and bone.

Lymph-node metastases are frequent, commonly the pelvic lymph nodes. Hematogenous metastases are rare.[8] In contrast, uterine sarcomas rarely have nodal metastases but frequently have blood-borne metastases.

Staging

The standard staging system for endometrial carcinoma is based on the clinical examination. Clinical staging consists of a pelvic examination to assess cervical, vaginal and parametrial spread. Endoscopic examination includes cystoscopy and sigmoidscopy. Histologic assessment includes the histologic differentiation of tumor, and assessment of the extent of uterine invasion and cervical involvement.

The staging of endometrial carcinoma is based on the recommendations of the FIGO[10,11] which has recently been updated to take into account lymph-node involvement (Table 17.3).

Table 17.3 FIGO staging of uterine carcinoma.

Stage	I	Carcinoma confined to corpus
	Ia	Tumor limited to endometrium
	Ib	Invasion to less than half of the myometrium
	Ic	Invasion to more than half of the myometrium
Stage	IIa	Endocervical glandular involvement only
	IIb	Cervical stromal invasion
Stage	IIIa	Tumor invades serosa and/or adnexa, and/or positive peritoneal cytology
	IIIb	Vaginal metastases
	IIIc	Metastases to pelvic and/or para-aortic lymph nodes
Stage	IVa	Tumor invasion of bladder and/or bowel mucosa
	IVb	Distant metastases including intra-abdominal and/or inguinal lymph nodes

Prognosis[19]

The main prognostic factors are as follows.

- The depth of myometrial penetration:[20] Patients with superficially invasive tumor have a 93.8% 5-year survival rate, while those with deeply invasive tumor have a 41% survival rate.
- Initial staging: the 5-year survival rates for stages I, II, III and IV are 80, 50, 30 and less than 10% respectively.
- Lymphatic involvement: only 2.8–10.0% of patients with stage I endometrial cancer have pelvic lymph node metastases.[21–23] Lymphatic involvement is closely interrelated with initial staging.

Imaging features

The main role of imaging in endometrial malignancies is to diagnose abnormalities in a post-menopausal woman referred for gynecologic bleeding. Histologic diagnosis is the most accurate in all cases, but MR can be helpful in the pre-operative assessment of myometrial invasion and during follow up.

Conventional radiography

For a long time, hysterography was performed because it was the only radiologic examination available for endometrial carcinomas. Tumors were shown as lacunae, but there was no information about the depth of myometrial penetration (Figure 17.3A). At present we prefer not to perform this examination for two reasons: (1) post-menopausal bleeding indicates cytological evaluation of exfoliated cells from the uterus, and biopsy or curettage, which make the diagnosis; and (2) US, MR and hysteroscopy provide better information than hysterography.

Ultrasonography

US is often performed for post-menopausal bleeding. Intrauterine fluid collection is a good sign of active carcinoma involving the uterine corpus, with a sensitivity of 94%.[24] Uterine fluid collections appear centrally with a high or low echogenicity compared with the myometrium. US can depict primitive tumor as a central intrauterine mass or as an eccentric mass invading the myometrium (Figure 17.3B). The accuracy of US in the evaluation of myometrial invasion is controversial, even though some studies have yielded good results.[25,26] The demonstration of a subendometrial halo is usually considered as superficial invasion. Unfor-

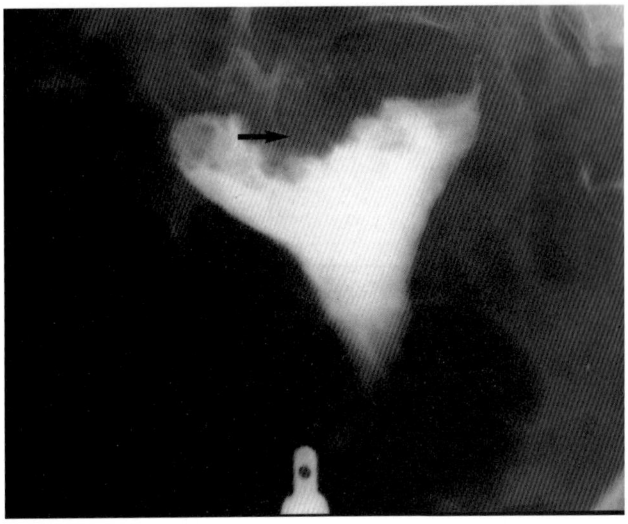

A

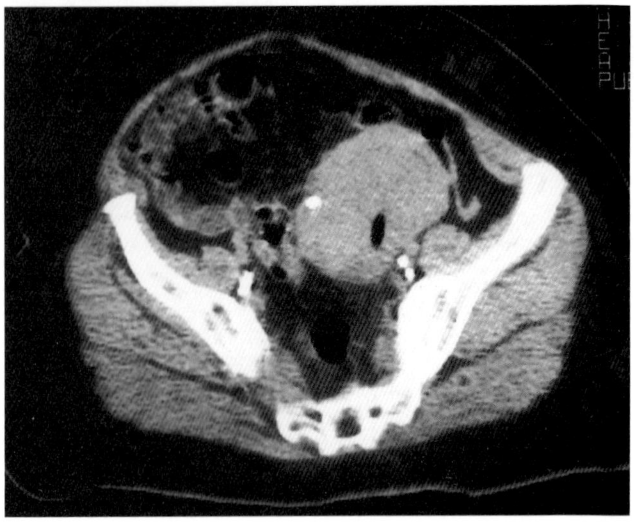

C

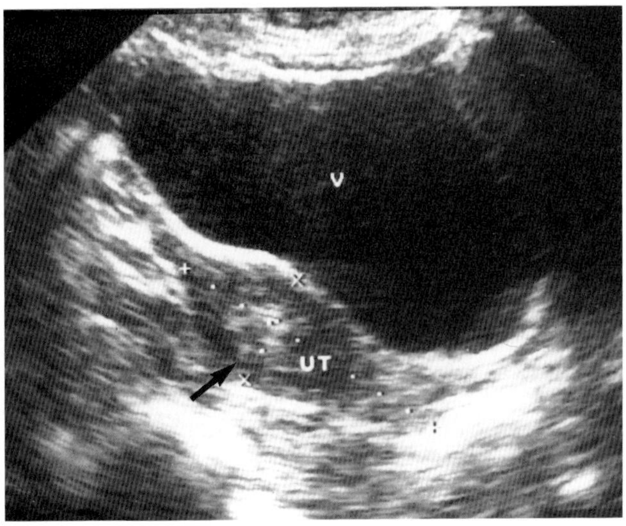

B

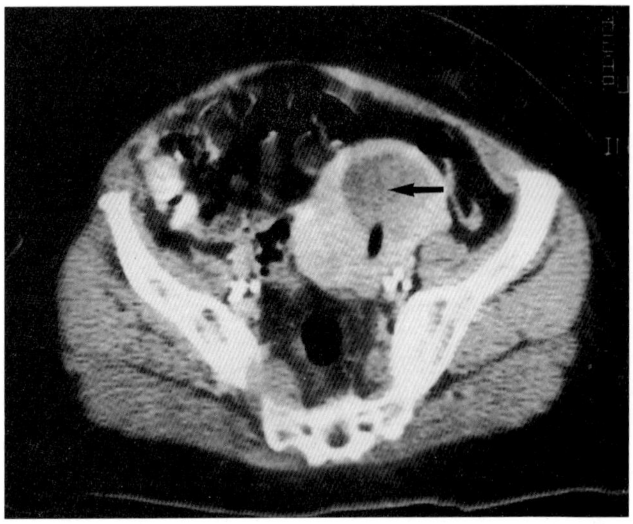

D

Figure 17.3

Endometrial carcinoma.

A Hysterography shows endometrial carcinoma as a lacuna with irregular margins (arrow).

B US in sagittal plane shows intrauterine hyperechoic mass, and the posterior extension into the myometrium (arrow).

C CT scan before bolus injection. The lesion is ill defined.

D CT scan during bolus injection shows endometrial tumor with well-defined margins (arrow). The lack of enhancement of the tumor permits assessment of the extent of myometrial involvement.

tunately, we have observed that the contiguity of the demarcating subendometrial halo can remain intact in patients with deeply invasive tumors. Furthermore, an overestimation of the depth of myometrial invasion occurs when a tumor has considerable intraluminal polypoid extension.

US is considered a front-line examination for uterine carcinoma.

Computed tomography

CT can depict primary tumor only if a sufficient volume alters the normal endometrium. Its accuracy in the assessment of the depth of myometrial invasion is controversial. We consider CT as unable to diagnose endometrial carcinoma confined to the uterus (stages I and II) on a precontrast examination (Figure 17.3C). However after intravenous injection of contrast medium, CT can demonstrate tumor involving one-third or more of the myometrium as hypodensity in a markedly enhanced myometrium[27] (Figure 17.3D). Nevertheless, in a prospective study carried out at the Institut Gustave-Roussy, such hypodensity was noticed in only 36% of cases. This is why we believe that CT cannot predict accurately the depth of myometrial invasion;[28] hypodense areas in the uterine corpus are non-specific CT findings (small carcinomas cannot usually be differentiated from retained blood in the uterine cavity).

As does US, CT depicts endometrial tumors as fluid-filled uterus due to tumor obstruction of the endocervical canal.

In conclusion, most of the time, CT is unable to add further information to that obtained with conventional clinical staging. Since surgery is the treatment of choice in stages I and III, we believe that CT is of no interest before staging laparotomy.

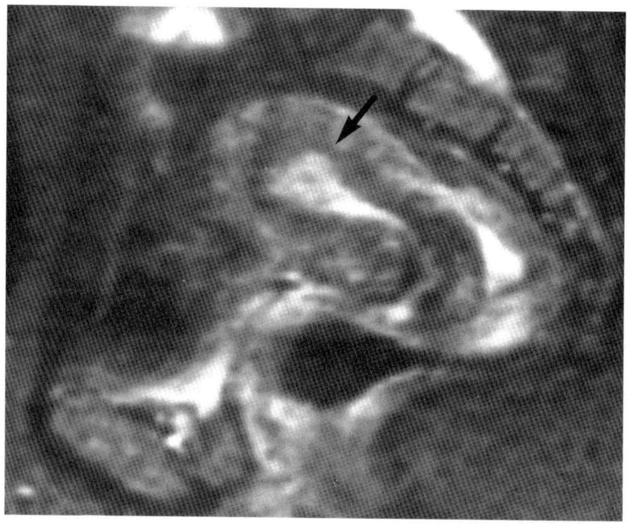

Figure 17.4

Endometrial carcinoma. MR T2-weighted sagittal image (SE: 2000/80) with high signal-intensity extending posteriorly to the myometrium. Disruption of the junctional zone is seen (arrow).

Magnetic resonance imaging

MR is considered a procedure of choice in the assessment of myometrial extension of endometrial carcinoma. However, in any sequence, MR is unable to differentiate endometrial carcinoma from hyperplasia and endometriosis, and it therefore has no place in the diagnosis per se of endometrial carcinoma. The use of gadolinium-DTPA facilitates differentiation of viable tumor from necrosis and intrauterine fluid collection.[29] Once the diagnosis of endometrial carcinoma is established, MR can demonstrate deep myometrial invasion as a disruption of the junctional zone with an accuracy of 94% on T2-weighted images[30, 31] (Figure 17.4). But in patients with superficial myometrial invasion, the sensitivity is only 69%.[31] Usually, the depth of myometrial infiltration is underestimated on MR. False negatives occur in the absence of a subendometrial low signal-intensity area in a postmenopausal woman.[32]

Extent

US has no contributary role in the diagnosis of bowel, omental and peritoneal involvement. We believe that US and TRUS are of no interest in the assessment of cervical involvement that is clinically diagnosed.

CT cannot differentiate stage Ia, Ib and II lesions.[33] Nevertheless, it is accurate in delineating stage III and IV endometrial carcinomas[34] and correctly indicates extrauterine tumor spread in 86% of stage III–IVb tumors.[33]

CT is valuable in stage III tumors, in showing extrapelvic metastases.[33]

MR is superior to contrast CT for the assessment of local extension of the lesions,[30] especially in bladder involvement.

Cervical carcinoma

Epidemiology

Carcinoma of the uterine cervix is currently the fourth most common cancer and the sixth most common cause of death from malignant disease in North American women. In recent years, the decline in the mortality rate has been due to the widespread use of Papanicolaou smears of the cervix in the identification of patients with dysplasia or carcinoma in situ, who are at high risk of developing invasive cancer. Dysplasias are significantly correlated with a history of genital herpes infection and positive serologic tests for HSV II. It has been suggested that the papillomavirus can originate the mutation or activation of oncogenes[35] and has an initiating role in cervical neoplasms.

Most newly diagnosed carcinomas of the cervix are pre-invasive. Invasive cervical neoplasms are more prevalent in women between 35 and 50 years old. However, they are being diagnosed with an increasing frequency in young women, at stages I or IIb.

Classification

Squamous-cell carcinomas represent 90% of cervical carcinomas. They originate in the metaplastic squamous cell epithelium and become atypical squamous metaplasias. Adenocarcinomas represent 9% and sarcomas less than 1% of cervical malignancies.

Mode of dissemination[36]

Cervical carcinomas can disseminate by:

- direct extension to local structures such as vagina, paracervical and paravaginal soft tissues, parametrium, bladder and rectum;
- via the lymphatic system, usually in the external iliac lymph nodes, and less commonly in the hypogastric lymph nodes (the involvement of common iliac and periaortic lymph nodes occurs secondarily);
- hematogenous route – hematogenous metastases are uncommon and later, and involve the bone, lungs, brain and liver.

Table 17.4 FIGO classification of cervical carcinoma.

Stage 0		Carcinoma in situ
Stage I		Carcinoma limited to cervix
	Ia	Microinvasive carcinoma
	Ib	Invasive carcinoma
Stage II		Extension beyond cervix, tumor involves the vagina but not as far as the lower third
	IIa	No parametrial involvement
	IIb	Parametrial involvement
Stage III		Extension to pelvic side wall or to lower third of the vagina
	IIIa	Extension to lower third of the vagina
	IIIb	Extension to pelvic side wall and/or hydronephrosis
Stage IV		Extension beyond true pelvis
	IVa	Spread to rectum and/or bladder
	IVb	Spread to distant organs

Staging[10]

The staging system for cervical carcinoma is based on clinical examination. Clinical staging consists of a bimanual pelvic examination under general anesthesia, and accurately determines vaginal and parametrial involvement. Radiologic examination consists in plain chest radiography and IVU. Cystoscopy and sigmoidoscopy are performed in symptomatic patients or in those with suspected advanced stage tumors. The staging system (Table 17.4) is based on the recommendations of the FIGO,[10] which does not take lymph-node involvement into account.

Clinical staging is fundamental to determine the main routes of treatment. Stage I and II tumors are surgically treated; more advanced tumors receive radiotherapy and/or chemotherapy.

Prognosis

Three main factors determining prognosis are:

- Clinical staging, the main prognostic factor:[37] the 5-year survival rates for stages I, II, III and IV are 80, 63, 33 and 12%, respectively.
- Lymph-node involvement: the 5-year survival rate varies from 82 to 96% in the absence of lymph-node involvement, and from 35 to 62% when pelvic lymph node involvement exists. In cases of common iliac lymph node involvement, 5-year survival is less than 10%.[38]
- Tumor volume: this correlates well with clinical staging, increased risk of regional spread and high risk of pelvic recurrence after radiation.

The importance of the histologic type is controversial.[39] It seems, however, to be less important in the prognosis of cervical carcinoma than ovarian or endometrial neoplasms.

Imaging features

Ultrasonography

US has a role in demonstrating fluid-filled uterine cavities that are suspected of being associated with cervical carcinoma. In the absence of fluid-filled uterine cavity, US can show the tumor as a hypoechoic or hyperechoic mass involving the cervix. TRUS seems to be more accurate than transabdominal US.

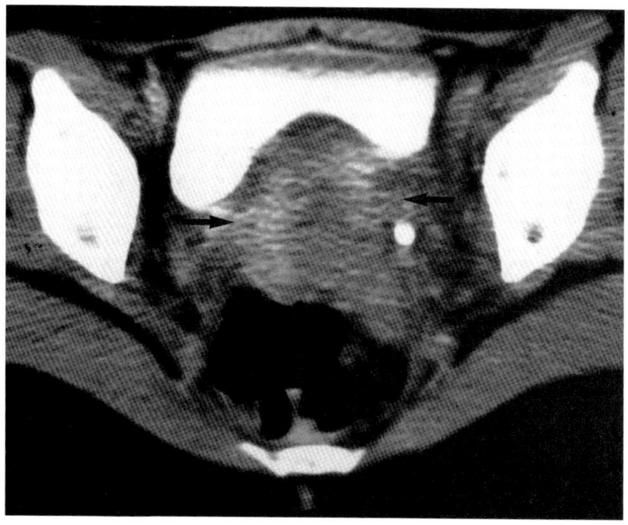

Figure 17.5

Cervical carcinoma. CT scan after contrast injection. Cervical carcinoma alters the contour of the cervix. The CT shows bilateral parametrial involvement (arrows).

Computed tomography

In our experience, CT is not generally indicated for stage Ib and IIa cervical neoplasm because it is less accurate than the clinical examination. CT shows cervical tumor only when its volume is sufficient to alter the contour of the cervix (Figure 17.5). The normal cervix and cervical carcinoma have similar densities.

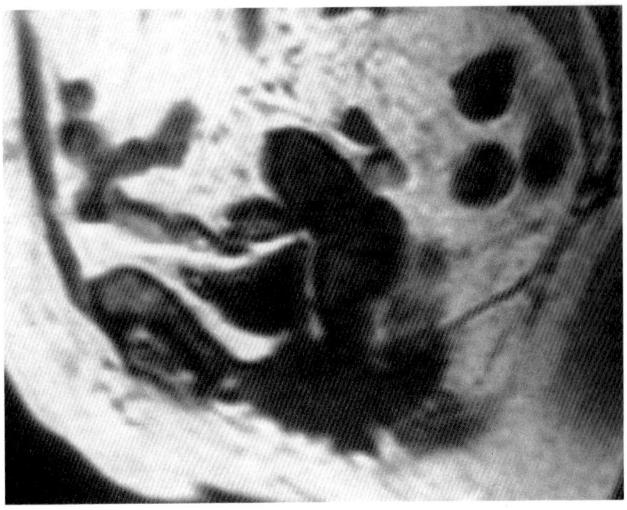

A

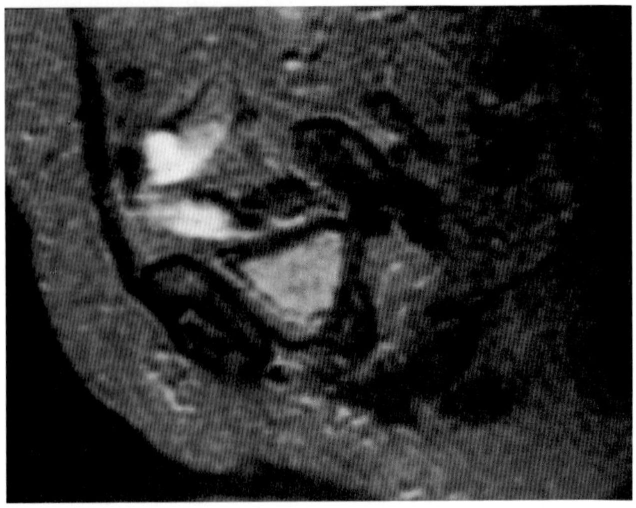

C

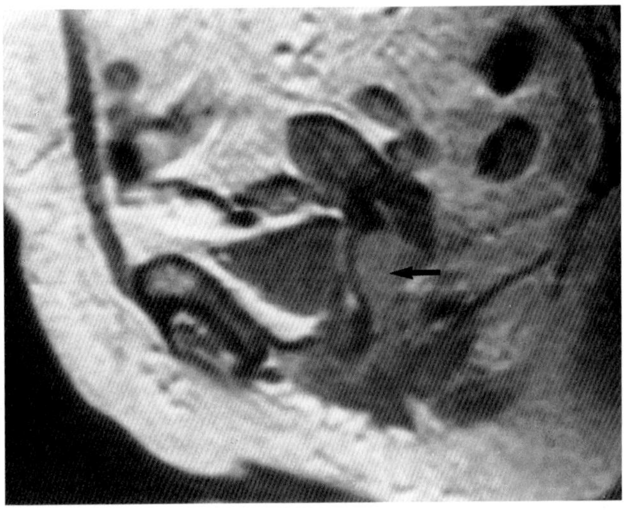

B

Figure 17.6

Cervical carcinoma.

A MR T1-weighted sagittal image (SE: 600/20) shows enlarged low signal-intensity cervix.

B MR spin-density-weighted sagittal image (SE: 2000/30) shows medium signal-intensity cervical mass corresponding to the tumor (arrow).

C MR T2-weighted sagittal image (SE: 2000/90) shows high signal-intensity cervical mass.

Magnetic resonance imaging

On T1-weighted images, the tumor is only visible when its volume causes cervical deformity (Figure 17.6A). On T2-weighted images, MR shows cervical tumor as a high signal-intensity mass (Figure 17.6B, C) with a high degree of accuracy. In a recent prospective study,[40] the sensitivity of T2-weighted images in the detection and determination of tumor location was 90% and specificity was 100%; the determination of tumor size was correct in 80% of cases. The tumor can be depicted when its size is over 15 mm[41] but sometimes, MR can be more accurate than the clinical examination in the assessment of the tumor size.[42] In some cases, on T2-weighted images, the tumor may have no high signal-intensity. In these cases, an indirect feature is the disappearance of the normal cervical low signal-intensity[30] that corresponds to the tumor sites.

Extent

It has been recently suggested that TRUS may have a role in the detection of parametrial involvement.[43] The TRUS findings for parametrium involvement have been described[44] as (1) disappearance of the normal hypoechoic parametrial flat area with internal heterogeneous echoes; and (2) irregular parametrial margins. These reports illustrate better accuracy for TRUS than for clinical examination.

IVU is performed for the assessment of urinary tract obstruction which correlates with a worse prognosis.

To improve diagnostic accuracy in the preoperative staging of cervical carcinoma, CT has been proposed as an adjunct to routine clinical staging procedures. CT can depict vaginal involvement in the event of wall thickening or an eccentric mass but is not accurate in the assessment of bladder or rectal involvement. We consider that CT is not indicated for clinical stage Ib and IIa tumors because clinical staging is far more accurate.[45] The role of CT in the detection of parametrial involvement is controversial. The accuracy of CT varies from 58%[46] to 88%.[47] These difference are due to the 'subtle' CT semiology of parametrial involvement.[48] Four main signs can be distinguished: (1) irregularity or poor definition of the lateral cervical margins, (2) disappearance of the periureteral fat plain, (3) eccentric parametrial soft tissue and (4) pre-eminent parametrial soft-tissue strands. Inaccuracy in the detection of parametrial involvement is usually due to the inability of CT to depict intraparametrial microscopic lymphatic or venous tumor spread. In advanced stage tumors, the extent of pelvic invasion shown by CT seems to correlate well with clinical findings but, in these inoperable cases, a surgical correlation cannot be established.

In our experience, MR is not accurate in the assessment of the extension of cervical carcinoma to the parametrium (Figure 17.7), vagina (Figure 17.8) and bladder (Figures 17.9 and 17.10), with sensitivities of only 38, 43 and 67%, respectively.[40] We consider the accuracy of MR to be disappointing even though some studies have shown encouraging results.[49] Recently, however, it has been reported that the preservation of the low intensity of normal cervical stroma correlates in all cases with the integrity of the parametrium.[50] This new feature has not been evaluated in our study.

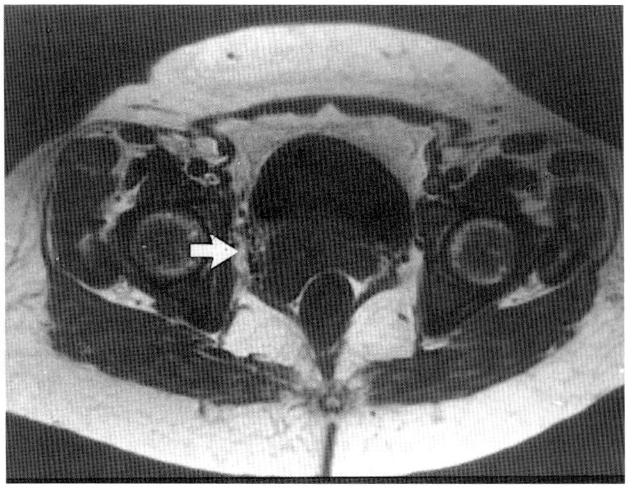

A

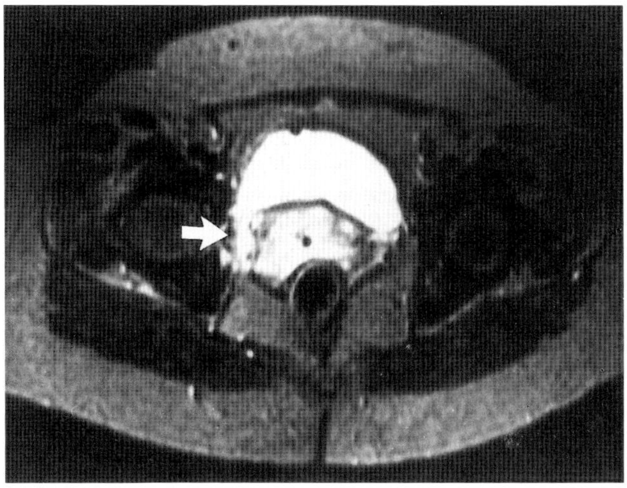

B

Figure 17.7

Cervical carcinoma.

A MR T1-weighted transverse image (SE: 600/20) shows right parametrial extension of cervical carcinoma and thickening of the right parametrium with a low signal-intensity (arrow).

B MR T2-weighted transverse image (SE: 2000/90). The right parametrial invasion is shown as a high signal-intensity area (arrow).

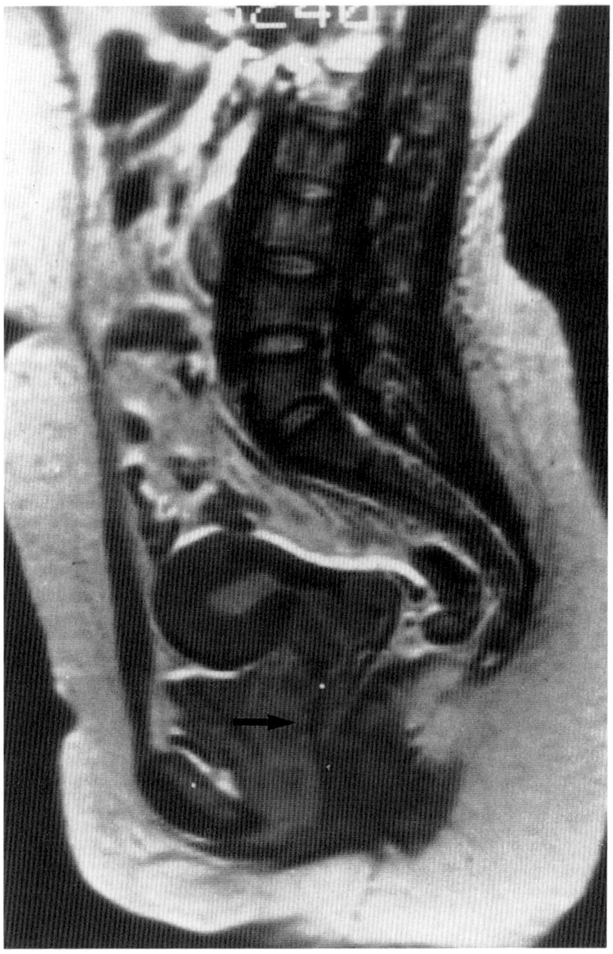

Figure 17.8

Cervical carcinoma. MR spin density-weighted sagittal image (SE: 2000/30) shows extensive tumor growth in both lips of the cervix, extending to the anterior wall of the vagina (arrow).

Figure 17.9

Cervical carcinoma. MR sagittal image shows extensive cervical carcinoma invading the vagina and the bladder (arrow). (Left) T1-weighted image (SE: 600/20). (Right) T2-weighted image (SE: 2000/90).

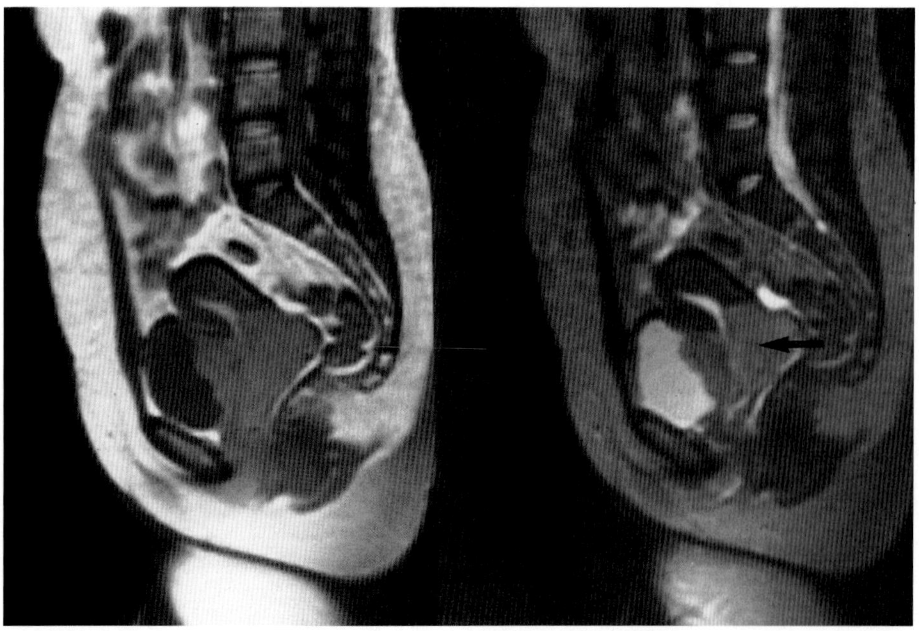

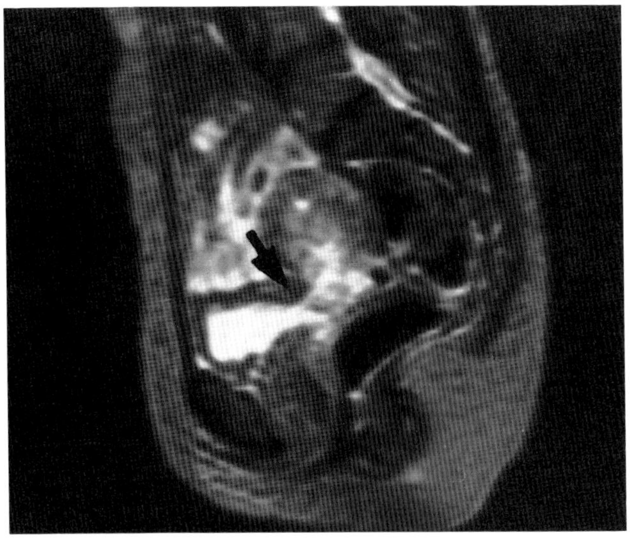

Figure 17.10

Cervical carcinoma. MR T2-weighted sagittal image shows extensive cervical tumor responsible for a cervicovesical fistula (arrow).

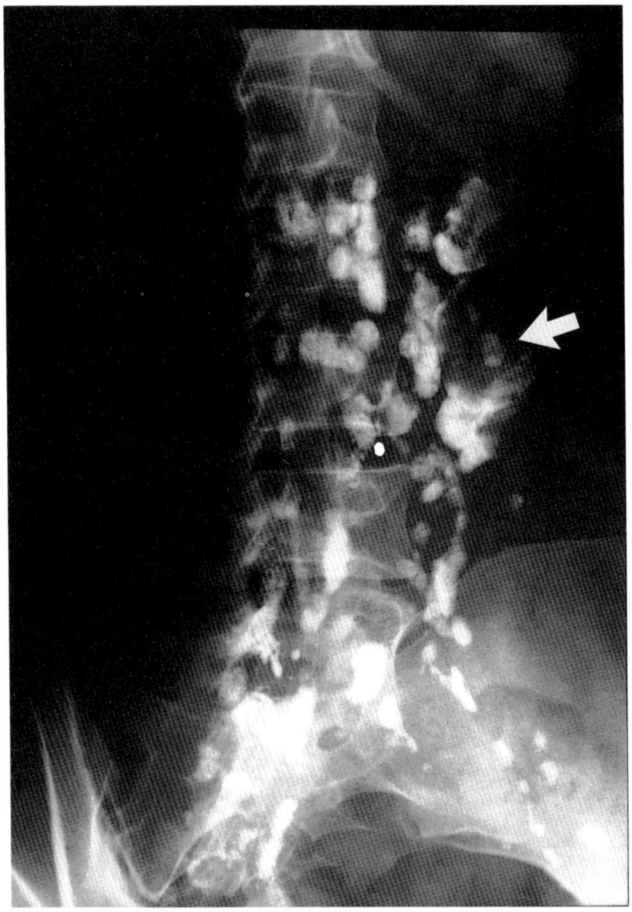

Figure 17.11

Cervical carcinoma. Lymphography on the second day shows metastatic involvement of lumboaortic lymph nodes as lacuna (arrow).

Lymph nodes

Imaging features of ovarian, endometrial and cervical lymph-nodes metastases are the same. For this reason, they will be presented together.

Lymphography

Lymphography is still the most accurate diagnostic technique in the assessment of pelvic or abdominal lymph-node metastases, having the advantage of being able to differentiate hyperplasia from metastatic involvement and to detect metastases in normal size nodes. Two semiologic aspects to be aware of are: (1) on the first day, a blockage in drainage channels with collateral circulation is a rare but typical sign; (2) on the second day, a lacuna is the most typical sign (Figure 17.11). A lacuna not traversed by lymphatics is of a metastatic nature whereas a lacuna traversed by lymphatics is of a lipomatous nature.[51] In fact, it is difficult to be sure of the real nature of a lacuna, especially when it is small. Radiographs can be repeated every 3 months while lymph-node opacification persists. Lymphography is a simple technique for follow up.

In the case of ovarian dysgerminomas, the radiological assessment of lymph-node invasion is obtained by lymphography. If lymphography shows no abnormality, a follow up or radiotherapy at a dose of 20 Gy is sufficient. If lymphography shows lymph-node involvement, post-operative radiation therapy must be given with a higher dose of about 45 Gy.

Computed tomography

CT can detect abdominal or pelvic lymphadenopathy but the diagnosis of malignant lymphadenopathy can only be based on the demonstration of nodal enlargement. CT is of value in detecting para-aortic lymph-node recurrence and shows, most of the time, a mass of more than 4 cm in size. CT is extremely useful for an assessment of the density of the lacuna. The lipomatous lacuna has the density of fat, but if there is still any doubt, a percutaneous biopsy of the suspect lymph node can be performed under CT guidance.

Magnetic resonance imaging

Early reports were optimistic and it has been established that MR is equal in accuracy to CT in the detection of pelvic or abdominal lymph-node involvement.[52, 53] The overall accuracy of MR in the detection of pelvic lymph-node metastasis is 78%.[50] The diagnosis of lymph-node involvement is based only on the demonstration of nodal enlargement; the measurement of T1 and T2 relaxation times and relative spin density does not differentiate between non-specific lymphadenopathy and lymph-node metastases.[53] The advantage of MR is in distinguishing blood vessels from lymph nodes without the need for contrast injection (Figure 17.12).[52] On the other hand, CT offers better spatial resolution and permits safe biopsy guidance.

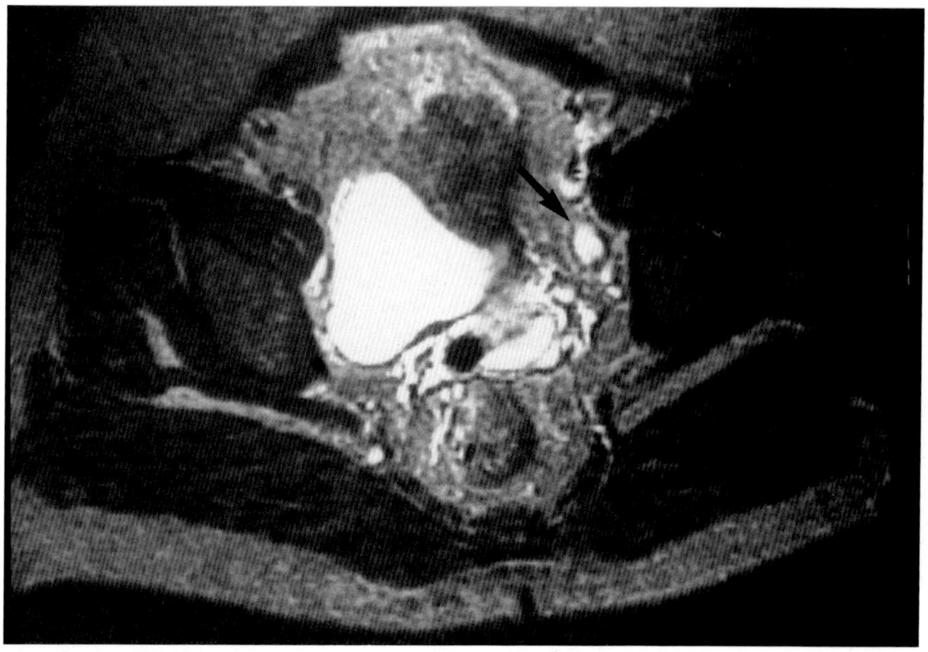

Figure 17.12

Cervical carcinoma. MR T2-weighted transverse image (SE: 2000/90). Enlarged lymph node with high signal intensity (arrow).

Follow up

Ovarian carcinoma

TRUS is highly sensitive in the detection of recurrences of ovarian neoplasms, while US has little diagnostic value.[54] TRUS is the procedure of choice in the evaluation of patients with a risk of recurrent ovarian carcinoma.

After surgery or before a second-look operation, CT findings are subtle and easily confused with peritoneal reaction and scarring.[55] Thin sections increase the level of confidence of diagnosing peritoneal metastases.[56]

The utility of MR is well established in suspected recurrent tumor.[57] MR demonstrates residual tumor as a pelvic mass in 89% of cases. One great hope of MR is that it may differentiate recurrence from fibrosis after radiation on T2-weighted images. After disappointing initial results,[57] more promising results were reported in a series of 21 patients with irradiated tumors of different types.[58] More recently, a recurrence was shown as a higher signal intensity mass than fibrosis.[59] In practice, however, MR like CT is of little help as a routine technique in distinguishing recurrent tumor from radiation necrosis, inflammation or fibrosis. In this setting, CT has a real advantage over MR in permitting biopsy guidance. Nevertheless, MR can be helpful on T2-weighted images when recurrence is suspected: the absence of a high signal-intensity mass eliminates a recurrence.

Uterine carcinoma

TRUS seems to differentiate pelvic tumor recurrence from endometrial carcinoma with a high degree of accuracy.[54] CT plays an important role in planning radiation therapy and assessing the response to treatment in showing persistent pelvic tumor,[33] having a sensitivity of 88%.

Endometrial carcinoma recurrences are uncommon but, when a recurrence is suspected, CT is of value. The CT features of recurrent endometrial carcinoma are usually those of a central pelvic mass. CT thus supplements the clinical examination.[60] Endometrial carcinoma recurrences have a high signal intensity on T2-weighted images.

MR is undoubtedly superior to contrast CT for the detection of recurrent tumor.[30] After radiotherapy, when recurrence exists, MR shows an abnormal increased signal intensity on T2-weighted images.

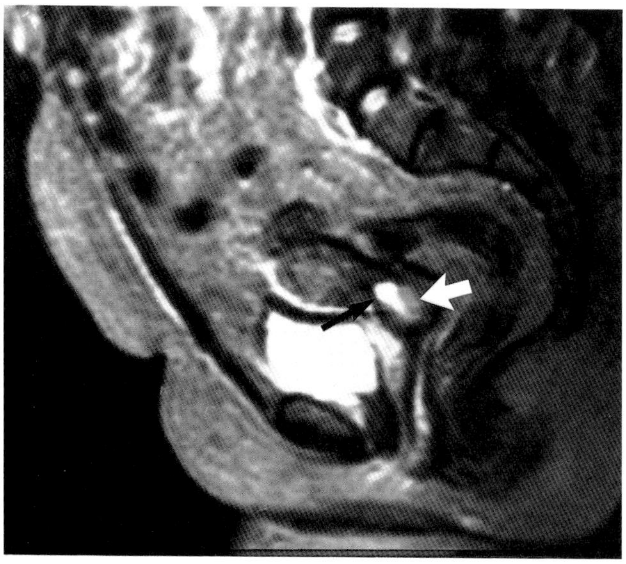

Figure 17.13

Cervical carcinoma. MR T2-weighted sagittal image (SE: 2000/90) shows recurrence of cervical carcinoma on the posterior lip of the cervix as a high signal-intensity area (white arrow). Hyperintense intracavital retention is seen (black arrow).

Cervical carcinoma

Clinical examination is the most accurate and the least expensive follow-up procedure. TRUS can be of interest in showing recurrent cervical neoplasms.[54] Even though hepatic metastases are uncommon, US is a regular feature of follow up. At the least, US can detect distention of the urinary tract at initial staging or during the follow up in the event of a recurrence. MR may have a particular role in the follow up of cervical carcinomas in depicting recurrences after radiotherapy[32] (Figure 17.13).

Imaging strategy

Ovarian carcinoma

US and CT can depict incidentally an ovarian mass. The pre-operative diagnosis of malignancy can be established when metastases exist and/or when the CA 125 is elevated.

In cases of operable patients, staging is performed during the laparotomy.

After surgery, two possibilities exist: (1) in cases of complete surgical tumor reduction, imaging is useless as there is no residual tumor; (2) in cases of incomplete surgical tumor reduction, we believe that CT should be performed to evaluate the residual tumor before adjuvant therapy. After adjuvant therapy (which is usually chemotherapy) a CT examination is performed to evaluate tumor response. If CT shows no obvious residual disease, a second-look operation can be performed.

For the follow up, we perform annually chest radiography and US of the abdomen and pelvis. When a recurrence is suspected we perform a CT examination to confirm the diagnosis.[61]

Uterine carcinoma

Before therapy, we perform chest radiography and IVU. The imaging strategy is based on the surgical protocol followed: (1) in cases of hysterectomy with systematic bilateral pelvic lymphadenectomy, we believe that imaging is of no interest; (2) in cases of lymphadenectomy only performed when myometrial invasion exists, we use MR, which because of its accuracy, should be performed before surgery. The results of MR are of value to predict myometrial invasion.[15]

During follow up, we perform six-monthly chest radiography and US or TRUS. When a recurrence is clinically suspected, MR is the most reliable examination for confirming the diagnosis.

Cervical carcinoma

Before therapy, chest radiography and IVU are of value. US is undertaken in case of renal obstruction and permits guidance for a urinary interventional procedure. Furthermore, US is of value in the assessment of the right position of the source in intracavitary therapy.[62]

The imaging strategy is based on staging and therapeutic. In cases of radiation therapy alone (inoperable cases), the assessment of lymph-node involvement is important because lymph-node metastases receive boosted therapy. In these cases, we perform CT examination. If CT shows lymph-node enlargement we consider that they are lymph-node metastases. If CT shows no obvious lymph-node enlargement, then lymphography, which has better sensitivity and specificity, is of real value.[1] In cases of surgical therapy (stages 0, I, II), we believe that, pre-operatively, lymphography is of no interest. Pelvic or abdominal lymph-node metastases are assessed peri-operatively.

During follow up, we perform chest radiography and abdominopelvic US, twice a year.

When a recurrence is suspected, we perform MR, which is of value in depicting a centropelvic or local recurrence, especially after radiation therapy.

References

1. Galakhoff C, Masselot J, Dam N et al, Lymphography in the initial evaluation of endometrial carcinoma, *Gynecol Oncol* (1988) **31:**276–84.
2. Mendelson EB, Bohm-Velez M, Joseph N et al, Gynecologic imaging: comparison of transabdominal and transvaginal sonography, *Radiology* (1988) **166:**321–4.
3. Sikora K, Imaging with radiolabelled monoclonal antibodies, *Clin Radiol* (1989) **40:**332–4.
4. Mach JP, Buchegger F, Forni M, Use of radiolabelled monoclonal anti-CEA antibodies for the detection of human carcinomas by external photoscanning and tomoscintigraphy, *Immunol Today* (1981) **6:**239–47.
5. Granowska M, Sheperd J, Britton KE, Ovarian cancer: diagnosis using I-131 monoclonal antibody in comparison with surgical findings, *Nucl Med Commun* (1984) **5:**485–99.
6. Bast RC, Klug TL, ST John E, A radio-immunoassay using monoclonal antibody to monitor the course of epithelial ovarian cancer, *N Engl J Med* (1983) **309:**883–7.
7. Fishman-Javitt MC, Loveshio JL, Stein HL, Imaging strategies for MRI of the pelvis, *Radiol Clin N Am* (1988) **26:**633–51.
8. Balfe DM, Heikein JP, Clennan BL, Oncologic imaging carcinoma of the cervix, ovary and endometrium. In: Bragg DG, Rubin P, Youker JE, eds, *Oncologic imaging* (Pergamon Press: New York, 1985) 439–75.

9. Di Saia PJ, Morrow CP, Townsend DE, *Synopsis of gynecologic oncology* (John Wiley: New York 1975) 136–202.
10. International Federation of Gynecology and Obstretrics, Classification and staging of malignant tumors in the female pelvis, *Acta Obstet Gynecol Scand* (1971) **50:**1–7.
11. Creasman WT, New gynecologic cancer staging, *Obstet Gynecol* (1990) **75:**287–8.
12. Nguyen-Tan T, Tumeurs ovariennes: critères échographiques de malignité et de bénignité (à propos de 100 cas), (36èmes Journées Françaises de Radiologie: Paris 1987).
13. Lande IM, Hill MC, Cosco FE et al, Adnexal and cul-de-sac abnormalities: transvaginal sonography, *Radiology* (1988) **166:**325–32.
14. Kormano M, Alamen A, Granroos M, Predicting malignancy of suspected ovarian tumors by CT, *Eur J Radiol* (1984) **4:**61–4.
15. Santoni R, Villari N, Bisin L et al, The role of lymphography in the staging and treatment of ovarian dysgerminoma. Report on 27 cases, *Acta Radiol (Oncol)* (1987) **26:**23–5.
16. Silverman PM, Osborne M, Dunnick NR et al, CT prior to second-look operation in ovarian cancer, *AJR* (1988) **150:**829–32.
17. Stern, J, Buscema J, Rosenhein N et al, Can computed tomography substitute for second-look operation in ovarian carcinoma, *Gynecol Oncol* (1981) **11:**82–8.
18. Thorvinger B, Samuelsson L, Skjaerris J, Computed tomography of malignant ovarian disease, *Acta Radiol* (1987) **28:**739–42.
19. Poulsen MG, Roberts SJ, Prognostic variables in endometrial carcinoma, *Int J Radiat Oncol Biol Phys* (1987) **13:**1043–52.
20. Boutselis JG, Endometrial carcinoma: prognostic factors and treatment, *Surg Clin N Am* (1978) **58:**109–19.
21. Piver MS, Para-aortic node biopsy in staging women with cervical ovarian and endometrial carcinoma: a review, *J Surg Oncol* (1979) **12:**365–70.
22. Novak ER, Woodruff SD, *Novak's gynecologic and obstetric pathology*, 8th edn (WB Saunders: Philadelphia 1978) 380–4.
23. Dunnick NR, Fischer RI, Chu E et al, Percutaneous aspirations of retroperitoneal in ovarian and endometrial cancer, *AJR* (1980) **135:**109–13.
24. Breckenridge JW, Kurtz AB, Ritchie WGM et al, Postmenopausal uterine fluid collection: indicator of carcinoma, *AJR* (1982) **139:**529–34.
25. Fleischer AC, Dudley BS, Entman SS et al, Myometrial invasion by endometrial carcinoma: sonographic assessment, *Radiology* (1967) **162:**307–10.
26. Lehtovirta P, Cacciatobe B, Wahlstrom T et al, Ultrasonic assessment of endometrial cancer invasion, *J Clin Ultrasound* (1987) **15:**519–24.
27. Hamlin DJ, Burgener FA, Beecham JB, CT of intramural endometrial carcinoma: contrast enhancement is essential, *AJR* (1981) **137:**551–4.
28. Legrand I, Masselot J, Girinski T et al, Tomodensitométrie des cancers du corps utérin (stades I et II). Confrontations anatomopathologiques. A propos de 25 cas, *J Radiol* (1984) **65:**776–81.
29. Hricak H, Hamm B, Wolf KJ, Use of Gd-DTPA in MRI of the female pelvis. In: Bydder G, Felix R, Bucheler E, eds, *Contrast media in MRI* (Medicom: Bussum 1990) 351.
30. Worthington JL, Balfe DM, Lee JKT et al, Uterine neoplasms: MR imaging, *Radiology* (1986) **959:**725–30.
31. Chen SS, Rumancik WM, Spiegel G, Magnetic resonance imaging in stage I endometrial carcinoma, *Obstet Gynecol* (1990) **75:**274–7.
32. Michel G, Galakhoff C, Masselot J et al, Intérêt de l'imagerie par résonance magnétique des cancers du col et du corps de l'utérus, *J Radiol* (1987) **68:**167–75.
33. Walsh JW, Goplerud DR, Computed tomography of primary, persistent, and recurrent endometrial malignancy, *AJR* (1982) **139:**1149–54.
34. Balfe DM, Van Dyke J, Lee JKT et al, Utility of CT in staging endometrial carcinoma, *J Comput Assist Tomogr* (1983) **7:**677–81.
35. Riou G, Barrois M, Le M et al, C-*myc* proto oncogene expression and prognosis in early carcinoma of the uterine cervix, *Lancet* (1987) 761–3.
36. Pujol H, Prade M, Extension anatomique des carcinomes infiltrants du col utérin, *Bull Cancer (Paris)* (1979) **66:**503–14.
37. Pejovic MH, Wolff JP, Kramar A et al, Cure rate estimation and long term prognosis of uterine cervix carcinoma, *Cancer* (1981) **47:**203–6.
38. Van Bommel PJF, Van Lindert ACM, Kock HCLV et al, A review of prognostic factors in early-syage carcinoma of the cervix (FIGO Ib and IIa) and implications for treatment strategy, *Eur J Obstet Gynecol Reprod Biol* (1987) **26:**69–84.
39. Prade M, Weill S, Sancho H et al, Indice histologique de pronostic dans les cancers du col utérin stades I et II proximal, *Rev Fr Gynecol* (1974) **69:**223–8.
40. Soyer PH, Rigaud C, Masselot J et al, Evaluation of the role of MR at 1.5T in staging of carcinoma of the uterine cervix, *J Belge Radiol* (1991) **74:**85–90.
41. Hricak H, Lacey CG, Sandles LG et al, Invasive cervical carcinoma: comparison of MR imaging and surgical findings, *Radiology* (1988) **166:**623–31.
42. Rubens D, Thornbury JR, Angel C et al, Stage IB cervical carcinoma: comparison of clinical, MR, and pathologic staging, *AJR* (1988) **150:**135–8.
43. Yuhara A, Akamatsu N, Sekiba K, Use of transrectal radial scan ultrasonography in evaluating the extent of uterine cervical cancer, *J Clin Ultrasound* (1987) **15:**507–17.
44. Aoki S, Hata T, Senoh D et al, Parametrial invasion of uterine cervical cancer assessed by transrectal ultrasonography: preliminary report, *Gynecol Oncol* (1990) **36:**82–9.
45. Villasanta U, Whitley No, Haney PJ et al, Computed tomography in invasive carcinoma of the cervix: an appraisal, *Obstet Gynecol* (1983) **62:**218–24.

46. Grumbine FC, Rosenheim NB, Zerhouni EA et al, Abdominopelvic computed tomography in the preoperative evaluation of early cervical cancer, *Gynecol Oncol* (1981) **12:**286–90.

47. Kilcheski TS, Arger PH, Mulhern CB et al, Role of computed tomography in the presurgical evaluation of carcinoma of the cervix, *J Comput Assist Tomogr* (1981) **5:**378–83.

48. Vick CW, Walsh JW, Wheelock JB et al, CT of the normal and abnormal parametria in cervical cancer, *AJR* (1984) **143:**597–603.

49. Greco A, Mason P, Leung AWL et al, Staging of carcinoma of the uterine cervix: MRI surgical correlation, *Clin Radiol* (1989) **40:**401–5.

50. Kim SH, Choi BI, Lee HP et al, Uterine cervical carcinoma: comparison of CT and MR findings, *Radiology* (1990) **175:**59–1.

51. Piver MS, Wallace S, Castro JR, The accuracy of lymphangiography in carcinoma of the uterine cervix, *AJR* (1971) **111:**278–83.

52. Lee JKT, Heiken JP, Ling D et al, Magnetic Resonance Imaging of abdominal and pelvic lymphadenopathy, *Radiology* (1984) **153:** 181–8.

53. Dooms GC, Hricak H, Moseley ME et al, Characterization of lymphadenopathy by magnetic resonance relaxation times: preliminary results, *Radiology* (1985) **155:**691–7.

54. Squillaci E, Salzani MC, Grandinetti ML et al, Recurrence of ovarian and uterine neoplasms: diagnosis with transrectal US, *Radiology* (1988) **169:**355–8.

55. Megibow AJ, Bosniak MA, Ho AG et al, Accuracy of CT in detection of persistent or recurrent ovarian carcinoma: correlation with second-look laparotomy, *Radiology* (1988) **166:**341–5.

56. Giwerc M, Masselot J, George M et al, Intérêt de l'examen tomodensitométrique dans la surveillance des cancers de l'ovaire. A propos de 69 observations, *J Radiol* (1986) **67:**769–74.

57. Bies JR, Ellis JH, Kopecky KK et al, Assessment of primary gynecologic malignancies: comparison of 0.15T resistive MRI with CT, *AJR* (1984) **143:**1249–57.

58. Glaze HS, Lee JKT, Levitt RG, Radiation fibrosis: differentiation from recurrent tumor by MR imaging, *Radiology* (1985) **156:**721–6.

59. Ebner F, Kressel HY, Mints MC et al, Tumor recurrence versus fibrosis in the female pelvis: differentiation with MR Imaging at 1.5T, *Radiology* (1988) **166:**333–40.

60. Franchi M, Lafianza A, Babilonti L et al, Clinical value of computerized tomography in assessment of recurrent uterine cancer, *Gynecol Oncol* (1989) **35:**31–7.

61. Masselot J, Galakhoff C, George M et al, La tomodensitométrie dans les cancers de l'utérus et de l'ovaire, *Rev Fr Gynecol Obstet* (1987) **82:**70–84.

62. Granai CO, Ellee P, Doherty F et al, Intraoperative real-time ultrasonography during intrauterine tandem placement, *Obstet Gynecol* (1986) **67:**112–14.

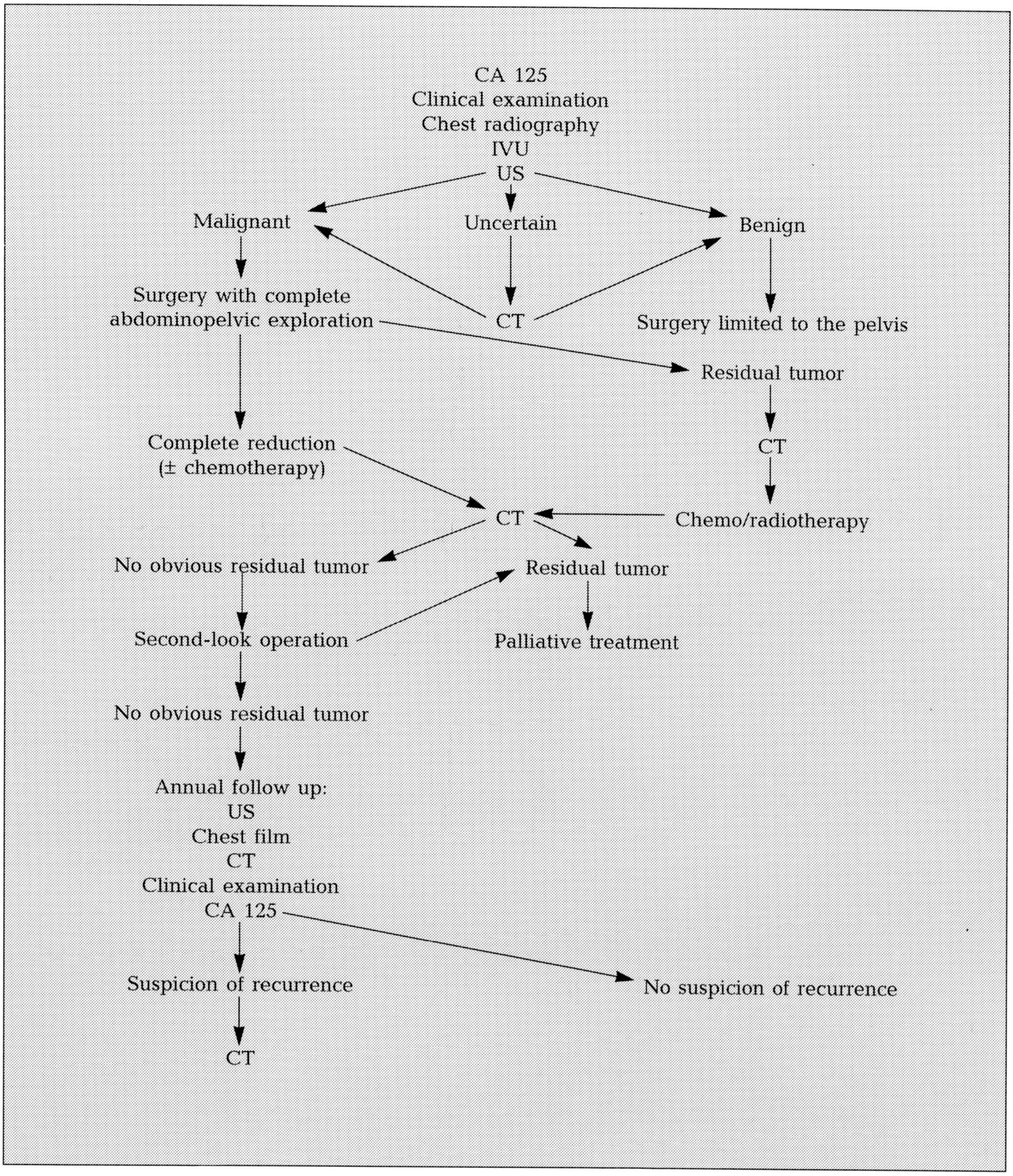

Diagram 17.1

Imaging strategy in epithelial ovarian carcinoma. CA 125, carcinogen antibody 125.

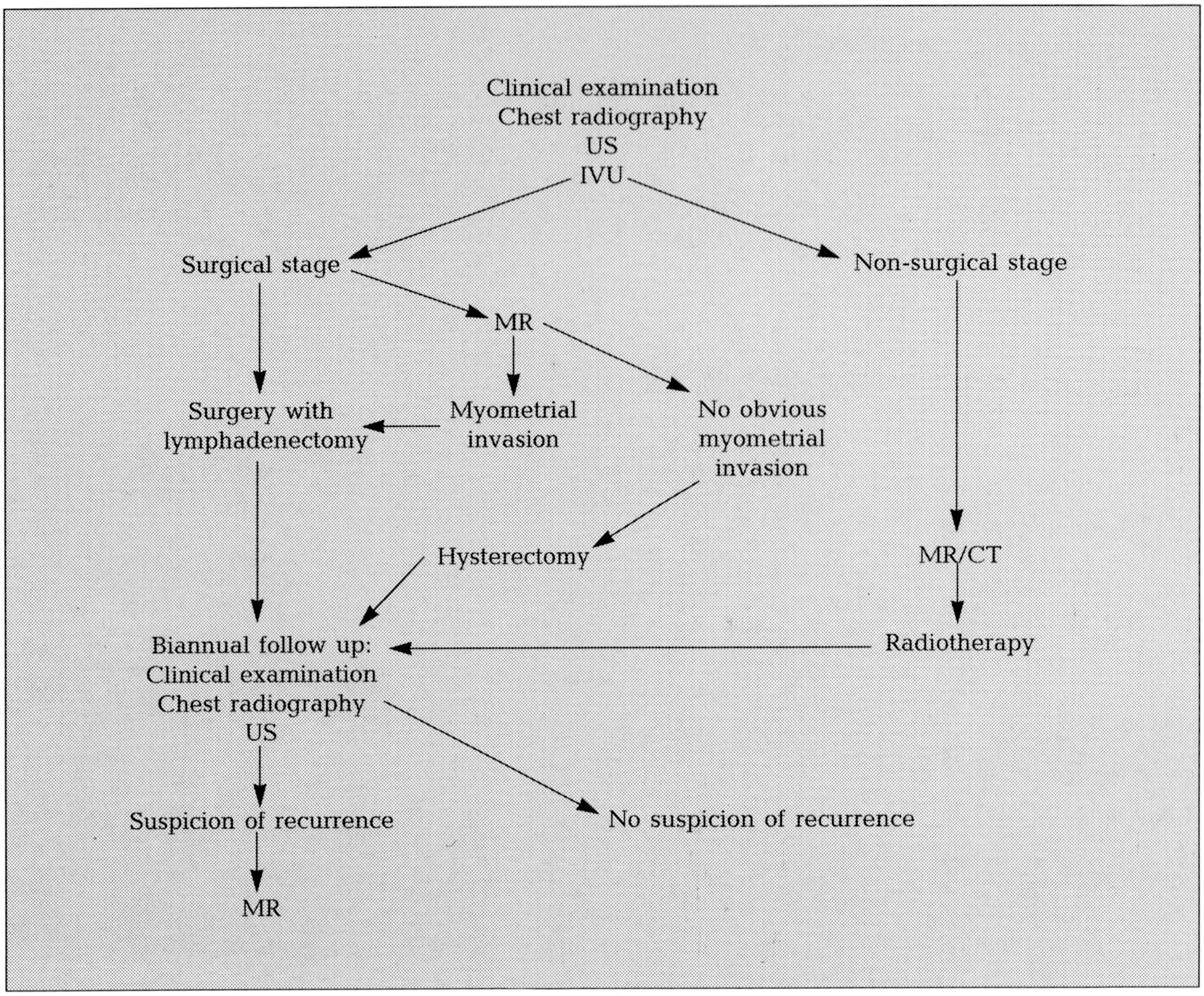

Diagram 17.2

Imaging strategy in uterine carinoma.

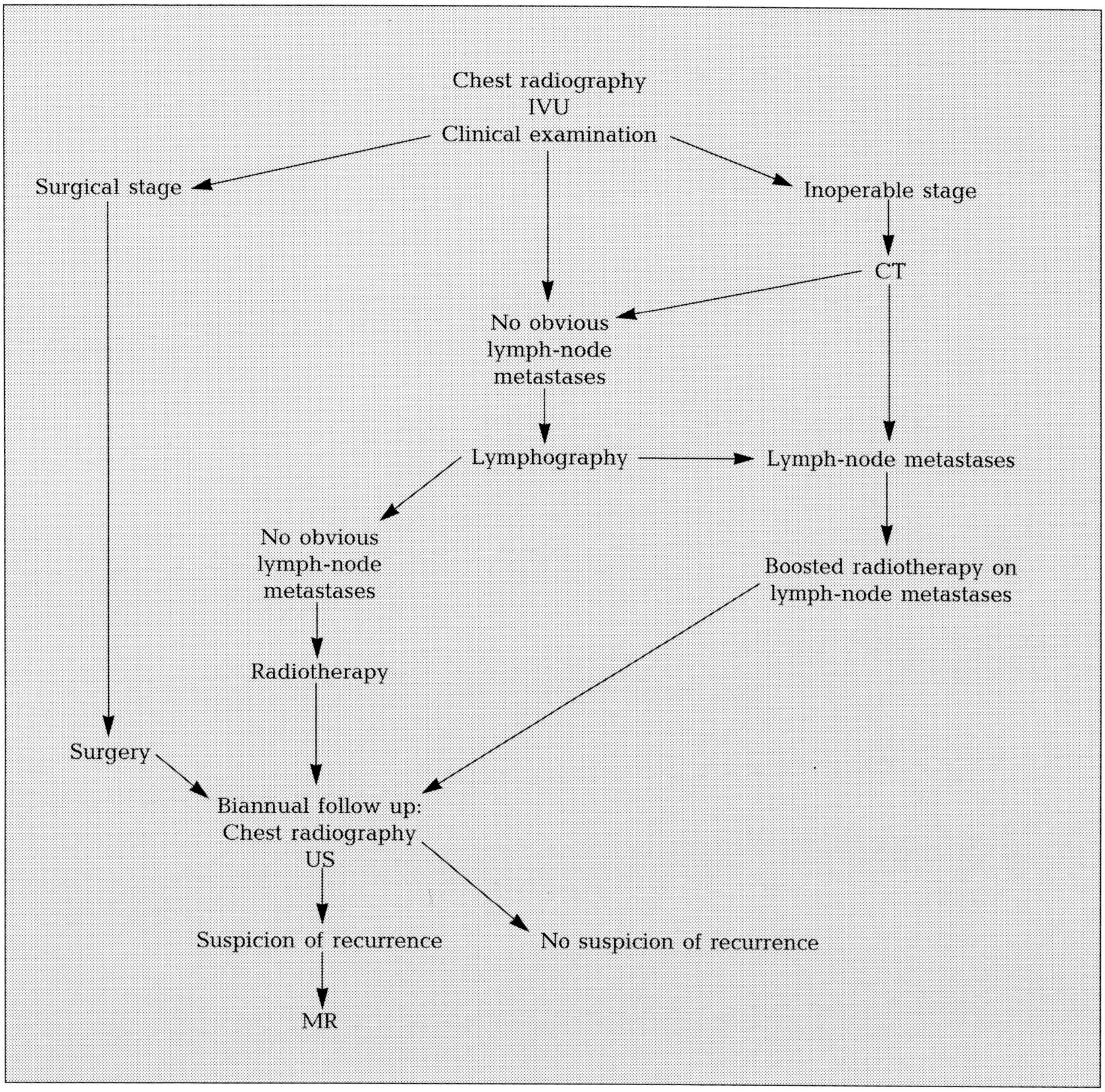

Diagram 17.3

Imaging strategy in cervical carcinoma.

18

Soft tissue

Lorraine G. Shapeero and Daniel Vanel

Introduction

Malignant soft-tissue sarcomas comprise 1% of cancers and 1–2% of cancer deaths each year and are twice as common as their skeletal counterparts. According to hospital studies, about 1% of soft-tissue neoplasms are malignant.[1–2] Because they are often mistaken for benign tumors, most malignant soft-tissue tumors are inadequately staged and incompletely resected with disastrous results. Fifty to a hundred per cent of soft-tissue malignancies recur locally. Optimal pre-operative evaluation is therefore essential to reduce their morbidity and mortality.[1–2]

Most soft-tissue tumors (75–85%) develop in adults, but some do occur in children. Although there is a slight male predominance in adults, the sex ratio varies with the particular histologic type.[1] On presentation, soft-tissue sarcomas are usually painless and palpable masses that measure more than 5 cm in diameter and are located in the deep soft tissues. They are derived from fat, synovium and neurovascular, muscular and undifferentiated tissue, and can develop at any location in the body. The most frequent sites are the lower extremities (40%), followed by the trunk (30%), upper extremities (20%), and head and neck (10%).[1]

The most common soft-tissue malignancies are malignant fibrous histiocytomas in adults and rhabdomyosarcomas in children. Other common soft-tissue tumors are, in decreasing order of frequency, liposarcoma, fibrosarcoma and synovial sarcoma. Although soft-tissue malignancies are usually single, multiple lesions may be found, particularly in Kaposi's sarcoma, angiosarcoma, neurofibrosarcoma, synovial sarcoma, T-cell lymphoma, and, of course, metastases.[1,3,4]

Even with adequate pre-operative staging, tumors that arise in the trunk, retroperitoneum, head, neck and axillae are more difficult to cure because of late detection, involvement of vital structures and complicated surgical excision.[1,5,6] At presentation, 5–10% of patients with soft-tissue sarcomas have metastases; these develop most frequently in the lungs and less commonly in the lymph nodes, other parts of the skeleton and the liver. Approximately 80% of all local recurrences and metastases will become manifest evident within 5 years of presentation. The overall 5-year survival rate of soft-tissue sarcomas is 50%.

To select the appropriate imaging procedure and sequence for evaluating soft-tissue sarcomas, one must understand their pattern of growth. Soft-tissue sarcomas grow centrifugally and produce a pseudocapsule with an inner 'zone' of compressed normal tissue and an outer 'zone' of reactive, neovascularized granulation tissue. High-grade sarcomas rapidly infiltrate the pseudocapsule, producing 'satellite' nodules, and spread into the adjacent normal tissue as 'skip' metastases. Awareness of the incomplete nature of the pseudocapsule is important for appropriately extensive surgical excision.[1,2,5] Although there are a large number of different histologic types and subtypes, these seem to have no prognostic value. The only histologic criterion of prognostic value is the grade.

Tumors are classified as intracapsular or extracapsular (extension outside the capsule), and intracompartmental or extracompartmental (extension outside the anatomic compartment, or development in poorly defined anatomic spaces such as the axillae).[2,5] High-grade tumors are usually extracompartmental and extracapsular, and destroy rather than erode adjacent joints, fascia and bone. They metastasize more readily. In contrast, the low-grade malignancies, usually intracompartmental, slowly invade locally, erode rather than destroy the adjacent structures, and infrequently metastasize. With recurrences and repeated surgery, a low-grade neoplasm may become more aggressive and may produce extensive local invasion and distant metastases.[5]

At present, imaging modalities can neither differentiate benign from malignant soft-tissue neoplasm nor diagnose the specific tumor type in many cases. The major role of imaging is to define the local and metastatic tumor extent, to evaluate the response to therapy, and to detect recurrences.

Radiography

In contrast to its primary role in diagnosing bone cancer, conventional radiography has more limited utility in evaluating soft-tissue malignancy. Radiography can sometimes confirm the presence of a mass suspected clinically, and it may identify calcifications and adjacent skeletal involvement (Figure 18.1).

Although radiographic findings are not diagnostic, several radiographic features, in the absence of inflammation, suggest malignancy: an ill-defined mass with obliteration of fat planes, an irregular interrupted periosteal reaction, cortical destruction, and lytic medullary lesions. However, some malignant sarcomas, such as synovial sarcoma, may stimulate a more benign process and present as well-defined masses that do not obliterate fat planes and produce erosive rather than destructive bony change.[6–10] In contrast, a benign tumor, the desmoid, characteristically obliterates fat planes and produces a spiculated periosteal reaction, features compatible with a more aggressive tumor.[8,11] On radiographs, CT and MR, the exact origin of the tumor, whether soft tissue or skeletal, may be difficult to ascertain when the tumour is extensive. Generally, the center of greatest volume denotes the origin.[7]

Both radiographs and CT are useful for defining calcifications in soft-tissue sarcomas, particularly in areas of hemorrhage or necrosis. These calcifications are usually irregular and faint; they are seen in 30% of synovial sarcomas and in some malignant fibrous histiocytomas[8–10] (Figure 18.2). The rare extraskeletal chondrosarcoma and osteosarcoma may show characteristic ring-shaped chondroid and stippled ossific calcifications, respectively.[12,13] One should also be aware that the pattern of calcification in the benign process, myositis ossificans,[14–18] can mimic soft-tissue sarcoma both on radiographs and CT and at histopathology. Initially (3–4 weeks after clinical onset), myositis ossificans appears as a soft-tissue mass with amorphous calcification on radiography and CT. Histopathology demonstrates a soft-tissue mass with central calcification and uncalcified periphery (the reverse zonal pattern), simulating soft-tissue malignancy. After 4–6 weeks, the

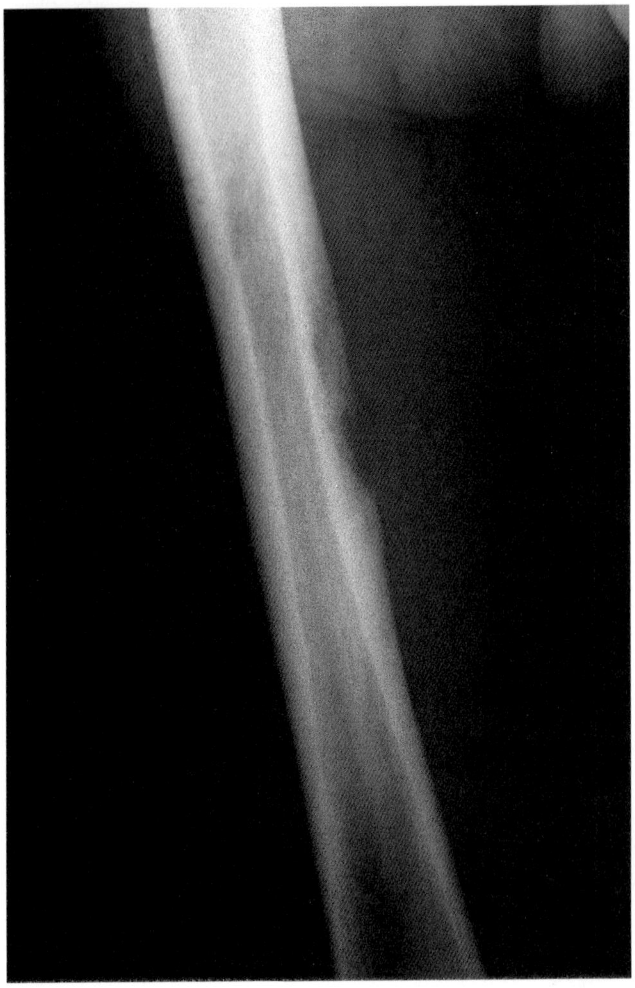

Figure 18.1

Plain radiograph: AP view of of the left femur. Leiomyosarcoma in a patient with pain for 3 months. The medial cortical bone is eroded by a mass of the soft tissue, which is not well seen. The mass contains few calcifications. Histology demonstrated leiomyosarcoma.

myositis ossificans matures, and CT and plain radiographs depict the characteristic zonal pattern with central lucency and peripheral calcification, corresponding to the central cellular tissue and peripheral immature bone at histopathology.

A primary role for radiography in soft-tissue malignancy is to define the areas of abnormal uptake on bone scan screening.[19] Metastases to bone from soft-tissue sarcoma develop in 7.3–19.0% of patients[20–22] and appear osteolytic in 88% of patients and osteoblastic in 12%. Most lesions (55%) display a moth-eaten pattern, but approximately 29% are geographic and 12% permeative.[19] In one study, all osteoblastic lesions were well defined and geographic in outline and were positive on radionuclide imaging. Osteolytic lesions may partially remineralize with chemotherapy. The axial skeleton is the most common site of metastatic involvement, with an incidence of 72%. Metastases in the long bones are usually diaphyseal in location, frequently invading the cortex with the development of extraskeletal soft-tissue masses and, sometimes, pathologic fractures. Periosteal reaction is uncommon.

For both initial evaluation and surveillance of soft-tissue malignancy, chest radiography should be performed, followed by CT if plain films are abnormal, to screen for pulmonary metastases.

Xeroradiography

Xeroradiography with its excellent edge-contrast enhancement and wide latitude displays both osseous and soft tissues in a single exposure. This technique, which requires higher radiation exposure than conventional radiography and special equipment, is not readily available or widely used for studying soft-tissue tumors,[23,24] particularly since the advent of cross-sectional imaging.

Scintigraphy

Scintigraphy[25–28] has low spatial resolution and therefore does not adequately define the primary tumor and its extent. Its principal function is to provide a global evaluation of the skeleton and the soft tissues and to detect non-palpable skip lesions and metastases. The abnormal areas of increased radionuclide uptake are then evaluated by plain radiography and MR. In one tumor, neurofibromatosis, gallium-67 scintigraphy has been shown to be promising for identifying malignant degeneration in generalized neurofibromatosis:[29] increased gallium-67 uptake was present in five malignant lesions of neurofibromatosis, whereas benign lesions demonstrated no uptake.

Angiography

Prior to the advent of CT and MR, angiography was the principal imaging modality for staging soft-tissue sarcomas, for following their response to therapy, and for identifying satellite and skip lesions.[30–32] At present, however, the primary role of angiography is interventional, for placement of chemotherapeutic catheters and pre-operative embolization of vascular tumors.

Angiographic studies display a varied vascular pattern in soft-tissue malignancy, from hypervascular flow with puddling and tumor blush to a hypovascular or even avascular flow. Within a particular tumor, the highly vascular areas tend to correlate with more malignant regions.[8,30] When vascular tumors respond significantly to chemotherapy, the hypervascular tumors become necrotic and less vascular. The vascularity, however, defines unequivocally neither the aggressiveness of the malignancy nor the tumor type. For example, a benign glomus tumor may be highly vascular, whereas an aggressive fibrosarcoma may show little vascularity.[30]

Sonography

Before the development of CT and MR, sonography was used for identifying the presence of superficial soft-tissue sarcomas and their recurrences.[33,34] The limited field of view and the inability to visualize bone and penetrate bowel has negated its usefulness. At present, ultrasonography serves for detecting parenchymal metastases, particularly to the liver.

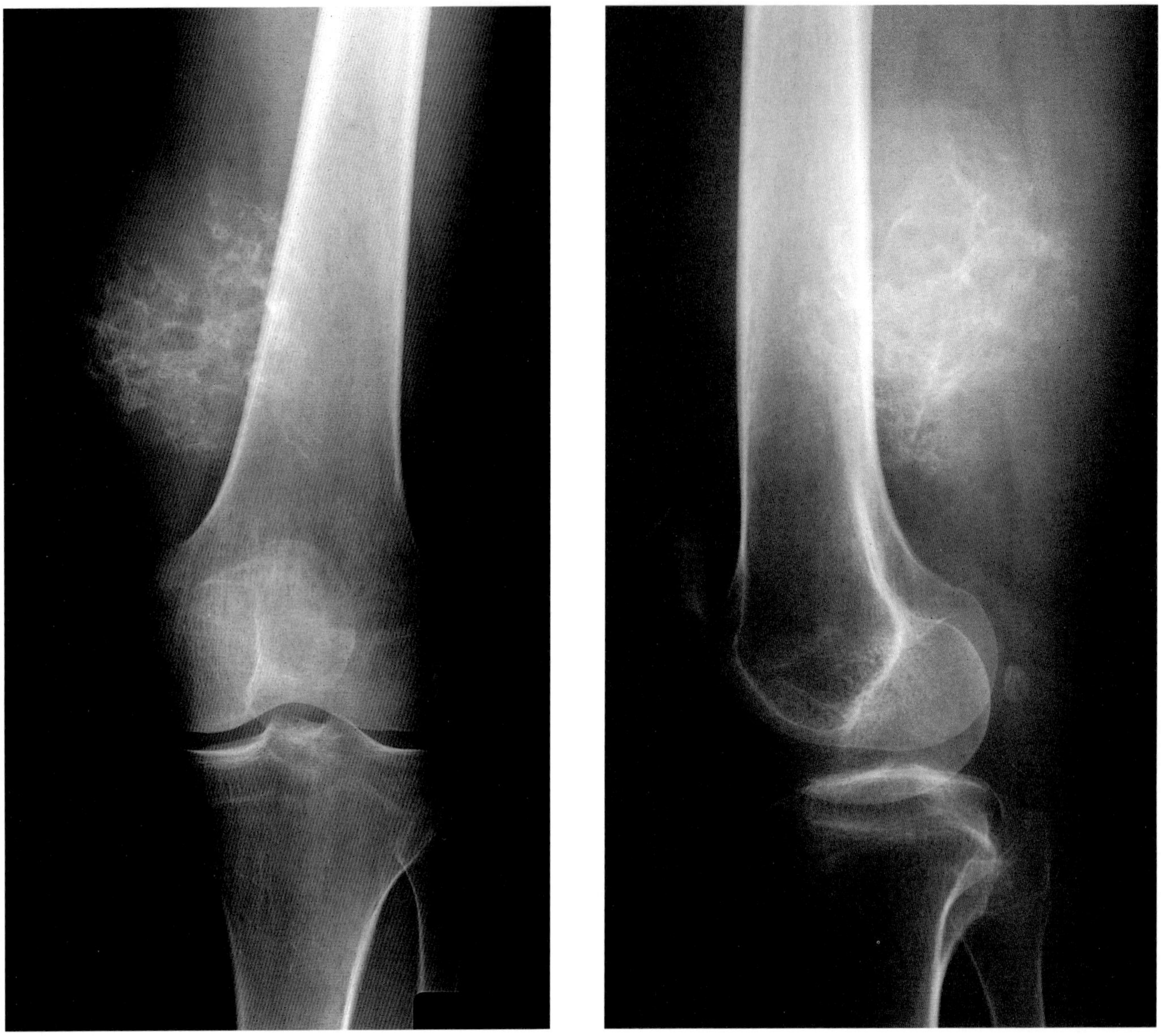

A B

Computed tomography

Prior to MR, CT along with angiography was the main modality for evaluating soft-tissue sarcomas and their response to chemotherapy.[33, 25–41] Poor soft-tissue contrast, good resolution limited to one plane, the need for contrast media and bone hardening artifacts limited its efficacy. Furthermore, CT may overestimate tumor size because of vessel displacement secondary to muscle edema.[36] Even with contrast enhancement, CT may not be able to distinguish between simple compression of neurovasular structures by tumor from actual entrapment. The addition of contrast media improves the demarcation of only the highly vascular tumors.

The main advantages of CT are in detecting calcifications, ossification and cortical bone destruction, although plain radiography may better define the specific type of calcification or ossification.

The major role of CT is for guiding percutaneous biopsies of metastatic or recurrent tumor. For

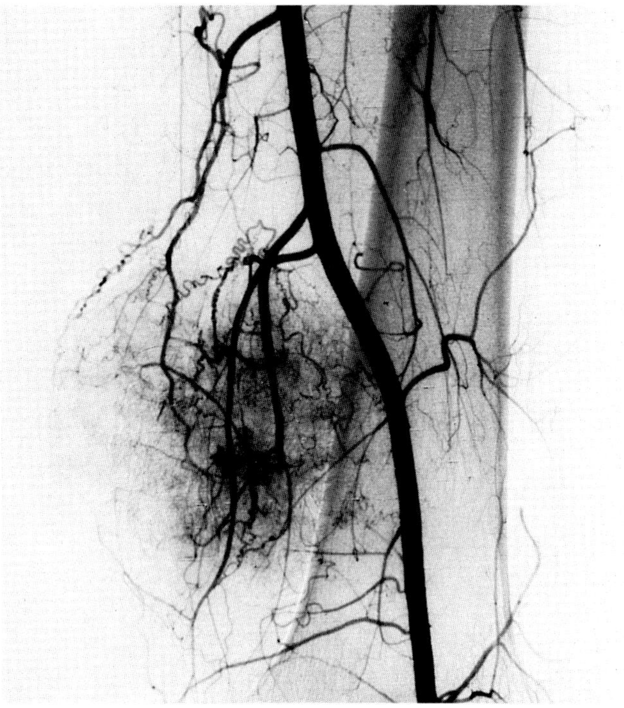

C

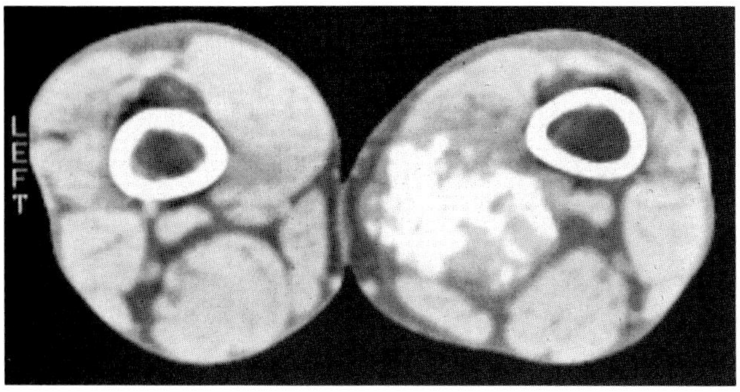

D

Figure 18.2

Initial evaluation of malignant fibrous histiocytoma.

A and **B** Plain radiography: AP (**A**) and lateral views (**B**), of the distal left femur.

C Angiography.

D CT.

The tumor contains irregular calcifications, and is highly vascular. The bone is not invaded.

initial diagnosis, however, open biopsies should be performed to assure adequate sampling and to prevent tumor spread.

Magnetic resonance imaging

In the past 5 years, MR has emerged as the most significant advance in the imaging of soft-tissue tumors because of its excellent soft-tissue contrast and multiplaner imaging.[28,40–49] Nevertheless, in contrast to CT, MR may fail to depict abnormalities of cortical bone, calcification and ossification because of the lack of mobile protons.[40] In addition, chemical shift artifacts may produce confusing images.

For the initial staging of soft-tissue sarcomas, MR should be performed prior to intervention[45] because biopsies can produce hemorrhage and edema and obscure the extent of the tumor. The protocol should include both T1- and T2-weighted sequences obtained in orthogonal planes (Figure 18.3). Soft-tissue extension is best delineated on T2-weighted images and intramedullary extension best defined on T1-weighted images. Contrast media are not usually used because contrast between tumor and fat and between tumor and soft tissues is lower than on pre-contrast scans.

MR depicts the 'characteristic' malignant soft-tissue tumor as an ill-defined inhomogeneous mass that encases neurovascular structures and invades bones.[44] Edema in adjacent muscles is another MR feature that has been strongly associated with malignant soft-tissue neoplasms, with 100% specificity and 95% sensitivity in the pristine tumor.[45] In contrast, the well-defined homogeneous lesion that respects the boundaries of adjacent bone and neurovascular structures and maintains soft-tissue planes speaks of a more benign process. However, there is considerable overlap. The well-demarcated synovial sarcoma is the malignancy most commonly misdiagnosed as benign, whereas desmoid tumors locally infiltrate adjacent tissue and mimic malignancy.[44] Misdiagnosis leads to inadequate surgical excision, which is the leading cause of recurrence.

Signal intensity does not differentiate benign from malignant lesions because, in most instances, both show low signal intensity on T1-weighted images and high signal intensity on T2-weighted images. However, tumors containing fibrous tissue,

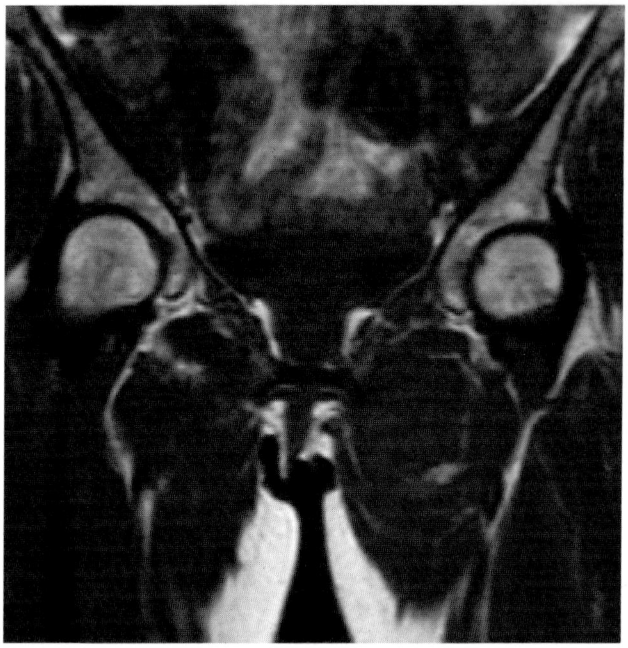

A

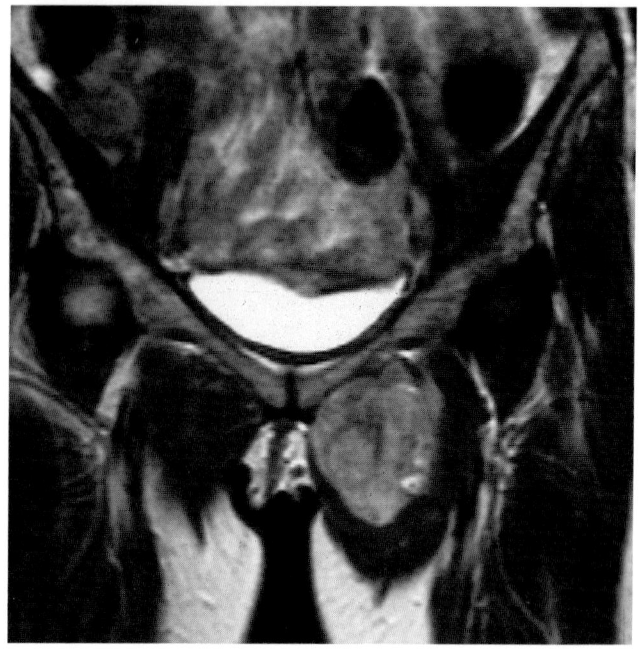

B

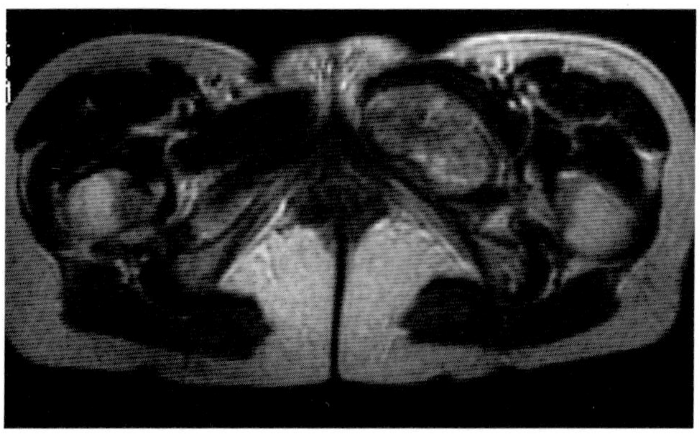

C

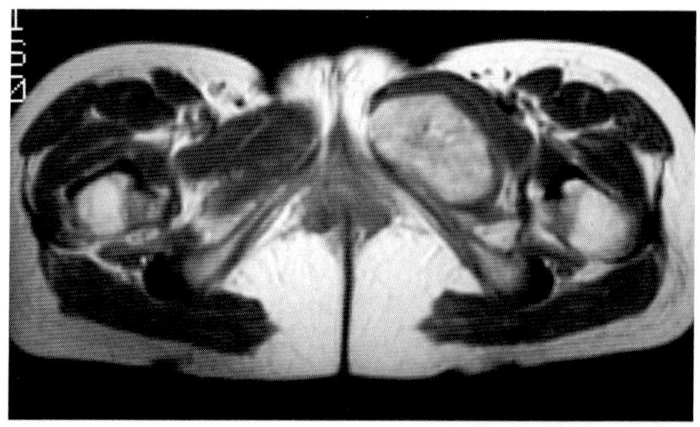

D

Figure 18.3

Initial evaluation by MR of malignant soft-tissue tumor (sarcoma).

A,B Coronal views before (**A**) and after (**B**) injection of contrast medium.

C,D Axial views: T1-weighted (**C**: TR 600/TE 20, after injection of contrast medium) and T2-weighted (**D**: TR 2000/TE 100) images.

The mass is poorly seen on the T1-weighted image contrast, and much better defined on T2-weighted images, and after injection of contrast medium. It is rather well limited inside the adductor muscles, and heterogeneous.

such as malignant fibrous histocytoma and desmoid tumors, can show low signal intensity on both T1-weighted and T2-weighted images: at histopathology, the low signal intensity correlates with relative acellularity and abundant collagen.[46] On the other hand, fat-containing tumors, such as benign lipoma and the uncommon well-differentiated lipoblastic liposarcoma, both show high signal intensity on T1- and intermediate signal on T2-weighted images because of the mature fat. In contrast, the more common myxoid liposarcoma demonstrates the more typical pattern of low signal intensity on T1-weighted images because of the paucity of fat.[4] Measurements of relaxation times show considerable overlap between different

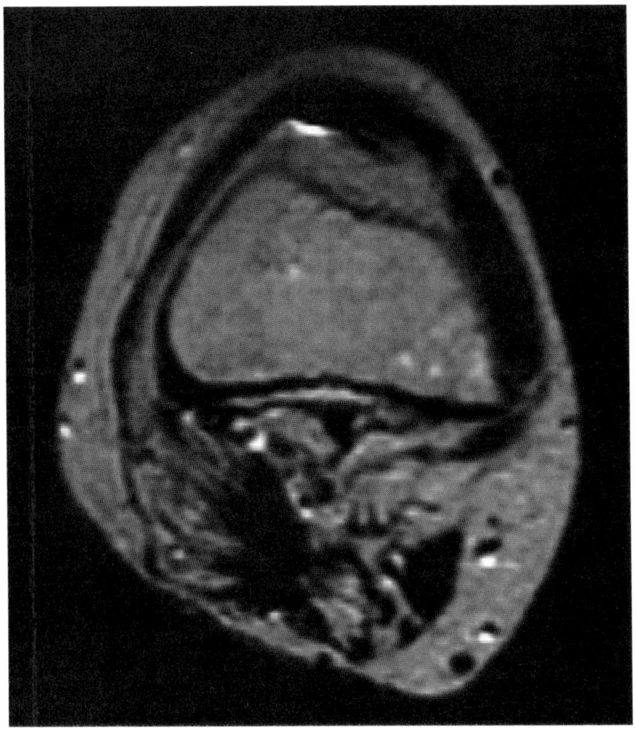

Figure 18.4

Aggressive fibromatosis followed after surgery and radiation therapy. On T2-weighted (TR 2000/TE 100) axial MR, the scar has a low signal intensity. It indicates no residual tumor.

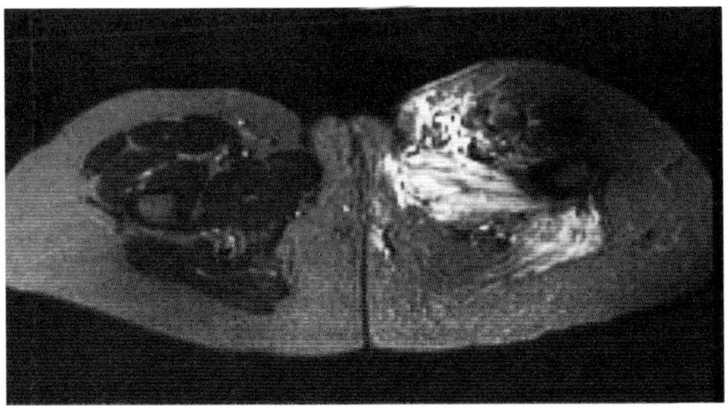

Figure 18.5

Malignant soft-tissue tumor followed after surgery and radiation therapy. On T2-weighted (TR 2000/TE 80) axial MR, the inflammatory changes have a widespread high signal with no mass, which indicates the radiotherapy portals.

tumors, and even benign and malignant tumors can not be differentiated.

Non-metastatic disseminated disease, such as neurofibromatosis, exemplifies a problem, in that neither CT nor MR distinguishes malignant from benign lesions. Tumor inhomegeneity may be present in either benign or malignant tumors. An irregular infiltrative tumor margin may occur in benign plexiform neurofibromas as well as in the more aggressive neurofibrosarcoma. Nevertheless, neurofibrosarcoma may appear well marginated and smooth in outline.

The main treatment is surgical, with radiation therapy if excision is incomplete or if there is recurrence. The usefulness of chemotherapy has not yet been proved. After radiation therapy and chemotherapy and/or surgery, MR scans should be utilized in the detection of recurrent or residual tumor.

In a recent study we evaluated 110 soft-tissue malignancies.[47] The T2-weighted sequence was the most useful for excluding recurrent or residual tumor.

- *Absence of high signal intensity* on T2-weighted images in a mass excluded tumor in 99% of our patients (Figure 18.4). Only one patient with a T2-weighted sequence that showed no high signal intensity had foci of active tumor at histopathology – two 1 mm foci.
- *Generalized high signal intensity without mass* in an area of previous tumor on T2-weighted images, signifies post-therapy change or infection. In patients who have had surgery and radiation therapy for soft-tissue tumors, the high signal intensity signal is usually localized to the radiotherapy portals (Figure 18.5).
- *High signal intensity mass* on T2-weighted images should promote one to consider a differential diagnosis. Although recurrent active tumor commonly presents with these findings, inflammatory and post-inflammatory masses, residual hematoma, hygroma, seroma, and necrosis may all simulate tumor with low signal intensity on T1-weighted images and high signal intensity on T2-weighted images.[43,47,50,51]

Addition of contrast medium usually permits differentiation between the enhancing active tumor or inflammation and the non-enhancing hematoma, hygroma or necrosis lesions (Figure 18.6).[47,51,52] However some mucus-containing tumors (certain chondrosarcomas, liposarcomas and chordomas) may show focal areas of non-enhancement, similar to necrosis. At histopathology these areas of low signal intensity are mucus-filled malignant cells.

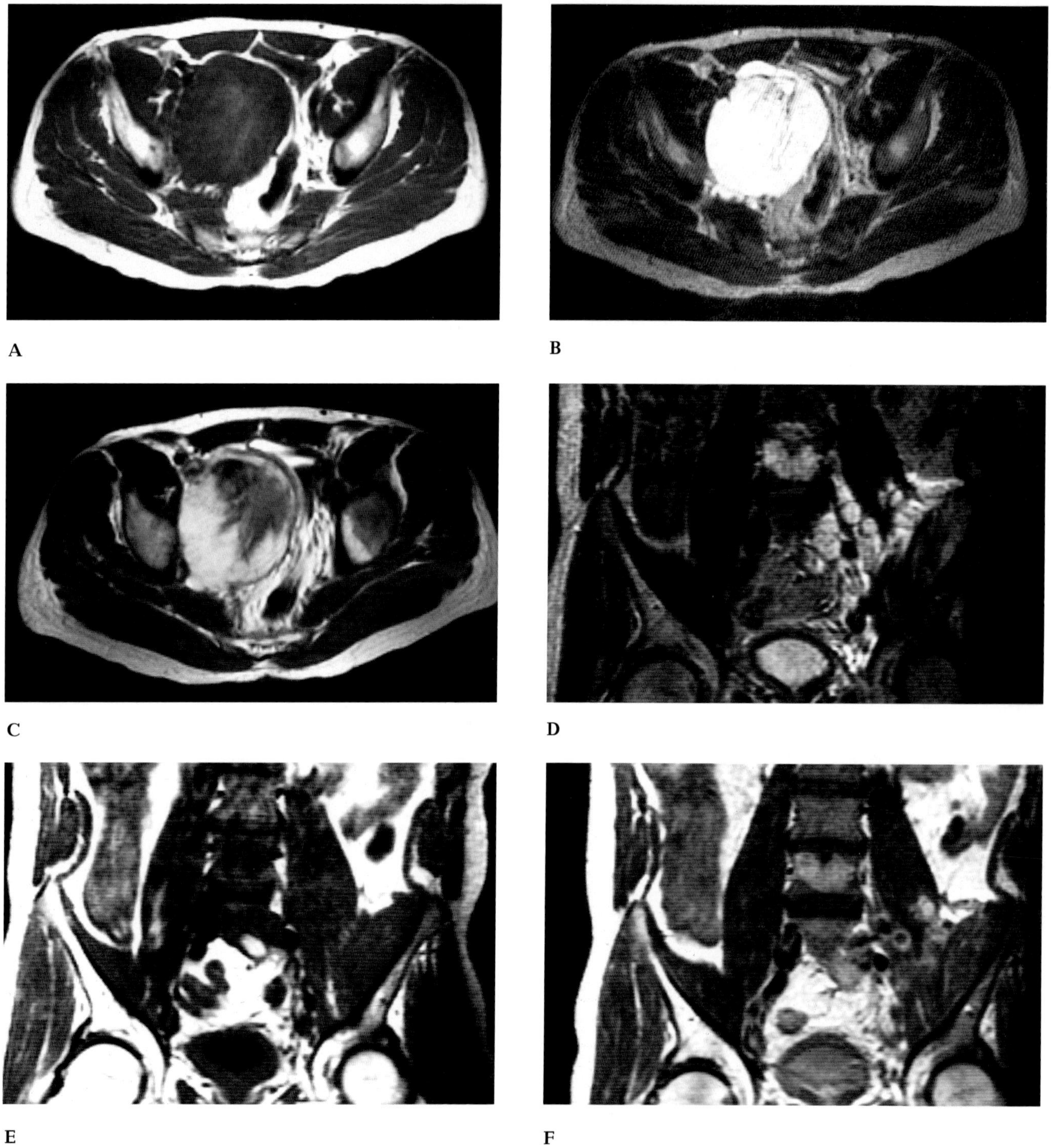

Figure 18.6

Initial evaluation of soft-tissue sarcoma.

A–C Axial views: T2-weighted image (**B**: TR 2000/TE 90) without contrast medium, and T1-weighted images (**A**, **C**: TR 600/TE 20) before (**A**) and after (**C**) injection of contrast medium, demonstrate a pelvic mass, close to the iliac vessels, and the piriformis muscle. There was high signal intensity on T2- and T1-weighted images after contrast. The partial low signal after contrast corresponds to necrotic areas.

A follow-up examination 6 months later was prompted by sciatica.

D–F Coronal views: T2-weighted image (**D**: TR 2000/TE 100) without contrast medium, and T1-weighted images (**E**, **F**: TR 600/TE 200) before (**E**) and after (**F**) injection of contrast medium. The recurrence is of multiple nodules involving the left iliac and psoas muscles. They have a high signal on T2- and T1-weighted post-contrast images.

A metastasis to L4 is easily diagnosed.

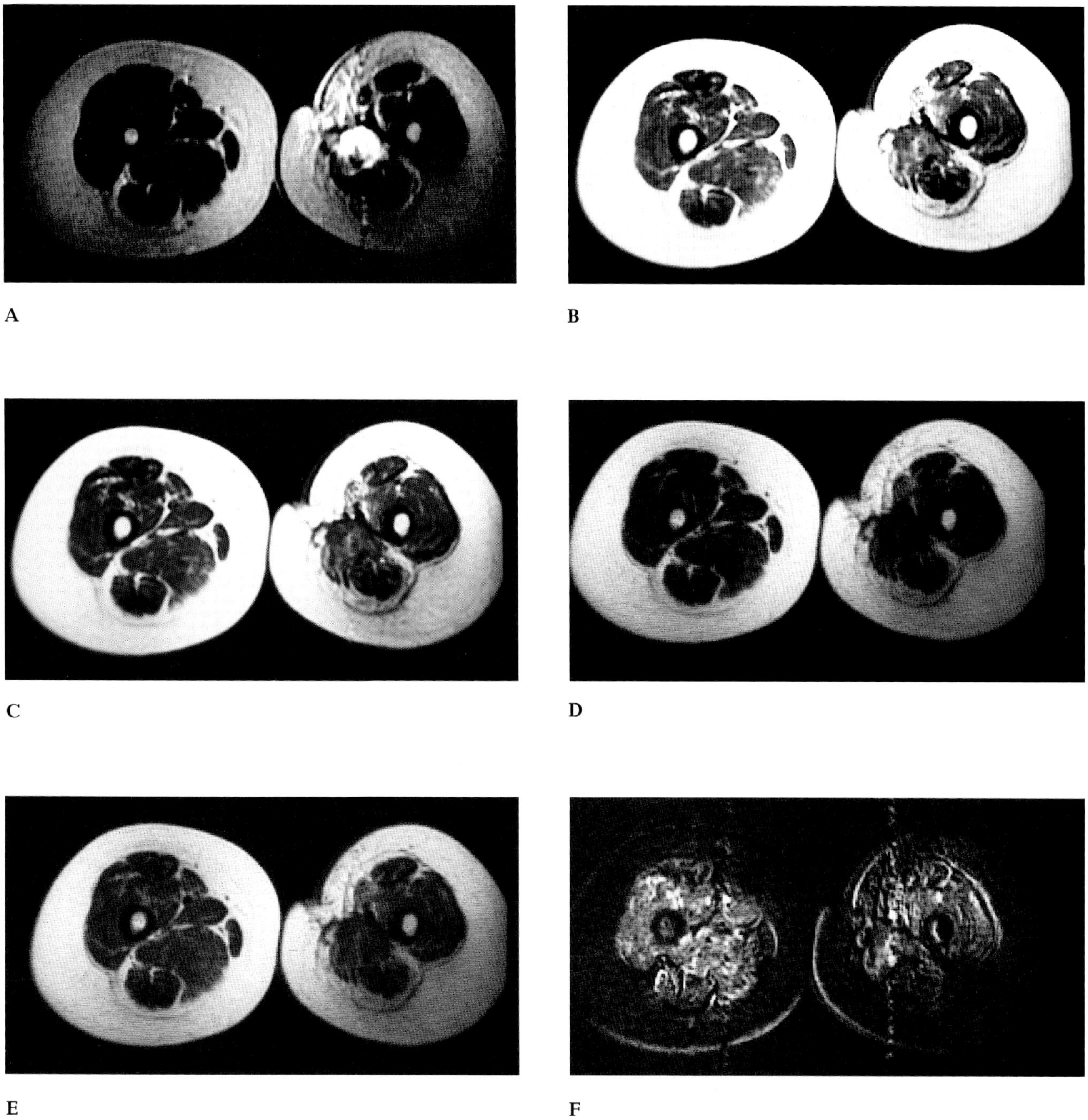

Figure 18.7

Systematic follow up of a malignant soft-tissue tumor after surgery and radiation therapy.

A–C Axial views: T2-weighted image (**A**: TR 2500/TE 100) without contrast medium, and T1-weighted images (**B**: TR 300/TE 20; **C**: TR 600/TE 20) before (**B**) and 10 minutes after (**C**) injection of contrast medium, show high signal intensity on the T2-weighted image: a poorly defined mass taking up contrast medium.

D–F On T1-weighted images (TR 300/TE 20) performed before (**D**) and 1 minute after (**E**) bolus injection and subtraction (**F**), there is no early enhancement.

This was an inflammatory pseudotumor.

However, contrast-enhanced static MR scans cannot distinguish the high signal intensities of active tumor from inflammatory, post-chemotherapeutic or post-radiotherapeutic change. Post-radiation enhancement may persist in inflammatory masses for more than 5 years after surgery. In a specific group of patients who received intra-arterial chemotherapy for musculoskeletal sarcomas, there develop additional MR findings related to their route of treatment.[49,50] Patients can show an intensification of the peritumoral edema after initial doses of cisplatin. With continued course of intra-arterial chemotherapy, soft tissues adjacent to the tumors may display areas of intermediate signal intensity on T1- and high signal intensity on T2-weighted images in a segmental arterial perfusion pattern. Furthermore, the chemotherapy-induced changes in muscle occasionally produce high signal intensity mimicking progression of the sarcoma: areas of myonecrosis may be found.[53]

After removal of the tumor, inflammatory changes very rarely mimic a mass. In these cases, subtraction MR enhanced imaging is very useful: tumor takes up contrast medium early (within 2 minutes of injection), whereas inflammatory reactions only take up contrast medium later[54] (Figure 18.7).

The follow up of soft-tissue sarcomas after radiation therapy and surgery is outlined in Diagram 18.1.

Conclusion

The imaging of soft-tissue malignancy, whether by conventional radiography, cross-sectional CT or MR, does not definitively differentiate benign from malignant lesions and usually cannot specify the particular tumor type. Plain radiography is useful predominantly for detecting calcifications and ossifications and to rule out a bone tumor. It is MR, however, that has become the most effective modality both for primary staging of soft-tissue malignancy and for following its response to therapy.

References

1. Enzinger FM, Weiss SW, eds, *Soft tissue tumors* (CV Mosby: Washington DC, 1988).
2. Conrad EV, Enneking, WF, Common soft tissue tumors, *Clin Symp* (1990) **42**: 1–32.
3. Shapeero LG, Young S, Mycosis fungoides: manifestations on computed tomography, *Radiology* (1983) **148**: 202.
4. Sundaram M, McLeod RA, MR imaging of tumor and tumor like lesions of bone and soft tissue, *AJR* (1990) **155**: 817–24.
5. Enneking WF, Spanier SS, Malamer MM, Effect of the anatomic setting on the results of surgical procedures for soft parts sarcomas of the thigh, *Cancer* (1981) **47**: 1005–22.
6. Madewell JE, Moser RP, Radiologic evaluation of soft tissue tumors. In: Enzinger FM, Weiss SW, eds, *Soft tissue tumors* (CV Mosby: Washington, 1988) 43–82.
7. Martel W, Abell MR, Radiologic evaluation of soft tissue tumors: a retrospective study, *Cancer* (1973) **32**: 352–65.
8. Resnick D, Niwayama G, Soft tissues. In: Resnick D, Niwayama G, eds, *Diagnosis of bone and joint disorders* (WB Saunders: Philadelphia, 1980) 4171–286.
9. Horowitz AF, Resnick D, Watson RC, The roentgen features of synovial sarcomas, *Clin Radiol* (1973) **24**: 481–4.
10. Feldman F, Norman D, Intra- and extraosseous malignant histiocytoma (malignant fibrous xanthoma), *Radiology* (1972) **104**: 497–508.
11. Abramowitz D, Zornoza J, Ayala AG et al, Soft-tissue desmoid tumors: radiographic bone changes, *Radiology* (1983) **146**: 11–13.
12. Shapeero L, Vanel D, Contesso G, Extraskeletal mesenchymal chondrosarcoma (abstr) *Radiology* (in press).
13. Vanel D, Shapeero L, Contesso G, Extraskeletal osteosarcoma *Eur J Radiol* (in press).
14. Norman A, Dorfman HD, Juxtacortical circumscribed myositis ossificans. Evaluation and radiographic features, *Radiology* (1970) **96**: 301–6.
15. Goldman AB, Myositis ossificans circumscripta: a benign lesion with malignant differential diagnosis, *AJR* (1976) **126**: 32–40.
16. Ackerman L, Ramamurthy S, Jablokow V et al, Case Report 488, *Skeletal Radiol* (1988) **17**: 310.
17. Amendola MA, Glazer GM, Faroog PA et al, Myositis ossificans circumscripta: computed tomographic diagnosis, *Radiology*, (1983) **149**: 775–9.
18. Ackerman LV, Extraosseous localized non-neoplastic bone and cartilage formation (so-called myositis ossificans), *J Bone Joint Surg (Am)* (1958) **40**: 279–98.
19. Wong WS, Kaiser LRR, Gold RH et al, Radiographic features of osseous metastases of soft tissue sarcomas, *Radiology* (1982) **143**: 71–4.
20. Ariel IM, Briceno M, Rhabdomyosarcoma of the extremities and trunk: analysis of 150 patients treated by surgical resection, *J Surg Oncol* (1975) **7**: 269–87.
21. Hajdu SI, Shui MH, Fortner JG, Tendosynovial sarcoma: a clinicopathological study of 136 cases, *Cancer* (1977) **39**: 1201–17.

22. Kindblom LG, Angervall L, Svendsen P, Liposarcoma. A clinicopathologic, radiographic, and prognostic study, *Acta Pathol Microbiol Scand* (1975) **253**: (suppl): 1–71.
23. Wolfe N, Xeroradiography of the bone, joints, and soft tissues. *Radiology* (1969) **93**: 583–7.
24. Otto RC, Pouliadis GP, Kungue DA, The evaluation of pathologic alterations juxtaosseous soft tissues by xeroradiography, *Radiology* (1976) **120**: 297–302.
25. Kirchner PT, Simon MA, The clinical value of bone and gallium scintigraphy for soft tissue sarcomas of the extremities, *J Bone Joint Surg (Am)* (1984) **66**: 319–27.
26. Chew FS, Hudson TM, Enneking WE, Radionuclide imaging of soft tissue neoplasms, *Semin Nucl Med* (1981) **11**: 266–76.
27. Hudson TM, Schakel M, Springfield DS et al, The comparative value of bone scintigraphy in determining bone involvement by soft tissue sarcomas, *J Bone Joint Surg (Am)* (1984) **66**: 1400–7.
28. Aisen AM, Martel W, Braunstein EM et al, MRI and CT evaluation of primary bone and soft-tissue tumors, *AJR* (1986) **146**: 749–56.
29. Levine E, Huntrakoon M, Wetzel LH, Malignant nerve-sheath neoplasms in neurofibromatosis: distinction from benign tumors by using imaging techniques, *AJR* (1987) **149**: 1059–64.
30. Herzberg DL, Schreiber MH, Angiography in mass lesions of the extremities, *AJR* (1971) **111**: 541–5.
31. Cockshott P, Evans KT. The place of soft tissue arteriography, *Br J Radiol* (1964) **37**: 367–75.
32. Hudson TM, Hass G, Enneking WF et al, Angiography in the management of musculoskeletal tumors, *Surg Gynecol Obstet* (1975) **141**: 11–21.
33. Bernardino ME, Jing BS, Thomas JL et al, The extremity soft-tissue lesion: a comparative study of ultrasound computed tomography, and xeroradiography, *Radiology* (1981) **139**: 53–9.
34. Yeh HC, Rabinowitz JG, Ultrasonography of the extremities and pelvic girdle and correlation with computed tomography, *Radiology* (1982) **143**: 519–25.
35. Weekes RG, McLeod RA, Reiman HM et al, CT of soft-tissue neoplasms, *AJR* (1985) **144**: 355–60.
36. Egund N, Ekelund L, Sako M et al, CT of soft tissue tumors, *AJR* (1981) **137**: 725–29.
37. Weinberger G, Levinsohn EM, Computed tomography in evaluation of sarcomatous tumors of the thigh, *AJR* (1978) **130**: 115–18.
38. Soye I, Levine E, De Smet A et al, Computed tomography in the preoperative evaluation of masses arising in and near joints of the extremities, *Radiology* (1982) **143**: 727–32.
39. O'Keeffe F, Lorigan JG, Wallace S, Radiological features of extraskeletal Ewing's sarcoma, *Br J Radiol* (1990) **63**: 456–61.
40. Tehranzadeh J, Mnaymneh W, Ghavam C et al, Comparison of CT and MR imaging in musculoskeletal neoplasm, *J Comput Assist Tomogr* (1989) **13**: 466–72.
41. Demas BE, Heelan RT, Lane J et al, Soft-tissue sarcomas of the extremities: comparison of MR and CT in determining the extent of disease, *AJR* (1985) **150**: 615–20.
42. Totty WG, Murphy WA, Soft-tissue tumors: MR imaging, *Radiology* (1986) **160**: 135–41.
43. Vanel D, Di Paola R, Contesso G, Magnetic resonance imaging in musculoskeletal primary malignant tumors. In: Kressel H, ed, *Magnetic resonance annual 1987* (Raven Press: New York, 1987) 237–61.
44. Berquist TH, Ehman RLL, King BF et al, Value of MR imaging in differentiating benign from malignant soft-tissue masses: study of 95 lesions, *AJR* (1990) **155**: 1251–5.
45. Beltran J, Simon DC, Katz W et al, Increased MR signal intensity in skeletal muscle adjacent to malignant tumors: pathological correlation and clinical relevance, *Radiology* (1987) **162**: 251–5.
46. Sundaram M, McGuire MH, Schajowicz F, Soft-tissue masses: histologic basis for decreased signal (short T2) on T2-weighted MR images, *AJR* (1987) **148**: 1247–50.
47. Vanel D, Shapeero LG, Michel G, The use of contrast medium in MR imaging of primary musculoskeletal tumors. In: Katayama H, Brasch RC, eds, *New dimensions of contrast media* (International Congress Series, Elsevier: New York, 1991) 274–9.
48. Wetzel LH, Levine E, Soft-tissue tumors of the foot: value of MR imaging for specific diagnosis, *AJR* (1990) **155**: 1025–30.
49. Shapeero LG, MRI of the foot and ankle. In: Gooding CR, ed, *Diagnostic Radiology 1990* (University of California Press: San Francisco, 1990) 454–66.
50. Vanel D, Lacombe MJ, Couanet D et al, Musculoskeletal tumors: follow-up with MR imaging after treatment with surgery and radiation therapy, *Radiology* (1987) **164**: 243–5.
51. Erlemann R, Reiser MF, Peters PE et al, Musculoskeletal neoplasms: static and dynamic Gd-DTPA-enhanced MR imaging, *Radiology* (1989) **171**: 767–73.
52. Pettersson H, Eliasson J, Egund N et al, Gadolinium-DTPA enhancement of soft tissue tumors on magnetic resonance imaging: preliminary clinical experience in five patients, *Skeletal Radiol* (1988) **17**: 319–23.
53. Sanchez RB, Quinn SF, Walling A et al, Musculoskeletal neoplasms after intraarterial chemotherapy: correlation of MR images with pathologic specimens, *Radiology* (1990) **174**: 237–40.
54. De Baere T, Vanel D, Shapeero LG et al, Osteosarcoma after chemotherapy: evaluation with contrast material-enhanced subtraction MR imaging, *Radiology* (1992) **185**: 587–92.

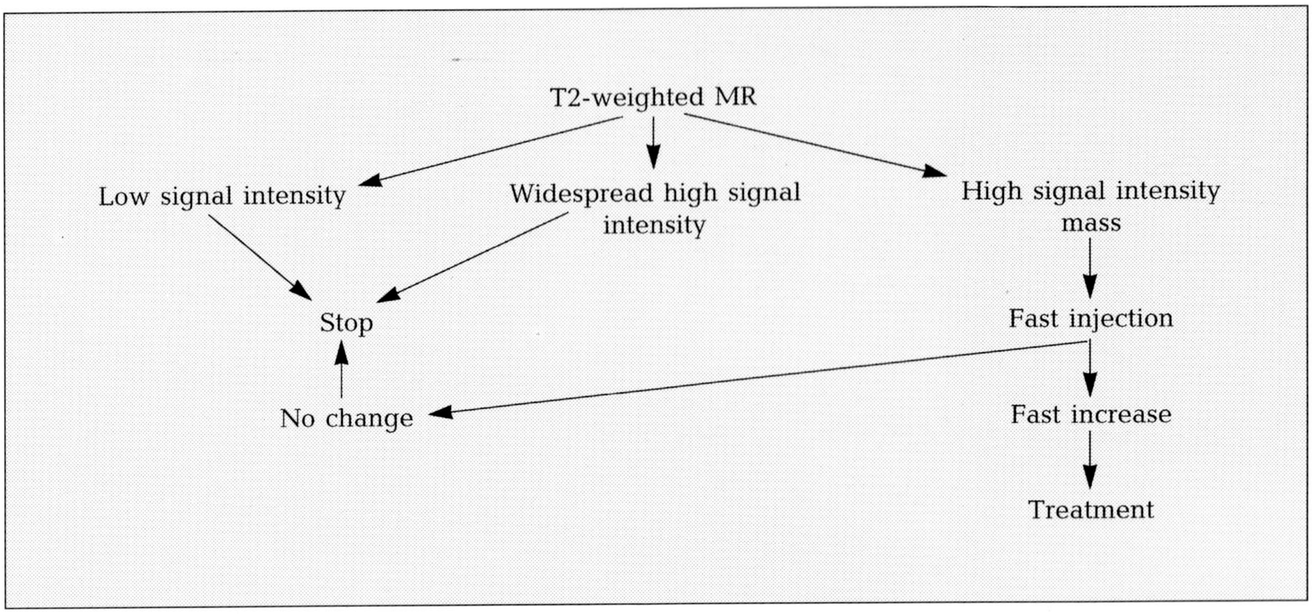

Diagram 18.1

MR in the follow up of aggressive soft-tissue tumors.

19

Bone

Daniel Vanel and Lorraine Shapeero

Introduction

Bone imaging techniques have undergone significant changes during the last decade. Ultrasonography, computed tomography (CT), and recently magnetic resonance (MR), have been added to arteriography, bone scanning and conventional radiology, the latter still being the primary examination. At the same time, survival in those diagnosed as having malignant primary bone tumors has improved with chemotherapy,[1,2] and conservative surgery continues to give improved results. Imaging plays a major role in diagnosis, local and distant staging, monitoring of the treatment's effectiveness and detection of recurrences.

General considerations

Diagnosis

The diagnostic approach is statistical,[3,4] and consists of evaluating various clinical and imaging data in order to select the most probable diagnosis. Age is an important factor: before 5 years of age, a malignant tumor is almost always a metastatic neuroblastoma; between 5 and 15 years of age, it is often an osteosarcoma or Ewing's sarcoma; after 40 years of age, it tends to be a metastasis or a myeloma.

Clinical symptoms show little variation; most often they are pain and swelling. Although fever suggests infection, it may also present in Ewing's sarcoma or more rarely in osteoblastoma. Laboratory examination is usually normal.

The first step in tumor evaluation is the determination of the aggressiveness of the tumor by conventional radiology. It is sometimes necessary to carry out multiple projections in order to evaluate the different characteristics of the tumor.

Important parameters include tumor size (most malignant tumors are over 6 cm at presentation), type of matrix, type of periosteal reaction when present, margination and cortical disruption. New bone formation and lack of margination, limited by a thin intact periosteum, both suggest a slower evolution and the presence of a benign mass. When the tumor crosses the periosteum, the periosteum reacts by provoking the addition of multiple layers. In benign lesions, the periosteal response is, typically, longitudinal and thick; in malignant lesions, it is lamellar interrupted and perpendicular to the bone axis.

Particular tumors are more commonly associated with particular bones, for example adamantinoma – usually found in adults – involve selectively the tibia and the ulna; chondroblastoma is the most common epiphyseal tumor in childhood. In addition, tumors may be more or less aggressive depending on their location in the axial or appendicular skeleton: in the hand, cartilaginous tumors are almost always benign, whereas, in the pelvis, they are often malignant.

If necessary, presence of multiple lesions can be estimated by bone scanning. Such multiple lesions are seen in chondromas, osteochondromas, histiocytosis X, metastases, and more rarely in multifocal osteosarcomas and metastatic Ewing's sarcomas.

The first step that must be taken is to definitively diagnose benign lesions based on clinical and radiologic signs; for this, biopsy is not necessary. The lesions that could be found are given below.

Fibrous cortical defect

A fibrous cortical defect is a benign bone lesion frequently found in children, being most common between the ages of 6 and 11 years; it is always an accidental finding. If the lesion is painful, then other lesions should be considered. The sites that are most commonly involved in these lesions are: the posteromedial side of the distal femoral metaphysis, the superior portion of the tibia, the fibula and, more rarely, the humerus, ribs and iliac bone. Radiographs should be evaluated in multiple projections, and should show the following typical finding: a metaphyseal lesion centered on the cortex of a long bone that is in contact with the cartilaginous growth plate. The lesion usually shows the following features: it measures less than 3 cm, it is oriented along the bone axis, it is oval in shape, it is lytic and it has well-defined margins which sometimes have a thin sclerotic border. Fibrous cortical defects may expand, but they do not disrupt the outer margin of the cortex. There is neither periosteal reaction nor soft tissue mass; there are also no problems with bone growth. The radiologic findings and absence of pain are so typical as to be diagnostic. Often fibrous cortical defects resolve spontaneously. Rarely, they become non-ossifying fibromas with filling in of the medullary cavity.

Non-ossifying fibroma

A non-ossifying fibroma may appear spontaneously or it may develop through transformation of a fibrous cortical defect. Children with this lesion are usually more than 8 years old. The lesion is usually asymptomatic but it produces pain when fractured (this happens in one-third of cases, particularly in the distal tibia). On radiographs, a non-ossifying fibroma is usually larger than the corresponding fibrous cortical defect, measuring 2–7 cm in size. Its location is metaphyseal and it is adjacent to cartilaginous growth plates. Non-ossifying fibromas appear as well-defined cortical lesions, centered on the cortex and oriented along the long axis of the bone. The internal border is well defined. The external border expands the cortex – the latter being thinned but often intact.

The lesion is lytic, although sometimes dense bone formation occurs in the older portion of the lesion, this segment being more distant from the cartilaginous growth plate. The prognosis is frequently favourable, and disappearance can be spontaneous; there is no malignant degeneration. Once again, as with fibrous cortical defects, radiologic findings and absence of symptoms are diagnostic.

Periosteal desmoid (Figure 19.1)

Periosteal desmoid is a common benign tumor in children, particularly in boys aged between 10 and 15 years. Although usually asymptomatic, it is frequently discovered following trauma.

Radiologically, its location is characteristic: it is found in the posterior part of the medial femoral condyle, just beneath the adductor tubercle. One-third of cases are bilateral. The lesion is similar to the fibrous cortical defect, with erosion of the cortex and peripheral sclerosis. It is difficult to differentiate from a periosteal sarcoma when the outer part of the lesion is lytic, with perpendicular periosteal reaction and soft tissue masses, although its typical location is suggestive. If there is any doubt, close follow up is needed to confirm its benign nature and to avoid more aggressive treatment.

Fibrous dysplasia

This lesion is frequent in children and adolescents. The monostotic form occurs more frequently and is often asymptomatic unless deformity or focal symptoms develop. The radiologic appearance depends on the degree of ossification of the lesions and on their expansile nature. Typically fibrous dysplasia is a homogeneous, slightly opaque, medullary lesion which obscures the trabeculation and extends to the cortex. It sometimes expands bone and shows a 'ground glass' appearance, contrasting with adjacent normal bone. Lesions can be either purely radiolucent or very dense, with the border disappearing between the cortex and the medullary cavity. In addition, they can be inhomogeneous with multiple sites of calcification. There can be varying combinations of these appearances. There is no periosteal reaction or soft tissue mass without a coexistent fracture.

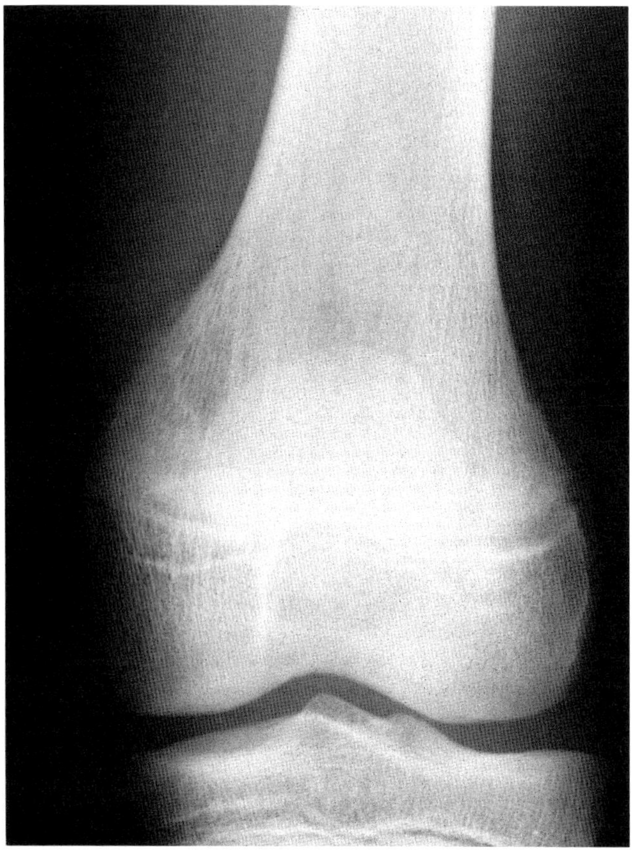

Figure 19.1

Plain radiograph of a periosteal desmoid. The radiologic pattern is aggressive with osteolysis of the cortex and periosteal bone formation. The location (posterior aspect of the medial condyle of the femur) gives a correct diagnosis. No biopsy is necessary.

Osteochondromas or exostoses

Osteochondromas or exostoses are frequent in children and teenagers. Patients usually present with an asymptomatic firm mass which develops in bone with endochondral growth. It is usually revealed by palpation of such a mass.

On radiographs, the findings are typical: the lesion is metaphyseal in location, but projects to the distal end of the long bones (most commonly the distal femur and the proximal humerus). Multiple projections are needed to evaluate the base of the lesion. The key to diagnosis is to show continuity of the cortex of the normal bone with that of the osteochondroma.

Chondroma

Chondromas are also frequent lesions, found in the hand in half of the cases. They are discovered fortuitously, pain and swelling only appearing after fracture. On radiographs, although usually centered on the bone, the chondroma is occasionally eccentric or periosteal in location. It is round or oval, lytic and it contains areas of cartilaginous calcification. Borders are well defined and the cortex can be thinned and expansile. There is no periosteal reaction or lesion in soft tissues where there is no fracture.

Simple bone cysts

Of all the benign lesions of the peripheral skeleton these lesions occur most frequently. Eighty to ninety per cent of the patients are aged between 3 and 19 years, boys being more often involved than girls. Simple bone cysts are asymptomatic until fractured: 50% are located in the proximal humerus and 25% in the femur.

Radiologically, simple bone cysts develop in the metaphysis and do not cross the cartilaginous growth plate. They are centrally located in the medullary cavity. The lesion is oriented along the bone axis, becoming wider when it contacts the metaphysis and narrower towards the diaphysis; it is lytic and well defined and it sometimes has localized dense bone when found in the extremities, especially on the diaphyseal side. The cortex is expansile and thinned, but not destroyed.

During growth, the cyst migrates into the diaphysis and is separated from the cartilaginous growth plate by normal bone. When growth ceases, it becomes ovoid. Fracture of bone cysts occurs in two-thirds of patients; they present with a typical radiologic appearance of a bone fragment within the cyst cavity.

Vertebral angiomas

Vertebral angiomas can occur in any age group. Radiologically, there is enlargement of vertebrae and striations within the vertebral body. Sometimes these angiomas can bleed and produce bowing of the paravertebral stripe on radiographs and soft tissue masses on CT.

Myositis ossificans

This lesion must be recognized (Figure 19.2), because biopsy is not necessary and can be harmful, and because histologic diagnosis can be very difficult. Patients are less than 30 years of age and trauma is found in two-thirds of cases. Swelling of the soft tissues appears with maximal pain during the second and third weeks; there is also redness of the skin, limitation of movement, fever and increase in erythrocyte sedimentation rate. Most commonly the lesion is located in the arm, the thigh, the pelvis, and the first and second metacarpals. Initial radiographs are normal, but within 3–4 weeks, areas of ossification appear in the soft tissues. Thus myositis ossificans, when first radiologically apparent, resembles a soft tissue mass (see Chapter 8). The lesion progressively ossifies and appears as a mass with a lucent center and a calcified periphery; this is diagnostic, particularly when previous images are available. The lesion evolves progressively to spontaneous regression.

Figure 19.2

Myositis ossificans: (**A,C**) plain radiographs; (**B,D**) CT scans. There is initially pain at presentation. Three weeks later (**A,B**), a calcified mass of the soft tissues is seen with periosteal reaction. The centre of the lesion is not calcified, suggesting the diagnosis. (**C,D**) One month later the lesion is much more calcified, with a typical pattern. Again the clear center is the key of the diagnosis. The lesion has disappeared without any treatment.

Others

In other cases, evidence favours a malignant lesion. Examination for metastases, and MR examination before biopsy, must be performed.

Finally, where certain diagnoses are involved, CT should be used to resolve difficulties. Problems can result from particular bone locations that are difficult to evaluate on conventional radiography (this happens with short, flat bones, especially the pelvis, sacrum, sternum and vertebrae). Sometimes, study of the tumor matrix can provide the necessary diagnostic features and these can include fluid density, small areas of calcification which allow diagnosis of cartilaginous tumor, osteoid matrix or fat.[5] Axial study and high contrast allow diagnosis of certain conditions: small lytic regions of the cortex, localized involvement of the soft tissues, and thin peripheral periosteal reaction (Figure 19.3); in addition, lesions with slow evolution, which displace and expand the cortex peripherally, can be distinguished from more aggressive lesions that cross the cortex. Before destruction, tumor on both sides of the cortex can be visualized on CT scan, and this is true of Ewing's sarcomas and osteosarcomas. If a tumor of this type is not ossified, it is probably Ewing's sarcoma; if ossified, it is probably an osteosarcoma.[6] CT allows measurement of the thickness of a non-calcified cuff on a cartilaginous tumor: the cuff is thin in benign lesions and thick (more than 3 cm) in chondrosarcoma.[7,8] CT is the examination of choice in the diagnosis of a nidus of osteoid osteoma in dense bone.[9]

Staging examination

Local

Focal extent and staging are based on magnetic resonance imaging (MR) (Figures 19.4 and 19.5).[10–22] The main advantages are high contrast and the ability to choose the plane of examination without moving the patient (Figure 19.3). However, MR is rarely useful for diagnosis. T1- and T2-weighted measurements are not reliable and reproducible and most large tumors are inhomogeneous and have a variable signal intensity. Therefore, it is impossible to characterize such tumors and to distinguish benign from malignant lesions.[23] MR is rarely useful in the diagnosis of fluid levels in blood-filled cavities, especially aneurysmal bone cysts.[24,25]

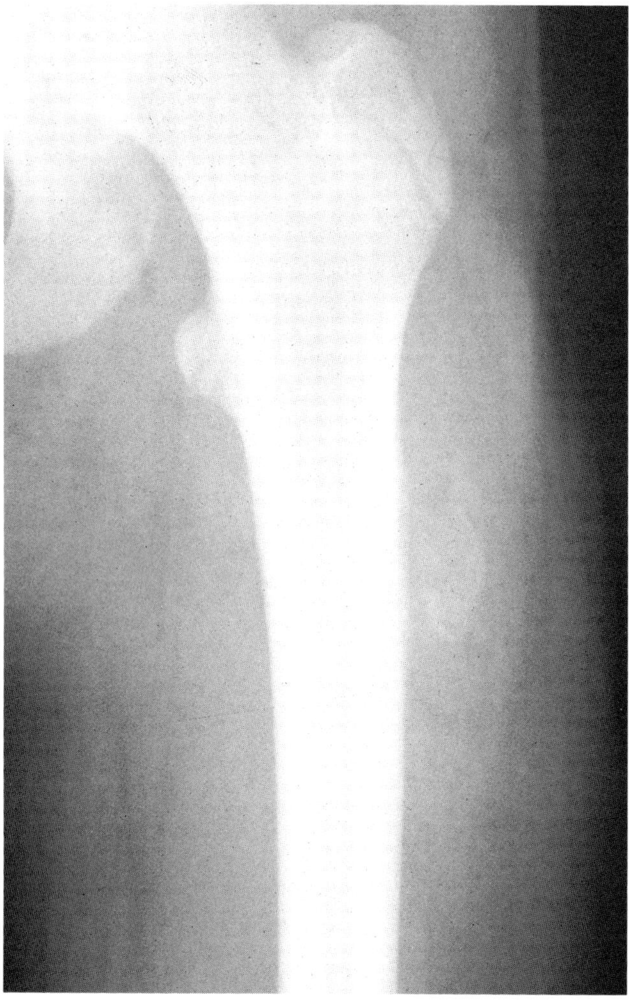

A

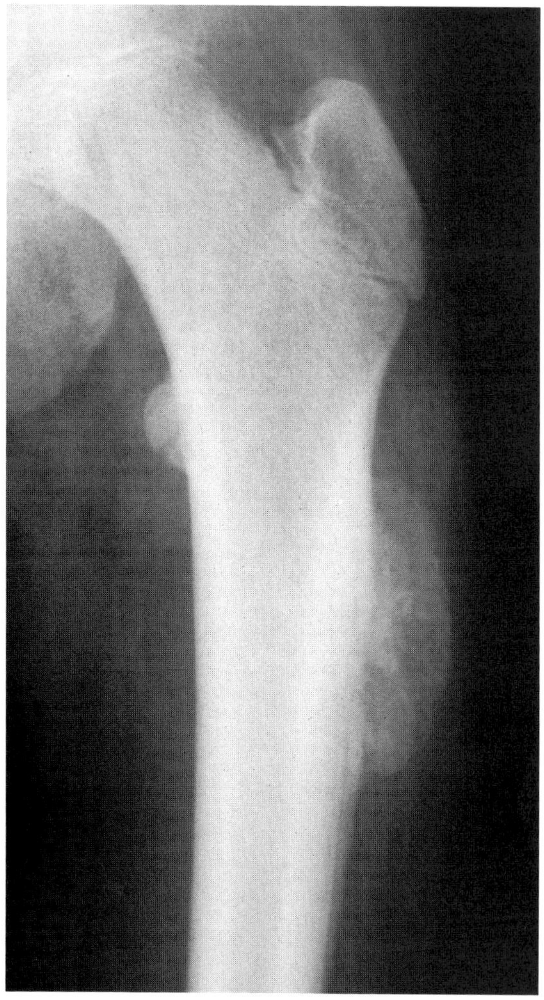

C

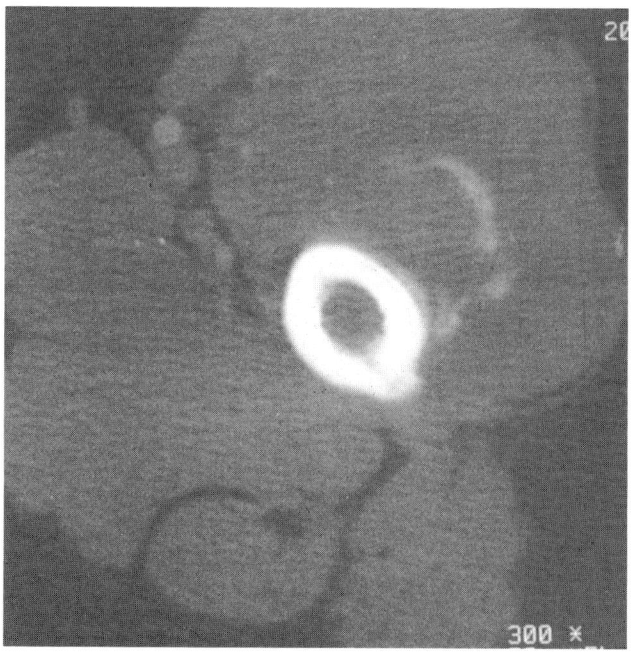

B

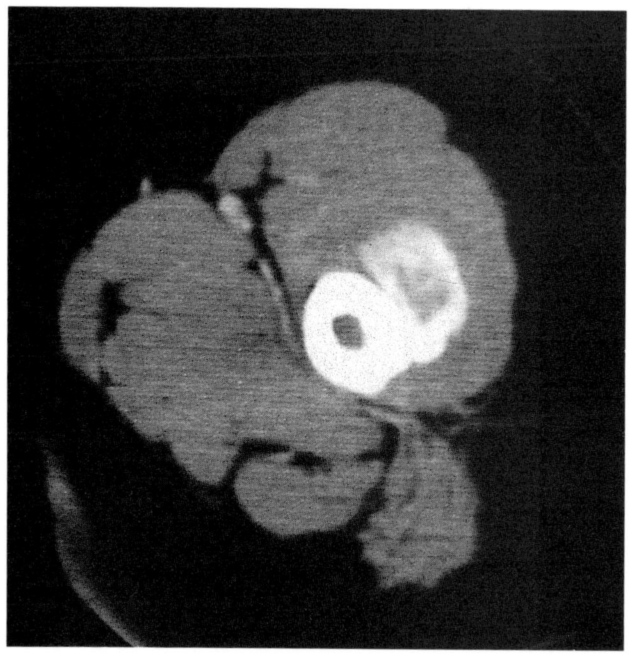

D

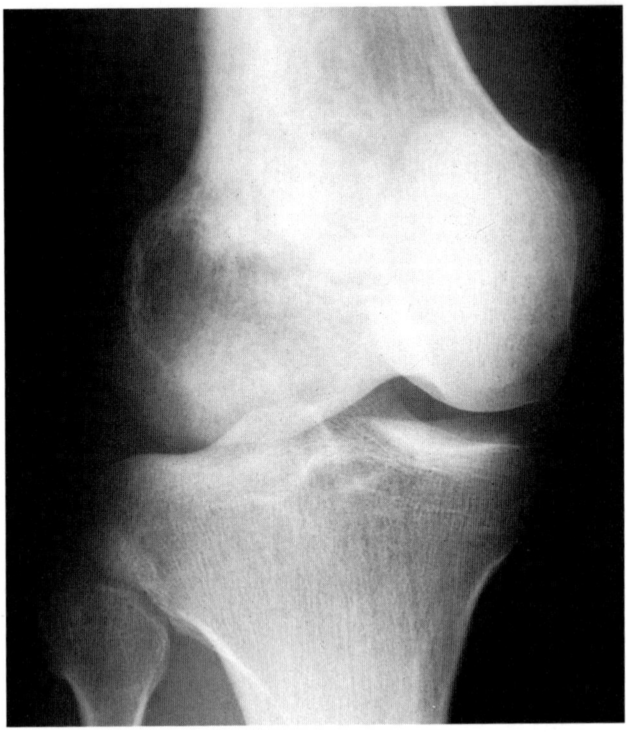

A

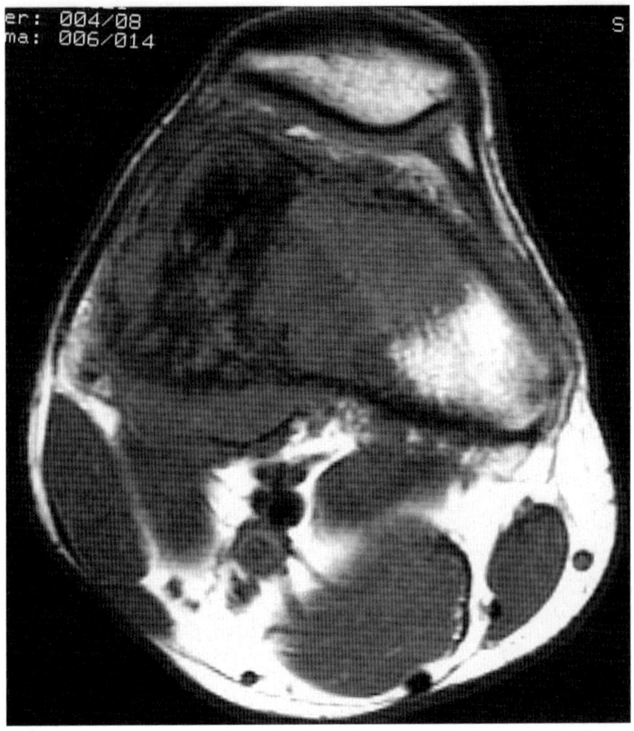

C

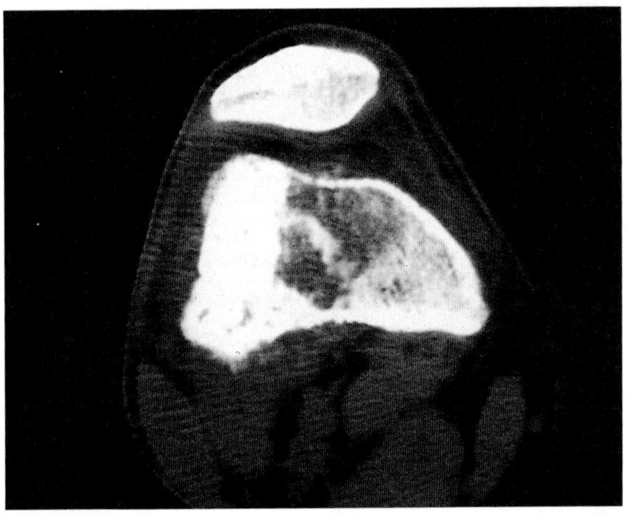

B

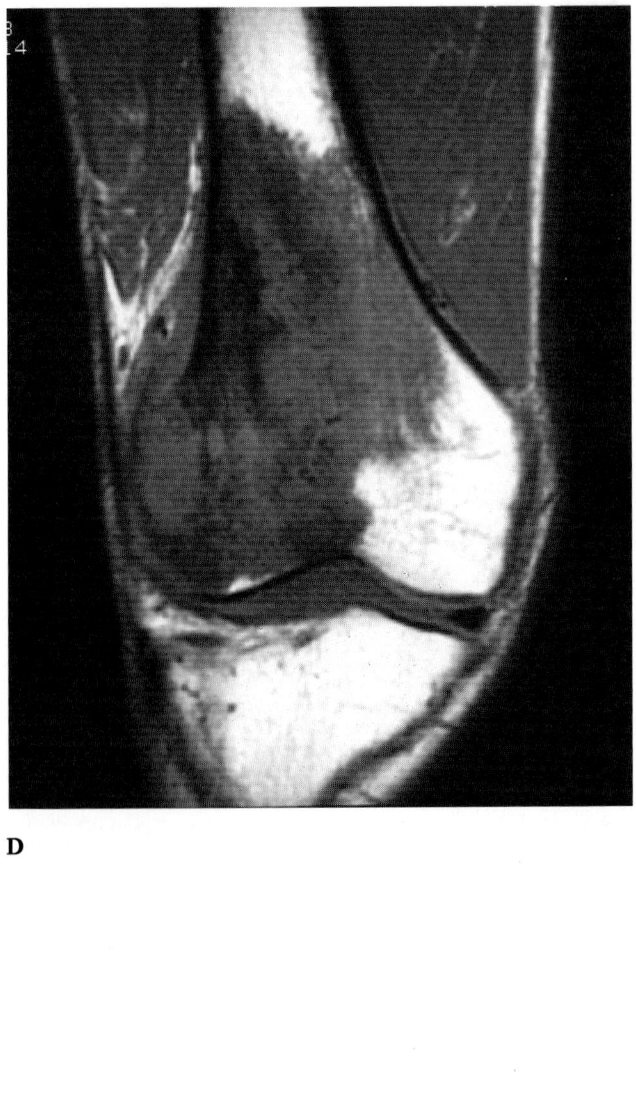

D

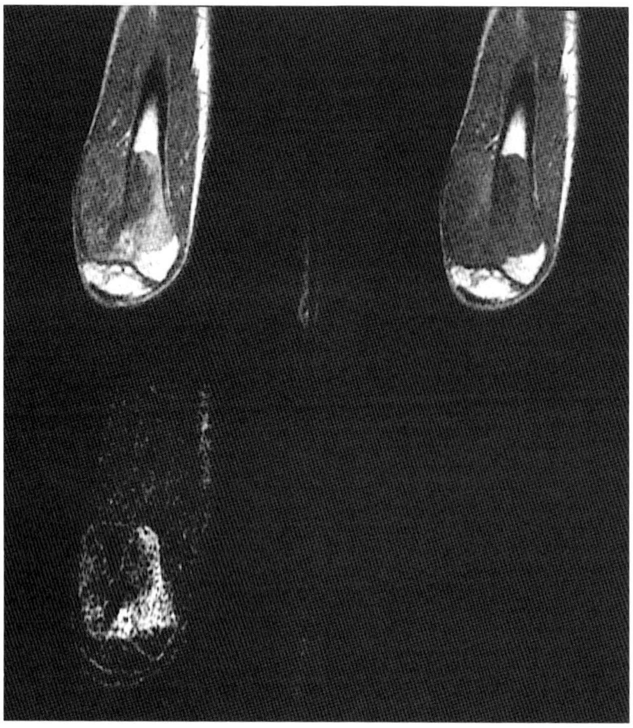

E

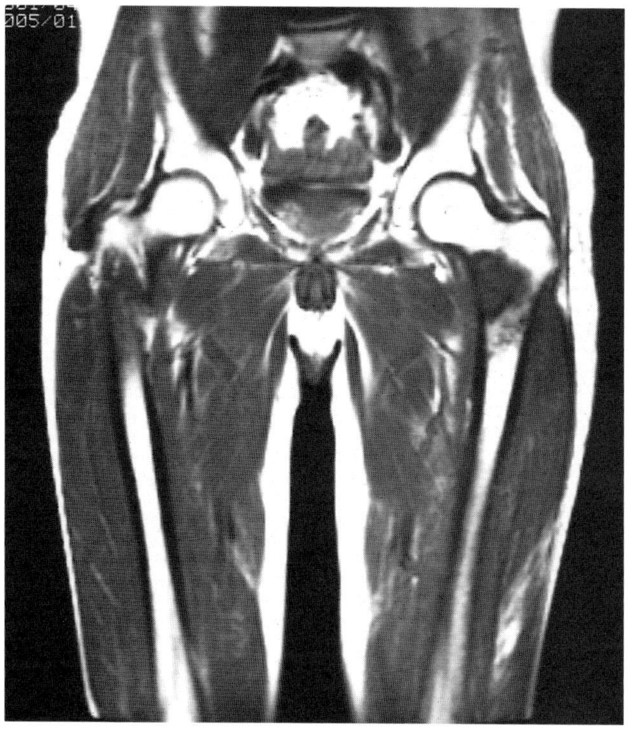

A

Figure 19.3

This is from a 35-year-old man with pain of the knee. (**A**) On plain films there is a sclerotic, poorly limited, metaphyseal lesion. (**B**) Thin perpendicular periosteal bone formations and soft tissue involvement are well detected on CT. MR T1-weighted (TR 600, TE 20): (**C**) axial and (**D**) frontal views. The extension into the marrow, soft tissue and the joint are well localized. Periosteal bone formations are better studied on CT. (**E**) After initial chemotherapy the tumor of the soft tissue has increased, indicating a poor response. The image below is the subtraction of two images, made before and just after a bolus injection of contrast medium (above) (TR 300, TE 20). The part that has taken contrast medium early, which is white on the subtraction, accurately indicates the active tumor.

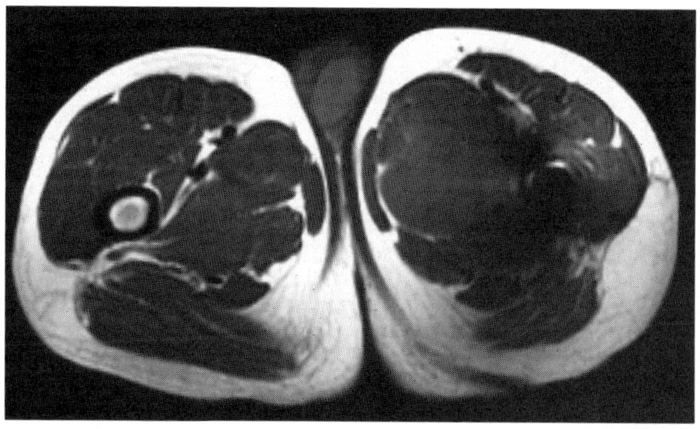

B

Figure 19.4

Osteosarcoma of the left femur: (**A**) T1-weighted coronal spin echo image (TR 600, TE 20). Low signal intensity lesion of the proximal metaphysis. Nine months later, there is a new pain, and a mass in the adductor muscles, well visualized on axial T1-weighted views (TR 600, TE 20) both before (**B**) and after (**C**) contrast medium. There are almost no artifacts from the titanium prosthesis.

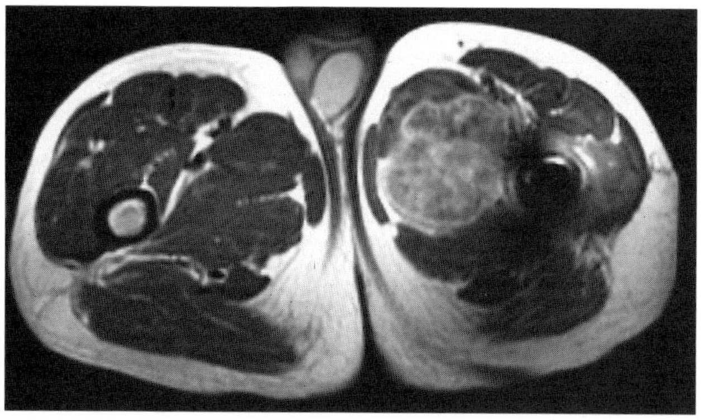

C

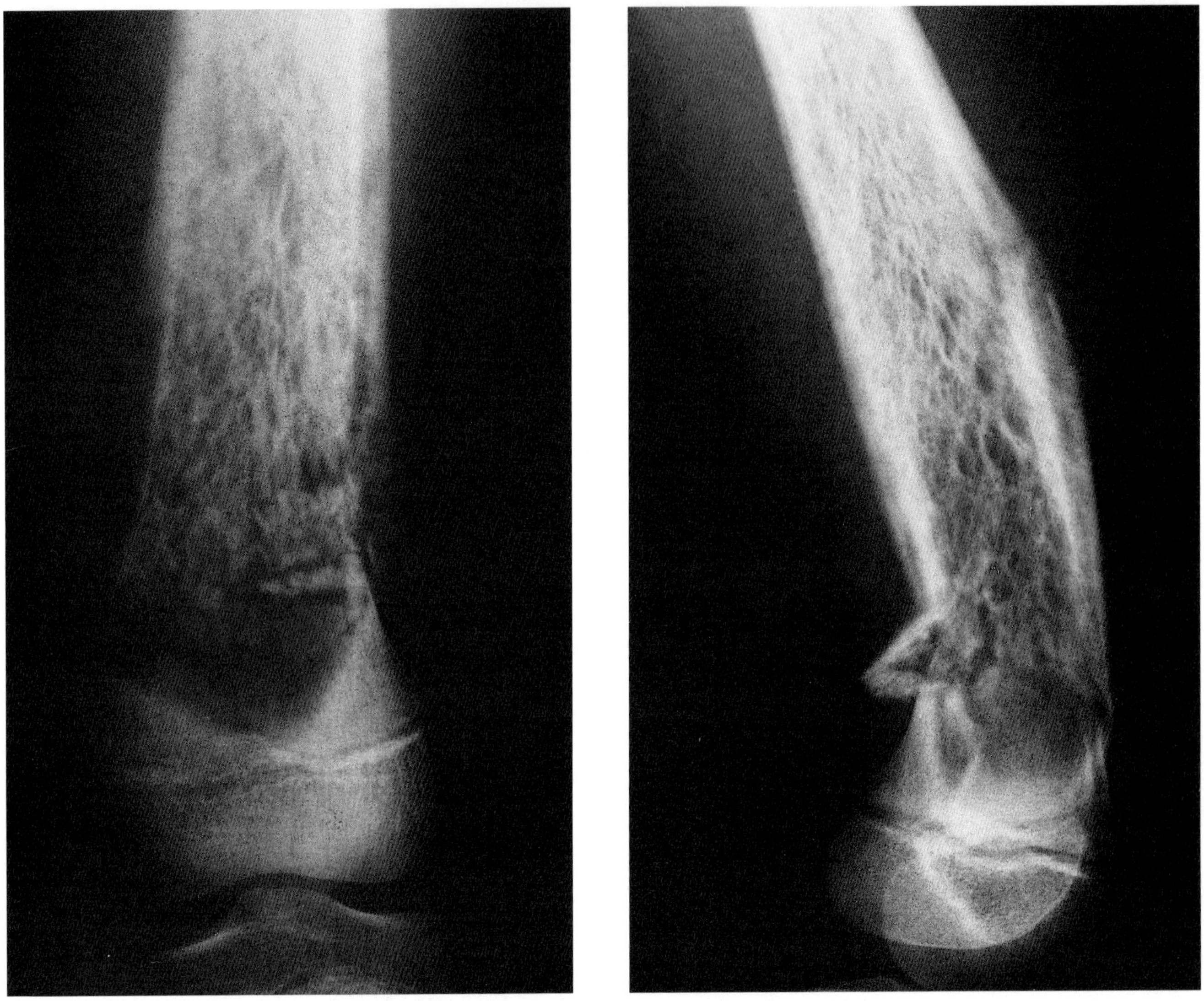

A B

Figure 19.5

Telangiectatic osteosarcoma: anteroposterior (**A**) and lateral (**B**) views on plain radiograph. Purely lytic tumor with a typical 'striation'.

Intramedullary extension

In medullary bone tumors, diaphyseal and metaphyseal extension in both adults and children, and extension across the growth plate in children, are best demonstrated on MR images, this is a result of the excellent contrast obtained in the longitudinal plane, and the lack of cortical bone signal. Although CT can also evaluate extension, it is limited to the axial plane.[26–29] Both CT and MR have other limitations: these include inability to detect very small lesions and overestimation of tumor volume on T2-weighted sequences due to peri-tumoral edema.[30,31] With accurate evaluation of tumor extent, the surgeon can determine the level of bone resection and the size of the prosthesis. The growth plate in children and the joints in adults can sometimes be preserved when they are not involved.

In periosteal tumors, MR demonstrates the periosteal location, the tumor's extension into the cortex and the medullary cavity.[32] CT can also define the extent of diaphyseal periosteal lesions, but not of metaphyseal periosteal tumors. Intra-articular extension can be detected with a much greater sensitivity than found in any other imaging technique due to the direct visualization of joint cartilage. Skip lesions (small metastases separated from the main tumor by healthy tissue) are easily detected on MR scans parallel to the long axis of the bone. MR also shows excellent demonstration of vessels and their relationship to the tumor without injecting contrast media. Finally, both CT and MR can show skin and subcutaneous extension.

In summary, MR should be used as the principal test for evaluating any extension of malignant tumors.

Examination of distant spread

Bone metastases are best detected on radionuclide bone scans, but pulmonary metastases are evaluated on conventional chest radiographs and chest CT.[3]

Effectiveness and follow up of treatment

Most primary malignant tumors are treated with preoperative chemotherapy before removal. At surgery, histological study of the tumor can be carried out and the effectiveness of treatment can be estimated. If effective, treatment will be continued postoperatively; if not, treatment should be changed.

As with the preoperative patient, plain radiographs and CT can provide information on the size of the tumor, its margins and degree of ossification.[34] However, MR provides a more accurate study of tumoral volume than other imaging tests or clinical examination. A signal decrease on T2-weighted sequences suggests increased ossification or the presence of more fibrous tissue in the tumor.[35] If there is no increase in the signal intensity of the lesion following injection of the contrast agent there could be necrosis present.[36–38]

MR using dynamic, contrast-enhanced images and subtraction may be useful for differentiating post-chemotherapeutic change from viable tumor, because viable tumor enhances rapidly, and the post-chemotherapeutic change enhances slowly.

Conclusion

Imaging should start with the plain radiograph, which can define a lesion as benign, in which case no treatment is necessary. CT should be performed when the type of matrix needs to be clarified. However, MR should be the primary study for staging of the extent of the tumor (Diagram 19.1).

Tumor types

Osteosarcoma

After multiple myeloma, osteosarcoma is the most frequent primary bone tumor. Its prognosis has greatly improved with the use of aggressive chemotherapy, more than 70% of patients being cured.[2] Limb-sparing surgery can also be performed in more than 70% of patients. Preoperative evaluation is important because local recurrences are almost invariably fatal.

Osteosarcoma is a malignant bone tumor that makes bone, and can be classified into several different lesions as follows.

Conventional osteosarcoma

This mainly involves patients in the second decade of life, and occurs more in men than in women. Long bones are affected in 90% of cases and the knee in 66%, the metaphysis being the most frequent location. A very poor survival rate is indicated when an open epiphyseal plate is crossed.[38] Radiologically, it is a very aggressive tumor, with periosteal bone formations, destruction of the cortex and involvement of soft tissues. The tumor may be purely lytic, sclerotic (Figure 19.6) or

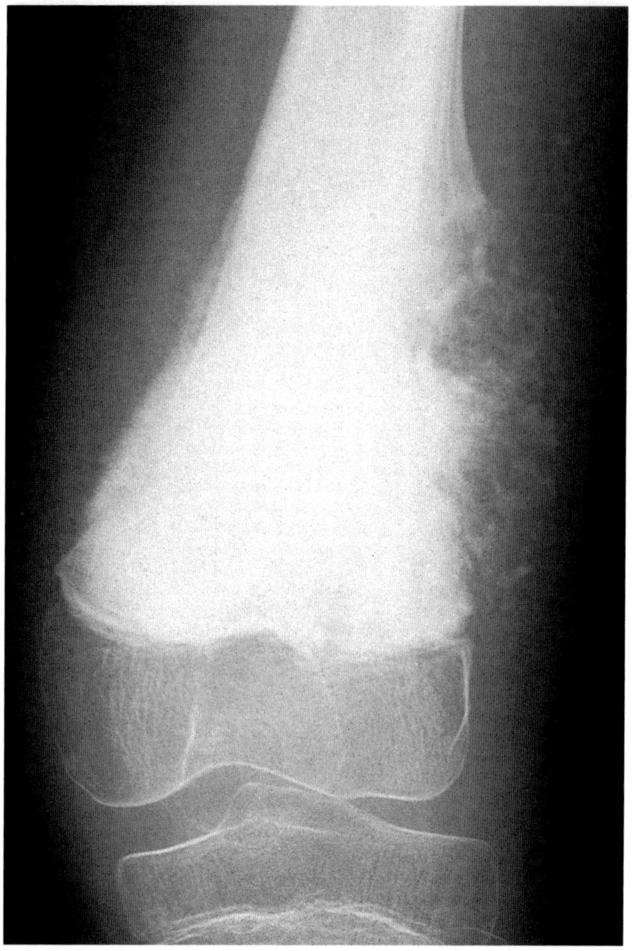

Figure 19.6

Conventional osteosarcoma, on a plain radiograph: anteroposterior view of the knee. The tumor is sclerotic, metaphyseo-diaphyseal, with destruction of the cortex, periosteal formations, involvement of soft tissues with ossification. The epiphysis is spared.

as is most often the case, mixed. The surgeon should use MR to decide whether to open the joint and for the best evaluation of local extension – the decision of where to cut the bone and what length the prosthesis should be. At presentation studies should include bone scans to exclude bone metastases, and chest radiographs and chest CT to search for pulmonary metastases. In fact, 20% of patients present with pulmonary metastases – these are important prognostic factors for osteosarcoma and the primary cause of death. Chemotherapy is performed before surgery, and its effectiveness evaluated on plain radiographs and CT;[34] good signs of effectiveness are a better limitation, increased ossification and a decrease in tumor volume. On MR indirect signs can be used:[39] increases in tumor volume and peri-tumoral edema are predictive of a poor histopathologic response, but a decrease in volume and edema are poor predictors.[39] Direct visualization of the active tumor is probably a more reliable sign; this can be evaluated by visualization of the regions of interest,[40] by factor analysis of dynamic structures[41] and, most recently, by contrast-enhanced subtraction MR imaging in which tumors enhance rapidly with contrast medium and any inflammatory reaction enhances more slowly[42] (see Figure 19.3).

After surgery, patients are followed up with chest radiographs and CT for pulmonary metastases. Local pain can be evaluated on plain radiographs or predominantly on MR, because there are few artifacts with non-paramagnetic prostheses (titanium or vitallium) (Figure 19.4).

The strategy is outlined in Diagram 19.2.

Telangiectatic osteosarcoma

This is a very aggressive type of osteosarcoma. It is purely lytic and can show a characteristic radiological pattern (Figure 19.5) with multiple parallel striations of the diaphysis.[43] Its prognosis, which used to be very poor, is now as good as for conventional osteosarcoma treated with chemotherapy.

Multicentric osteosarcoma

This is rare and involves mainly children between 6 and 9 years of age. The multiple lesions are usually sclerotic (Figure 19.7) and often involve epiphyses. The survival rate is very poor.

Low-grade osteosarcoma

This often presents as a slowly growing, less aggressive tumor (Figure 19.8). Even histologically the diagnosis may be difficult. A wide resection seems to be adequate as treatment.[44]

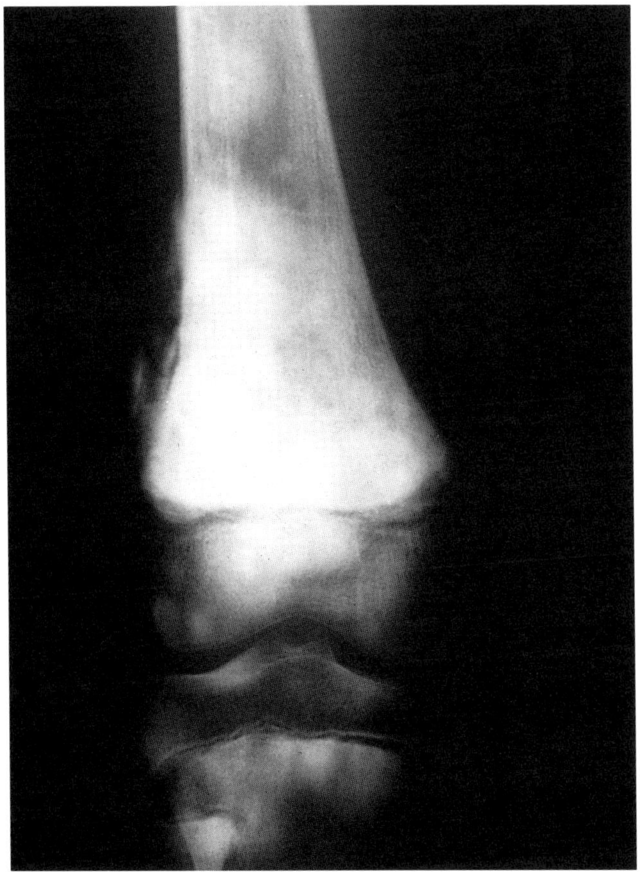

A

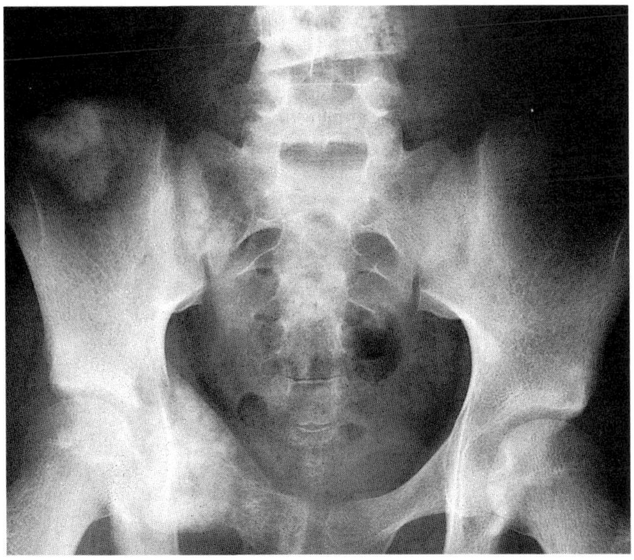

B

Figure 19.7

Multicentric osteosarcoma: multiple sclerotic lesions are seen simultaneously. The epiphyseal involvement is very typical: (**A**) knee and (**B**) pelvis.

Surface osteosarcoma

This shares the same prognosis as conventional osteosarcoma.[45]

Periosteal osteosarcoma

This produces 'saucerization' of the cortex on radiographs (Figure 19.9).[46] Histologically, it is composed mainly of cartilage and it may be difficult to differentiate from periosteal chondrosarcoma.

Parosteal or juxtacortical osteosarcoma

This usually occurs in adults with the most frequent location being the posterior aspect of the distal metaphysis of the femur. The radiological pattern is very suggestive (Figure 19.10): a large calcified mass is attached in a sessile fashion to the cortex. Non-involvement of the medullary cavity seems to provide a reliable sign of a local disease without metastases,[32] and this must be evaluated on MR. Histologically the tumor consists of mainly fibrous tissue.

Secondary osteosarcomas

These occur in Paget's disease, fibrous dysplasia and after radiotherapy. Radiologically, it is mainly a lytic lesion, with destruction of the cortex and soft tissue mass. The survival rate is very low.

Ewing's sarcoma

Ewing's sarcoma[47] is the most frequent primary bone tumor in children. It may represent one end of the spectrum of neuroectodermal tumors. More than half of the cases are cured with chemotherapy and local treatment, surgery or radiotherapy. Radiologically, it is a very aggressive tumor, poorly limited, with destruction of the cortex, periosteal bone formation and involvement of soft tissues (Figure 19.11). Although the tumors do not produce bone, they are sclerotic on CT in about

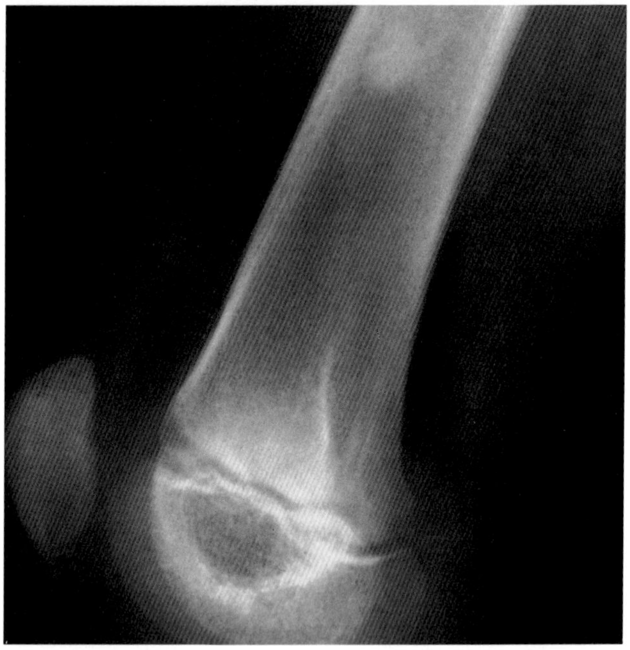

A

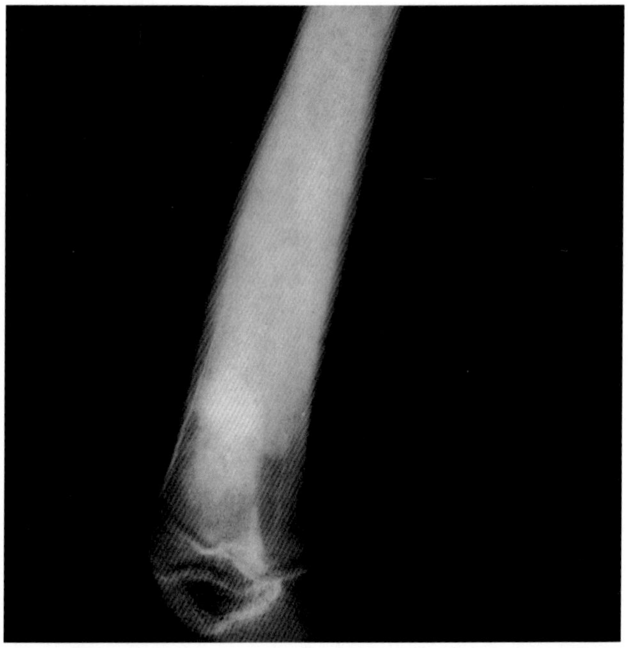

B

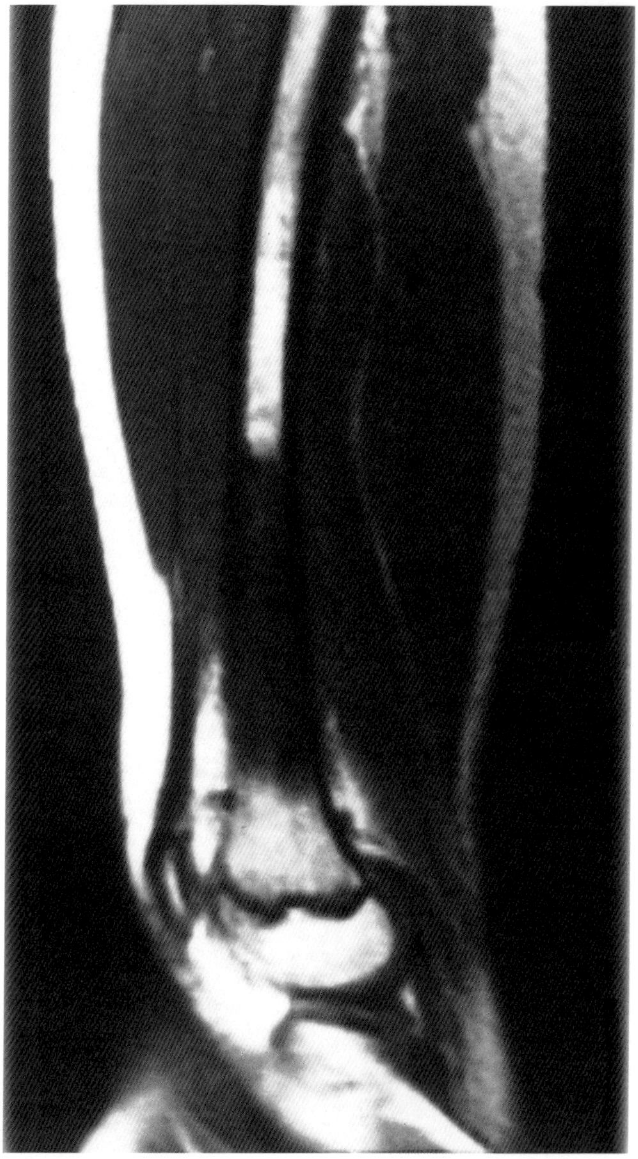

C

Figure 19.8

Low-grade osteosarcoma: an isolated sclerotic lesion is discovered systematically (sprain of the other knee) (**A**). No biopsy is performed. (**B**) 2 years later there is an obvious sclerotic lesion of the distal shaft of the femur. (**C**) The involvement of the marrow is obvious on MR (TR 600, TE 20).

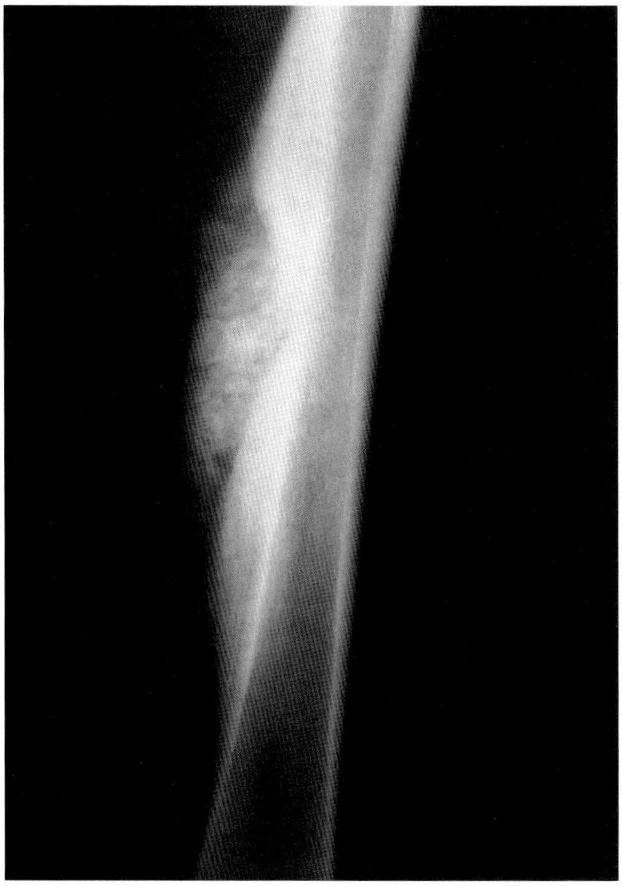

Figure 19.9

Periosteal osteosarcoma of the shaft of the femur: plain radiograph. Saucerization of the cortex has occurred, and an ossified tumor has developed in the soft tissue. The involvement of the medullary cavity was evaluated on MR.

half of cases due to secondary deposits of calcium on the remaining trabeculae. The soft tissue component is massive and may obscure a small primary bone lesion, especially in the pelvis and ribs (Figure 19.12).

Ewing's sarcoma is different from osteosarcoma in the following ways:

1. The age of the patient. Most patients are younger (between 5 and 15 years old) during the stage of active growth.
2. The location of involvement: central sites are more frequent (50%) in patients with Ewing's sarcoma (Figure 19.13).

Surgery may not be feasible as a result of factors (1) and (2). Radiotherapy combined with chemotherapy may be the only local therapy possible, although the local recurrence rate is 33%.

3. Ewing's sarcoma is not as well marginated as an osteosarcoma. Although Ewing's sarcoma often shrinks after chemotherapy, nests of tumor cells may remain in the muscles and adequate resection may be difficult.
4. Periosteal tumors, which are usually found in boys, are rare but the subjects have a better survival rate (Figure 19.14).

Primary neuroectodermals tumor (PNET)

This tumor[48] seems to be a well-differentiated form and is from the same family as Ewing's sarcoma. Clinical and radiologic patterns are similar. Pulmonary metastases are found in 50% of patients at presentation, in contrast to only 15% in Ewing's sarcoma. The survival rate is very poor.

Chondrosarcoma

This cartilaginous malignant tumor, usually found in adults, grows slowly and is treated by surgical resection. Various forms of chondrosarcoma have been described, as indicated below.

Conventional chondrosarcoma

This is a medullary lesion which contains typical annular or popcorn-like areas of calcification and endosteal scalloping of the cortex. The cortex may be destroyed and the adjacent soft tissues invaded.

Clear-cell chondrosarcoma

This is a rare tumor, involving the epiphysis; it is of low-grade malignancy.

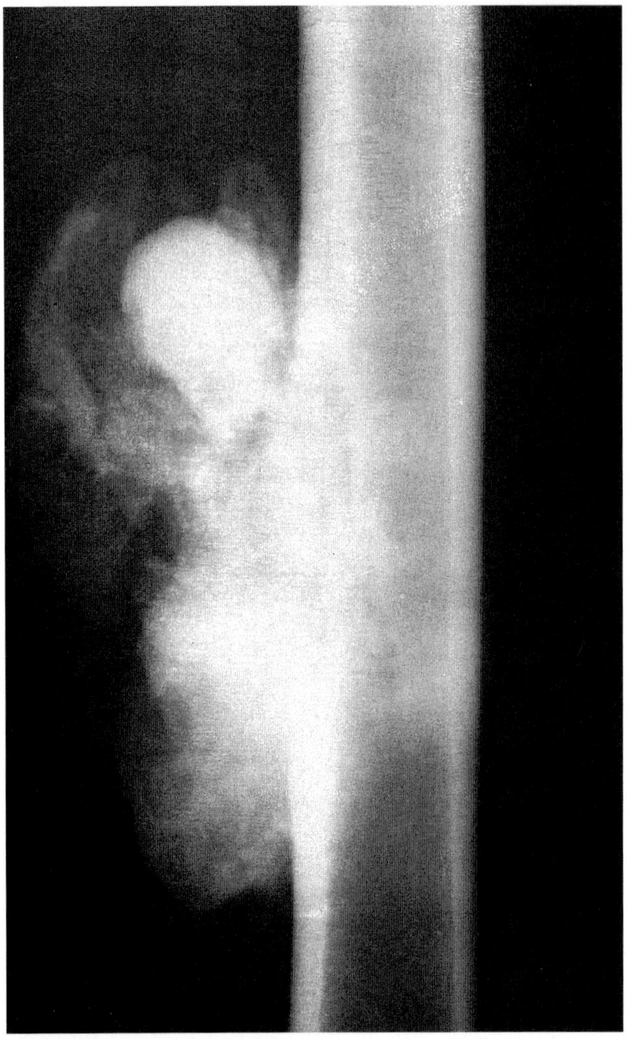

A

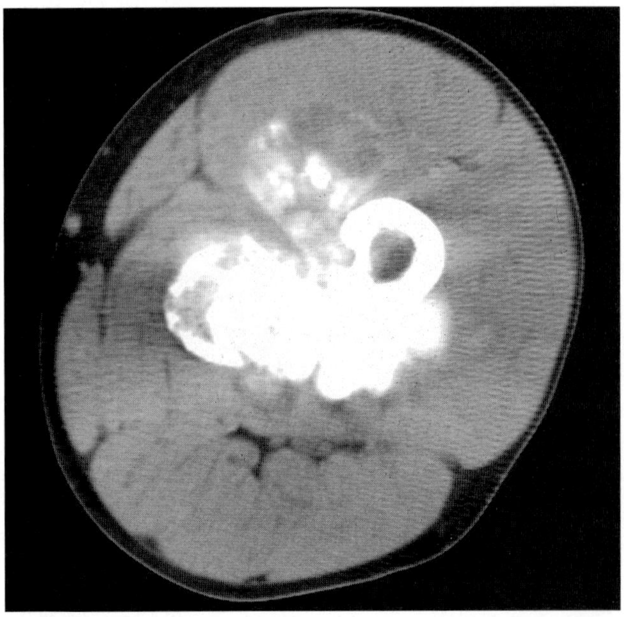

B

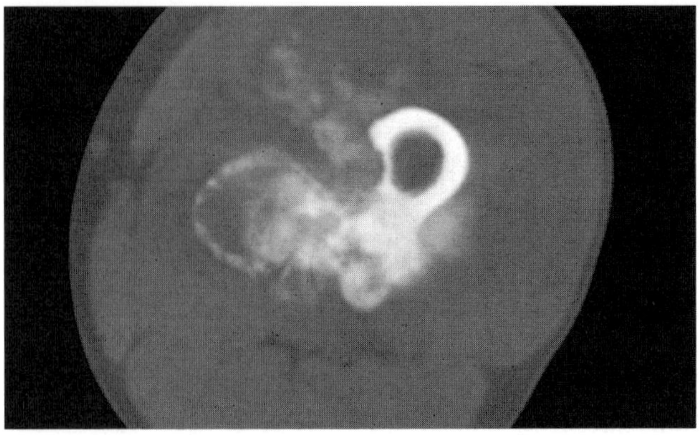

C

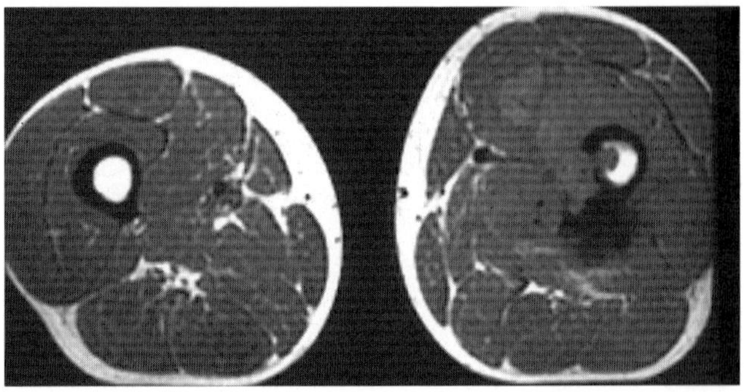

D

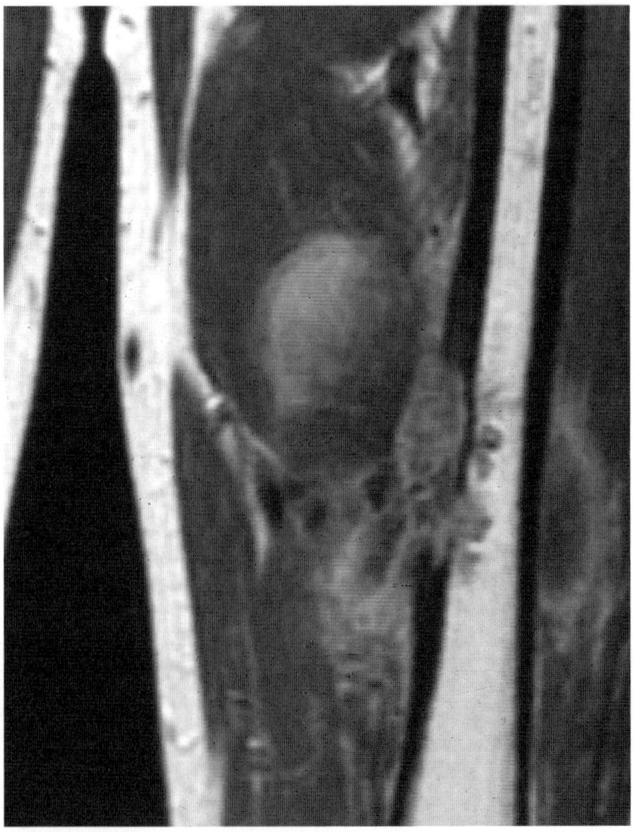

E

Figure 19.10

Parosteal osteosarcoma: ossified mass mainly developed outside the shaft of the left femur. (**A**) Plain radiograph; CT with (**B**) a soft tissue and (**C**) a bone window; MR T1-weighted (TR 600 TE 20) (**D**) axial view before injection, and (**E**) coronal view after injection of contrast medium. Ossifications are better studied on plain radiographs and CT; the involvement of the medullary cavity, visible on CT, is much better studied on MR.

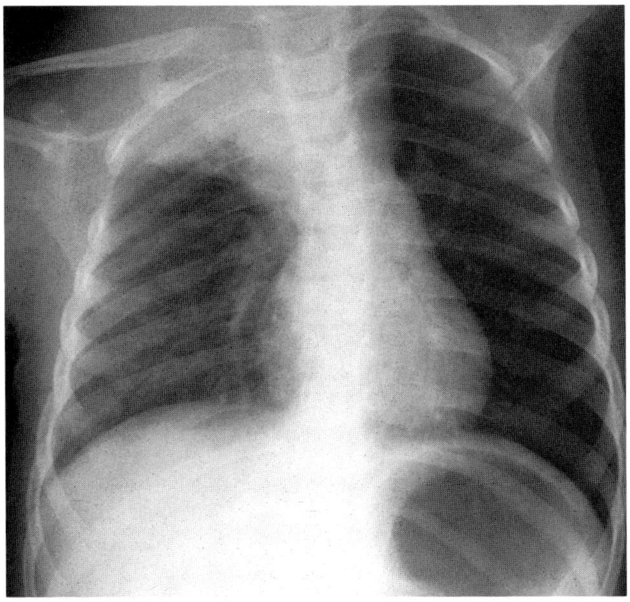

A

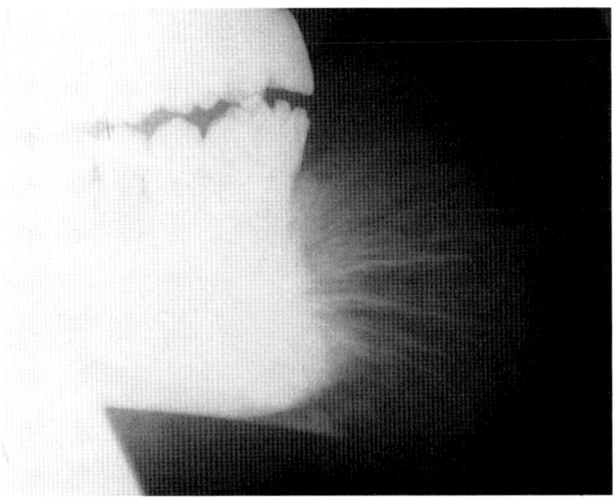

Figure 19.11

Ewing's sarcoma of the mandible, with typical perpendicular periosteal bone formations.

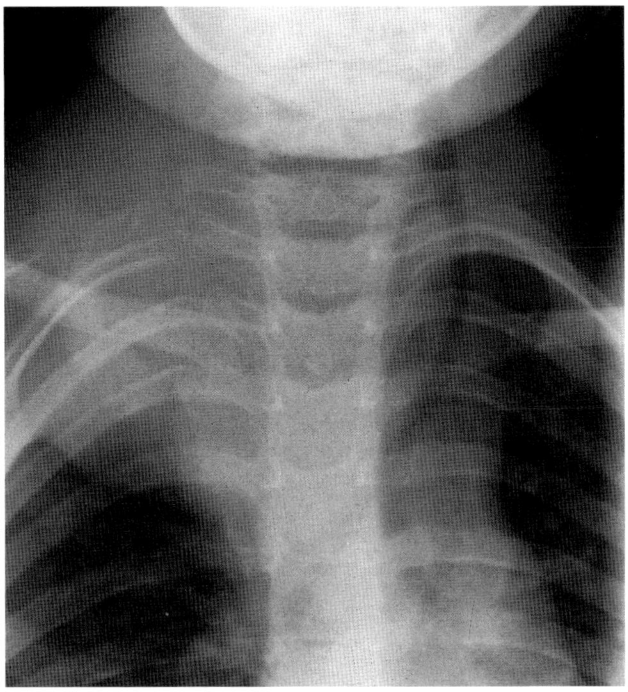

B

Figure 19.12

Ewing's sarcoma of the right first rib. The soft tissue mass can hide the small bone lesion: (**A**) anteroposterior view of the chest; (**B**) localized radiograph.

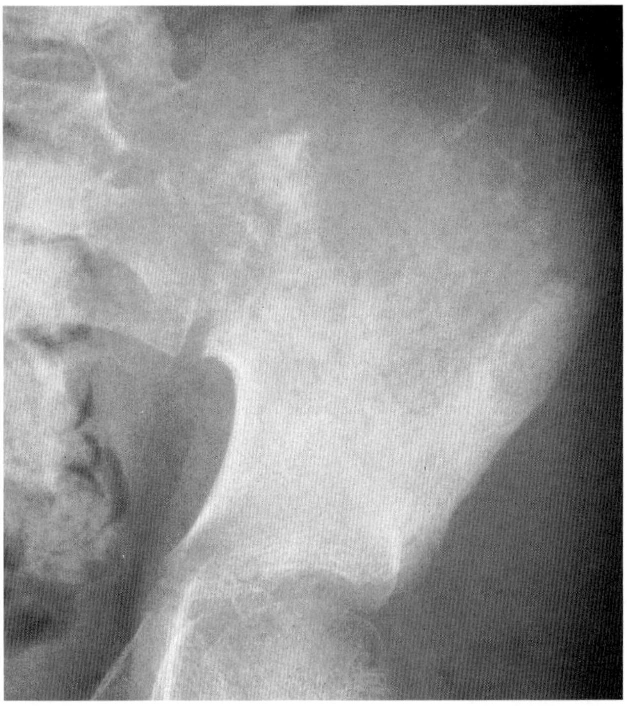

A

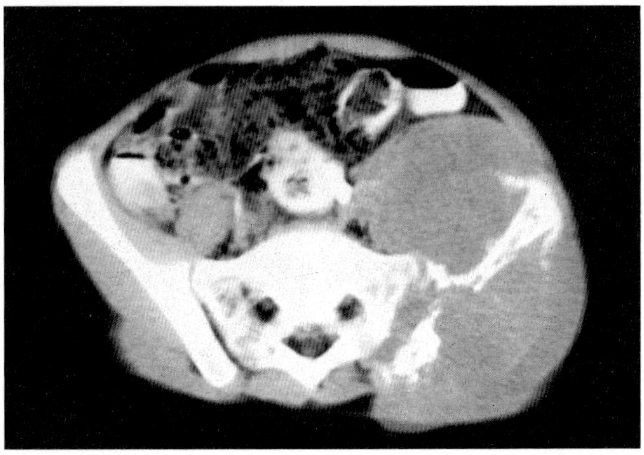

B

Figure 19.13

Ewing's sarcoma of the left iliac wing. (**A**) Mixed lesion on plain film. (**B**) The involvement of the soft tissues is well evaluated on CT.

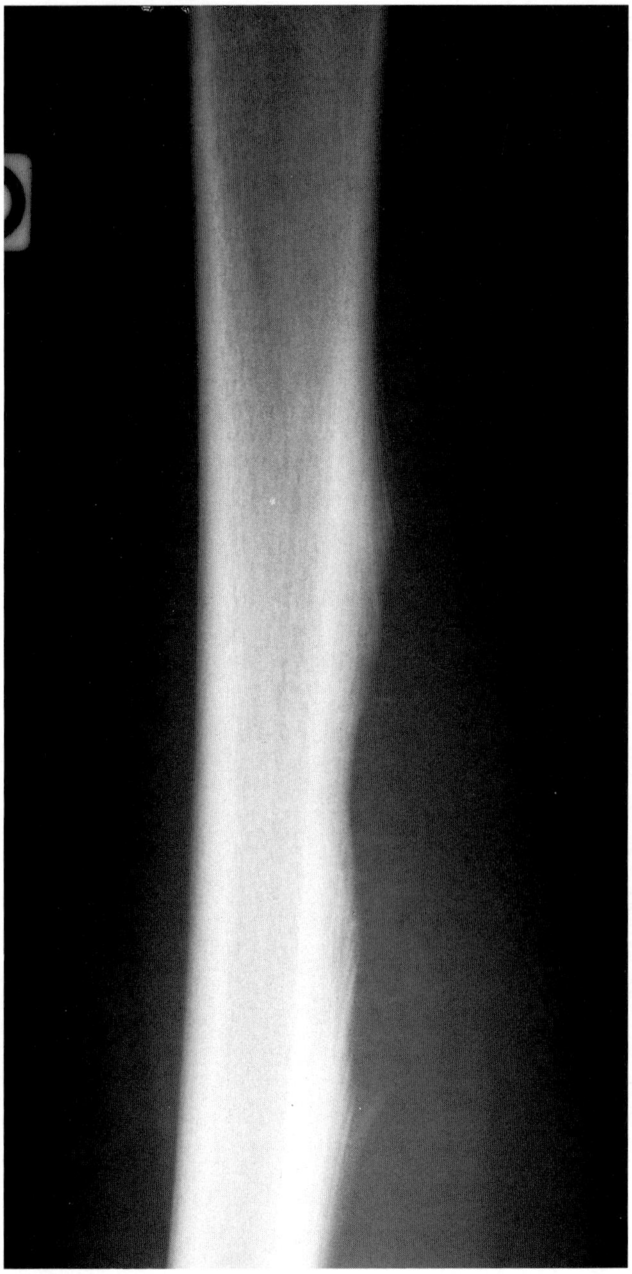

Figure 19.14

Periosteal Ewing's sarcoma of the shaft of the right femur. The 'saucerization' is typical, with longitudinal and perpendicular periosteal bone formations.

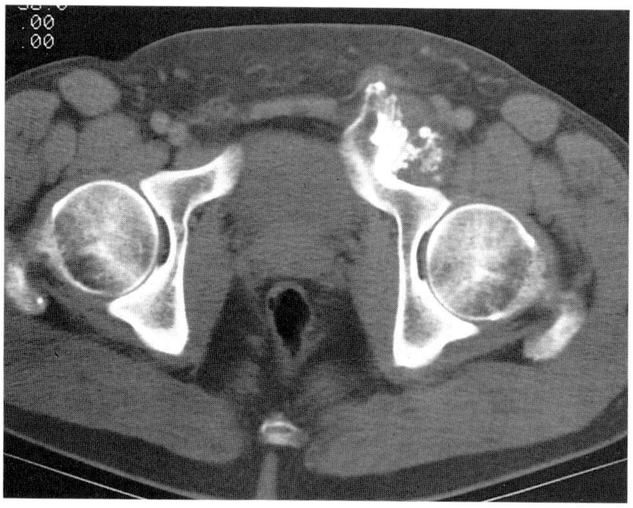

A

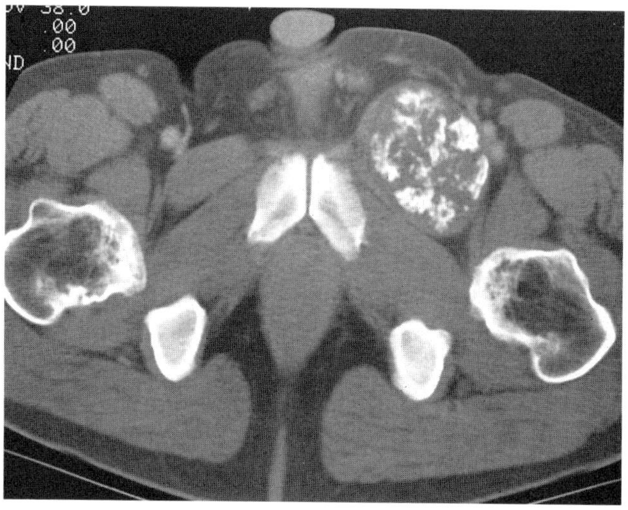

B

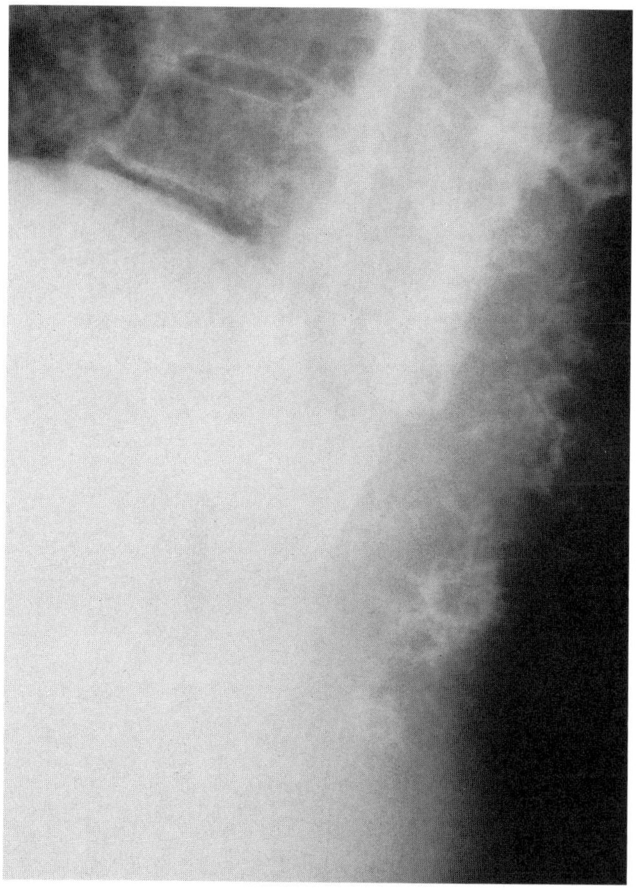

C

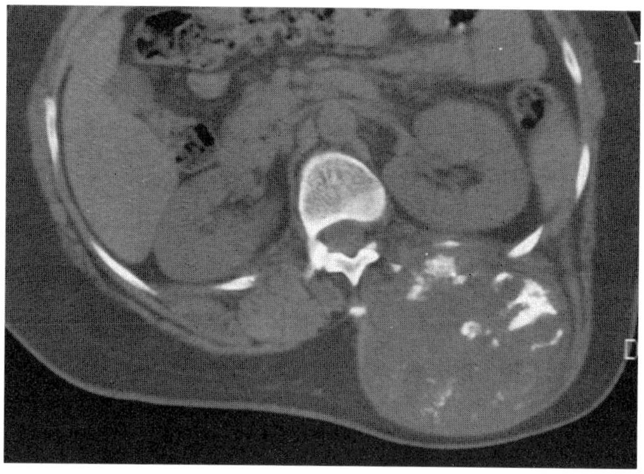

D

Figure 19.15

Exostosis and chondrosarcoma: (**A**) the pedicle of the exostosis is clearly visible. (**B**) The non-calcified cap is thin (CT images). In another patient with a chondrosarcoma the typical arciform calcifications are well studied on the lateral view of the thoracic film: (**C**) plain radiograph; (**D**) on CT the non-calcified cap is very thick, suggesting malignancy.

Mesenchymal chondrosarcoma

This is a rare, highly malignant tumor.

De-differentiated chondrosarcomas

These have a very poor survival rate and are tumors in which a low-grade chondrosarcoma de-differentiates into a highly malignant bone tumor (osteosarcoma or malignant fibrous histiocytoma). The survival rate for patients is poor. Radiologically, an aggressive tumor develops on a well-limited cartilaginous lesion.

Secondary chondrosarcoma

This develops on an exostosis. The thickness of the cartilaginous cap is a good sign of aggressiveness (caps > 3 cm thick suggest malignancy) (Figure 19.15). It can be evaluated on CT, MR or even ultrasonography.[49]

As with osteosarcoma, the main role of imaging in chondrosarcoma is to diagnose the lesion on plain radiographs, and sometimes with CT, to determine local extent on MR and to detect the local recurrences, which are frequent, on plain radiographs, CT and MR.

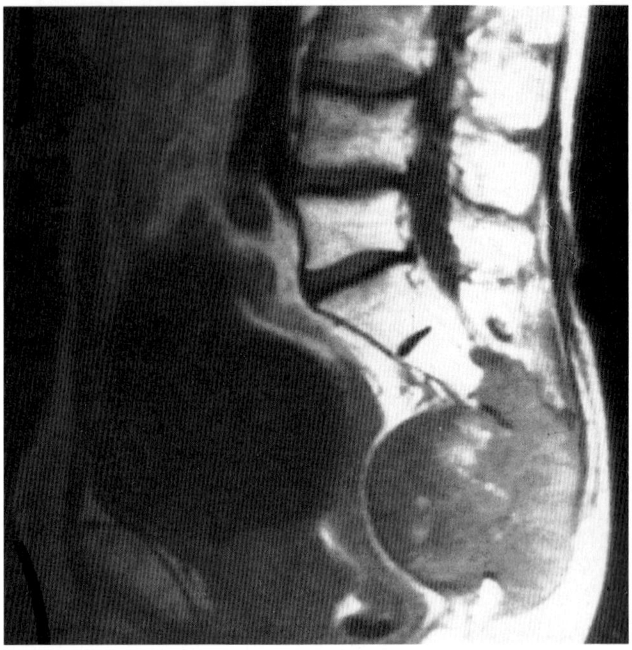

Figure 19.16

Recurrence of a chordoma of the sacrum after radiation therapy: sagittal T1-weighted (TR 600, TE 20) MR image. The first two sacral vertebrae are not involved. The third sacral vertebra and those below are involved. The anterior soft tissue mass displaces the rectum (note the post-radiation changes of the marrow of L5 and the sacrum).

Chordoma

Chordoma is a malignant bone tumor arising from developmental remnants of the notochord, and is found in adults, usually older than 40 years. The most frequent sites of involvement are the spheno-occipital and the sacral regions of the spine. Because surgery is the only curative treatment, imaging must accurately demonstrate this tumor (Figure 19.16). For example, for sacral tumors evaluation of invasion of the sacral canal and nerve roots is mandatory. Radiologically, a chordoma demonstrates a lytic tumor, with a large soft tissue mass, and areas of calcification that correspond to incomplete destruction of bone.

MR using sagittal and coronal oblique views is the best technique for showing the initial tumor and its recurrences.

Fibrosarcoma and malignant fibrous histiocytoma (MFH)

These share the same clinical, radiologic and prognostic patterns, and they usually affect the long bones in adults. Treatment is preoperative chemotherapy, surgery and postoperative chemotherapy. Radiologically, the tumors are lytic and usually not very aggressive (Figure 19.17). Imaging is useful in diagnosis of the lesion, for local evaluation before surgery and for general evaluation (bone scan and chest radiograph).

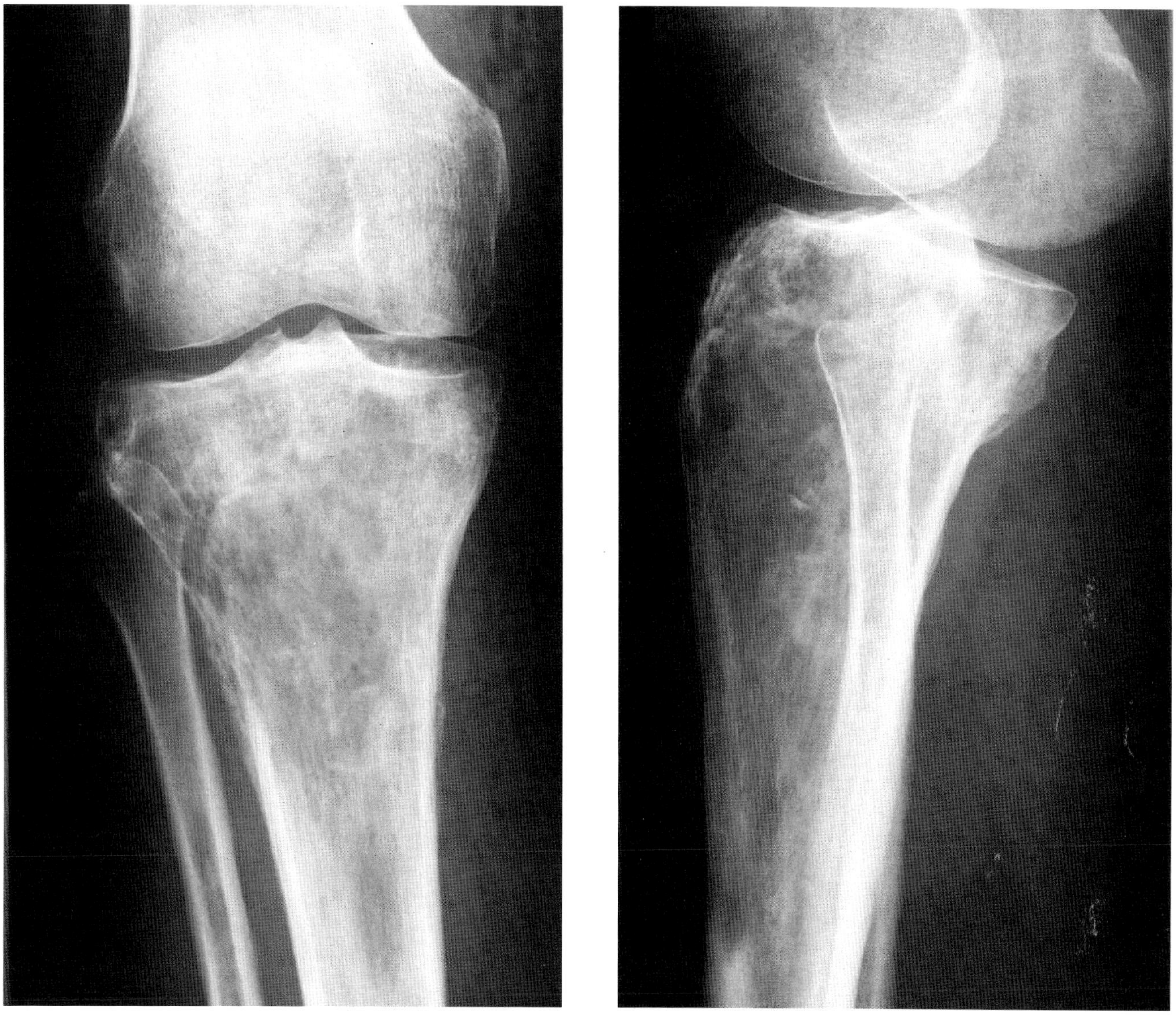

A B

Figure 19.17

Malignant fibrous histiocytoma of the proximal right tibia: plain films, radiographs with (**A**) anteroposterior and (**B**) lateral views. Lytic tumor involving the metaphysis and epiphysis, with little periosteal bone formation.

Adamantinoma

This is a rare malignant tumor in adults which involves the tibia. It is a locally aggressive tumor, with local recurrences. Metastases are rare and late.

The radiologic pattern is usually suggestive of the diagnosis with limited areas of osteolytic defects involving the shaft (Figure 19.18). Imaging is useful for diagnosis on plain radiographs, and for local evaluation using MR before surgery.

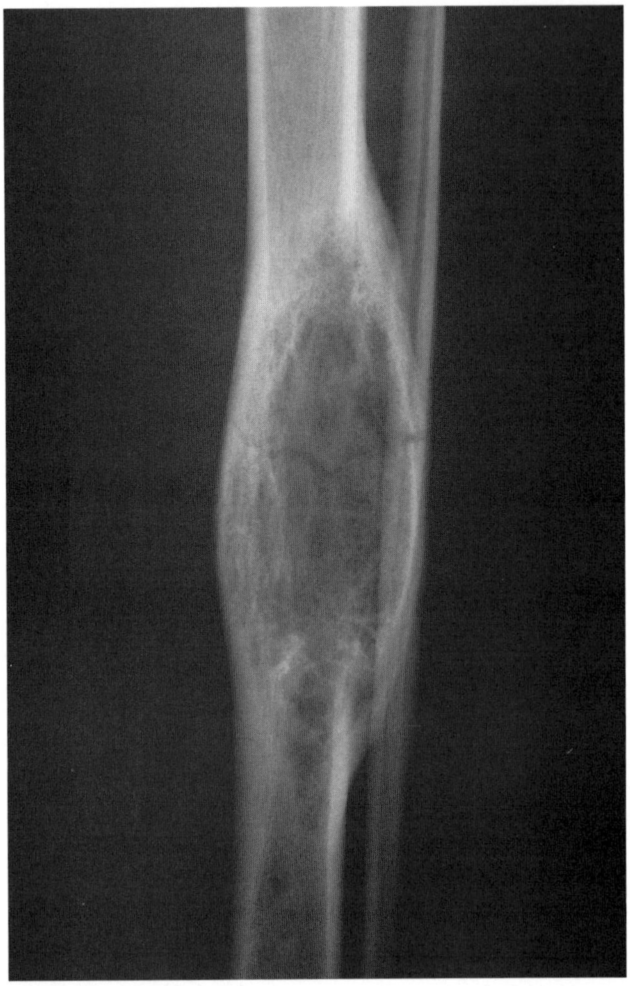

Figure 19.18

Adamantinoma of the tibia: anteroposterior view, plain radiograph. Well-marginated lytic lesion, expanding the bone, with a horizontal fracture. Satellite lesions are easily diagnosed, and very suggestive of the diagnosis.

Metastatic bone disease

Introduction

Bone metastases are frequent and jeopardize the length and quality of survival in cancer patients. Early detection is necessary so that treatment can be modified appropriately.

General information

Frequency

Metastases occur mainly in adults and the elderly. The most common metastases in men (60%) are from the prostate and in women (70%) from breast cancers. Although the exact incidence of metastases from various tumors is difficult to determine, autopsy statistics give the following values:[50,51] 50–80% of breast cancers, 30–50% of cancers of the kidneys or the lungs, 30–40% of melanomas, 50–70% of cancers of the prostate and approximately 40% of thyroid cancers; in children 80% of cases of neuroblastoma, 60% of Ewing's sarcoma and 25% of osteosarcoma.

Location

Metastases occur mainly in the axial skeleton, the spine, mainly in the lumbar region, the pelvis, the ribs, the sternum, the skull and the proximal part of the long bones, in decreasing order of frequency. The high incidence of metastases to the spine, sometimes in the absence of other metastases, notably pulmonary, emphasizes the importance of Batson's perivertebral venous system in the dissemination of metastases.[52]

Characteristics of lesions

Standard radiographs

These are not particularly sensitive, but they are characteristic when positive. Metastases can be lytic (Figure 19.19), as is the case in cancer of the kidneys, lungs, thyroid, breast or digestive tract. In the long bones, metastases will not be seen unless the cortex is affected. In the short bones, they can only be detected when there is considerable destruction. They may also be sclerotic (Figure 19.20) or mixed, especially in the case of breast cancer.[53] Sclerosis consists of either direct calcification of the fibrous tumoral stroma (especially in cases of cancer of the prostate), or, as is more often the case, purely reactive calcification. Cortical destruction occurs frequently, and fracture is possible. Extension to the soft tissues is usually minimal.

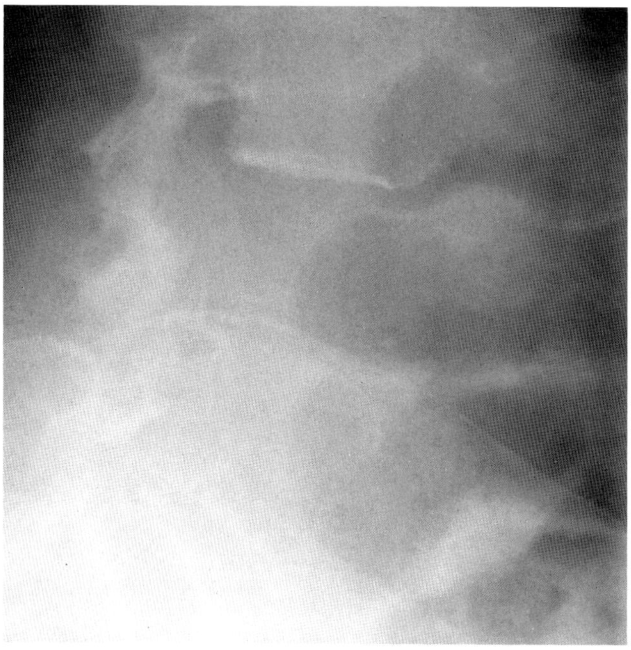

Figure 19.19

Purely lytic metastasis of the body of L4 (cancer of the breast). The posterior arch is spared (plain film, lateral view).

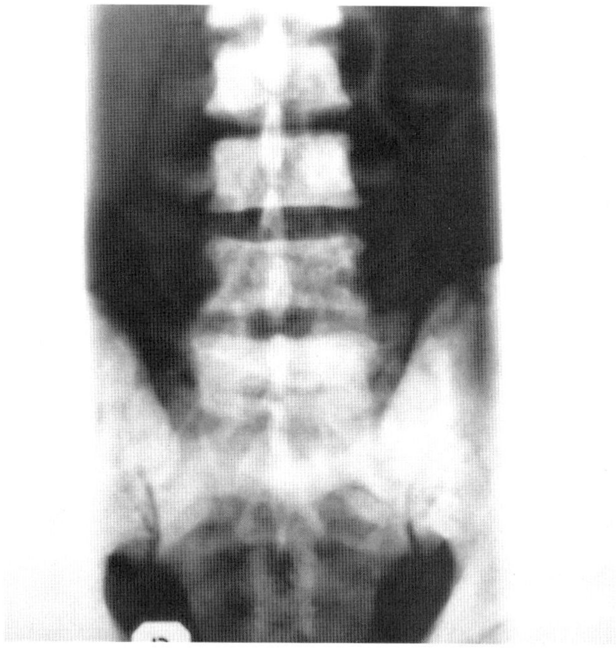

A

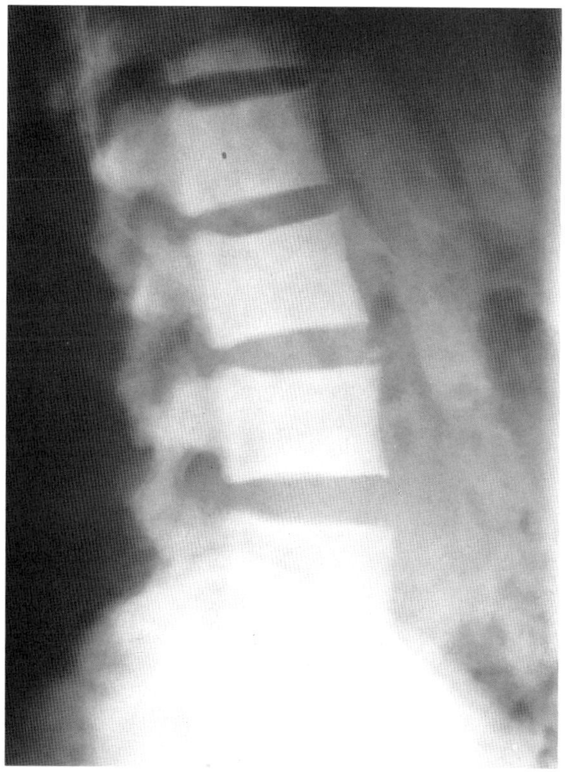

B

Figure 19.20

Sclerotic metastases of the lumbar spine and the pelvis on plain radiographs: (**A**) anteroposterior and (**B**) lateral views. All the vertebrae, the sacrum and iliac bones are involved.

Bone tomography

This was often used to detect lesions of the short bones, especially the vertebrae, but has been completely replaced by CT, which has better spatial resolution and better contrast.

Computed tomography

This demonstrates the character of the lesions (sclerosis or lysis) and cortical destruction, and it can detect extension into the soft tissues and minimal changes in medullary density. Its sensitivity is nevertheless inferior to that of MR, which has completely replaced it in the detection of tumor extent. However, CT is often useful for guiding biopsies.

Bone scintigraphy

This technique uses technetium-99m-labelled pyrophosphate or diphosphonate, and is extremely sensitive in the detection of the turnover of osteoid (Figure 19.21). It reaches the whole body and most abnormalities show up as areas of increased radioactive uptake. Correct interpretation necessitates examination of the patient and of the clinical file in order to ascertain the etiology of the radioactive hot spot. Several different types of bony abnormalities can produce increased accumulation of radioactivity. In a series of 301 patients with cancers and no known metastases, one or two new abnormalities appeared in the follow up: 11% of patients had one, and 24% had two metastases – which were more frequent in the sternum and pelvis.[54] Typically metastatic disease affects the pedicles of the vertebrae, the areas of ribs that have not suffered traumatic fractures, eg the costovertebral junction, and the skull and the proximal shafts of long bones. The pelvis is also a common site of involvement.

The 'superscan' (Figure 19.22) is an unusual phenomenon related to widespread metastatic disease where skeletal activity is so intense that the whole skeleton avidly takes up the tracer; this can easily be confused with a normal scan. However, there is usually some heterogeneity in the appearance and no renal activity is seen in such patients.

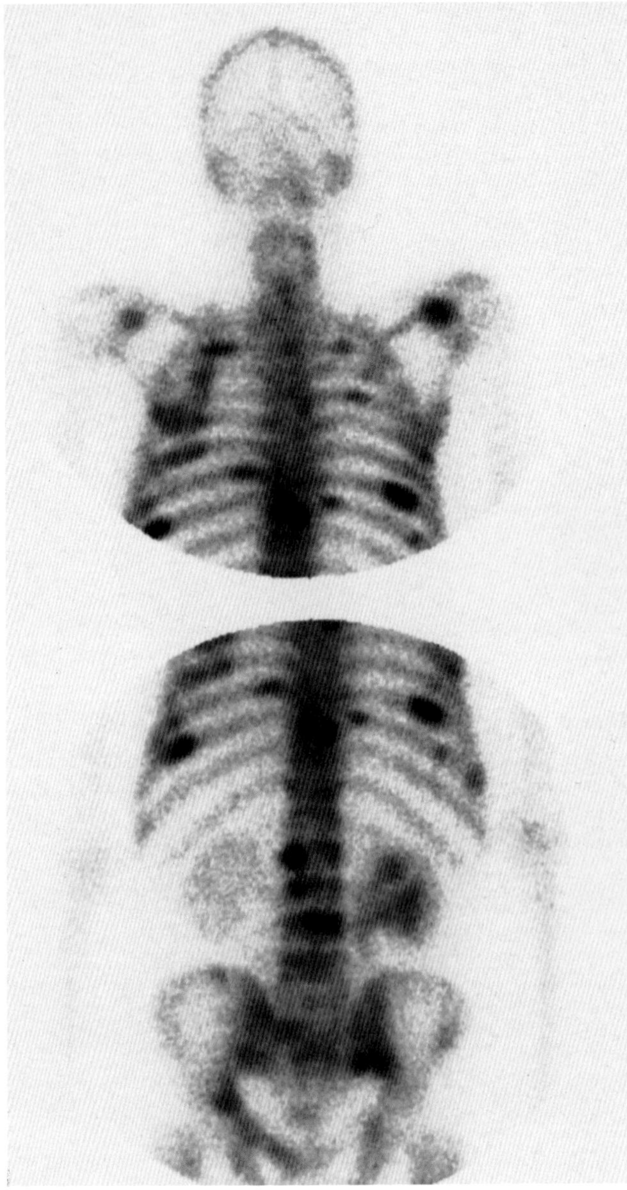

Figure 19.21

Bone scan: cancer of the prostate. Multiple hot spots of the ribs, spine and pelvis indicate metastases.

Magnetic resonance imaging

This is probably the most sensitive technique (Diagram 19.3), as it can detect an intramedullary abnormality before there is sufficient osteoblastic activity to be detected on bone scans.[55] Its main limitation is that MR can only be performed on part of the skeleton. The thoracolumbar spine and the pelvis are most frequently evaluated on routine screening. The basic sequence is a spin echo T1-weighted sequence in which the normal fatty marrow appears bright (high signal intensity) and metastases are darker (low signal intensity), making interpretation relatively simple in the adult. When the marrow is hemopoietic, particularly in the child, it may appear inhomogeneous and darker (low signal intensity) as a normal variant. Metastases may not be as apparent on T1-weighted images in the child or in the adult with this marrow pattern.

On T2-weighted sequences, metastases may show high or low signal intensity or be isointense with marrow; therefore this sequence is not very useful in the adult.

Other sequences may be helpful in visualizing metastases. Gradient echo sequences profit from magnetic susceptibility: the vertebral trabeculae

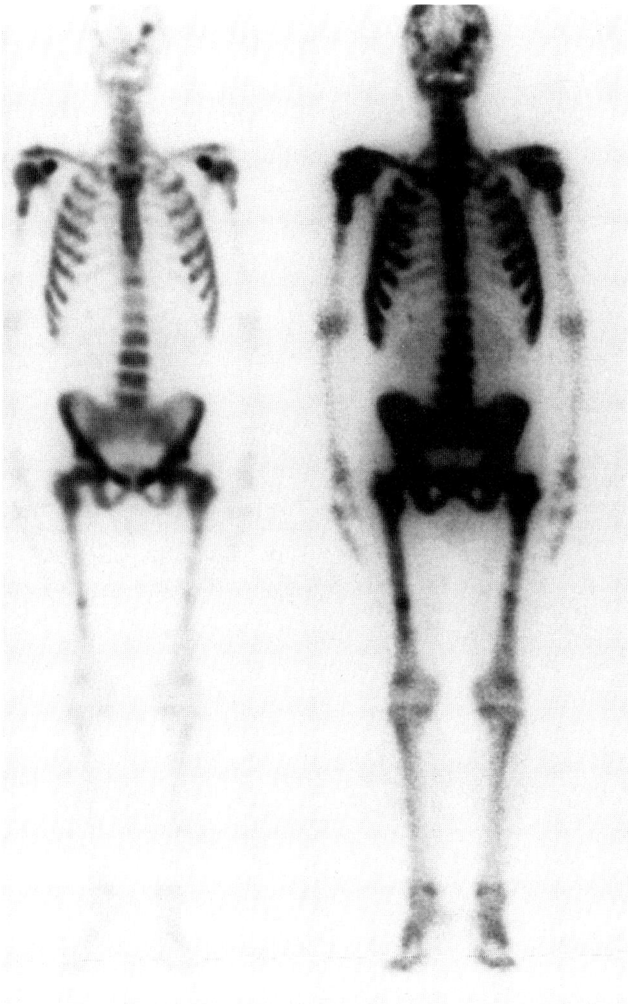

Figure 19.22

Bone scan: superscan. Cancer of the bladder (usually this image is seen in prostatic cancers) on an anteroposterior view. The contrast between the axial and distal skeleton is too high, the kidneys are not visible, and the skeleton is a little heterogeneous.

make the local field inhomogeneous, causing a reduction in the overall signal. This interference is compensated for in the spin echo sequence, but not in the gradient echo sequence, and the normal vertebrae appear black. Metastases that cause local destruction are bright (Figure 19.23).

Water–fat subtraction may be used to visualize the disappearance of fat in metastatic sites. Short inversion time inversion recovery (STIR) sequences show metastases as high signal intensity whereas normal fat is black. These sequences are, however, time-consuming and can be performed at only a limited number of levels. The injection (Figure 19.23) of a contrast medium can help: the signal from normal marrow only changes slightly or not at all following an injection, whereas metastases absorb the contrast medium (Figure 19.23).

In summary, the basic sequence for MR is a T1-weighted sequence with the addition of other sequences in equivocal cases (Diagram 19.3).

Unusual metastases

Distal metastases

Such metastases (Figure 19.24)[56,57] are rare. When metastases to the fingers and toes occur, lung and gastrointestinal cancers should be considered.

Cortical metastases[58]

These cause well-defined lysis (Figure 19.25) and are most frequently due to lung cancer.

Expanding 'bubbly' metastases

These are often highly vascularized lesions (Figure 19.26) and usually result from primary cancers of the kidneys and the thyroid.

Metastases with soft tissue involvement and periosteal bone formation

Metastases with extensive soft tissues, and calcified components, and with considerable periosteal

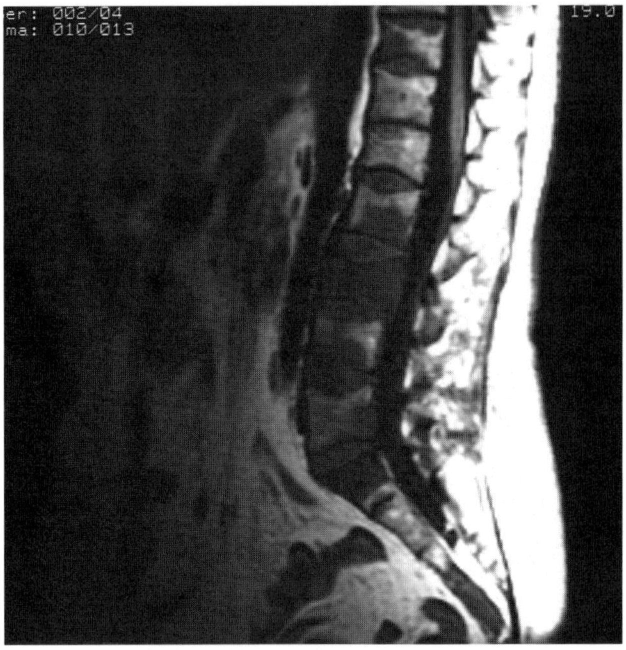

A

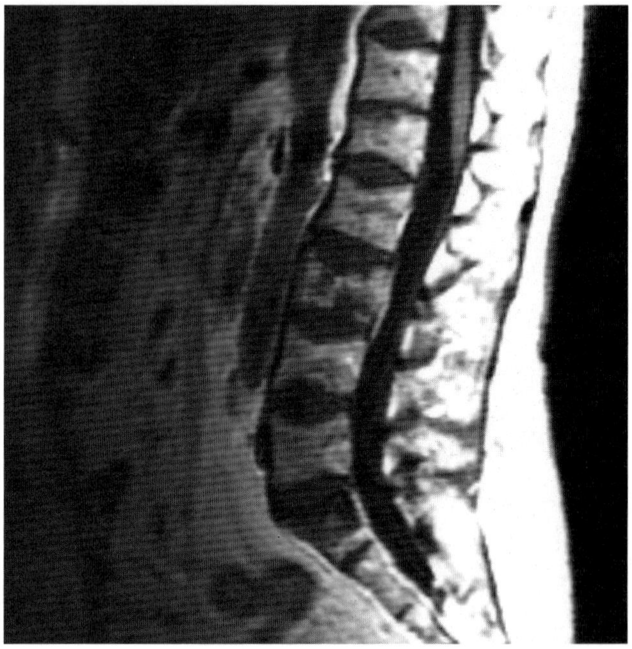

C

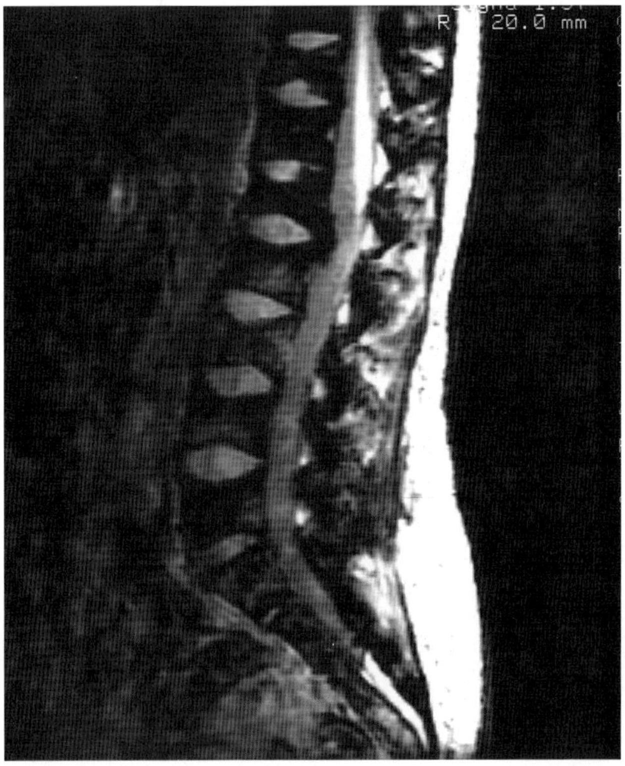

B

Figure 19.23

Lumbar spine metastases of a breast cancer. Sagittal MR images, T1-weighted spin echo (TR 500, TE 10), before (**A**), and after (**C**) contrast medium, and gradient echo (**B**) (TR 500, TE 30, flip angle 90°). There is a collapse of T11, L1, L2, L3, L5. Low density areas of T11, L2, L3, L4, L5 and S1, S4 and S5 indicate metastases (**A**). On gradient echo (**B**), they have a high signal indicating destruction of bone trabeculae. After injection (**C**) the signal of metastases increases, making the contrast with fatty marrow lower: some metastases are no longer visible.

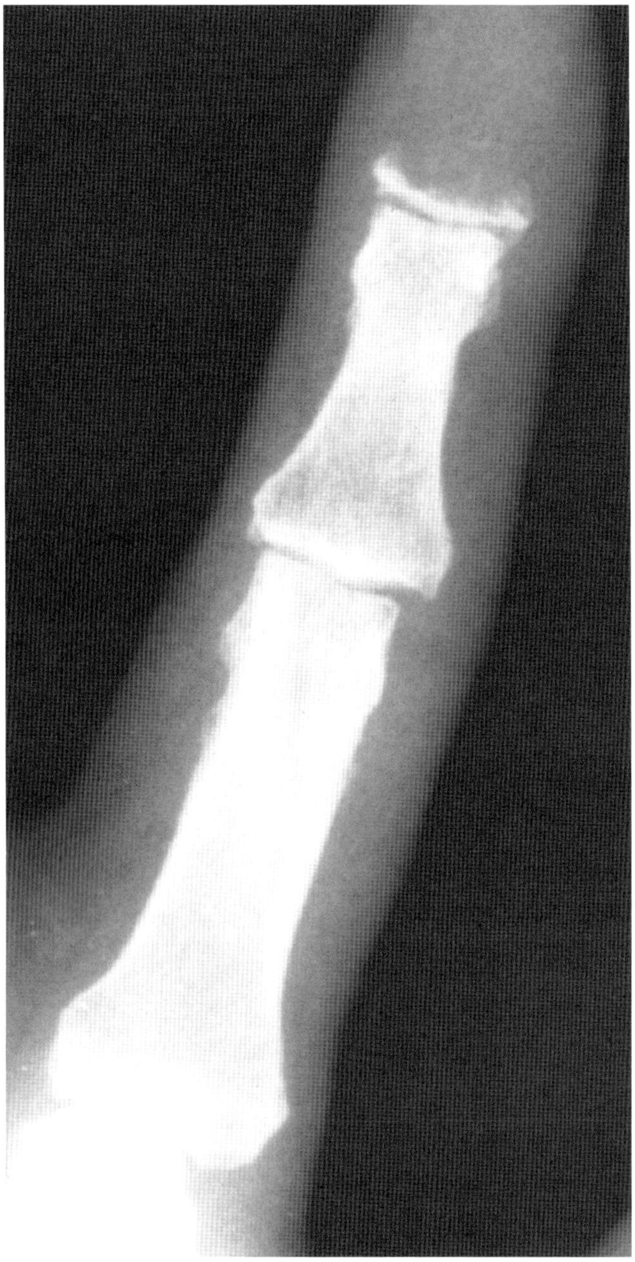

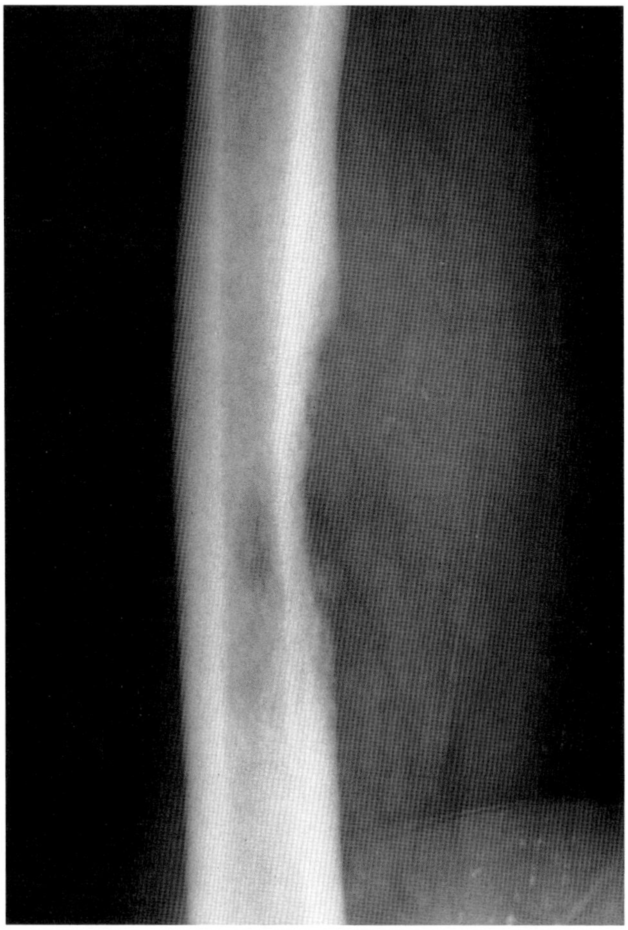

Figure 19.25

Cortical metastasis of the shaft of the femur, plain radiograph (chest cancer).

Figure 19.24

Plain radiograph of a finger: distal metastasis from lung cancer.

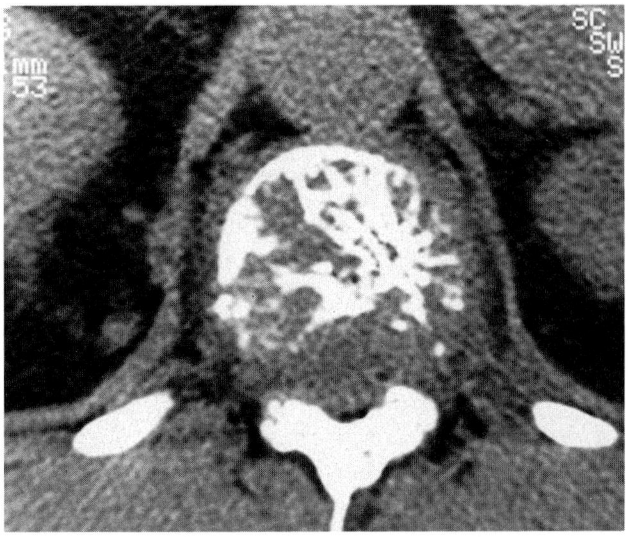

A

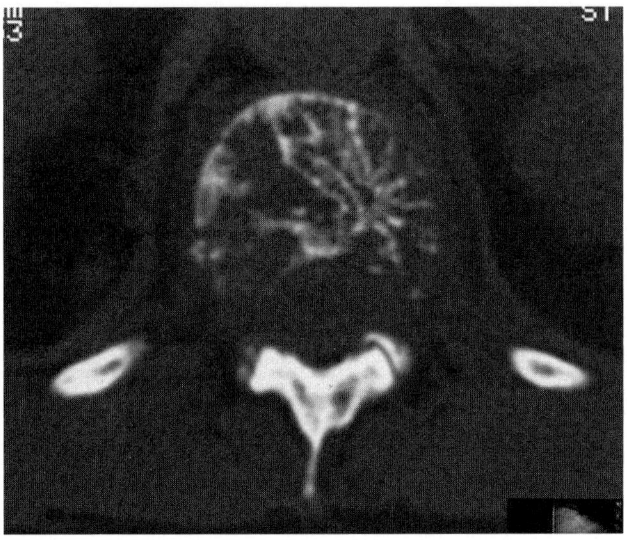

B

Figure 19.26

Pseudoangiomatous metastasis from renal cancer, revealing the disease. CT of T12 with soft tissue (**A**) and bone (**B**) windows. The lesions suggest an aggressive angioma. A cancer of the kidney was discovered 6 months later.

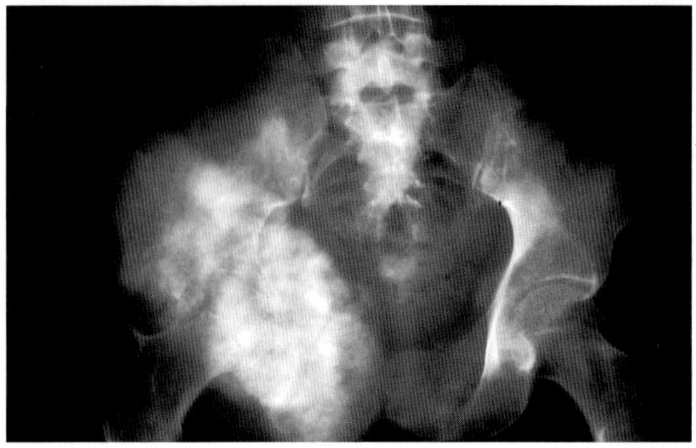

A

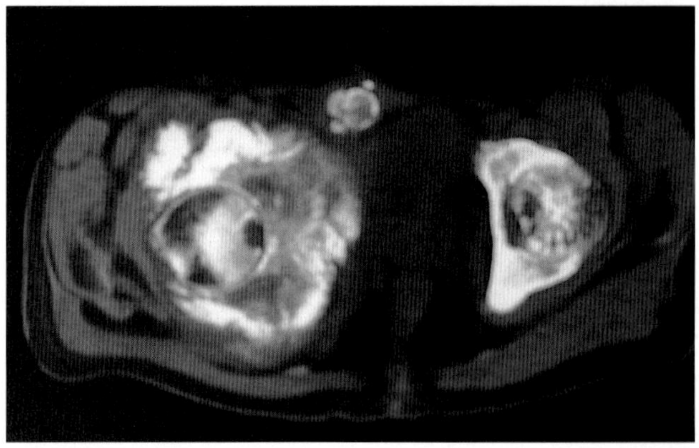

B

Figure 19.27

Metastasis of a cancer of the bladder mimicking a primary tumor of the pelvis: there is a soft tissue ossified mass, visible on (**A**) plain radiograph and (**B**) CT.

bone formation (Figure 19.27)[59,60] may resemble primitive bone tumors, and occur most frequently with cancers of the prostate; less frequently they occur with cancer of the bladder or the digestive tract.

Revealing metastases

Metastases can be synchronous, appearing at the same time as the primary tumor. They are often observed quite late on and are, rarely, revealing. In the event of such metastases, neuroblastomas should be investigated in children, especially in those under 5 years of age; in young adults, cancer of the kidney or thyroid should be looked for, whereas in older adults, it is rather more likely to be cancer of the prostate, the breast or melanomas.

Surveillance of metastases

The follow up of bone metastases can be made by skeletal scintigraphy. An interesting phenomenon which can lead to serious confusion is the so-called 'flare' reaction, in which the bone scan apparently worsens and then improves or becomes stable. The flare occurs as a result of increased isotope uptake secondary to healing, and it is usually seen within the first 3 months of therapy, disappearing within 6 months. On plain radiographs, for lytic lesions, the reossification of all foci, without the appearance of new lesions, suggests that healing is taking place, but osteolysis on a previously sclerotic lesion suggests progression. MR should be performed in cases of spinal compression, plus normal or equivocal plain radiographs and bone scans for new pain. When the marrow becomes completely fatty, eg after radiotherapy, it is easy to evaluate the result. However, if a lesion persists after treatment the difference between fibrous sequelae and active metastasis cannot be identified.

Choice of examination technique[61] (Diagram 19.4)

Standard radiographs

In case of localized pain conventional radiology should be performed on the painful areas and for confirmation of scintigraphic abnormalities. Skeletal survey is only used as a screening examination in rare cases, when scintigraphy may not be available or when patients are suspected of having purely osteolytic metastases.

Scintigraphy

This is the key examination, because it facilitates the study of the whole skeleton and is very sensitive in detection of lesions.

Magnetic resonance imaging

This is used if scintigraphy is positive and conventional radiographs are normal; it may show up other seats of involvement that are not shown on scintigraphs. A negative local result rules out metastases.[62]

In case of further doubt, a biopsy should be carried out. This is safe, simple, rapid and reliable. Metastases are usually easy to diagnose, even with cytology. It is often sufficient to perform a biopsy with a fine needle, guided by the most simple imaging procedure – either fluoroscopy or CT for more complicated areas such as the vertebrae.[63,64]

Strategy

The problem is different for each type of cancer, due to the variation in incidence of the individual cancer and to variation in the aggressive nature of the treatment. During the initial examination of the primary tumor, the patient should be evaluated for metastases: whether the treatment is changed, eg extensive surgery or radiotherapy, or whether complementary chemotherapy should be added to the treatment plan. In a series of 429 patients with bone metastases, the average survival was 5 months[65] (33% after 1 year, 17% after 2 years, 5% after 5 years). Tumors such as gastrointestinal, ENT and chest tumors are unresponsive to hormone and chemotherapy: the survival average was 2 months. In those cases, treatment regimens should be as mild as possible. In other tumors the survival may be better: in hormone-sensitive cancers (breast, prostate) or slowly growing tumors (adenoid cystic carcinoma, thyroid cancer).

In revealing metastases, the average survival is usually between 6 and 12 months, so the strategy must prevent the treatment of the patient with costly, aggressive and useless examinations. Biopsy of the metastasis should be performed when it is isolated and before chemotherapy is started. Investigation of the primary is only useful if chemotherapy has been decided upon or if the metastasis seems to be isolated. Ultrasonography and/or CT of the abdomen are the best choices of investigation.

Conclusion

The basic examination used in the detection of metastatic bone disease is bone scintigraphy, which is both sensitive and non-specific. Standard radiographs are used for painful areas, or for checking abnormalities observed on scintigraphy, because they improve on specificity. The exact role of and the best sequences for MR are not yet clear. However, MR should be used in cases of doubtful diagnosis, or when bone scintigraphy is normal and extensive surgery is being considered.

Myeloma

This is the most common primary malignant tumor of bone. It is more frequent in men than in women, and it usually presents between the fifth and the seventh decades. The tumor originates from the plasma cells of the bone marrow. In 90% of patients an immunoglobulin/protein produced by the tumor can be detected on serum electrophoresis: IgG (30%), IgA (25%), light chains (30%), others (5%). In 10% of the patients no abnormal protein is observed (non-secretory myeloma). Plasmacytosis is detected in the marrow by biopsy or aspiration. The lesions are usually located in bones that harbor hemopoietic marrow in adult life (spine, ribs, skull, pelvis, more rarely long bones). The radiologic patterns can be one of the following:

- Diffuse osteolytic lesions of the skeleton, with multiple well-defined lesions, and with no osteosclerosis (Figure 19.28).
- Diffuse osteoporosis, predominantly in the spine, with multiple compression fractures.
- Very rarely sclerotic lesions. These may be associated with polyneuropathy (P), endocrinopathy (E), M proteins (M) and skin changes (S), making the acronym POEMS[66] (Figure 19.29).

Radionuclide examination is often negative. MR of the spine[67] may reveal foci of tumor as low-signal-intensity lesions on T1-weighted images, and high-signal-intensity lesions on T2-weighted sequences, which are more reliable. Other MR findings are the absence of fatty replacement or a generalized decrease in signal intensity on T1-weighted images. There is no correlation between MR findings and laboratory or bone marrow findings.

The Durie–Salmon staging is used to classify myelomas. It uses biological markers, and skeletal radiographs.

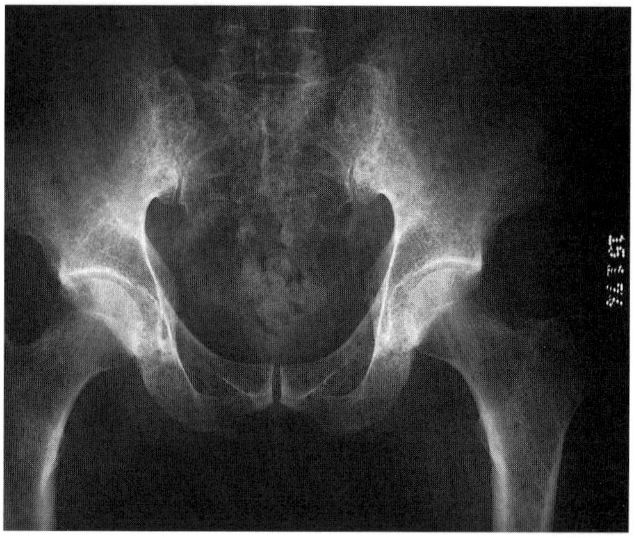

A

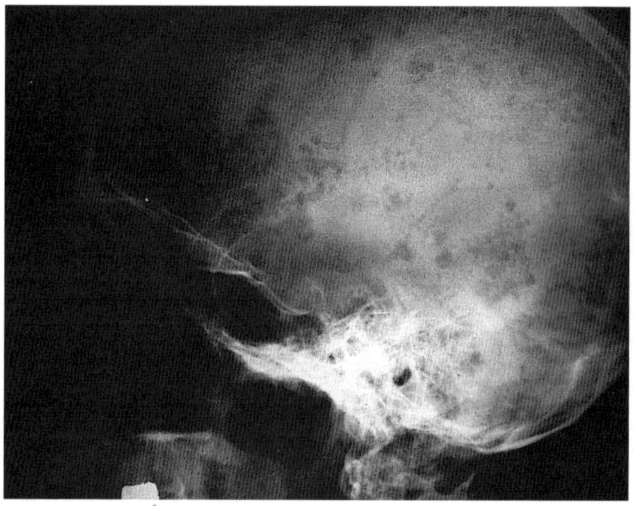

B

Figure 19.28

Myeloma: plain radiographs, (**A**) anteroposterior view of the pelvis and (**B**) lateral view of the skull. Multiple, small, well-limited lytic lesions.

The treatment consists of chemotherapy, and its efficacy is evaluated by pain and serum markers. Unless there is a new localized pain, or non-secretory forms, imaging is not necessary on follow up.

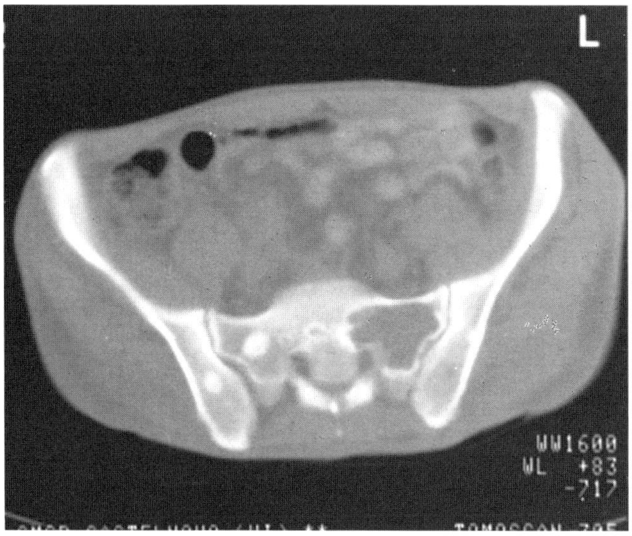

A

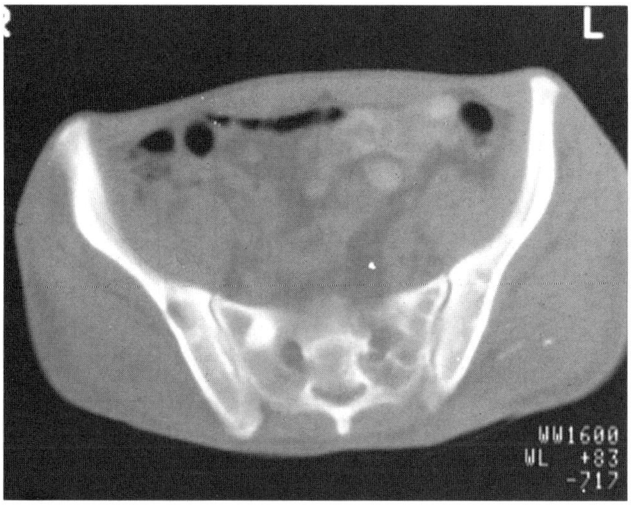

B

Figure 19.29

POEMS syndrome: (**A,B**) well-limited lytic and sclerotic lesions of the sacrum and iliac bones, visible on CT.

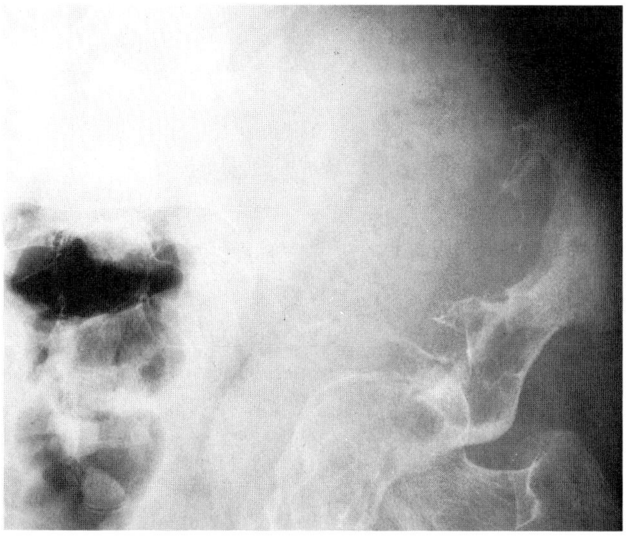

A

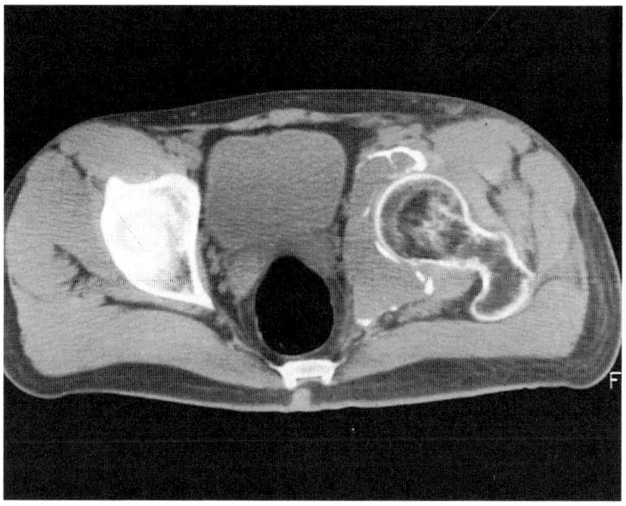

B

Figure 19.30

Solitary plasmocytoma of the pelvis: well-limited, purely lytic lesion on (**A**) plain radiograph and (**B**) CT.

Myeloma can occur as a solitary bone lesion called a plasmacytoma[68] (Figure 19.30). Patients are 10 years younger than those with myeloma. The most frequent site of involvement is the spine (50%). Radiologically, plasmacytoma may expand or destroy bone and produce a trabecular pattern. Radiotherapy is effective; however, local recurrences and generalized disease occur in 75% of cases.

References

1. Kalifa C, Mlika N, Dubousset J et al, Expérience du protocole T10 dans le Service de Pédiatrie de l'Institut Gustave-Roussy, *Bull Cancer* (1988) **75**: 207–11.
2. Rosen G, Caparros B, Huvos AG et al, Preoperative chemotherapy for osteogenic sarcoma: selection of postoperative adjuvant chemotherapy based on the response of the primary tumor to preoperative chemotherapy, *Cancer* (1982) **49**: 1221–30.
3. Lodwick GS, Wilson AJ, Farrel C et al, Estimating rate of growth in bone lesions: observer performance and error, *Radiology* (1980) **134**: 585–90.
4. Madewell JE, Ragsdale BD, Sweet DE, Radiology and pathology analysis of solitary bone lesions, *Radiol Clin N Am* (1981) **19**: 715–48.
5. Regent D, Tamisier JN, Fery A et al, Intérêt du traitement de l'information dans l'exploration scanographique des lésions focales bénignes de l'os, *Rev Rhum Mal Osteoartic* (1986) **53**: 77–82.
6. Brown KT, Kattapuram SSV, Rosentahl DI, Computed tomography analysis of bone tumors: patterns of cortical destruction and soft tissue extension, *Skeletal Radiol* (1986) **15**: 448–51.
7. Hudson TM, Springfield DS, Spanier SS et al, Benign exostoses and exostosis chondrosarcomas, evaluation of cartilage thickness by CT, *Radiology* (1984) **153**: 595–9.
8. Kenney PJ, Gilula LA, Murphy WA, The use of CT to distinguish osteochondroma and chondrosarcoma, *Radiology* (1981) **138**: 129–37.
9. Glass RB, Poznanski AK, Fisher MR et al, MR imaging of osteoid osteoma, *J Comput Assist Tomog* (1986) **10**: 1065–7.
10. Aisen AM, Martel W, Braunstein EM et al, MRI and CT evaluation of primary bone and soft tissue tumors, *AJR* (1986) **146**: 749–56.
11. Berquist Th, Magnetic resonance imaging: preliminary experience in orthopedic radiology, *Magn Reson Imag* (1984) **2**: 41–52.
12. Bloem JL, Bluemm RG, Taminiau AHM et al, MRI of primary malignant bone tumors, *Radiographics* (1987) **7**: 425–45.
13. Bloem JL, Taminiau AHM, Eulderink F et al, Radiologic staging of primary bone sarcoma. MRI, scintigraphy, angiography and CT correlated with pathologic examination, *Radiology* (1988) **169**: 805–10.
14. Bohndorf K, Reiser M, Lochner B et al, Magnetic resonance imaging of primary tumors and tumor like lesions of bone, *Skeletal Radiol* (1986) **15**: 511–17.
15. Boyko OB, Cory DA, Cohen MD et al, MR imaging of osteogenic and Ewing's sarcoma, *AJR* (1987) **148**: 317–22.
16. Brady TJ, Rosen BR, Pikett IL et al, NMR imaging of leg tumors, *Radiology* (1983) **149**: 181.
17. Hudson TM, Hamlin DJ, Enneking WF et al, MRI of bone and soft tissue tumors. Early experience in 31 patients compared with CT, *Skeletal Radiol* (1985) **13**: 134.
18. Reiser M, Rupp N, Biehl T et al, MRI in the diagnosis of bone tumors, *Eur J Radiol* (1985) **5**: 1–7.
19. Rosentahl DI, Scott JA, Mankin HJ, Sacrococcygeal chordoma: MRI and CT, *AJR* (1985) **145**: 143–7.
20. Sundaram M, McGuire MH, Herbold DR et al, Magnetic resonance imaging in planning limb-salvage surgery for primary malignant tumors of bone, *J Bone Joint Surg (Br)* (1986) **68**: 809–19.
21. Vanel D, Di Paola R, Contesso G, Magnetic resonance imaging in musculoskeletal primary malignant tumors. In: HY Kressel, ed, *Magnetic Resonance Annual* (Raven Press: New York 1987) 237–61.
22. Zimmer WD, Berquist TH, McLeod RA et al, Bone tumors: magnetic resonance imaging versus CT, *Radiology* (1985) **155**: 709–18.
23. Petterson H, Slone RM, Spanier S et al, Musculoskeletal tumors: T1 and T2 relaxation times, *Radiology* (1988) **167**: 783–5.
24. Beltran X, Simon DC, Levy M et al, Aneurysmal bone cysts. MR imaging at 1.5 T, *Radiology* (1986) **158**: 689–90.
25. Hudson TM, Hamlin DJ, Fitzsimmons JR, MRI of fluid levels in aneurysmal bone cysts and in anticoagulated human blood, *Skeletal Radiol* (1985) **13**: 267–70.
26. Azouz EM, Esseltine DW, Chevalier L et al, Radiologic evaluation of osteosarcoma, *J Cancer Assoc Radiol* (1982) **33**: 167–71.
27. Ginaldy S, De Santos LA, CT in the evaluation of small round cell tumors of bone, *Radiology* (1980) **134**: 441–6.
28. Hudson TM, Schieber LM, Springfield DS et al, Radiologic imaging of osteosarcoma. Role in planning surgical treatment, *Skeletal Radiol* (1983) **10**: 37.
29. Vanel D, Contesso G, Couanet D et al, CT in evaluation of 41 Ewing's sarcomas, *Skeletal Radiol* (1982) **9**: 8–13.
30. Coffre C, Vanel D, Contesso G et al, Problems and pitfalls in the use of CT for the local evaluation of long bone osteosarcoma, *Skeletal Radiol* (1985) **13**: 147–153.
31. Beltran J, Simon DC, Katz W et al, Increased MR signal intensity in skeletal muscle adjacent to malignant tumors: pathologic correlation and clinical relevance, *Radiology* (1987) **162**: 251–5.
32. Campanacci M, Middi P, Gherlinzoni F et al, Parosteal osteosarcoma, *J Bone Joint Surg (Br)* (1984) **66**: 313–21.
33. Vanel D, Henri-Amar M, Lumbroso J et al, Pulmonary evaluation of patients with osteosarcoma: roles of standard radiography, tomography, CT, scintigraphy and tomoscintigraphy, *AJR* (1984) **143**: 519–23.
34. Smith J, Heelan RT, Huvos AG et al, Radiologic changes in primary osteogenic sarcomas following intensive chemotherapy, *Radiology* (1982) **143**: 355–60.

35. Vanel D, Lacombe MJ, Couanet D et al, Musculoskeletal tumors: follow-up with MR imaging after treatment with surgery and radiation therapy, *Radiology* (1987) **164**: 243–5.
36. Vanel D, Coffre C, Tumeurs primitives des os et des parties molles. In: Vanel D, ed, *IRM corps entier* (Springer-Verlag: Paris 1989) 315–26.
37. Reiser MF, Erhardt W, Bauer R et al, Gd DTPA enhance magnetic resonance imaging in the diagnosis of inflammatory and neoplastic musculoskeletal lesions, *Excerpta Medica* (1986) 170–6.
38. Vanel D, Valenty M, Henry-Amar M et al, Radiologic prognostic factors in osteosarcomas: report of 102 cases, *Radiology* (RSNA scientific program 1990) **177**: 146.
39. Holscher HC, Bloem JL, Vanel D et al, Osteosarcoma: chemotherapy-induced changes at MR imaging, *Radiology* (1992) **182**: 839–44.
40. Erleman R, Reiser M, Peters PE, Time dependent changes in signal intensity in neoplastic and inflammatory lesions of the musculoskeletal system after IV administration of Gd DTPA, *Radiology* (1988) **28**: 269.
41. Bonnerot V, Charpentier A, Frouin F et al, Factor analysis of dynamic MR imaging in predicting the response of osteosarcoma to chemotherapy, *Invest Radiol* (1992) **27**: 847–55.
42. De Baere T, Vanel D, Shapeero LG et al, Osteosarcoma after chemotherapy: evaluation with contrast material-enhanced subtraction MR imaging, *Radiology* (1992) **185**: 587–92.
43. Vanel D, Tcheng S, Contesso G et al, The radiological appearances of telangiectatic osteosarcoma, *Skeletal Radiol* (1987) **16**: 196–200.
44. Kurt A, Unni KK, McLeod RA et al, Low grade intraosseous osteosarcoma, *Cancer* (1990) **65**: 1418–28.
45. Wold LE, Unni KK, Beabout JW et al, High grade surface osteosarcoma, *Am J Surg Pathol* (1984) **8**: 181.
46. Unni KK, Dahlin DC, Beabout JW, Periosteal osteogenic sarcoma, *Cancer* (1976) **37**: 2476.
47. Frouge C, Vanel D, Coffre C et al, The role of magnetic resonance imaging in the evaluation of Ewing sarcoma, *Skeletal Radiol* (1988) **17**: 387–92.
48. Rousselin B, Vanel D, Terrier-Lacombe MJ et al, Clinical and radiologic analysis of 13 cases of primary neuroectodermal tumors of bone, *Skeletal Radiol* (1989) **18**: 115–20.
49. Malghem J, Van De Berg B, Noel H et al, Benign osteochondromas: evaluation of cartilage cap thickness by ultrasound, *Skeletal Radiol* (1992) **21**: 33–7.
50. Abrams HL, Spiro R, Goldstein N, Metastases in carcinomas. Analysis of 1000 autopsied cases, *Cancer* (1950) **3**: 74.
51. Willis, RA, A review of 500 consecutive cancer autopsies, *Med J Aust* (1941) **2**: 258.
52. Batson OV, The function of the vertebral veins and their role in the spread of metastases, *Ann Surg* (1940) **112**: 138.
53. Galasko CSB, Mechanisms of lytic and blastic metastatic disease of bone, *Clin Orthop Rel Res* (1982) **169**: 20.
54. Jacobson AF, Cronin EB, Stomper PC et al, Bone scans with one or two new abnormalities in cancer patients with no known metastases: frequency and serial scintigraphic behavior of benign and malignant lesions, *Radiology* (1990) **175**: 229–232.
55. Avra Hami E, Tadmor R, Dally O et al, Early MR demonstration of spinal metastases in patients with normal radiographs and CT and radionuclide bone scans, *J Comput Assist Tomog* (1989) **13**: 598–602.
56. Fragiadakis EG, Panayotopoulous G, Metastatic carcinoma of the hand, *Hand* (1972) **4**: 268.
57. Kerin R, Metastatic tumors of the hand, *J Bone Joint Surg (Am)* (1958) **40**: 263.
58. Deutsch A, Resnick D, Eccentric cortical metastases to the skeleton from bronchogenic carcinoma, *Radiology* (1980) **137**: 49.
59. Vilar J, Lezana AH, Pedrosa CS, Spiculated periosteal reaction in metastatic lesion of bone, *Skeletal Radiol* (1979) **3**: 230.
60. Wyche LD, De Santos LA, Spiculated periosteal reaction in metastatic disease resembling osteosarcoma, *Orthopedics* (1978) **1**: 215.
61. Gold RJ, Seeger LL, Bassett LW et al, An integrated approach to the evaluation of metastatic bone disease, *Radiol Clin N Am* (1990) **28**: 471–83.
62. Ramsey RG, Zacharias CE, MR imaging of the spine after radiation therapy: easily recognizable effects, *AJR* (1985) **144**: 1131.
63. Hardy DC, Murphy WA, Gilula LA, Computed tomography in planning percutaneous bone biopsy, *Radiology* (1980) **134**: 447.
64. Mink J, Percutaneous bone biopsy in the patient with known or suspected osseous metastases, *Radiology* (1986) **161**: 191.
65. Stines J, Conroy T, Bey P et al, L'imagerie dans les metastases osseuses, *Feuillets de Radiologie* (1992) **32**: 95–116.
66. Bardwick PA, Zwaifler NJ, Gill GN et al, Plasma cell dyscrasia with polyneuropathy, organomegaly, endocrinopathy, M protein, and skin changes: the POEMS syndrome, *Medicine* (1980) **59**: 311.
67. Libshitz HI, Malthouse SR, Cunningham D et al, Multiple myeloma: appearance at MR imaging, *Radiology* (1992) **182**: 833–7.
68. Bataille R, Sany J, Solitary myeloma. Clinical and prognostic features of a review of 114 cases, *Cancer* (1981) **48**: 845–51.

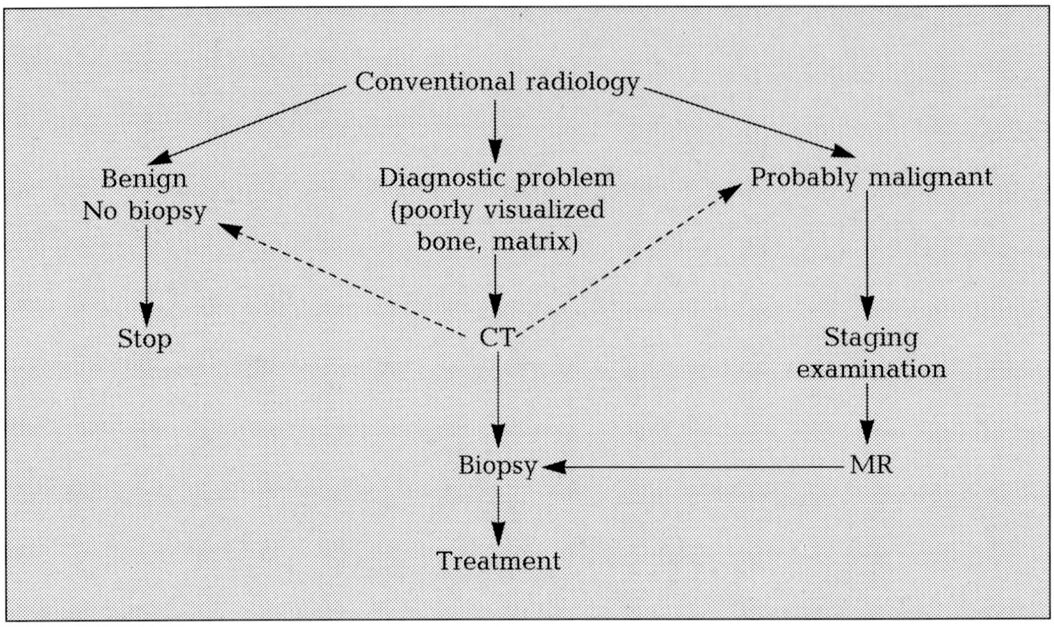

Diagram 19.1

Strategy for local evaluation of bone tumors.

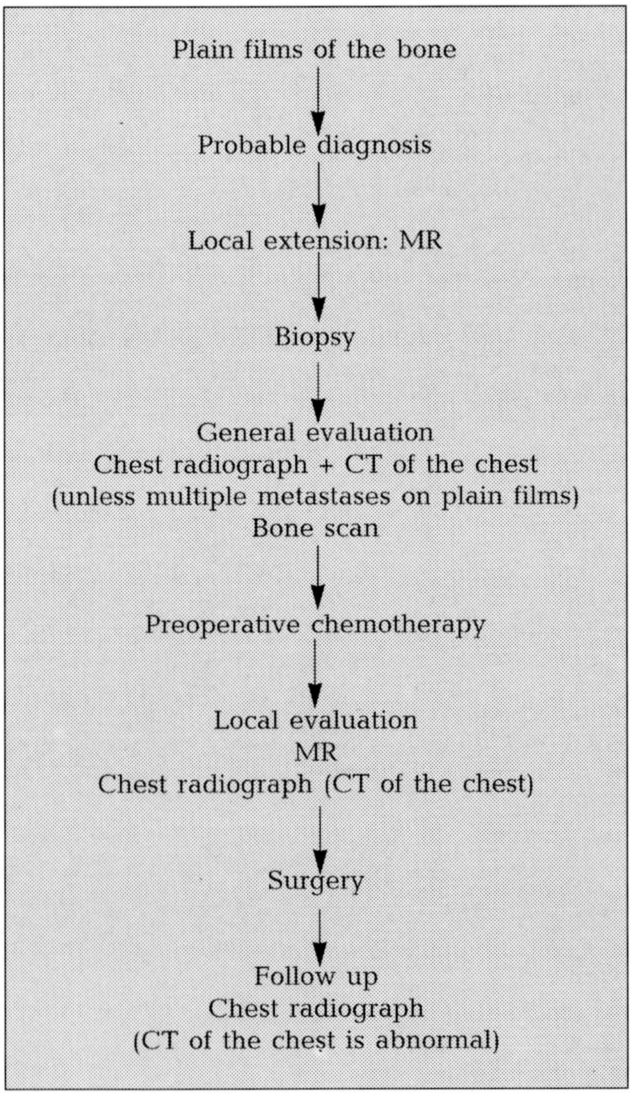

Diagram 19.2

Strategy for imaging a conventional osteosarcoma.

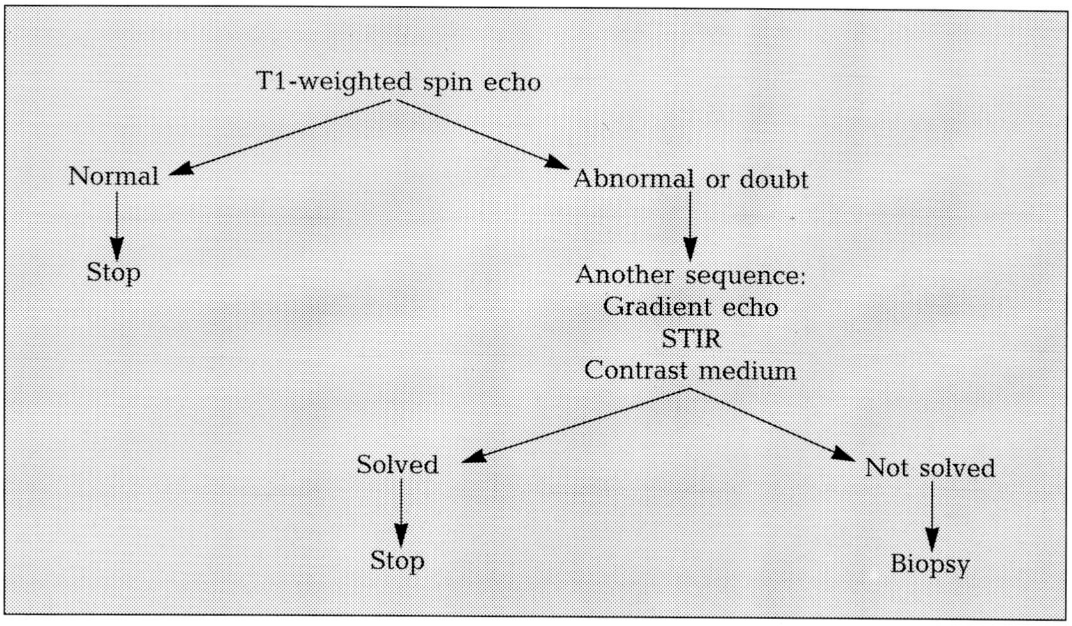

Diagram 19.3

MR strategy for detection of bone metastases.

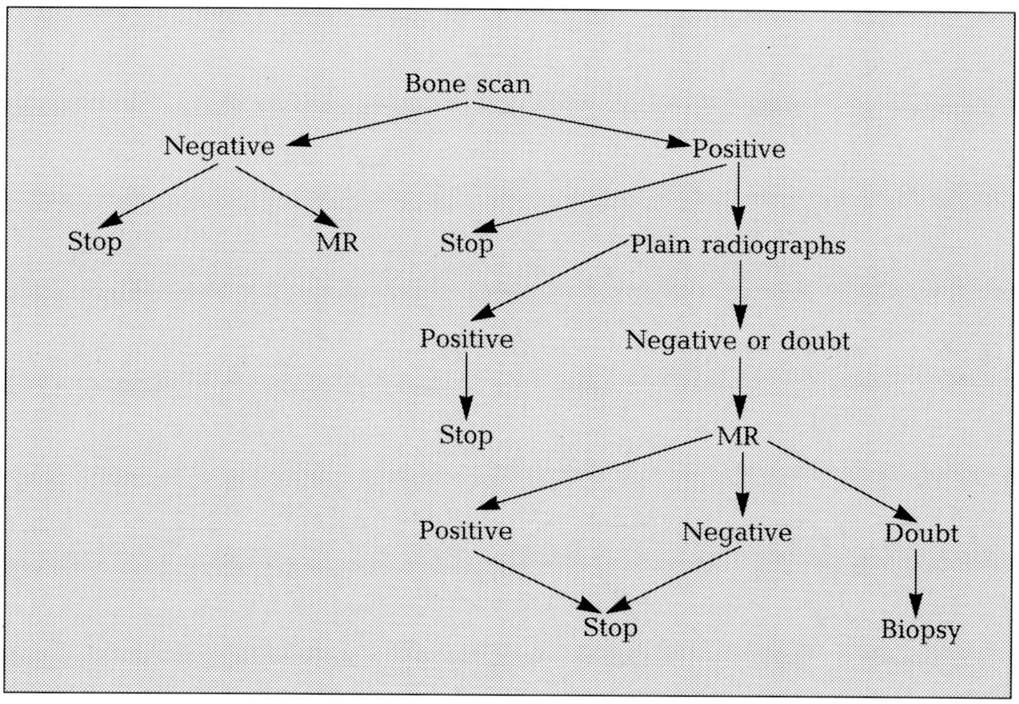

Diagram 19.4

Detection of bone metastases.

20

The skin

Philippe Soyer, Alvaro Margulis, Jacques Masselot

Introduction

Accurate staging of skin tumors is useful in selecting the best therapy. A wide range of options is available for diagnostic imaging of skin tumors. Recently, high-resolution ultrasonography (US), and magnetic resonance imaging (MR) raise the possibility of modifying the imaging strategies for skin tumors. The purpose of this chapter, which is focused on malignant melanoma, is to present basic concepts of imaging strategies for staging and follow up of skin tumors.

Techniques

Skeletal radiography

For a long time, radiography was the sole method for the assessment of local bone involvement in advanced malignant skin tumor and the diagnosis of skeletal metastases.

Lymphography

Malignant melanoma frequently metastasizes to regional lymph nodes. Lymphography has been applied to the detection of lymph-node metastases,[1,2] but it produces too many false-negative and false-positive reports. In a recent study[2] in which lymphography was performed prior to lymphadenectomy, the sensitivity and the specificity were, respectively, 57 and 56% for the upper extremity (axillary lymphography), and 77 and 73% for the lower extremity (bipedal lymphography). In the same study, CT had a high accuracy. For these reasons, lymphography is rarely indicated in a clinical setting; it is no longer performed at our institute.

Chest radiography

Chest radiography is performed to look for thoracic metastases of melanoma and squamous-cell carcinomal. In a carcinologic setting, we commonly perform anteroposterior and lateral view films.

Computed tomography

CT is the front-line examination in malignant skin tumors, providing an assessment of the local extent and identifying distant metastases.

Before pelvic and abdominal examination, patients receive oral contrast medium to outline the small bowel. CT slices are carried out during bolus injection of contrast medium followed by drip infusion. Contrast enhancement differentiates lymph nodes from vascular structures. The abdominal survey is performed from the dome of the diaphragm to the iliac crests, with 10–15 mm contiguous slices. The pelvic survey is performed from the iliac crests to the pubic symphysis with

10 mm contiguous slices. Thoracic examination explores both lungs and mediastinum. CT slices are carried out during bolus injection which permits differentiation of lymph-node enlargement from mediastinal vessels. Cranial examination is performed after injection of contrast medium.

Ultrasonography

Ultrasonography (US) provides an evaluation of squamous-cell carcinomas and melanomas at initial presentation and assesses the presence of residual, recurrent or progressive disease after therapy. Real-time scanners equipped with a 3.5 or 5.0 MHz sector transducer are utilized. US, when indicated, explores the liver, the retroperitoneal space, the pelvis and the pelvic lymph-node areas; a fully distended urinary bladder is required for this.

For basal cell carcinomas, US is rarely indicated. Recently, high-resolution linear transducers have been proposed to evaluate the depth of malignant melanoma.[3–5]

Radioscintigraphy

In advanced stages of squamous-cell carcinoma and melanoma, scintigraphy of bone with ^{99m}Tc-diphosphonate is performed before surgery. This technique provides a total body exploration, permitting the assessment of the local and distant extent of bone involvement.[6] Recently, lymphoscintigraphy with ^{99m}Tc-rhenium sulfide colloid has been shown to be a reliable technique for the demonstration of the regional lymphatic drainage of malignant melanoma.[7]

Magnetic resonance imaging

MR is a well-established technique in the diagnosis of intracranial metastatic melanoma[8] and squamous-cell carcinoma. MR is also indicated in the evaluation of the local extent of malignant skin tumors. Rapid developments in surface-coil technology have made MR suitable for studies of cutaneous structures.

Malignant melanoma

Epidemiology

The incidence of malignant melanoma is rising rapidly: there has been an 80% increase in the USA between 1973 and 1980[9] and it accounts for approximately 1% of all cancers. Increased exposure to sun and ultraviolet light is an important etiological agent. Heredity and racial factors have also been advocated.

Classification

There are three major clinicopathologic types of malignant melanoma:[10] (a) superficial spreading melanoma, accounting for 64% of cases; (b) nodular melanoma, the most malignant, 28%; and (c) lentigo maligna melanoma, the least malignant, 7%.

Mode of dissemination

Metastases from malignant melanoma may occur anywhere in the body. It has an elective lymph-node dissemination, and, in 80% of cases with metastases, the spread is primarily to regional lymph nodes via the cutaneous lymphatic system. It also metastasizes by direct extension to the skin or by hematogeneous spread to the lung and the liver.

Malignant melanoma has a very clear predilection for spread to the central nervous system. It is the third most common neoplasm to metastasize to the brain, after lung and breast carcinomas.[11] Over 50% of patients dying of malignant melanoma have cerebral metastases.[12] Adrenal glands, kidney, small bowel and bone are common sites of metastatic disease.

Staging

The standard staging[13] system for malignant melanoma is based on clinical and histologic examination (Table 20.1).

Histologic classification takes into account two parameters which assess the depth of invasion. The thickness of malignant melanoma (Breslow thickness)[14] permits distinction of five groups: ≤0.75 mm, 0.75–1.50 mm, 1.51–2.25 mm, 2.26–3.00 mm and >3.00 mm in thickness. The anatomic level of invasion (Clark's level)[15] allows the distinction of five levels (Table 20.2).

Table 20.1 Clinical staging of malignant melanoma.

Stage I	Localized primary melanoma, local recurrence or satellites
Stage II	Metastases in regional lymph nodes or 'in-transit' metastases
Stage III	Distant metastases

Prognosis

The Breslow thickness and Clark's level of invasion are important prognosic factors[13] in malignant melanoma, but their prognostic values are overshadowed by the presence of lymph-node metastasis (clinical stage II).

In stage I malignant melanoma patients, thickness is the most important prognosis factor. Mortality increases in steps with respect to thickness in stain (Table 20.3).[16]

In stage II, virtually all patients die, the 10-year survival rate being between 0 and 3%.

In stage III, virtually all patients die of disease. Patients with resectable distant metastases have a median survival time of 16 months, versus 5 months for patients with unresectable metastases.

Table 20.2 Clark's levels: invasion of malignant melanoma.

Level 1	Tumor confined to the epidermis (in-situ tumor)
Level 2	Tumor invading the papillary dermis but not the reticular dermis
Level 3	Extension to the interface between papillary and reticular dermis
Level 4	Infiltration into the reticular dermis
Level 5	Infiltration of the subcutaneous tissue

Table 20.3 8-year survival rate (±SD) related to thickness of malignant melanoma.

Thickness (mm)	*8-year survival rate (%)*
<0.85	99±1
0.85–1.69	93±2
1.70–3.60	69±5
>3.60	38±6

Imaging features

In malignant melanoma, imaging techniques have a major role to play in follow up, evaluation of tumor response to therapy and in assessment of recurrence. Their most important role is in the assessment of the extent of the disease at initial presentation because of the wide variety of therapeutic managements, choice of which is related to stage. Diagnosis and depth are confirmed by gross examination.

Tumor

Ultrasonography

The use of high resolution and high frequency (more than 10 MHz) has been recently proposed in the evaluation of the thickness of the lesion.[5] The accurate measurement of the thickness of malignant melanoma should provide pre-operative information for local management. But, in its current form, US cannot replace gross examination.

Magnetic resonance imaging

High resolution MR provides a dramatic improvement of the spatial resolution. Thus it permits a clear delineation of the different layers of the skin.[17] It gives an accurate pre-operative assessment of depth invasion.

It has been suggested that MR may be helpful in differentiating benign from malignant pigmented skin lesions,[18] but further investigations must confirm this first report.

Extent

Conventional radiography

Chest radiography is performed for the assessment of pulmonary metastases, which correlate with a worse prognosis. Lung metastases are the most frequent, occurring in 70% of advanced stage malignant melanoma cases. Lung metastases present most commonly as multiple round nodular deposits,[19] but many non-specific features have been described (solitary nodule, disseminated miliary pattern, atelectasia). The chest film reveals pleural effusion and/or pleural metastases, and enlarged hilar or mediastinal lymph nodes.

Skeletal radiography has a low accuracy in detecting skeletal metastasis and, until the onset of cortical destruction, most medullary lesions remain radiographically invisible.[20] When they are visible, most skeletal metastases are non-specific, similar to other osteolytic metastases, but some particular (potentially misdiagnosing) findings have been described:[6] (a) subarticular location which can lead to a misdiagnosis of giant cell tumor, (b) periosteal reaction and (c) well-circumscribed lesion with sclerotic rim.

Small bowel enema is still the most useful examination in the assessment of small bowel involvement. Metastatic involvement of the small bowel can be found coincidentally or may be the cause of abdominal pain, melena and obstruction. Intussusception of polypoid metastasis is a frequent cause of bowel obstruction in patients with malignant melanoma.[19] Small bowel enema can also show multiple submucosal nodes as well-defined lacunae. Endoscopic examination provides further information[21] on upper gastrointestinal tract involvement.

Ultrasonography

US is commonly performed for the assessment of liver metastases. Depending on local practice, MR or CT can also be performed. An US exploration of the spleen, kidneys, adrenal glands and pancreas is also performed because of the possibilities of secondary localizations to those organs. Furthermore, US explores the retroperitoneal space, searching for adenomegaly.

Computed tomography

Malignant melanoma has a high propensity for metastases to the lung. To improve diagnostic accuracy in pretreatment staging, CT has been proposed as an adjunct to routine plain chest radiography, because of the discrepancy in plain chest film and post mortem findings. The chest CT findings are responsible for a modification of the therapeutic management in 26% of cases.[22] The CT appearance of lung metastases is variable and non-specific. Furthermore, CT provides an accurate detection of mediastinal or hilar adenopathy.

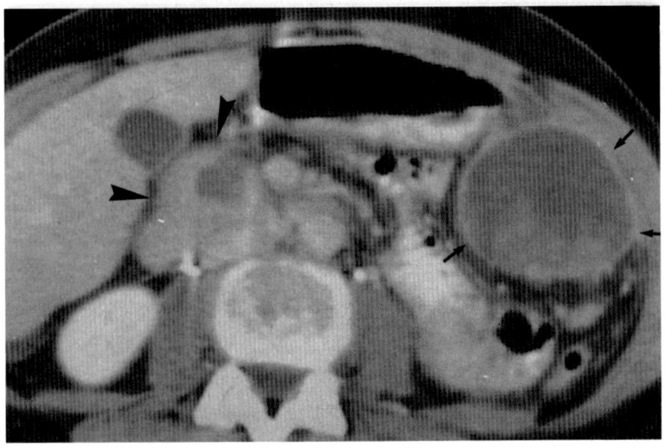

Figure 20.1

Stage III malignant melanoma. CT in the axial plane shows enlargement of the cephalic part of the pancreas (arrowheads), well-circumscribed pseudocystic lesion with highly enhanced wall (arrows). Surgery confirmed the diagnosis of intrapancreatic and epiploic metastases.

Abdominal CT scan permits an assessment of hepatic, pancreatic (Figure 20.1), splenic (Figure 20.2) and renal extent. Hepatic metastases are frequent, with variable appearance. Lesions can be single or multiple, and may be partly calcified[23] and hypervascular.

Bowel and mesenteric involvement by malignant melanoma has no particular features and is indistinguishable from any malignant tumor.

CT is particularly accurate in demonstrating lymph-node involvement. Extension to lymph node depends on the location of the primary tumor. This fact guides the CT examination when searching for lymph-node metastases.

CT features of intracranial metastases from malignant melanoma have been well described:[24]

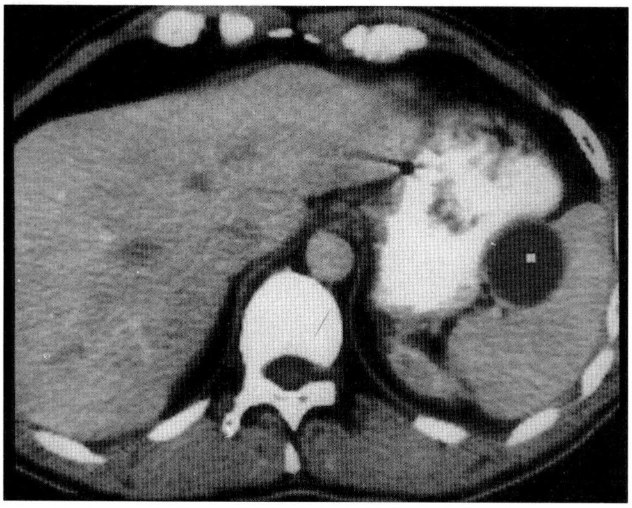

Figure 20.2

Stage III malignant melanoma. CT in the axial plane shows the cystic feature of a splenic metastasis.

(a) in all cases, there is an enhancement after injection and some lesions are only seen after injection, (b) enhanced lesions are surrounded by a hypodense area in 84% of cases with intracranial metastases, (c) the frontal lobe and temporoparietal region are the two most common locations, (d) intracranial metastases are hyperdense without injection when intratumoral hemorrhage occurs.

Magnetic resonance imaging
Liver metastases can be depicted by MR. Malignant melanoma can be distinguished without injection from normal liver parenchyma on T1-weighted spin-echo images because of the short T1 due to melanine or blood. This MR feature strongly suggests the diagnosis when a history of malignant melanoma is known. In cases of amelanotic lesions, the MR findings are non-specific.

Intracranial metastases are ideal lesions to study with MR due to their inherent paramagnetic effects, related to melanin and both hemoglobin and hemosiderin. The MR findings for intracranial metastatic malignant melanoma are:[8] (a) melanotic non-hemorrhagic malignant melanoma has a high signal intensity on spin-echo T1-weighted images and a low signal intensity on spin-echo T2-weighted images; (b) amelanotic non-hemorrhagic malignant melanoma has a moderate signal intensity on both T1- and T2-weighted images; (c) hemorrhagic malignant melanoma has a signal intensity depending on the stage of hemorrhage.

Bone metastases are accurately detected by MR, but the most important role of MR is in the evaluation of spinal cord compression before surgical decompression.

Scintigraphy
Radionuclide (^{99m}Tc-diphosphonate) bone scan provides a total body exploration and detects lesion earlier and in greater number than does radiography.[6] Scintigraphy shows non-specific hyperfixation. Ribs are the most frequent location.

Squamous-cell carcinoma

Epidemiology

Squamous-cell carcinomas (SCC) are more numerous than basal-cell carcinoma (BCC), at a 9:1 ratio, occurring mainly in males.[25] The incidence increases with age, correlating well with sun exposure: (a) 90% of SCCs are on exposed parts of the body; (b) SCC is more prevalent in outdoor people; (c) when skin pigmentation decreases, SCC incidence increases; (d) the incidence doubles with every 10° latitude decrease.

Something over half of SCCs occur on head and neck. Most of the remainder are found on hands and forearms. The lower lip is a common location.

Classification

Histologically, SCCs are classified as to relative malignancy according to the degree of cellular differentiation. Broders' classification distinguishes four grades (Table 20.4).

Table 20.4 Broders' classification of squamous-cell carcinoma, according to cellular differentiation.

Grade	*Percentage anaplastic cells*
Grade I	<25
Grade II	25–050
Grade III	50–75
Grade IV	>75

Mode of disseminations

SCC can disseminate by direct extension to local structure (hypodermis and bone), the lymphatic system and perineural spaces.[26]

Prognosis

Ulcerated forms, which tend to grow rapidly and may metastasize to regional lymph nodes promptly, have a bad prognosis.

Broders' classification is of value in prognosis with respect to rate of recurrence and metastases: only 10% of Broders' grade I tumors recur after excision, whereas 90% of Broders' grade IV do. The location has prognostic value: lesions of the lower extremity, lips and tongue metastasize the most frequently.

Imaging features

Imaging techniques have a less important role to play than in malignant melanoma.

Tumor

Imaging techniques have no purpose in diagnosis. The diagnosis is purely clinical and histologic.

Extent

Conventional radiography
Skeletal radiography can depict spread to the surrounding bone structures. Chest radiography shows lung metastases, which are rare and non-specific.

Ultrasonography
US easily depicts liver metastases, which are not frequent. US is often unable to analyze the retroperitoneal space and is not the procedure of choice for the assessment of lymph-node involvement.

Computed tomography
Usually, CT is the procedure of choice in the assessment of local extent, and especially of skeletal involvement. CT depicts osteolytic areas through 'bone-windows' (large windows to study bone structures) (Figure 20.3B and 20.4). In one study of 53 cases of advanced calvarian skin tumors, CT was the most reliable examination for the pre-operative assessment of the depth.[27]

Magnetic resonance imaging

MR is the best procedure for detecting invasion of perineural space from SCC located close to skull foramina (Figure 20.3C). MR can easily depict tumor spread along the facial nerve or the branches of the trigeminal nerve.

Basal cell carcinoma

Epidemiology

Basal cell carcinomas (BCCs) are less numerous than SCC. BCCs are often associated with history of trauma and chronic ulcer, occurring mostly in females.

The relationship of sun exposure and incidence of BCC is the same than for SCC. Nearly all BCCs occur on the head and neck, and mostly on the nose and circumocular region.

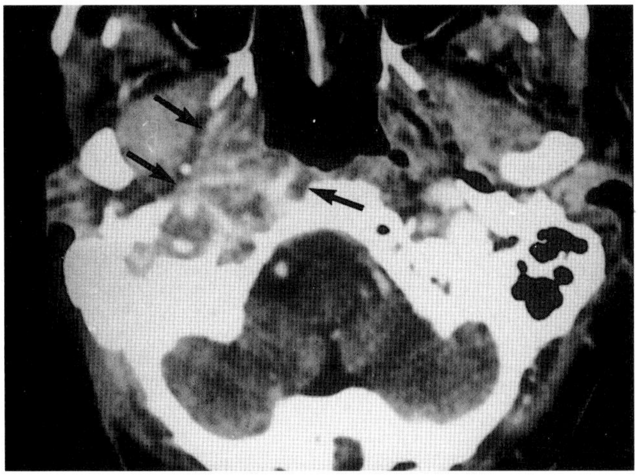

A

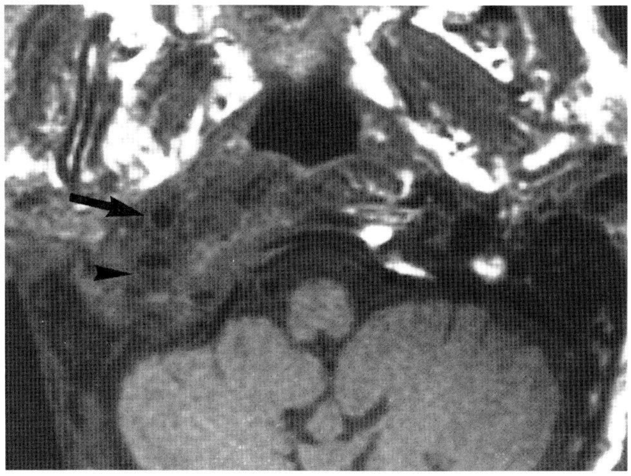

C

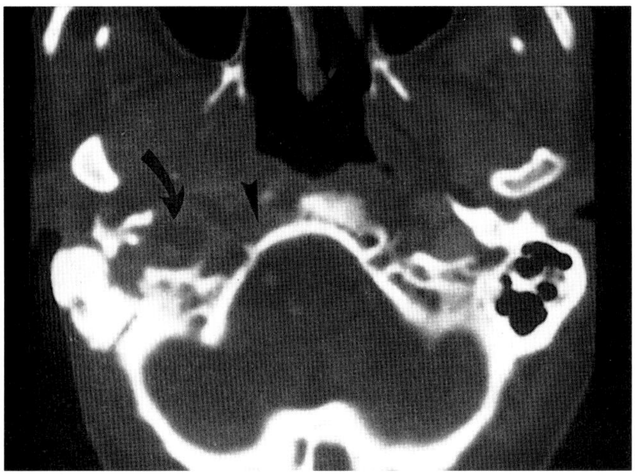

B

Figure 20.3

Recurrence of a right retroauricular squamous-cell carcinoma after surgery.

A After injection, CT shows heterogeneous enhanced mass invading the right pterygomaxillary fossa and parapharyngeal space (arrows).

B Bone window reveals extension to the basioccipital bone (arrowhead) and the petrous part of the temporal bone (curved arrow).

C T1-weighted MR reveals extension to the jugular foramen and hypoglossal canal; the right internal carotid artery (arrow) and jugular vein (arrowhead) are surrounded by the tumor.

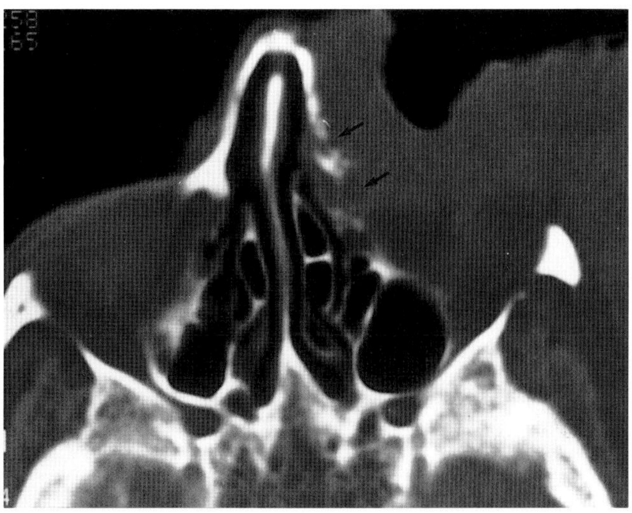

Figure 20.4

Advanced stage squamous-cell carcinoma of the face. CT in the axial plane shows extension into the orbitary fossa and involvement of bone structures. Bone window reveals lysis of the nasal and frontal processes of the maxilla (arrows).

Classification

Ten morphologic types are described: (a) solid type, (b) cystic, (c) adenoid, (d) keratotic, (e) pigmented, (f) multifocal, (g) sclerosing, (h) infiltrating, (i) basosquamous, and (j) premalignant fibroepithelial tumor of Pinkus.

Mode of dissemination

BCC rarely metastasizes. It is a localized malignancy which grows slowly but may cause serious local mutilation and bone invasion when neglected. Most commonly, as the BCC progresses, it ulcerates in its center and develops rolled edges. One type, which exhibits deeply extensive ulceration, is the rodent ulcer.

Metastases to regional lymph nodes are exceptional,[28] occurring with the metatypical or basosquamous types.

Prognosis

BCC has a good prognosis, only causing local damage. In 20% of cases, spontaneous regression has been shown.[29]

Imaging features

Tumor

Imaging techniques are of no interest. Clinical and histologic examinations provide the diagnosis.

Extent

Conventional radiography
Skeletal radiography shows local spread to skeletal structures. Skull radiography can be of interest in BCC of the head.

Computed tomography
CT is the procedure of choice for the assessment of the local spread to the bone. CT shows, more precisely than conventional radiography, bone erosion in cases of ulcerated deeply invasive BCC.[27]

Follow up

Malignant melanoma

Clinical examination is the most accurate and least expensive procedure for the assessment of local recurrences.

Follow-up examination after radical surgical treatment in clinical stage I is of great importance. Early identification of metastases will sometimes permit successful further treatment. Chest films are believed[30] to be essential in the follow up. The frequency of optimal radiographic follow-up examinations is controversial. We believe that chest radiography should be performed twice a year.

US and CT are highly sensitive in the detection of hepatic metastasis and are regularly performed during follow up.

CT is the most accurate imaging technique for the detection of lymph-node involvement.[2] Furthermore, CT can play an important role in the detection of brain metastases,[24] although MR is superior. For these reasons, abdominopelvic CT and intracranial MR are regular features of follow up.

Squamous cell carcinoma

Clinical examination is the most important means of follow up. Most SCCs that metastasize are large and aggressive tumors which recur locally.

CT and/or MR can be helpful in the evaluation of local bone extent when there is recurrence.

Basal cell carcinoma

Clinical examination is sufficient for demonstrating recurrence.

Imaging strategy

Malignant melanoma

When malignant melanoma is clinically suspected, the lesion is surgically excised with variable tumor-free margins. Before surgery, we commonly perform a chest radiography. The imaging strategy is based on the histologic report and particularly on the Breslow stage. In Breslow stage I (tumor thickness less than 0.75 mm), we perform only chest radiography and US or CT of the liver. In Breslow stages II–V (tumor thickness more than 0.75 mm), commonly we perform chest radiography, intracranial MR or CT, and abdominopelvic CT in the assessment of lymph-node involvement.

During the follow up we commonly perform chest radiography and US or CT of the liver. In case of doubt following chest radiography, thoracic CT is carried out. Intracranial metastases are most of the time clinically obvious (only 11% of patients with cerebral metastases are clinically free of disease), and we do not perform brain MR or CT routinely.[24] When tumor thickness is more than 2 mm, we commonly perform brain MR or CT, chest and abdominopelvic CT.

When a subcutaneous recurrence is clinically suspected, we perform CT or MR to assess the local involvement.

Squamous cell carcinoma

Before surgery, a chest radiography is still of value in every case. In locally advanced stages, we perform CT for the evaluation of bone involvement. When skeletal and/or hepatic metastases are clinically suspected, bone scintigraphy and/or US of the liver are undertaken.

During the follow up, according to the results of the clinical examination, we perform CT when local recurrence is suspected.

Basal cell carcinoma

Imaging techniques have little role to play in BCC. Before surgery, and only in advanced cases, we perform bone radiography and/or CT for the evaluation of the local skeletal involvement or other local involvement.

References

1. Musumeci R, Monica GL, Orefice S, Lymphographic evaluation of 250 patients with malignant melanoma, *Cancer* (1976) **38**:1568–73.
2. Abdi EA, Terry T, Lymphography and computed tomography in lymph node metastases from malignant melanoma, *Acta Radiol* (1988) **29**:391–4.
3. Fornage BD, Deshayes JL, Ultrasound of normal skin, *J Clin Ultrasound* (1986) **14**:619–22.
4. Kraus W, Schramm P, Hoede N, First experiences with a high-resolution ultrasonic scanner in the diagnosis of malignant melanomas, *Arch Dermatol Res* (1983) **275**:235–8.
5. Shafir R, Itzchak Y, Heyman Z et al, Preoperative ultrasonic measurements of the thickness of cutaneous malignant melanoma, *J Ultrasound Med* (1984) **3**:205–8.
6. Fon GT, Wong WS, Gold RH et al, Skeletal metastases of melanoma: radiographic, scintigraphic and clinical review, *AJR* (1981) **137**:103–8.
7. Lock-Anderson J, Rossing N, Drzewiecki KT, Preoperative cutaneous lymphoscintigraphy in malignant melanoma, *Cancer* (1989) **63**:77–82.
8. Atlas SW, Grossman RI, Gomori JM et al, MR Imaging of intracranial metastatic melanoma, *J Comput Assist Tomogr* (1987) **11**:577–82.
9. Greene MH, Clark WH Jr, Tucker MA et al, Acquired precursor of cutaneous malignant melanoma, *N Engl J Med* (1985) **312**:91–7.
10. Davis NC, Malignant melanoma. In: Emmett AJJ, O'Rourke MGE, eds, *Malignant skin tumors* (Churchill Livingstone: New York 1982).
11. Baker GS, Kernohan JW, Kiefer EJ, Metastatic tumors of the brain, *Surg Clin Am* (1951) **31**:1143–5.
12. Gottlieb JA, Frei E, Luce JK, An evaluation of the management of patients with cerebral metastases from malignant melanoma, *Cancer* (1972) **29**:701–5.
13. Harrist TJ, Day CL Jr, Malignant melanoma: prognostic factors. In: Nathanson L, ed, *Basic and clinical aspects of malignant melanoma* (Martinus Nijhoff: Boston 1987).
14. Breslow A, Thickness, cross-sectional areas, and depth of invasion in the prognosis of cutaneous melanoma, *Ann Surg* (1970) **172**:902–8.
15. Clark, WH, From L, Bernardino EA, The histogenesis and histologic behavior of primary human malignant melanoma of the skin, *Cancer Res* (1969) **29**:705–15.
16. Day CL, Lew RA, Mihm MC Jr, The natural break points for primary tumor thickness in clinical stage I melanoma, *N Engl J Med* (1981) **305**:1155.
17. Bittoun J, Saint-Jalmes H, Querleux BG et al, In vivo high-resolution MR imaging of the skin in a whole-body system at 1.5 T, *Radiology* (1990) **176**:457–60.
18. Schwaighofer BW, Fruehwald FXJ, Pohl-Markl H et al, MRI evaluation of pigmented skin tumors, *Invest Radiol* (1989) **24**:289–93.
19. Meyer JE, Radiographic evaluation of metastatic melanoma, *Cancer* (1978) **42**:127–32.

20. Lodwick GS, Reactive response to local injury in bone, *Radiol Clin Am* (1964) **2**:209–19.
21. Reintgen DS, Thompson W, Garbut J, Radiologic, endoscopic and surgical considerations of melanoma metastatic to the gastro-intestinal tract, *Surgery* (1984) **95**:635–9.
22. Kostrubiak I, Whitley NO, Aisner J et al, The use of computed body tomography in malignant melanoma, *JAMA* (1988) **259**:2896–7.
23. Fishman EK, Kuhlman JE, Schuchter LM et al, CT of malignant melanoma in the chest, abdomen and musculoskeletal system, *Radiographics* (1990) **10**:603–20.
24. Ginaldi S, Wallace S, Shalen P et al, Cranial computed tomography of malignant melanoma, *AJR* (1981) **136**:145–9.
25. Gordon D, Silverstone H, Worldwide epidemiology of premalignant and malignant cutaneous lesions. In: Andrade R, Gumport S, Popkin G, Rees T, eds, *Cancer of the skin* (WB Saunders: Philadelphia 1976).
26. Banerjee TK, Gottschalk PG, Unusual manifestations of multiple cranial nerve palsies and mandibular metastasis in a patient with squamous cell carcinoma of the lip, *Cancer* (1984) **53**:346–8.
27. Lang H, Kendrich J, Surgical management of advanced scalp cancer, *Head Neck Surg* (1983) **5**:299–305.
28. Domarus H, Stevens PJ, Metastatic basal cell carcinoma: report of five cases and review of 170 cases in the literature, *J Am Acad Dermatol* (1984) **10**:1043–60.
29. Curson C, Weedon D, Spontaneous regression in basal cell carcinomas, *J Cutan Pathol* (1979) **6**: 432.
30. Webb WR, Gamsu G, Thoracic metastasis in malignant melanoma: a radiographic survey of 65 patients, *Chest* (1977) **71**:176–81.

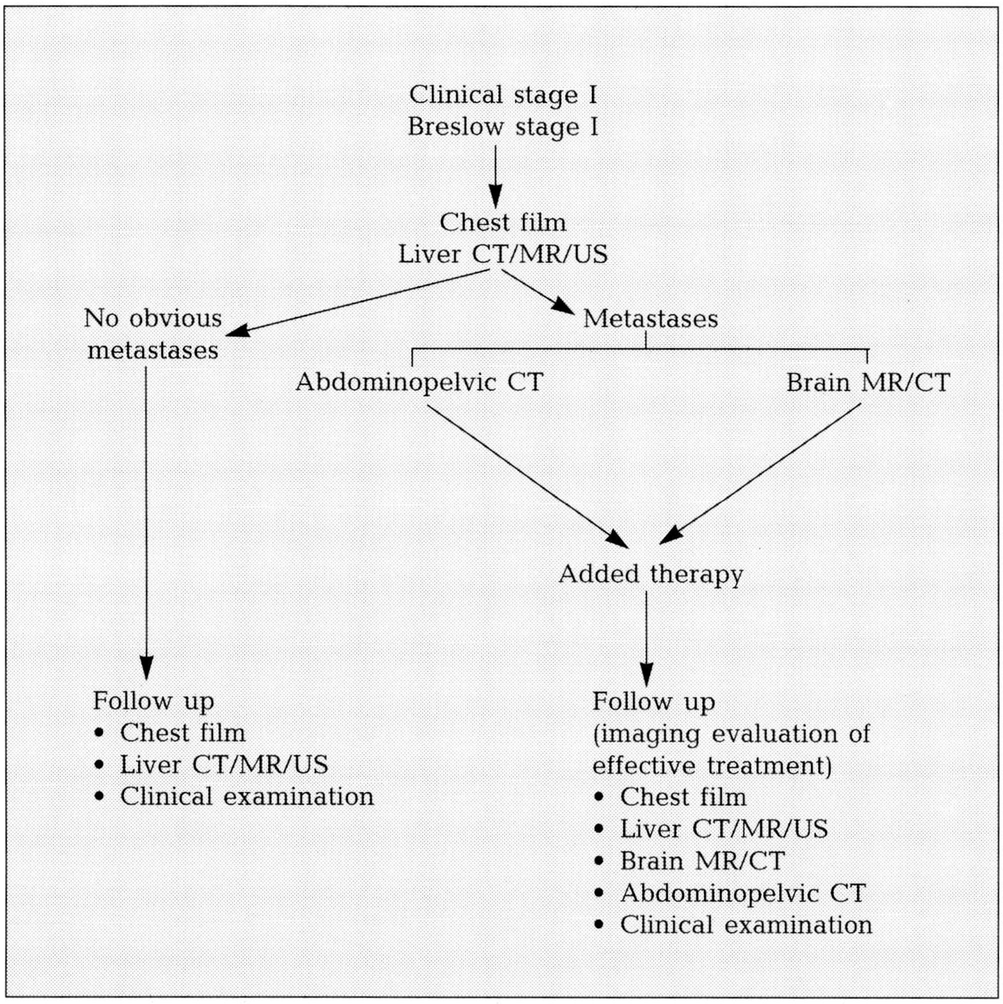

Diagram 20.1

Imaging strategies for minimal stage malignant melanoma.

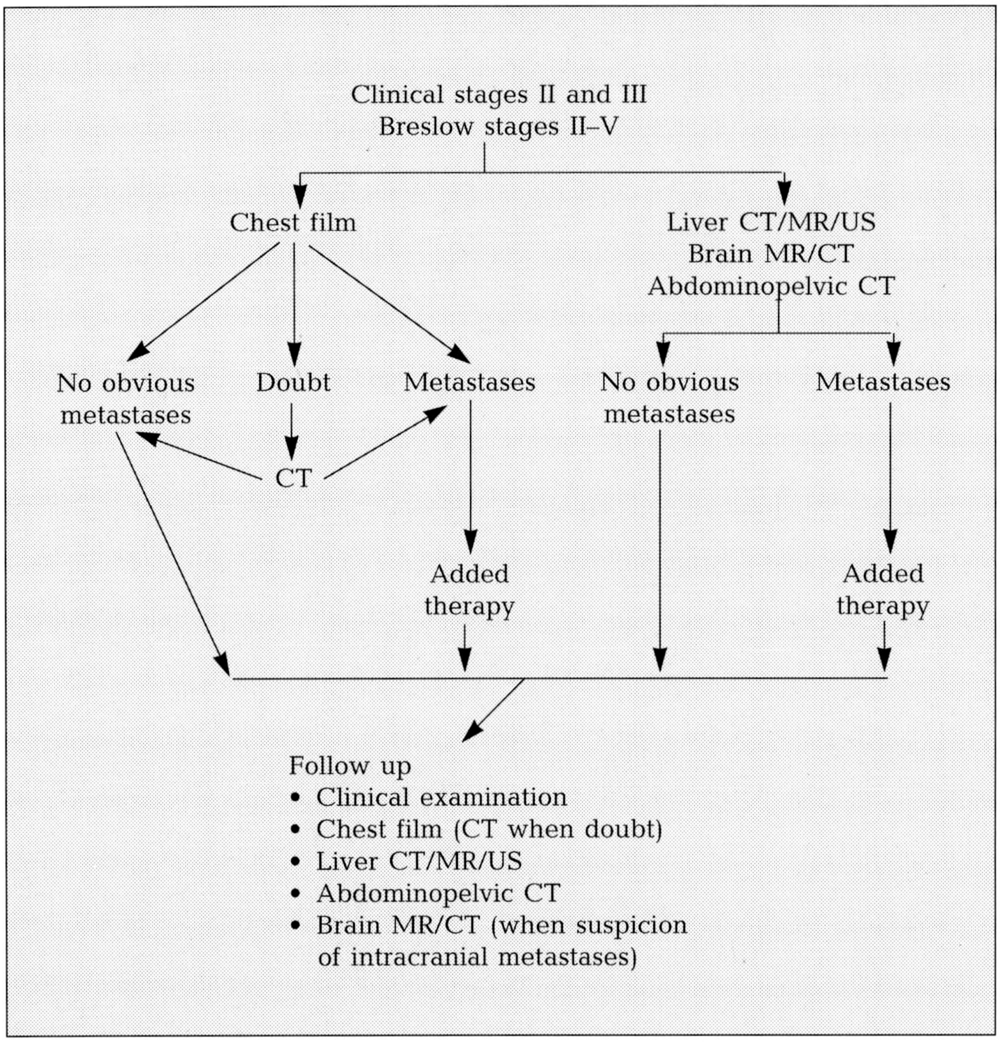

Diagram 20.2

Imaging strategies for advanced stage malignant melanoma.

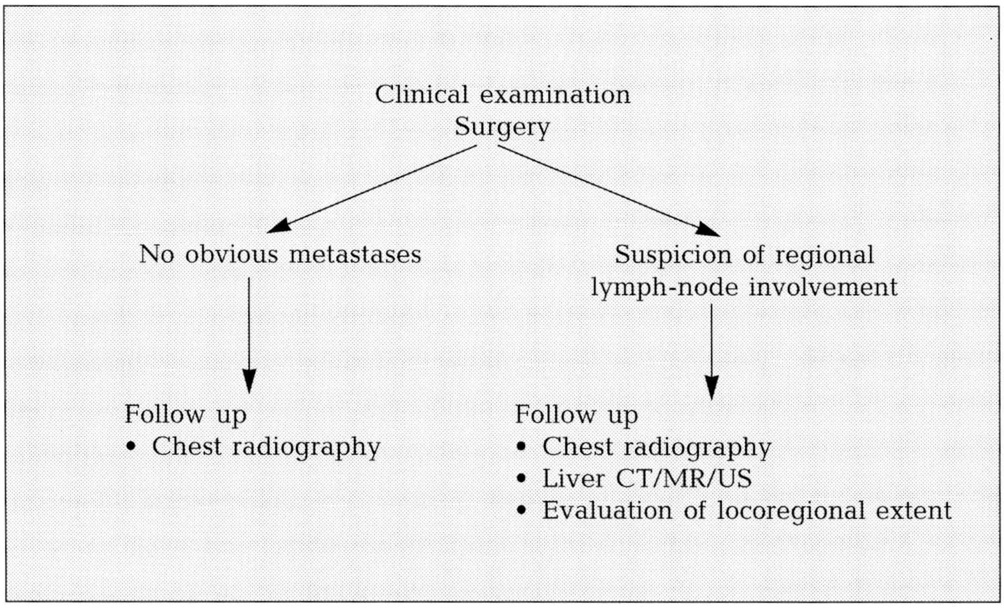

Diagram 20.3

Imaging strategy in squamous-cell carcinoma.

21

Lymphomas

Jean Noel Bruneton, Gérard Socie and Michel Y Mourou

Introduction

There have been few examples in oncology of such considerable progress in the past decades as has been made in the case of lymphomas. This has resulted from a better understanding of physio-pathogenesis, clinical management and modes of extension, as well as a multidisciplinary approach. The introduction of CT considerably modified the role of imaging, which is one of the cornerstones and a determining factor in the assessment of extensions, the estimation of the response to treatment and follow up. It also allows early detection of relapses or complications resulting from therapy.

Certain general characteristics of imaging should be emphasized:

- The optimum frequency of check ups in the follow up of malignant non-Hodgkin's lymphomas remains difficult to determine but seems to depend mainly on the histologic type.
- The choice of target zones for follow up using imaging techniques also depends on the type of lymphoma.
- Follow up using various imaging modalities is indispensable, firstly to evaluate the efficiency of treatment and secondly to diagnose relapses as soon as possible.[1]

It is imperative to differentiate between Hodgkin's disease and non-Hodgkin's lymphomas. They present certain differences, such as:

- Hodgkin's disease affects the mediastinal lymph nodes more frequently that non-Hodgkin's lymphomas (65% compared with 25%), but involvement of the mesenteric lymph nodes (51% compared with 4%) and bone marrow infiltration (20% compared with 3%) are more frequent in cases of non-Hodgkin's lymphomas.[2]
- Malignant non-Hodgkin's lymphomas are generally diagnosed at a more advanced stage, 64.7% already being stage III and IV.[3,4]

Finally, malignant non-Hodgkin's lymphomas correspond to diseases and different clinical patterns. Therefore a certain number of authors do not advocate a global approach, as far as imaging techniques are concerned.[2,5] Clinical manifestations and localizations of lymphomatous non-Hodgkin involvement depend mainly on histologic findings:

- Bone marrow involvement is frequent in low-grade lymphomas.[6]
- Hepatic involvement is observed in 15–20% of cases, according to the histologic type.[7]
- Mesenteric adenopathies are more frequent in malignant lymphomas of the follicular type than in diffuse forms.[5]

General characteristics of lymphomas

Hodgkin's disease

During the last few years, different therapeutic trials have been carried out to try to evaluate the risks and advantages of two fundamental types of treatment, chemotherapy and radiotherapy. The classification of Hodgkin's disease has not been greatly modified over the past few years (Table 21.1). However, an international committee recently brought up to date the Ann Arbor classification of extension (essentially because of recent progress in new imaging techniques).[8]

Exploratory laparotomy remains controversial in the assessment of extensions. Although it is widely used in the USA, it has more or less been abandoned in Europe. Diagnosis of splenic involvement depends on it. The therapeutic strategy of localized stages[9] has also been the object of different therapeutic trials comparing radiotherapy with a combination of chemo- and radiotherapy.

Favorable prognosis in Hodgkin's disease makes the long-term consequences of therapy even more important than usual.[10,12] Efforts are being made to reduce acute morbidity due to treatment. The major iatrogenic problem remains the increased incidence of malignant hemopathy and solid tumors.

The relative risk of acute leukemia in patients receiving chemotherapy of the MOPP type (mustine, oncovine, procarbozine and prednisone) seems to be increased a hundred-fold compared with the normal population. Moreover, this risk depends on, amongst other things, the age of the patient at the time of diagnosis. Non-Hodgkin's lymphomas have been observed following radiotherapy alone and radiotherapy in association with adjuvant chemotherapy. They are of intermediate

Table 21.1 Ann Arbor classification of Hodgkin's disease: stages and subclassification.

Stage I	Involvement of a single lymph node region or of a single extralymphatic organ or site
Stage II	Involvement of two or more lymph node regions on the same side of the diaphragm, or localized involvement of an extralymphatic organ or site and one or more lymph node regions on the same side of the diaphragm. Optionally, the number of node regions involved is indicated by a subscript
Stage III	Involvement of lymph-node regions on both sides of the diaphragm. This may or may not be accompanied by localized involvement of an extralymphatic organ or site, involvement of the spleen, or both
Stage III 1	Abdominal disease limited to spleen, splenic, celiac or portal nodes
Stage III 2	Abdominal disease involving para-aortic, iliac, or inguinal nodes
Stage IV	Diffuse or disseminated involvement of one or more extralymphatic organs or tissues, with or without associated lymph-node involvement. Extralymphatic organs are defined as those other than lymph nodes, spleen, thymus, Waldeyer's ring, appendix and Peyer's patches. Liver or bone marrow involvement always indicates stage IV disease
AB Subclassification	Unexplained fever with oral temperature over 38°C Night sweats Unexplained weight loss of 10% or more of body weight in the 6 months before admission 'A' refers to patients without, 'B' to patients with, these general symptoms

or high grades, perhaps related to immunosuppression inherent in the disease and aggravated by treatment. The relative risk of solid tumors after radiotherapy and/or chemotherapy is about 2; cancer of the lungs, stomach, breast, melanomas and tumors of the soft tissues or of the bone can occur, some of these (lungs, stomach, bone and soft tissues) appearing only in the the radiation field.[12] Other, non-tumor complications following radiotherapy have been observed, such as sterility, radiation-induced pneumonia, which has become rarer nowadays because of the improvement in radiotherapy techniques, and growth problems in children.[13]

Therapeutic strategies have been modified in order to reduce these complications: new associations of non-leukemogenic chemotherapy (ABVD – adriamycin, bleomycin, vinblastine and dacacarbazine), reduction in the total dose of MOPP, reduction in the area irradiated, use of a single type of treatment whenever possible and combined treatment to reduce the toxicity of chemo- and radiotherapy.

Non-Hodgkin's lymphomas

Progress has recently been made in histologic classification, prognostic factors and treatment.

Histologic classification[14 15]

Several histologic classifications were used up to the beginning of the 1980s, but the absence of any concordance between the different methods made any comparison of studies emanating from different centers extremely difficult. A new classification was therefore elaborated under the auspices of the the National Cancer Institute[16] (Tables 21.2 and 21.3). It differentiates between three groups of malignant non-Hodgkin's lymphomas: of a low degree of malignancy, of intermediate malignancy or of high malignancy. There is correspondance between this classification and that of Kiel–Lennert, which is widely used in Europe

Table 21.2 Working formulation of non-Hodgkin's lymphomas for clinical use.

Histological type	*Frequency (%)*	*Age (years)*	*Complete response rate (%)*	*5-year survival (%)*
Low grade				
Mixed cell, follicular	8.8	56	65	50
Small cleaved cell, follicular	25.5	54	73	70
Small lymphocytic	4.0	61	61	59
Intermediate grade				
Large cell, diffuse	22.4	57	59	35
Mixed cell, diffuse	7.6	58	69	38
Small cleaved cell, diffuse	7.8	58	56	33
Large cell, follicular	4.3	55	61	45
High grade				
Small non-cleaved cell	5.7	30	48	23
Lymphoblastic	4.8	17	69	26
Large cell, immunoblastic	9.0	51	53	32

Table 21.3 Working formulation of non-Hodgkin's lymphomas for clinical use.

Histologic type	*Stage I (%)*	*Stage II (%)*	*Stages III and IV (%)*	*Involvement of extranodal sites (%)*
Low grade				
Mixed cell, follicular	15	12	74	S,L,M (30)
Small cleaved cell, follicular	8	10	82	S,L,M (51)
Small lymphocytic	3	8	89	S,L,M (71)
Intermediate grade				
Large cell, diffuse	16	30	54	S,L,W,GI, Lung, M (10)
Mixed cell, diffuse	19	26	55	S,L,W,GI, Bone, M (14)
Small cleaved cell, diffuse	9	19	72	S,L,W,GI, Skin, M (32)
Large cell, follicular	15	12	73	S,L,W,GI,M (34)
High grade				
Small non-cleaved cell	13	21	66	GI, Lung, M (14)
Lymphoblastic	7	20	73	L,S, Lung, Skin, M (50)
Large cell, immunoblastic	23	29	48	L,S,W,GI,M (12)

Abbreviations: S, spleen; L, liver; M, bone marrow; W, Waldeyer's ring; GI, gastrointestinal tract.

(Table 21.4). However, the latter classification does not use immunological criteria such as the use of monoclonal antibodies, which identify lymphomas developed at the expense of B or T lymphoid chains, or the distinction of new entities like the Ki1 lymphoma.

Molecular biology makes a useful contribution to a better understanding of the physiopathogenesis of lymphomas (specific rearrangement of certain genes) and allows the detection of residual tumor cells that escape detection by other methods. However, highly specialized techniques are involved and so this approach is not routinely employed.

Assessment of extensions

An accurate assessment of extensions of lymphomatous disease is mainly based on Ann Arbor classification, which was elaborated for Hodgkin's disease, but is a little less exact for malignant non-Hodgkin's lymphomas; it is nevertheless extremely useful, as the stage of extension is always a decisive prognostic factor.

Prognostic factors

In addition to including the size of the tumor and biological data such as lactate dehydrogenase levels, the value of the working formulation lies in the essential prognostic role of the histopathological diagnosis.

Low-grade malignant lymphomas have a complete remission rate approaching 60%, and a 5-year survival rate of between 50 and 70%. Relapses are frequent, usually occurring after 2 or 3 years. The tumor usually remains chemosensitive and a second complete remission can be expected,

Table 21.4 Correspondence between the working formulation (Ann Arbor classification) and the Kiel–Lennert classification.

Working formulation	*Kiel–Lennert*
Low grade	
Small lymphocytic	Chronic lymphoctyic leukemia
	Lymphocytic
	Lymphoplasmocytoid
Small cleaved cell, follicular	Centroblastic–centrocytic, small cell (follicular)
Mixed cell, follicular	
Intermediate grade	
Large cell, diffuse	Centroblastic–centrocytic, large cell (diffuse)
	Centrocytic, large cell
	Centroblastic
Mixed cell, diffuse	Centroblastic–centrocytic, small cell (diffuse)
	Lymphoplasmocytic
Small cleaved cell, diffuse	Centrocytic, small cell
Large cell, follicular	Centroblastic–centrocytic, large cell (follicular)
High grade	
Small non-cleaved cell	Lymphoblastic (Burkitt's type)
	Other lymphoblastic B
Lymphoblastic	Lymphoblastic, convoluted cell type
Large cell, immunoblastic	Immunoblastic
Miscellaneous	
Composite	
Mycosis fungoides	Mycosis fungoides
Histiocytic	
Extramedullary plasmocytoma	Plasmocytic
Unclassifiable	

but only during a limited time. The main factors of unfavorable prognosis in this type of lymphoma are: the size of the tumor, especially bulky subdiaphragmatic nodal masses, general signs and the stage of extension. More than 60% of cases are stage IV, and, in almost 50%, bone marrow is invaded at the time of diagnosis. Stage I cases represents less than 10% of all cases.[16,17] In these, evolution is slow and treatment is often not aggressive; imaging assessment is infrequent and carried out on request.

Lymphomas with intermediate and high-grade malignancy are generally bracketed together as aggressive lymphomas.[3,18] It is in this category that therapeutic progress has been the most spectacular: the frequency of relapses is less considerable than in the 1970s, and the incidence of complete remission is 75–90%; relapses occur early on, usually in the 2 years following the completion of treatment and 3-year survival is almost 50%. However, the intensification of chemotherapy is the cause of increased iatrogenic complications, especially infections. Maximum aggressiveness is, therefore, only legitimate in forms with extremely poor prognosis.

The initial unfavorable elements in the assessment of a clinical extension are the invasion of the bone marrow, with extranodular involvement causing most concern, the multiplication of extra-lymphatic involvement and bulky tumor masses. Moreover, deterioration in general health is also associated with a lower rate of complete remission. Finally, two markers correlate with a reduction in the remission rate and 3-year survival: an increase in dehydrogenase lactates and, in the experience of certain authors, a reduction in albumin.[3] In these forms, follow up with imaging procedures should be strict during the first 2 years.

Evolution of treatment

In the case of lymphomas of low-grade malignancy, the most common attitude is to use only slightly aggressive treatment, which can vary from no treatment at all with regular check ups to polychemotherapy, according to the risk factor involved. In the case of aggressive lymphomas, recent progress seems to result mainly from an increase in doses of chemotherapy. The use of hematopoietic growth factors is also a new therapeutic possibility.

Imaging techniques

A number of techniques are available. Conventional techniques include chest radiography, lymphography and barium studies. More recently developed techniques are CT, ultrasonography, gallium scan and MR.

Chest radiographs

Hodgkin's disease

Sixty-seven per cent of patients with Hodgkin's disease present with intrathoracic involvement during assessment, and 90% of nodular lesions are situated in the upper mediastinum (anterior mediastinum, paratracheal and/or suprabronchial lymph nodes). The usual pattern is an anterosuperior mediastinal mass. On lateral-view films, the retrosternal space is filled in; occasionally margins are vertical, leading to a chimney-shaped view. An irregular line can be seen next to the azygous line; to the left, the supra-aortic region may appear enlarged, with the aortic-pulmonary window blocked. Lymph nodes situated below the carina and hilar nodes are often difficult to distinguish on standard radiographs.

The pattern observed in case of relapse is the same as that initially observed; relapses are considered by some to be more frequent in non-irradiated areas,[19] but by others to be more frequent in areas which had already been invaded,[21] and only in non-treated areas in 8% of relapses. During the evolution of residual masses, calcifications and conditions resulting from radiotherapy can be observed.

Pulmonary lesions are rare at the time of assessment (11.6%)[21] and are rarely solitary; in over half the cases, they are bilateral either due to bronchiovascular infiltration, subpleural diffusion or massive pulmonary infiltration.[22] Thus, different lesions can be seen: small or large nodules with well- or poorly-defined borders, cavitation with irregular margins and a fluid level, thickening of the bronchial walls, more or less coalescent infiltrates, respiratory difficulties secondary to endobronchial infiltration and causing atelectasis, or rare miliary lesions. Pleural involvement usually implies unfavorable prognosis, but it is often difficult to differentiate between pleural tumoral effusion and a mechanical obstruction due to abnormal lymphatic drainage.[23]

Non-Hodgkin's lymphomas

Patterns of intrathoracic involvement are the same as for Hodgkin's disease but the frequency differs, being less than 22% of cases.[24,25] The incidence of mediastinal involvement with non-Hodgkin's lymphomas varies from zero (for the diffuse and well-differentiated lympocytic type) to 35% (for the diffuse and only slightly differentiated lymphocytic type). Massive mediastinal involvement is more often observed in diffuse types with large cells and lymphoblastic types. Pleural involvement is not rare, but its origin is often mechanical, as is pericardial effusion.

Pulmonary paryenchymal involvement is observed in 20% of cases of histiocytic non-Hodgkin's lymphomas;[26] this usually takes the form of nodules of varying sizes, sometimes isolated, with no nodal involvement.[27] Primary pulmonary involvement is rare; the radiological view is that of lung cancer, that is, a badly defined mass, sometimes with a bronchogram; topography is central rather than peripheral, with extra-bronchial, extravascular and extra-alveolar lesions.[28]

Lymphography (Figure 21.1)

Hodgkin's disease

Lymphography allows the examination of the iliac and lumboaortic chains but not of the celiomesenteric sites. Its use depends on the size of lymphatic channels and the experience of the radiologist. Since it is used less and less frequently, there are fewer radiologists capable of using it correctly, except in specialized centers. Its main value is that it can be used on an unprepared abdomen and gives a result identical to that of CT in the diagnosis of lymph-node relapses.[29] Lipiodol slow resorption facilitates the follow up of the retroperitoneum during at least 1 year, but after 2 years only 12% of patients conserve sufficient opacity for this to be of any use.[30] Lymphography is especially useful in the assessment of Hodgkin's disease, as it allows the anatomical study of the distribution of lymph-node involvement and the analysis of each opacified lymph node (diameter, margins and appearance).[31]

The lymphographic patterns of Hodgkin's disease are remarkable because of their considerable heterogeneity. Usually only a fraction of the opacified lymph nodes are involved and radiological patterns can be observed. Initially, involvement includes lacunae which may be more or less regular, a moderate increase in the diameter of the node and an absence of stasis. This pattern is usually observed with different types of inflammation and is therefore not specific. However, the discovery of a normal-sized lymph node with a well-defined lacuna should lead to the analysis of earlier films in search of abnormalities in circulation, which can be observed in about 50% of cases. Diagnosis is easier in diffuse forms, in which abnormalities result from stasis, lymph-node enlargement and large irregular lacunae. In some serious lesions, lymph nodes may not be opacified, which can lead to underestimation of the size of the tumor.

A second series of lymphograms is not usually carried out, as relapses often occur in sites that are not opacified in the examination; CT is much more useful for follow up.

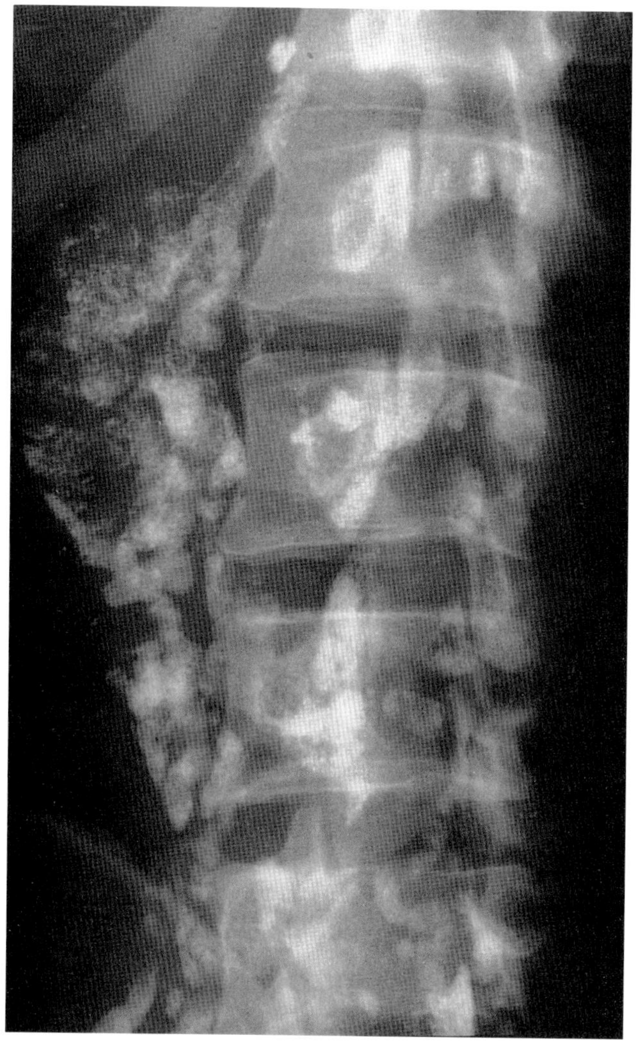

Figure 21.1

High retroperitoneal lymph-node localization of a non-Hodgkin's lymphoma.

The rare false negatives are due to microscopic lesions. Etiological diagnosis remains extremely difficult. Diffuse enlargement of lymph nodes can be observed in immunological deficiency, granulomatous disease or infection. Moreover, identical metastatic lacunae are always a possibility.

Despite its diagnostic limitations, lymphography remains an excellent technique for the assessment of extensions in Hodgkin's disease, as its overall sensitivity is between 69 and 97%.[32–34]

Non-Hodgkin's lymphomas

Lymphography has been replaced by CT because frequent involvement of the mesenteric lymph nodes is not shown by the former and pathological lymph nodes are almost always hypertrophied.

Barium studies

Barium studies are not necessary for assessment, as symptomatic lesions are exceptional.[35] However, clinical presentations do necessitate an investigation of the digestive tract; increasingly this is carried out by endoscopy and CT, with digestive opacification.

Primary involvement in Hodgkin's disease is unusual and only secondary presentations are usually observed, mainly in the stomach. In non-Hodgkin's lymphoma, a primary presentation affecting the digestive tract is not unusual in the stomach or small intestine, and can take multiple presentations.[36]

There is no fibroblastic stroma reaction with non-Hodgkin's lymphomas, as opposed to Hodgkin's disease. Thus lymphomatous non-Hodgkin's lesions are often bulky. These bulky lesions often have quite discrete clinical symptoms and stenosing forms are rare (Figure 21.2).

With Hodgkin's disease, gastric involvement, as well as involvement of the small intestine, are the most common localizations and their appearance is comparable with that of carcinomas.

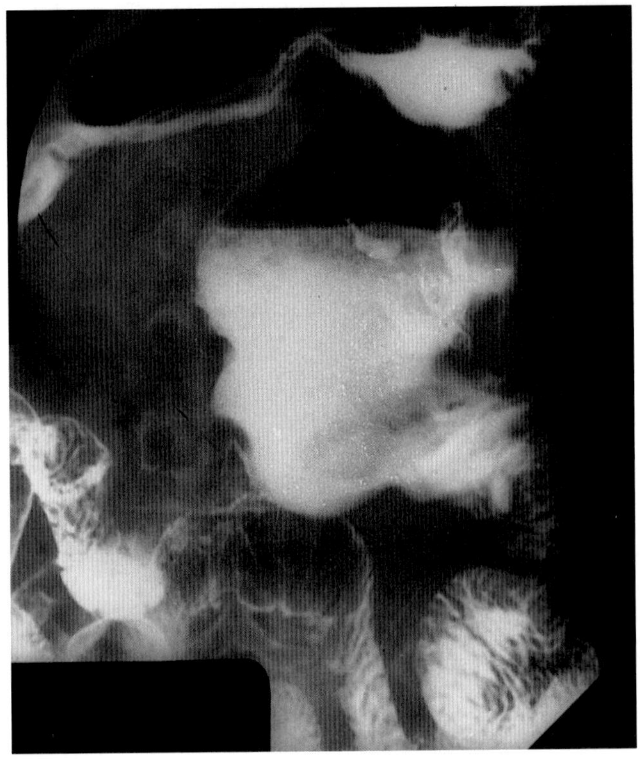

Figure 21.2

Pseudoaneurysmal form of a jejunal non-Hodgkin's lymphoma.

Other conventional techniques

Apart from clinical urological symptoms which necessitate urological investigation, renal and non-renal urological lesions are usually observed with abdominal ultrasound or CT.[37] In cases of urethral involvement, with no signs from the kidneys, CT is insufficient and antero- or retrograde opacification of the urethra may be necessary.

Bone involvement is not frequent and, as in the digestive tract, it is the presence of clinical signs which leads to skeletal investigation. Bone scintigraphy using technetium is not routinely used, as it does not usually modify treatment; it can be useful in cases of primary or secondary lesions which have already been observed and treated.[38]

Computed tomography (Figures 21.3–21.18)

This technique has completely modified the imaging of lymphomas. In general, nodal hypertrophy shows up well, which means that CT is very useful for cases of non-Hodgkin's lymphoma. However, this is not the case for Hodgkin's disease, where nodal hypertrophy is not the most common form. Moreover, the frequency of extranodal site involvement (spleen, liver, kidneys, digestive tract) leads to its use in the assessment and follow up of non-Hodgkin's lymphomas.

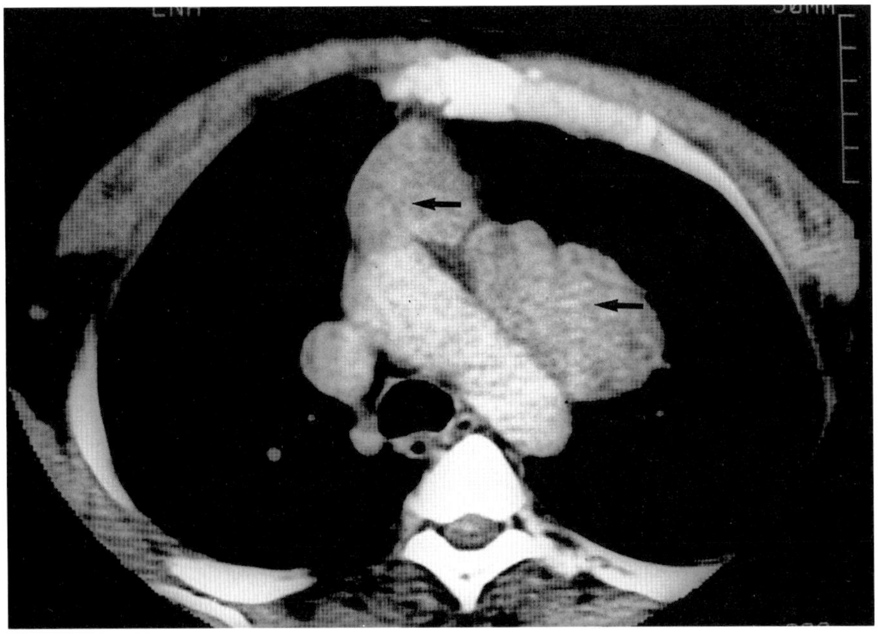

Figure 21.3

Thoracic lymph-node localization of a non-Hodgkin's lymphoma (arrows).

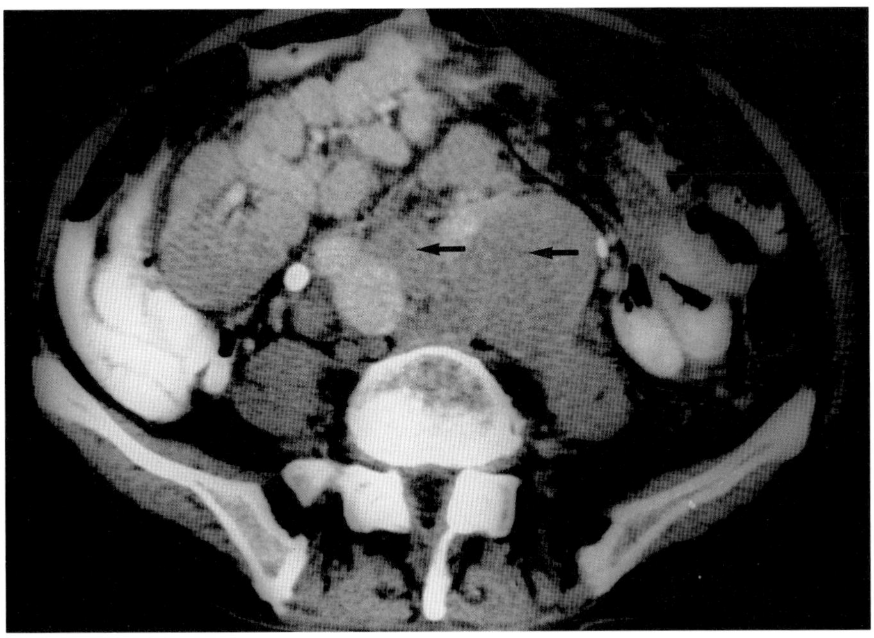

Figure 21.4

Intra- and retroperitonal lymph-node localization of a non-Hodgkin's lymphoma (arrows).

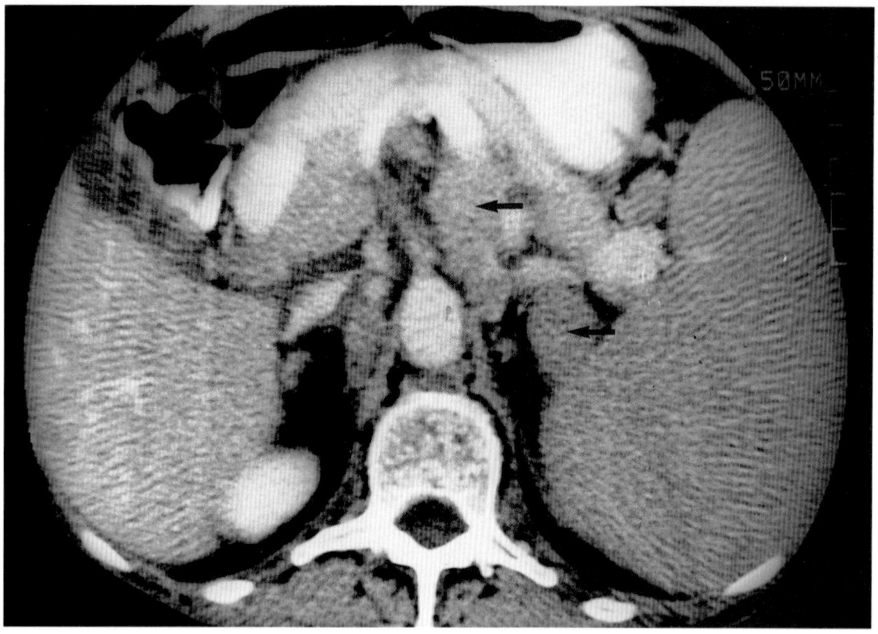

Figure 21.5

Retroperitoneal and splenic hilar adenopathies with splenomegaly in non-Hodgkin's lymphoma (arrows).

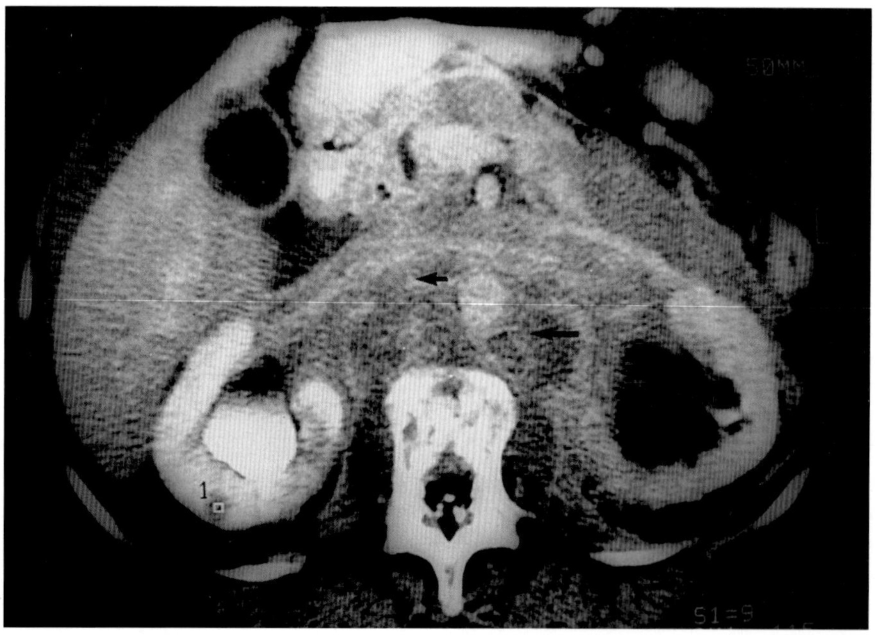

Figure 21.6

Widespread lymphomatous non-Hodgkin's infiltration of the retroperitoneum (arrows), causing bilateral urinary stasis, associated with right renal localization (115 HU in the white square marked at 1).

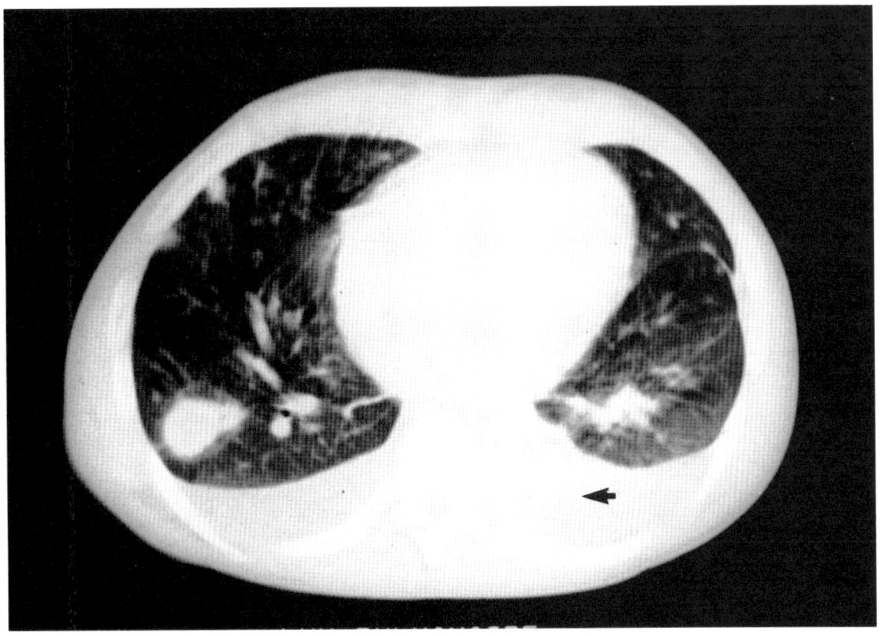

Figure 21.7

Pulmonary non-Hodgkin's lymphoma (arrows) with bilateral pleural effusion (arrow).

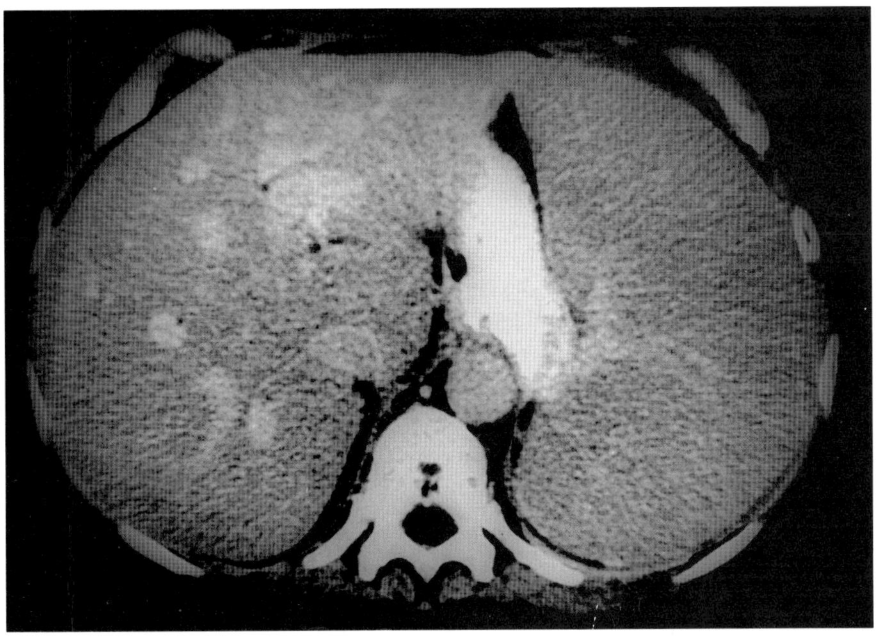

Figure 21.8

Splenomegaly with Hodgkin's disease.

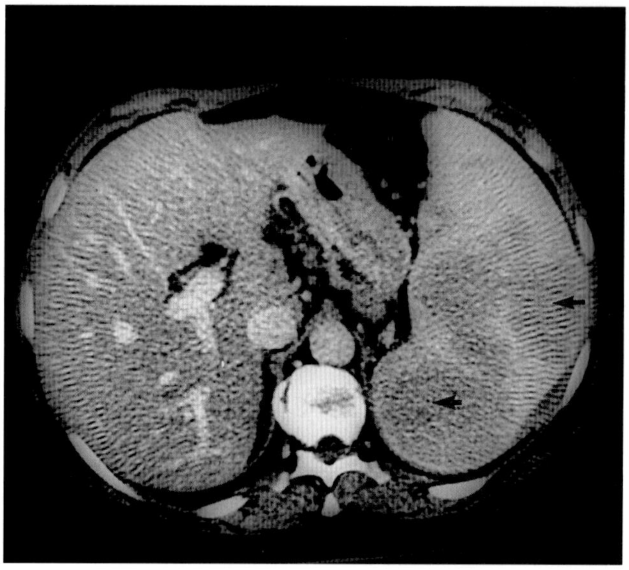

Figure 21.9

Intrasplenic nodular localization (arrows) with non-Hodgkin's lymphoma.

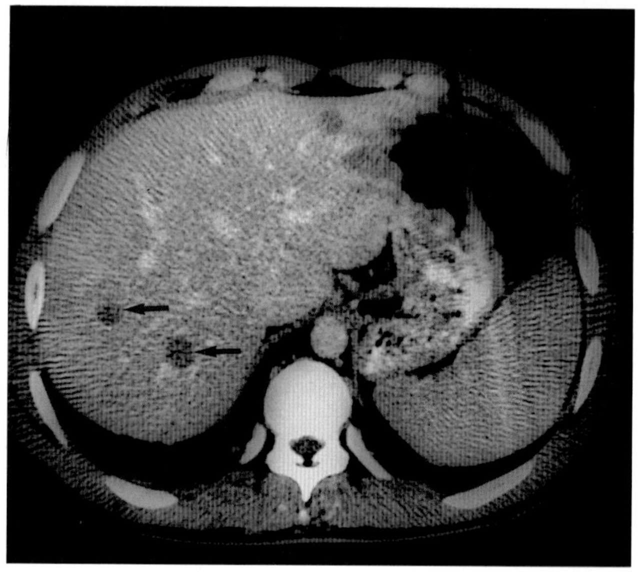

Figure 21.10

Intrahepatic nodular localization (arrows) with non-Hodgkin's lymphoma.

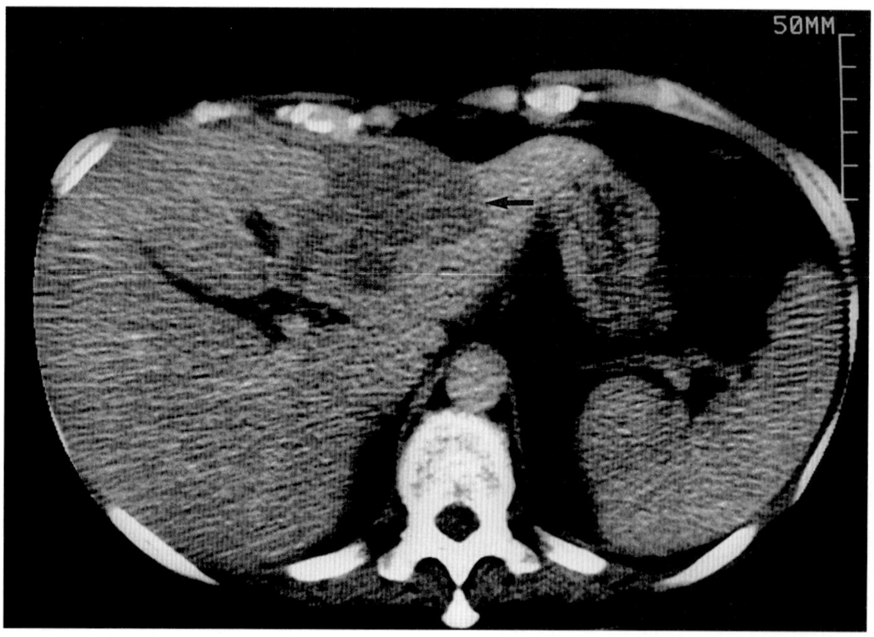

Figure 21.11

Lymphomatous non-Hodgkin's infiltration of the left liver (arrow).

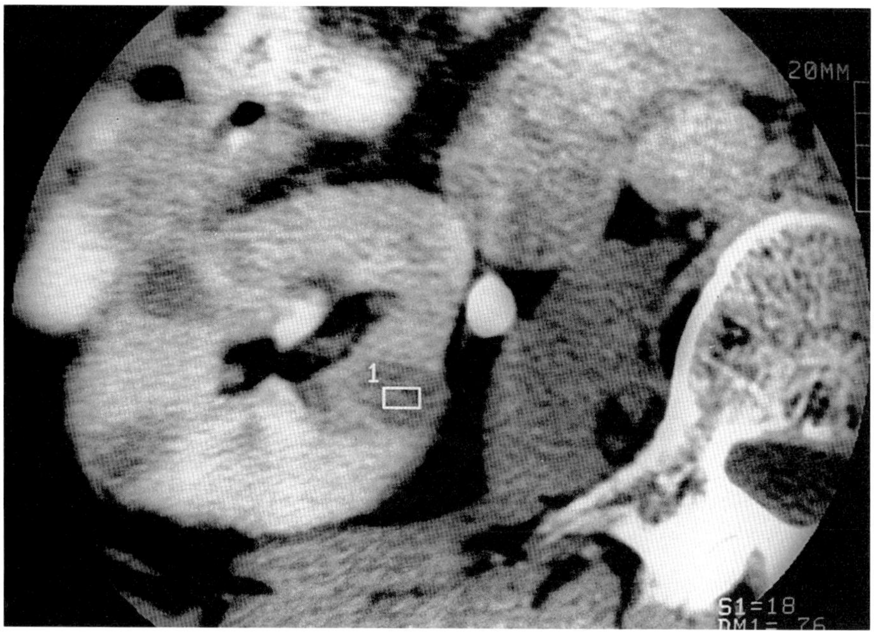

Figure 21.12

Lymphomatous nodular localization of the right kidney (76 HU in the white rectangle).

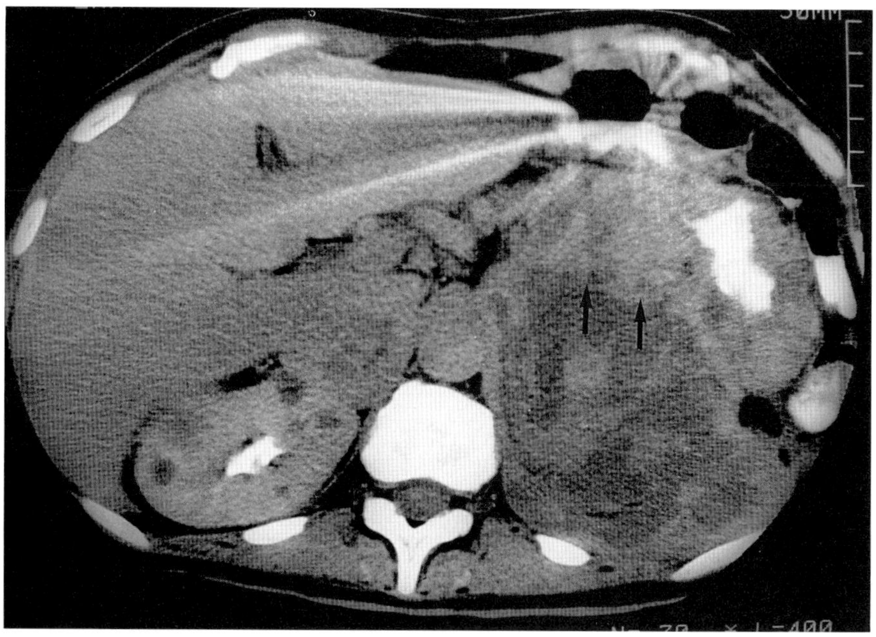

Figure 21.13

Widespread tumoral infiltration of the left kidney with anterior extension towards the stomach (arrows). Right renal nodular localization.

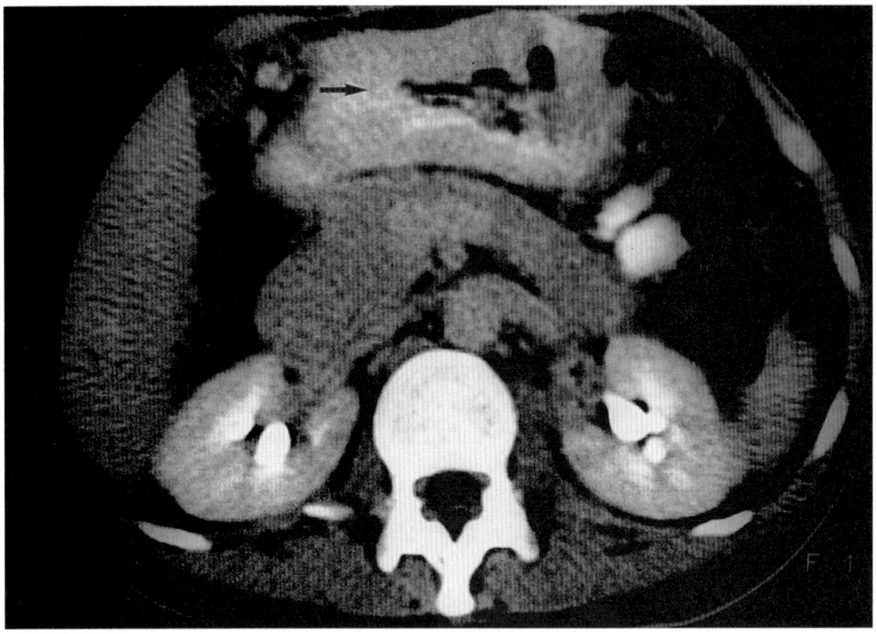

Figure 21.14

Parietal involvement of the gastric ansa (arrow) with non-Hodgkin's lymphoma.

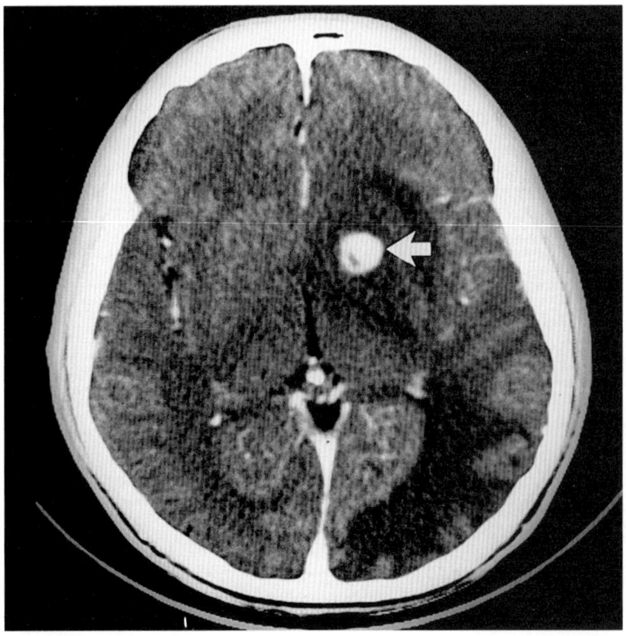

Figure 21.15

Intracerebral localization of a non-Hodgkin's lymphoma: hyperdense mass (arrow) with edema.

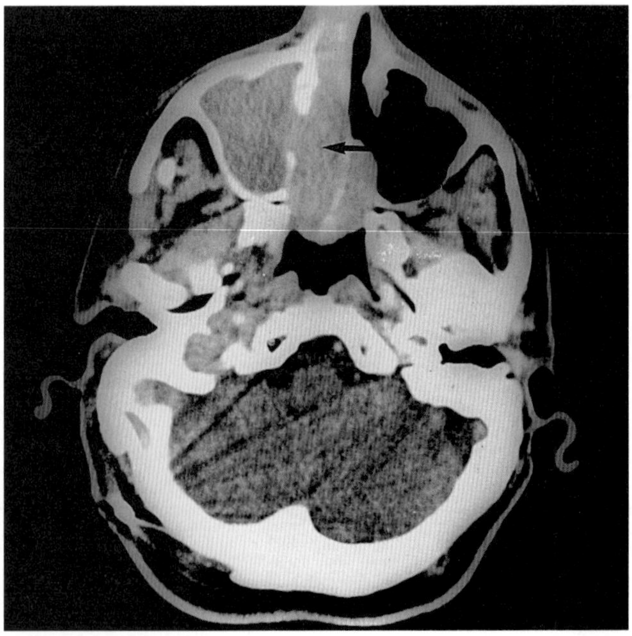

Figure 21.16

Maxillofacial localization of a non-Hodgkin's lymphoma. Recurrence after surgery (arrow).

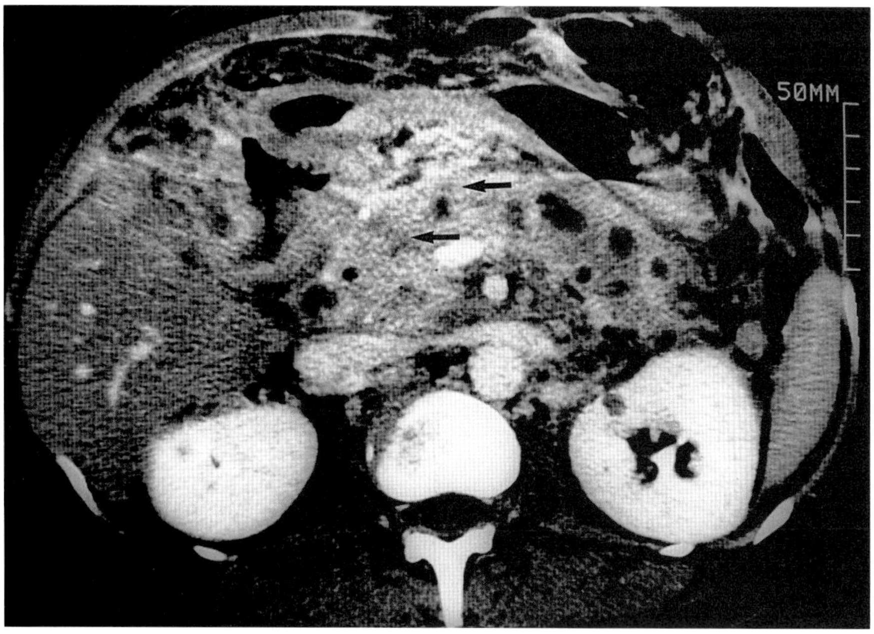

Figure 21.17

Lymphomatous non-Hodgkin's infiltration of the pancreas. Heterogeneous mass (arrows).

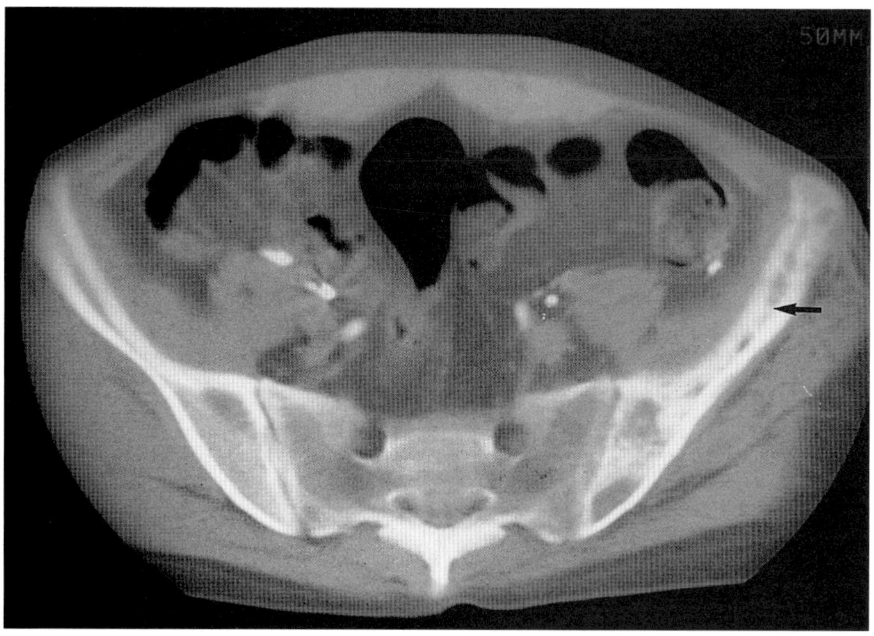

Figure 21.18

Left iliac localization with non-Hodgkin's lymphoma (arrow).

If one considers as suspect lymphomatous thoracic sites all node formations of more than 1 cm in a patient presenting with lymphoma, CT has a sensitivity of 95%, compared with 50% for standard radiographs.[39]

An isolated abdominal lymph node with a transverse diameter of more than 1.5 cm can be considered lymphomatous; whereas multiple involvement, with nodes of 1.0–1.5 cm, is also suspected of being lymphomatous. As with ultrasonography, only volumetric data can be used in the diagnosis of lymphomatous lymph nodes if there are no signs of benign reactional hyperplasia or residual nodal hypertrophy following infection. In spite of these reservations, CT can provide useful information in comparison with standard films. Thus in Hodgkin's disease of the thorax,[40] CT prompts modification of treatment in 9.4% of cases, which justifies its systematic use in the pretherapeutic examination. The frequency with which treatment is changed after examination with CT is between 6.5 and 62.5%, according to the stage and treatment plans.[41] Subcarinal and internal mammary adenopathies are mainly visible on CT but not on standard chest films. Pleural or anterior mediastinal involvement is similarly more visible on CT. Also, CT is more efficient for recognizing relapses, and the number of indeterminate cases in which there is doubt between sequela and relapses is smaller than with standard radiographs.

A modification to the treatment of thoracic non-Hodgkin's lymphoma is observed in almost 25% of cases.[43] In a third of cases in CT contributes information on nodal involvement in the subdiaphragmatic area complementary to that provided by lymphography.[5]

In addition to its contribution to lymph-node pathology, CT also contributes useful information on extranodal involvement. Primary involvement is, however, less frequent than secondary forms. Primary splenic involvement occurs in 1% of all lymphomas, whereas secondary involvement is observed in 37–39% of Hodgkin's disease and 32.8% of non-Hodgkin's lymphomas cases.[44]

Macroscopic involvement usually takes the form of a homogeneous or miliary lesion[1] (73% of cases), whereas multiple masses are rather rare (27%). Estimation of the volume of the spleen is possible using CT, and nodules of more than 1 cm are usually visible, either before or after the injection of a contrast medium. The use of material opacifying the reticuloendothelial system, which is injected intravenously, can improve the diagnosis of lymphomatous lesions by allowing visualization of nodules as small as 5 mm.[45]

Primary hepatic involvement is exceptional (0.4%) in extranodal non-Hodgkin's lymphomas.[27,46] Hepatic involvement is observed in 5–14% of Hodgkin's disease cases and 15–27% of non-Hodgkin's lymphoma during assessment.[47] Miliary forms are more frequent than nodular, and are the predominant forms in Hodgkin's disease. An association of hepatic and splenic involvement is not always observed and, in our series, only 51.6% of cases of hepatic involvement were associated with splenic involvement. In diagnosing lymphomatous hepatic involvement, CT has a sensitivity of 80% and a specificity of 84%, but the high occurrence of false-negative hepatic biopsies should be taken into account, as well as the therapeutic efficiency of chemotherapy in infraradiological lesions. Signs observed with CT are a normal appearance, which does not eliminate the diagnosis of lymphomatous hepatic involvement, hepatomegaly, multiple nodules, which are the most frequent form, or an isolated tumor form.

Urological involvement is mainly renal (68% of cases[48]). Primary forms are extremely rare, as opposed to secondary forms which represent the third cause of renal metastases after lung and breast cancer. CT usually shows homogeneous lesions that are less dense than normal paryenchema. These are most often multiple nodules of different sizes, or more rarely single nodules, renal infiltration with nephromegaly and renal infiltration from adjacent adenopathy. They are usually associated with retroperitoneal adenopathies.[49]

CT proves especially useful in pre-treatment assessment of the digestive tract, mainly the gastric region; infiltration of the wall is easily seen, even if its appearance is not specific – thickening (from 2 to 8 cm) of more than half of the gastric wall, parietal focalized thickening and ulcerated polypoid masses. It is less sensitive than barium studies in the detection of small lesions.[35] Similarly, in the small intestine, CT shows any thickening of the wall or adenopathies.

Other extranodal sites can be either primary or secondary and can be investigated with CT; they include the brain, orbit, cervical and maxillofacial regions,[50,51] pancreas,[15] female genital organs,[5] muscles.[10]

Ultrasonography (Figures 21.19–21.24)

The use of ultrasound in lymphomatous pathology is usually on the superficial lymph nodes or the abdomen, or else with endoscopy.

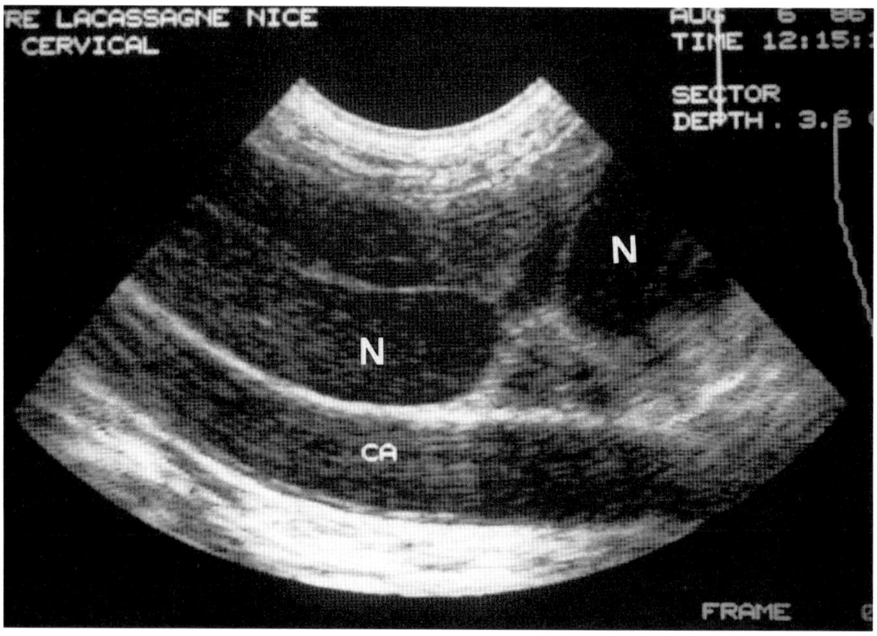

Figure 21.19

Precarotid cervical adenopathies. CA, carotid artery; N, lymph nodes.

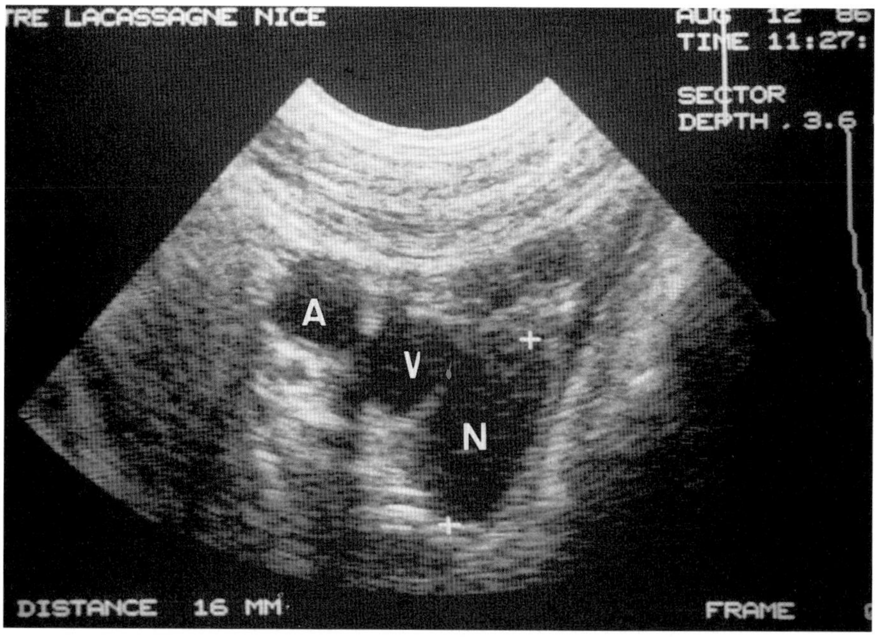

Figure 21.20

Axillary adenopathy with Hodgkin's disease. A, axillary artery; V, axillary vein; N, adenopathies; 16 mm between the two crosses.

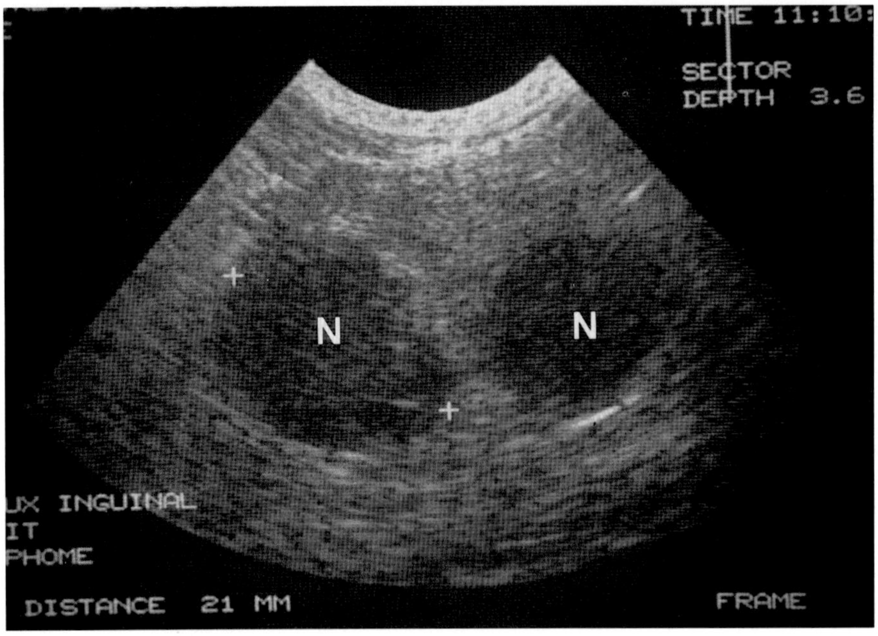

Figure 21.21

Inguinal adenopathies (N); 25 mm between the two crosses.

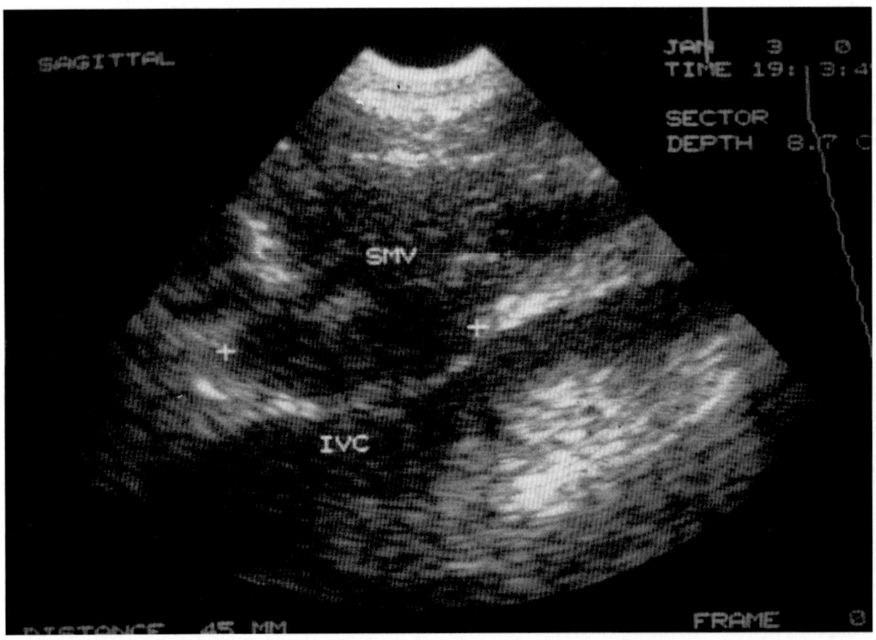

Figure 21.22

Retroperitoneal adenopathies with Hodgkin's disease. IVC: inferior vena cava; SMV, superior mesenteric vein; 45 mm between the two crosses.

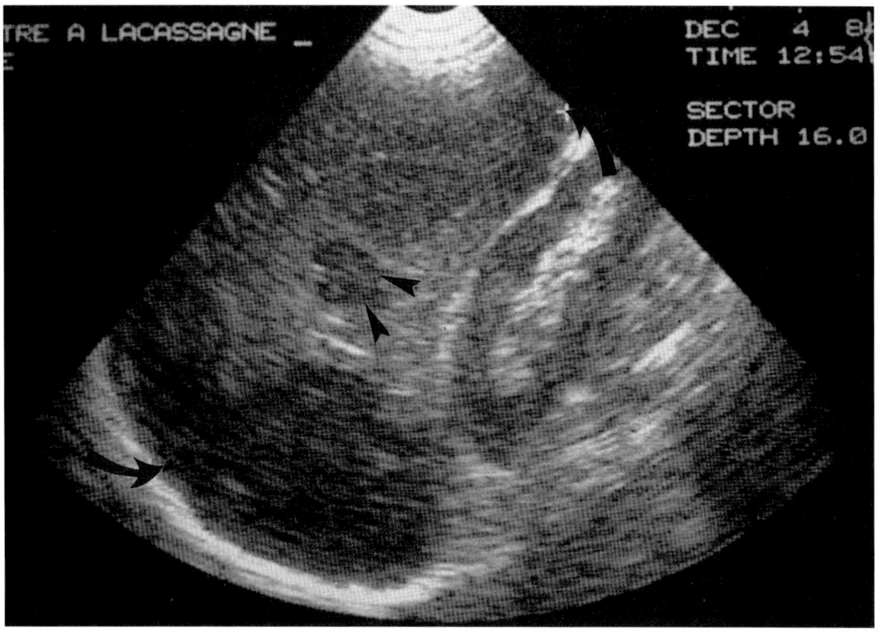

Figure 21.23

Lymphomatous nodular intersplenic localization (arrowheads) with moderate splenomegaly (154 mm between the two arrows).

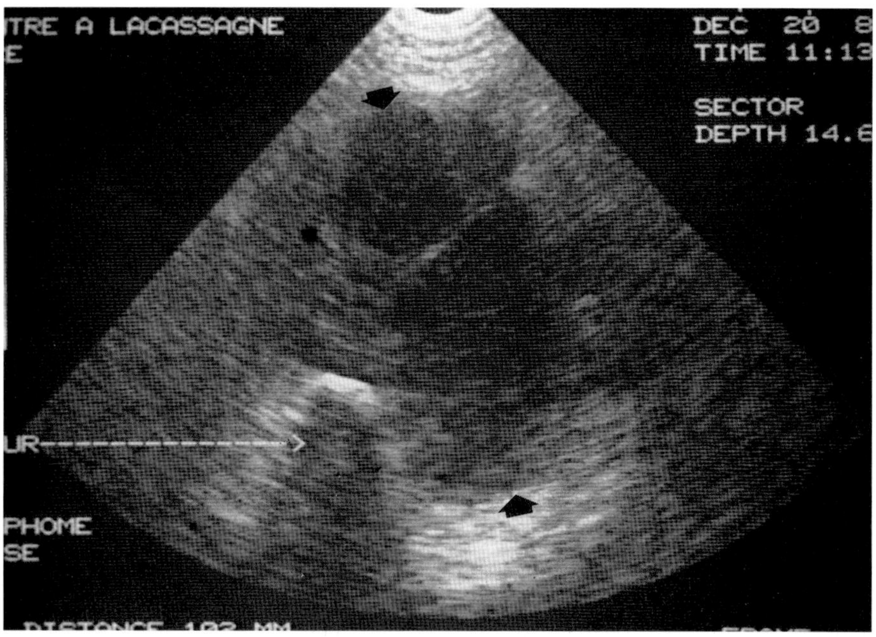

Figure 21.24

Lymphomatous localization of the quadriceps (102 mm between the two arrows).

Superficial adenopathies are the most frequent clinical localization in lymphoma, whether in cervical, supraclavicular, axillary or inguinal sites. Generally, node formations can be observed with ultrasonography, when the clinical examination is negative in 10.8% of cervical and subclavicular sites, 17.9% of axillary sites and 4.1% of inguinal sites.[50]

Ultrasonography of the abdomen is unfavorable in patients presenting with meteorism; the essential indication for its use is to analyse the liver or the spleen, in which case it has a similar value to CT. Lymphomatous lymph nodes are extremely hypoechoic and, sometimes, especially with non-Hodgkin's lymphomas, pseudocystic. If superficial or deep-seated lymph nodes have been irradiated, ultrasound examinations can detect a reduction in size and fibrous echoic areas.

The association of ultrasound and endoscopy allows a more accurate assessment of the digestive tract, since hypoechoic infiltration and thickening of the wall are easily visualized, as is a polypoid pattern.[52] The visualization of perigastric adenopathies is also facilitated with this method.

Gallium scan

This method is extremely controversial, especially in pre-treatment assessment, since sensitivity reported in the literature varies from 18 to 78%. Actually, sensitivity seems to depend on localization; in the parahepatic (because of hepatic activity) and iliac (because of colic radioactivity) regions, this method is often unsatisfactory. The analysis of the mediastinum is generally of better quality than that of the abdomen,[53] especially with the use of single photon emission computed tomography (SPECT). This technique seems to be useful mainly for the analysis of residual masses.[54]

Magnetic resonance imaging

At the present time, investigation of bone-marrow involvement is usually carried out by biopsy. Although MR seems extremely useful, it has not yet been sufficiently evaluated, either in the assessment or in the follow up of lymphomas. Normal fatty or hematopoietic bone marrow has a distribution which varies considerably according to age and from one patient to another, which makes the interpretation of results extremely difficult. T1 spin echo sequences are most often used. The study of bone marrow is an important factor in the assessment of non-Hodgkin's lymphomas, since biopsy reveals involvement in 30–40% of cases at the time of diagnosis.[55] Adenopathies can be easily recognized in relation to vessels and solid organs by MR of the mediastinum and abdomen.[56] Only size is useful, as signals are not specific. In the case of the liver and the spleen, MR appears more satisfactory than CT. The use of a contrast medium, such as ferrite, will probably lead to the detection not only of nodules, but also of diffuse infiltration which is not visible at present. In the future, MR will probably replace or complement CT for imaging of the spleen and bone marrow and in the assessment and follow up of lymphomas.

Imaging strategies for investigation

Hodgkin's disease (Diagram 21.1)

Assessment

For thoracic lesions, CT is useful even if standard radiographs appear sufficient when these lesions are evident. It allows visualization of abnormal lymph nodes, especially subcarinal or internal mammary nodes, not observed on chest radiographs. In cases of adenopathies that are already evident on standard films and are to be treated by chemotherapy, CT is not indispensable but does allow the optimization of the ultimate follow up, whatever the treatment (radiotherapy with determination of the field, or chemotherapy in case of diffuse lesions).

In the abdomen, apart from advanced cases where massive diffuse nodal infiltration exists, lymphography is justified because of its superior sensitivity; almost 10% of adenopathies observed with Hodgkin's disease have a normal diameter and are only recognized because of architectural alterations.[2,57] If it cannot be used, an abdominal CT is necessary.

Ultrasound allows the analysis of the liver and the spleen, if CT is not used. MR of the spleen using ferrite, when available, can be used to detect isolated supradiaphragmatic forms if laparotomy is not available. MR of the bone marrow is used for later stage II or for stage III lesions.

Follow up

Relapses are frequent during the first 2 years, but can occur later. In the supradiaphragmatic region, standard films are used;[58] if these are normal, it is not considered necessary to use the CT, but if a residual mass exists (14% of cases) then it becomes indispensable. Follow up of these residual masses is especially useful, since relapses occur here twice as frequently as in areas which have returned to normal.[58] Moreover, CT can prove useful in the evaluations of the topography of a relapse, as compared with the radiation field, as well as in the search for other sites, which are often poorly illustrated by standard films, as in the case of diaphragmatic, mammary or bony involvement.[59]

Subdiaphragmatic investigation is carried out using standard radiographs after lymphography. The value of lymphography in the detection of relapses decreases if lipiodol resorption is important. If follow-up films suggest an aggravation of lesions, then further examinations can be carried out using the scanner.[60] After opacification has disappeared, follow up is continued with CT.

Non-Hodgkin's lymphomas (Diagram 21.2)

Assessment

It is difficult to be unequivocal about non-Hodgkin's lymphomas, since different diseases, each with their own natural history and different clinical aspects, are bracketed together under this term;[2,5] 90% of non-Hodgkin's lymphomas are no longer stage I at the time of diagnosis and will therefore be treated with chemotherapy; in these cases an accurate clinical assessment is not necessary, only the distinction between a stage I or stage II tumor which can be treated by local treatment (radiotherapy), or another stage necessitating chemotherapy. For this reason, CT examination of the thorax and the abdomen is a vital element in the assessment of extensions. If the lesions appear to be stage I or II, MR of the bone marrow, liver and spleen, with ferrite opacification, confirms that the lesions are localized. Certain authorities[29,43] believe that CT should be reserved for patients with a stage I or II lesion and normal standard radiographs with no subdiaphragmatic abnormalities; however, 28% of normal standard films show abnormalities with CT,[43] which justifies an examination before treatment which can be then used as a reference. In addition to CT for examinations of the thorax and the abdomen, other techniques can be proposed, such as standard films of the chest and examination of the abdomen, for all stages beyond I.[2] Ultrasound and CT can also be used in association for the assessment and follow up of non-Hodgkin's lymphomas. In a stage I case of the cervical nodes, the facial mass can be examined with CT to investigate any involvement.

Follow up

Since the sites of non-Hodgkin's lymphomas have a variable evolution, follow up can be decided according to the localization of the lesions. For example, subdiaphragmatic involvement only could be followed up with CT and a chest radiograph. It is difficult to determine the frequency at which lymphomas should be followed up. Generally, the histologic type is the main factor in deciding the frequency of follow-up examinations. More especially, aggressive lymphomas necessitate examinations at shorter intervals during the first 2 years.

Special cases

AIDS and lymphomas (Figure 21.25)

Lymphomas occurring in conjunction with AIDS are extremely aggressive; renal, splenic and hepatic involvement are more frequent than in lymphomas in the absence of AIDS.[61] Similarly, mesenteric adenopathies, which are rare with Hodgkin's disease (5%), have an incidence of 20% with AIDS. A problem specific to non-Hodgkin's lymphomas associated with AIDS is the frequency of primitive lymphomas of the central nervous system, and the major differential diagnosis of cerebral toxoplasmosis.

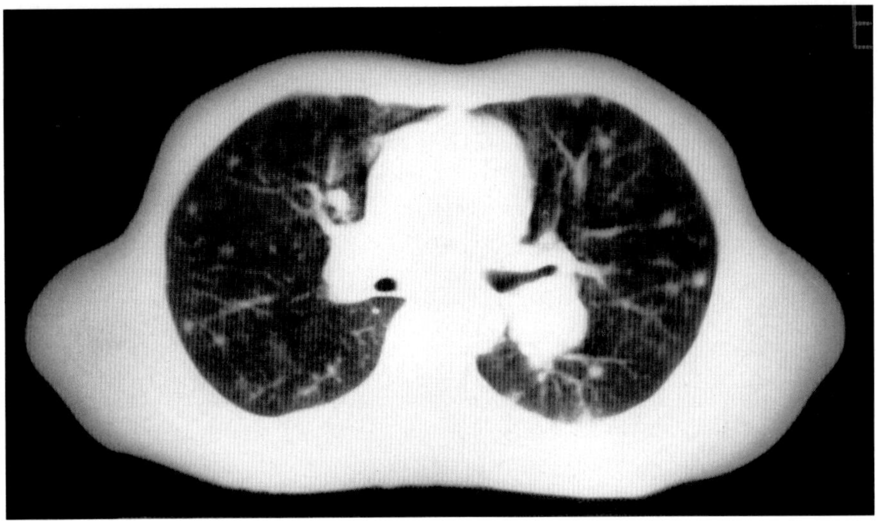

Figure 21.25

Hodgkin's disease with AIDS: intrapulmonary nodular localization.

Relapses and residual masses (Figures 21.26–21.28)

After thoracic radiotherapy, lesions remain whose size depends on the dose, the size of the radiation field, individual variations, and possibly adjuvant chemotherapy. The results of examinations carried out after 1 month and supplemented by others less than a year after completion of radiotherapy should not be confused with relapses.[42,62] In the thorax or the abdomen, whether with Hodgkin's disease or non-Hodgkin's lymphoma, sequelae consist of solid or cystic masses that are often calcified. It is impossible to propose a diagnosis of residual lesion or tumor remains solely on the basis of size. A percutaneous biopsy of residual masses guided by CT was not considered, until recently, as having any great diagnostic value, but the introduction of new histologic techniques has led to improvements that can influence the choice between follow up with CT or surgical exeresis.

Conclusion

The assessment and follow up of lymphomas have benefited from the introduction of CT which is now the main technique used. CT will probably be replaced sooner or later by MR, in view of the latter's efficiency and the increasing number of machines available.

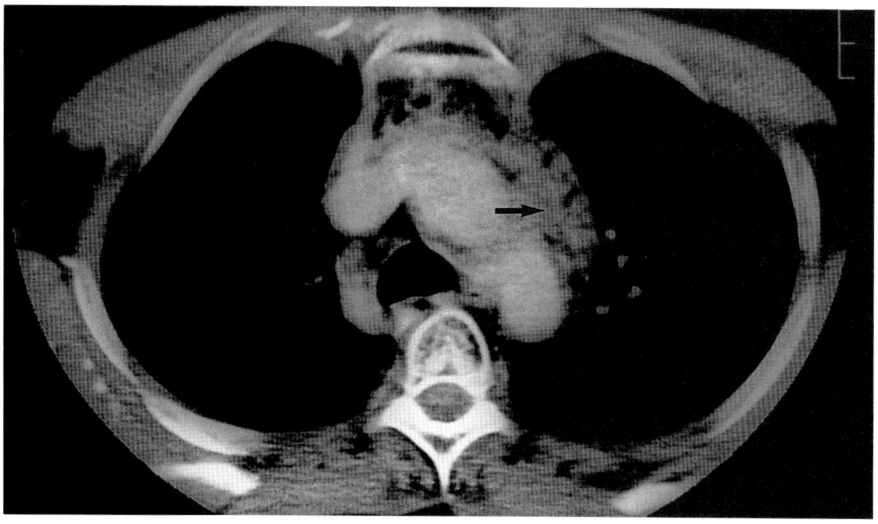

Figure 21.26

Residual mediastinal lesions with Hodgkin's disease (arrow).

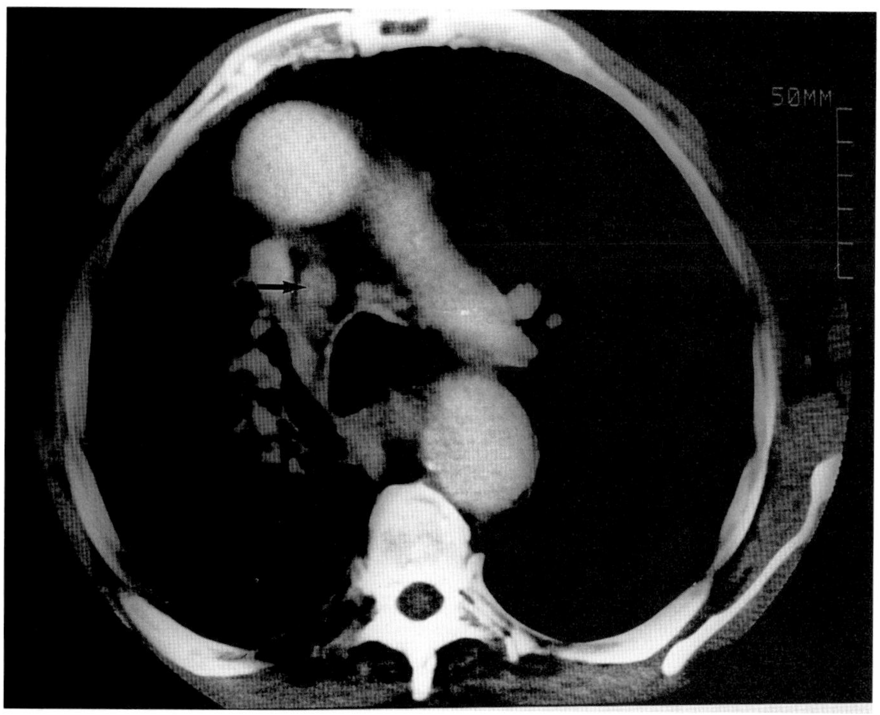

Figure 21.27

Residual lymph nodes after radiotherapy for Hodgkin's disease (arrow).

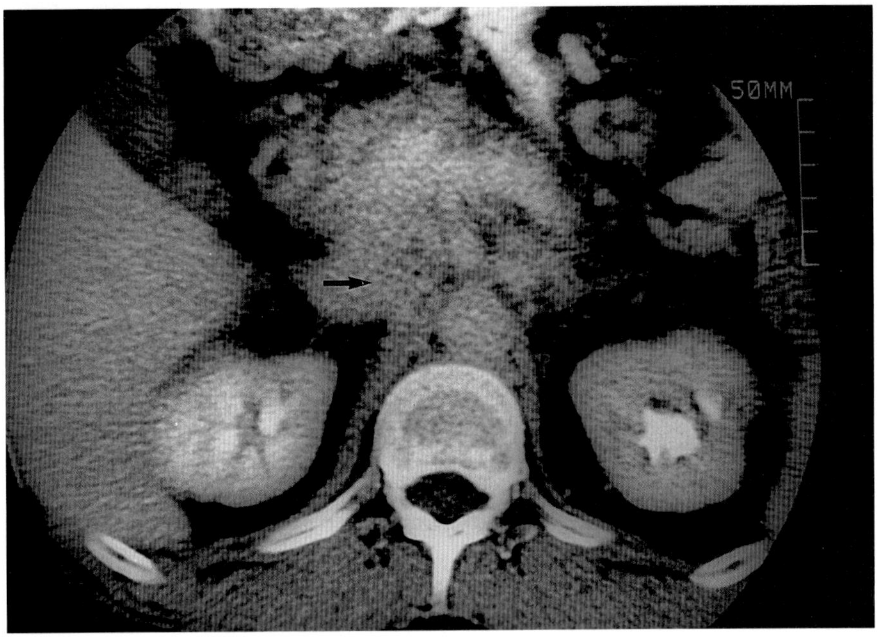

Figure 21.28

Sequelae (unchanged after 1 year) of lymphomatous non-Hodgkin's lymph-node involvement (arrow).

References

1. Cohen MD, Siddiqui A, Weetman R et al, Hodgkin's disease and non-Hodgkin's lymphomas in children: utilisation of radiological modalities, *Radiology* (1968) **158**:499–505.
2. Marglin S, Castellino RA, Selection of imaging studies for newly presenting patients with non-Hodgkin's lymphoma, *Semin Ultrasound CT MR* (1986) **7**:2–8.
3. Coiffier B, Gisselbrecht C, Herbrecht R et al, L.N.H. 84 regimen: a multicenter study of intensive chemotherapy in 737 patients with aggressive malignant lymphoma, *J Clin Oncol* (1989) **7**:1018–26.
4. Kaplan HS, *Hodgkin's disease*, 2nd edn (Harvard University Press: Cambridge 1980).
5. Moormeier JA, Williams SF, Golomb HM, The staging of non-Hodgkin's lymphomas, *Semin Oncol* (1990) **17**:43–50.
6. Dick F, Bloomfield CD, Brunning RD, Incidence, cytology and histopathology of non-Hodgkin's lymphomas in the bone marrow, *Cancer* (1974) **33**:1382–98.
7. Bruneton JN, Drouillard J, Balu-Maestro C et al, Lymphoma of the pancreas, *J Med Imag* (1988) **2**:137–42.
8. Lister TA, Crowther D, Sutcliffe SB et al, Report of the Committee convened to discuss evaluation and staging with Hodgkin's disease: Cotswolds meeting, *J Clin Oncol* (1989) **7**:1630–6.
9. Crnkovich MJ, Leopold K, Hoppe RT et al, Stage I to II B Hodgkin's disease: the combined experience at Stanford University and the Joint Center for Radiation therapy, *J Clin Oncol* (1987) **5**:1041–9.
10. Prosnitz LR, Radiation complications for Hodgkin's disease and seminoma: assessing the risk benefit rates, *Int J Radiat Oncol Biol Phys* (1988) **15**:239–41.
11. Tucker MA, Loleman CN, Cox RS et al, Risk of second cancers after treatment for Hodgkin's disease, *N Engl J Med* (1980) **318**:76–81.
12. Rosenberg SA, Kaplan HS, The evolution and

summary results of the Stanford randomized clinical trials of the management of Hodgkin's disease: 1962–1984, *Int J Radiat Oncol Biol Phys* (1985) **11**:5–22.

13. Kennedy B, Loeb V, Peterson V et al, National survey of patterns of case for Hodgkin's disease, *Cancer* (1985) **56**: 2547–6.
14. Lenhert K, Mohrin, Stein H et al, The histopathology of malignant lymphoma, *Br J Haematol* (1975) **31**(suppl):193–203.
15. Schneider M, Thyss A, Classification of malignant lymphomas. In: Bruneton JN, Schneider M, eds, *Radiology of lymphomas* (Springer-Verlag: Heidelberg 1986) 1–6.
16. The non-Hodgkin's lymphoma pathologic classification project, National Cancer Institute sponsored study of classification of non-Hodgkin's lymphomas. Summary and description of a working formulation for clinical usage, *Cancer* (1982) **42**:2112–35.
17. Young RC, Longo DL, Glatstein E et al, The treatment of indolent lymphomas: watchful waiting versus aggressive combined modality treatment, *Semin Hematol* (1988) **25**(suppl 2):11–16.
18. Miller TP, Dana BW, Weick JK et al, Southwest oncology groups clinical trials of intermediate and high grade non Hodgkin's lymphomas, *Semin Hematol* (1980) **25**(suppl 2):17–22.
19. Castellino RA, Blank N, Cassady JR et al, Roentgenologic aspects of Hodgkin's disease. II. Role of routine radiographs in detecting initial relapse, *Cancer* (1973) **31**:316–23.
20. Young RC, Canellos GP, Chabner BA et al, Patterns of relapse in advanced Hodgkin's disease: treatment with combination radiotherapy, *Cancer* (1978) **42**:1001–7.
21. Filly R, Blank N, Castellino RA, Radiographic distribution of intrathoracic disease in previously untreated patients with Hodgkin's disease and non-Hodgkin's lymphoma, *Radiology* (1976) **120**:277–81.
22. Stolberg HO, Patt NL, MacEwen KF et al, Hodgkin's disease of the lung. Roentgenologic–pathologic correlation, *AJR* (1964) **92**:96–115.
23. Weick JK, Kiely JM, Harrison EG et al, Pleural effusion in lymphoma, *Cancer* (1973) **31**:848–53.
24. Levitt LJ, Aisenberg AC, Harris NL et al, Primary non-Hodgkin's lymphoma of the mediastinum, *Cancer* (1982) **50**:2486–92.
25. Lichtenstein AK, Levine A, Taylor CR et al, Primary lymphoma in adults, *Am J Med* (1980) **68**:509–14.
26. Burgener FA, Hamlin DJ, Intrathoracic histiocytic lymphoma, *AJR* (1981) **136**:499–504.
27. Freeman C, Berg JW, Cutler SJ, Occurrence and prognosis of extranodal lymphomas, *Cancer* (1972) **29**:252–60.
28. Gebauer C, Primary lymphosarcoma of the lungs. A review of 121 cases, *Oncology* (1982) **39**:345–9.
29. Pera A, Capek M, Shirkhoda A, Lymphangiography and CT in the follow up of patients with lymphoma, *Radiology* (1987) **164**:631–3.
30. Steiner RM, Harell GS, Glatstein E et al, Repeat lymphography in Hodgkin's disease, *Radiology* (1970) **97**:613–18.
31. Hessel SJ, Adams DF, Abrams HL, Lymphography in lymphoma. In: Clouse ME, ed., *Clinical lymphography* (Williams and Wilkins: Baltimore 1977) 160–84.
32. Castellino RA, Billingham M, Dorfman RF, Lymphographic accuracy in Hodgkin's disease and malignant lymphoma with a note on the "reactive" lymph node as a cause of most false positive lymphograms, *Invest Radiol* (1974) **9**:155–65.
33. Castellino RA, Hoppe RT, Blank N et al, Computed tomography, lymphography, and staging laparotomy: correlations in initial staging of Hodgkin's disease, *AJR* (1984) **143**:37–41.
34. Marglin SI, Castellino RA, Lymphographic accuracy in 632 consecutive, previously untreated case of Hodgkin disease and non-Hodgkin lymphoma, *Radiology* (1981) **140**:351–3.
35. Megibow AJ, Gastrointestinal lymphoma: the role of CT in diagnosis and management, *Semin Ultrasound CT MR* (1986) **7**:43–57.
36. Bruneton JN, Valette PJ, Lymphomas. In: Bruneton JN ed., *Imaging of the gastrointestinal tract tumors* (Springer-Verlag: Heidelberg 1990) 193–211.
37. Bruneton JN, Drouillard J, Normand F et al, Non-renal urological lymphomas, *Fortschr Roentgenstr* (1987) **146**:42–6.
38. Anderson KL, Kaplan WD, Leonard RCF, et al, Role of 99 m Tc methylene diphosphate bone imaging in the management of lymphoma, *Cancer Treat Rep* (1985) **69**:1347–51.
39. Salonen O, Kivisaari L, Standertskjold-Nordenstam CG et al, Chest radiography and computed tomography in the evolution of mediastinal adenopathy in lymphoma, *Acta Radiol* (1987) **28**:747–50.
40. Castellino RA, Blank N, Hoppe RT et al, Hodgkin's disease: contributions of chest CT in the initial staging evaluation, *Radiology* (1986) **160**:603–5.
41. Hoppe RT, The contemporary management of Hodgkin disease, *Radiology* (1988) **169**:297–304.
42. Heron CW, Husband JE, Williams MP et al, The value of thoracic computed tomography in the detection of recurrent Hodgkin's disease, *Br J Radiol* (1988) **61**:567–72.
43. Khoury MB, Godevin JD, Halvorsen R et al, Role of chest CT in non Hodgkin lymphoma, *Radiology* (1986) **158**:659–62.
44. Bruneton JN, Caramella E, Manzino JJ, Nodal lymphomas of the abdomen. In: Bruneton JN, Schneider M, eds, *Radiology of lymphomas* (Springer-Verlag: Heidelberg 1986) 60–9.
45. Thomas JL, Bernardino ME, Vermess M et al, EOE-13 in the detection of hepatosplenic lymphoma, *Radiology* (1982) **145**:629–34.
46. Osborne BM, Butler JJ, Guarda LA, Primary lymphoma of the liver. Ten cases and a review of the literature, *Cancer* (1985) **56**:2902–10.
47. Bruneton JN, Mathieu D, Vasile N et al, Computed tomography of hepatic lymphoma, *J Med Imag* (1988) **2**:293–7.

48. Weimar G, Culp DA, Loening S et al, urogenital involvement by malignant lymphomas, *J Urol* (1981) **125**:230–1.

49. Jafri SZH, Bree RL, Amendola MA et al, CT of renal and perirenal non-Hodgkin lymphoma, *AJR* (1982) **138**:1101–5.

50. Bruneton JN, Normand F, Balu-Maestro C et al, Lymphomatous superficial lymph nodes: US detection, *Radiology* (1987) **165**:233–5.

51. Fierstein JT, Thawley SE, Lymphoma of the head and neck, *Laryngoscope* (1978) **88**:582–93.

52. Bolondi L, Casanova P, Caletti GC et al, Primary gastric lymphoma versus gastric carcinoma: endoscopic US evaluation, *Radiology* (1987) **165**:821–6.

53. Tumeh SS, Rosenthal DS, Kaplan WD et al, Lymphoma: evaluation with Ga-67 SPECT, *Radiology* (1987) **164**:111–14.

54. Anderson KC, Leonard RCF, Canellos GP et al, High dose gallium imaging in lymphoma, *Am J Med* (1983) **75**:327–31.

55. Jones SS, Rosenberg SA, Kaplan HS, Non-Hodgkin's lymphomas: I. bone marrow involvement, *Cancer* (1972) **29**:954–60.

56. Nyman R, Rehn S, Glimelius B et al, Magnetic resonance imaging, chest radiography, computed tomography and ultrasonography in malignant lymphoma, *Acta Radiol* (1987) **28**:253–62.

57. Koehler PR, Lymphography vs CT of lymphomas, *AJR* (1978) **131**:1116–17.

58. North LB, Fuller LM, Sullivan-Halley JA et al, Regression of mediastinal Hodgkin disease after therapy: evaluation of time interval, *Radiology* (1987) **164**:599–602.

59. Frija J, Bellin MF, Laval-Jeantet M et al, Role of CT in the study of recurrences of Hodgkin's disease on the chest wall. Report on 12 cases, *Eur J Radiol* (1987) **7**:229–34.

60. Hopper KD, Diehl LF, Lesar M et al, Hodgkin disease: clinical utility in initial staging and treatment, *Radiology* (1988) **169**:17–22.

61. Nyberg DA, Jeffrey RBJ, Federle MP et al, AIDS-related lymphomas: evoluation by abdominal CT, *Radiology* (1986) **159**:59–63.

62. Libshitz HI, Shuman LS, Radiation induced pulmonary change: CT findings, *J Comput Assist Tomogr* (1984) **8**:15–19.

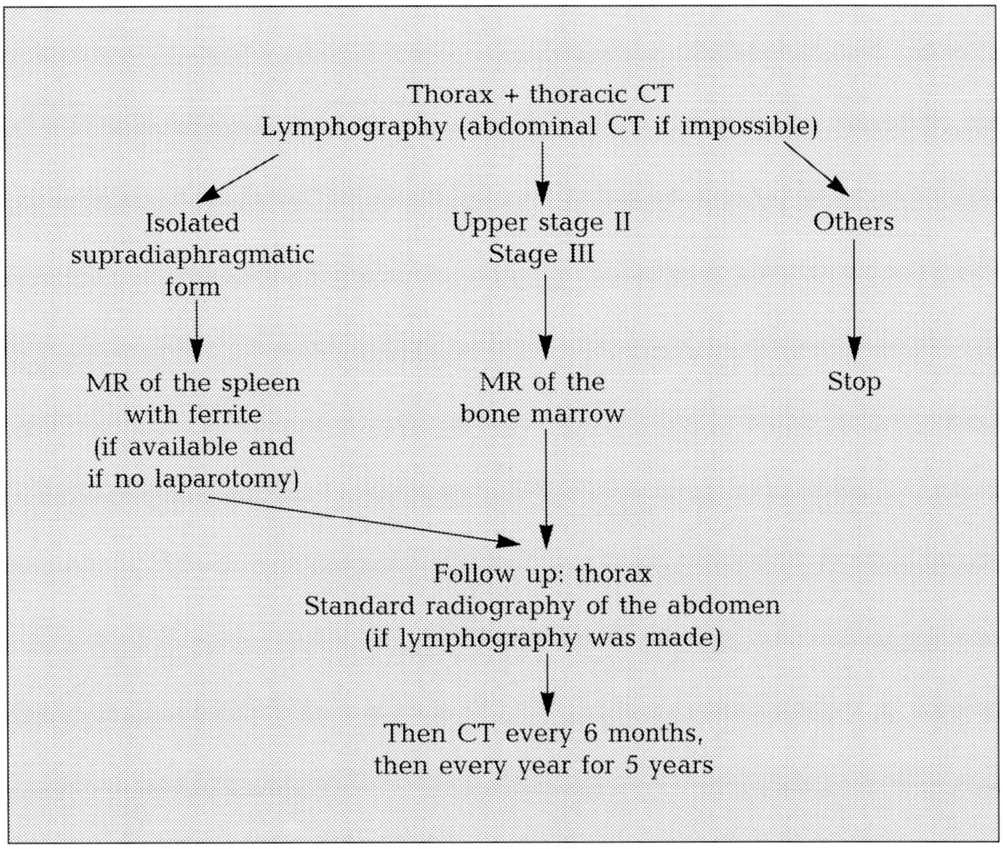

Diagram 21.1

Strategies for the radiological investigation of Hodgkin's disease.

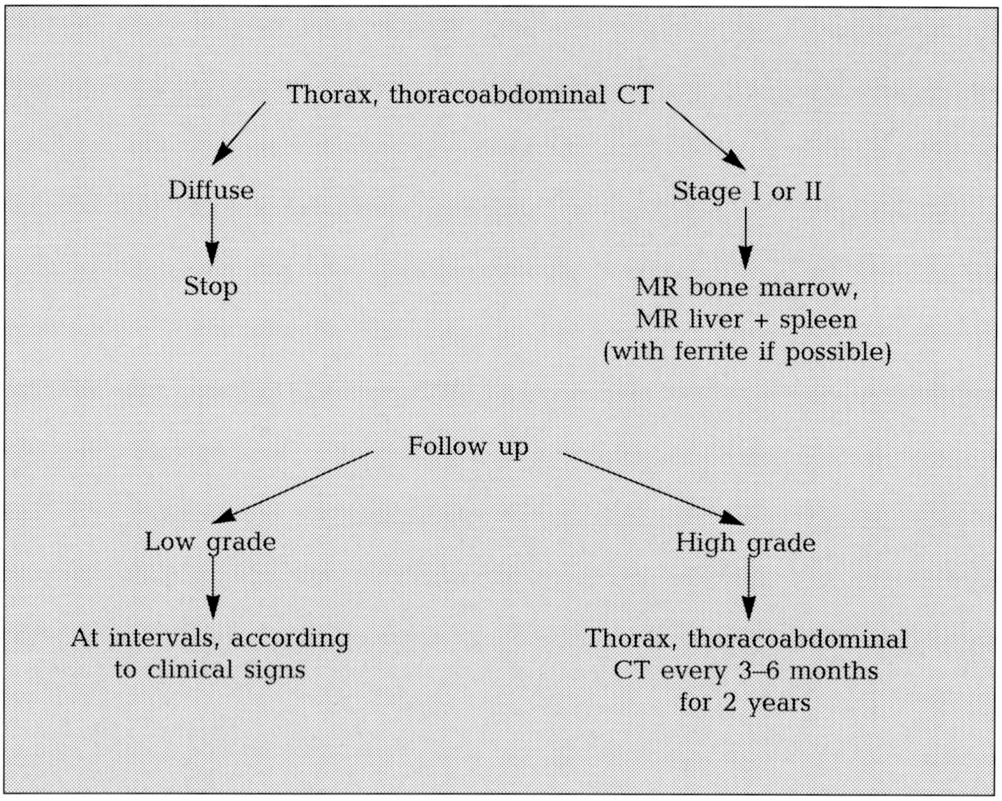

Diagram 21.2

Strategies for the radiological investigation of malignant non-Hodgkin's lymphoma of the lymph nodes.

22

Pediatrics

Dominique Couanet

Introduction

In the past decade, pediatric oncology has made great progress in three fields: first, in the means of investigation by imaging: ultrasound, CT scan, magnetic resonance imaging (MRI), ^{123}I-meta-iodobenzylguanidine (m-IBG) scintigraphy, which have all facilitated the detection of tumors and their extensions; second, in the development of biological markers and percutaneous fine-needle biopsies, which lead to more prompt diagnosis and facilitate follow up; and third, in the development of new drugs for chemotherapy, which have increased the survival of children with tumors considered to have an unfavorable histologic prognosis, such as osteosarcomas, non-Hodgkin's lymphomas or malignant teratomas.

At present, the requirements of imaging are a rapid diagnostic approach, an objective evaluation of the response to chemotherapy, which can be an important prognostic factor and early detection of an eventual recurrence. More rapid diagnosis speeds up the initiation of treatment, which will thus become more effective, because disease often evolves quickly and can impair the patient's vital functions.

General observations

Tumors in children have specific characteristics. From the histologic viewpoint, they are often slightly differentiated embryonal tumors. Two types of solid tumors can be distinguished: embryonal tumors related to an organ, such as nephroblastoma or Wilms' tumor of the kidney, and tumors related to tissues having multiple localizations (hence the various tumoral sites), for example non-Hodgkin's lymphoma, which can originate in the head and neck, the thorax, the abdomen or the limbs. Thus, solid tumors in children can be broadly classified according to the organ involved and their histologic type when they are found in a single localization (Table 22.1), and by the tissue from which they originate and their histologic type if they are found in various locations (Table 22.2). From a clinical point of view, growth is rapid, creating a certain therapeutic urgency. Circumstances leading to

Table 22.1 Histologic type of solid tumors related to specific organs.

Organ	*Histologic type*[a]
Nasopharynx	*Undifferentiated carcinoma*
Lung	Pneumoblastoma
Kidney	*Wilms' tumor (nephroblastoma)*
	Beckwith's tumor (sarcoma)
	Grawitz's tumor (adenocarcinoma)
	Nephroblastomatosis
Liver	Hepatoblastoma
	Hepatocarcinoma
Adrenal	Malignant corticosurrenaloma

[a]Italics indicate the most common histologies.

Table 22.2 Malignant solid tumors with variable location.

Histologic origin	*Cellular differentiation*[a]
Mesenchymal tissue	Myoblastic: *rhabdomyosarcoma* Osseous: *osteosarcoma* Conjunctive: fibrosarcoma synovial sarcoma Vascular: malignant hemangioendothelioma malignant hemangiopericytoma Undifferentiated
Neuroectodermal tissue	*Neuroblastoma* Pheochromocytoma *Ewing's sarcoma* Primary neuroectodermal tumor *Retinoblastoma* Esthesioneuroblastoma
Lymphoid tissue	*Non-Hodgkin's lymphoma* Malignant histiocytosis (Ki 1-lymphoma) Hodgkin's disease
Germinal tissue	Malignant teratoma Dysgerminoma

[a]Italics indicate the most common histologies.

discovery of tumors often arise from the effects of the mass, such as parietal deformation, pain, respiratory or urological disorders, or because of metastatic osteomedullar, hepatic or neuromeningeal involvement. Less often, discovery is incidental, due to investigation of another pathology.

The tumors are often chemo- and radiosensitive. The main way of treating them is to reduce the size of the tumor and any metastases with initial chemotherapy, followed by complementary surgery, if necessary, and sometimes followed by post-surgical radiotherapy, which should be used circumspectly because of the long-term consequences for growth.

An outline of diagnosis

In general, the diagnostic work up aims to locate the tumoral mass responsible for the clinical symptoms having led to its discovery by the most simple imaging technique, then to identify the lesion histologically or with the aid of specific markers, and finally to clarify any local or distant extension of tumoral disease.

Malignant tumoral pathology of the head and neck

Symptoms leading to the discovery of tumors of the head and neck in children depend on the site of the primary tumor: obstruction of the nasal fossae, nasal speech or otalgia for tumors of the cavum; neuralgia in the region of the trifacial nerve and trismus with lesions of the pterygomaxillary region; unilateral nasal obstruction, purulent rhinorrhea and epistaxis for tumors of the nasal fossae and the sinal cavities of the face; otorrhea and otalgia for tumors in the tympanic cavity; retromandibular tumefaction and peripheral facial

Table 22.3 Histology and site of malignant tumors of the head and neck.

Histology	*Orbit*	*Nasopharynx*	*Ear*	*Paranasal sinuses*	*Parotid*	*Neck*
Bone metastasis	✔					
Undifferentiated carcinoma of nasopharyngeal type		✔				
Rhabdomyosarcoma	✔	✔	✔	✔	✔	✔
Non-Hodgkin's lymphoma	✔	✔		✔	✔	✔
Hodgkin's disease						✔
Fibrosarcoma				✔		
Adenocarcinoma					✔	
Neuroblastoma						✔

paralysis in case of parotid involvement; exophthalmia and troubled vision for intraorbital disorders; Claude Bernard–Horner syndrome for lesions in the laterocervical regions. Metastatic cervical adenopathies can be revealed by deformation of the neck.

After a clinical ENT examination, the first investigation to be carried out, in response to suspicious symptoms that have gradually worsened and not responded to antibiotic treatment, is CT (Diagram 22.1).[1,2] The biopsy is guided by CT findings so as to obtain a significant pathologic sample. The main types of tumoral histology, according to the location of the lesion, are summarized in Table 22.3.

Malignant thoracic tumoral pathology

The circumstances leading to the discovery of malignant thoracic tumors are variable and depend on the size of the tumor, its growth rate and its location. Symptoms include thoracic pain, respiratory disorders, such as dyspnea or a cough, neurologic symptoms of the trunk or roots, such as intercostal neuralgia, motor deficiency in the lower limbs, intercurrent pathology, such as an infection, or incidental discovery. The initial examination in the face of such symptoms should be chest radiography (Diagram 22.2).

On the basis of the tumor's localization—in the anterior, middle or posterior mediastinum—it should be possible to suggest a diagnosis and the etiology. This will be all the easier if the tumor is small, which is not often the case for rapidly growing malignant tumors. Tumors of the anterior mediastinum are lymphomas (more often non-Hodgkin's lymphomas than Hodgkin's disease), germ-cell tumors (teratomas) and thymomas. The middle mediastinum may be invaded by Hodgkin's or metastatic adenopathies. The posterior mediastinum may reveal neurogenous tumors, such as neuroblastomas and ganglioneuroblastomas or, less frequently, malignant teratomas. The thoracic wall is the location of the malignant mesenchymal tumors (rhabdomyosarcomas) and Ewing's sarcoma (see Figure 22.1 and Table 22.4).

In the presence of clinical symptoms, the first examination to be carried out is a standard thoracic radiograph, anteroposterior (AP) and lateral views. If necessary, a lateral decubitus view can be taken in order to detect any pleural effusion; the puncture of any such effusion can contribute cytologic proof of a non-Hodgkin's lymphoma. Apart from these cases, the tumoral mass is either well localized in a given sector of the mediastinum, or else it is badly defined, at most showing as an opaque hemithorax. It is useful to complete assessment with CT in order to clarify the densitometric characteristics of the tumoral mass, and to investigate the possibility of calcifications and the relation with the vascular axis of the mediastinum for the anterior and middle portions. For all posterior

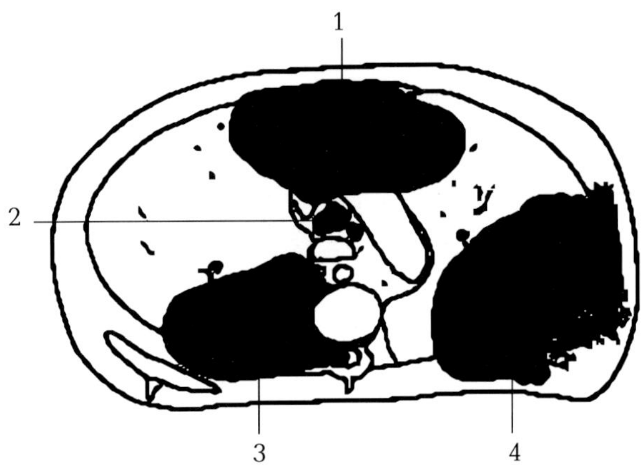

Figure 22.1

Sites of mediastinal tumors: 1, anterior mediastinum; 2, middle mediastinum; 3, posterior mediastinum; 4, thoracic wall.

Table 22.4 Histology related to site in mediastinal malignant solid tumors.

Histology	*Mediastinum*			*Thoracic wall*
	anterior	*middle*	*posterior*	
Non-Hodgkin's lymphoma	✔			
Hodgkin's disease	✔	✔		
Teratoma	✔		✔	
Metastatic adenopathy	✔	✔	✔	
Thymoma	✔			
Neuroblastoma			✔	
Ewing's sarcoma				✔
Mesenchymal soft-tissue tumor				✔

lesions, MR is indispensable, in order to detect any eventual intraspinal extradural extension.[3] The nature of the thoracic lesion is determined by biological markers such as urinary catecholamines or serous α-fetoproteins (AFPs), by peripheral sampling or by tumoral biopsy.

Tumoral pathology of the abdomen

Signs revealing the presence of an abdominal tumor in children are related either to the tumor or to metastatic diffusion. An abdominal mass palpable by the parents or the pediatrician is the most frequent reason for the discovery of a tumor. Signs of compression with abdominal pain and transit disorders may also be observed. Clearly evident, metastases are bony and painful or hepatic and palpable (hepatomegaly with Pepper's syndrome). Urologic disorders, such as dysurea or acute urine retention, reveal tumoral masses in the pelvic region. Occasionally, certain malformations which are often linked to the presence of a tumor lead to its discovery, for example corporal hemihypertrophia and a nephroblastoma.[4,5] Finally, a tumor may be discovered by ultrasound during antenatal assessment.

In children, the abdomen is especially easy to investigate by ultrasonography (US),[6] which should always be the initial investigation. It helps to locate the mass to an anatomic sector of the abdomen—retroperitoneal space, intraperitoneal space, pelvic extraperitoneal space—and sometimes to an organ—kidney, liver, etc. Ultrasonography also clarifies tumor characteristics: echogenicity, size, vascular links.

Table 22.5 The main malignant tumors of the abdomen.[a]

Retroperitoneal space
Renal tumors
Wilms' tumor
Beckwith's tumor
Grawitz's tumor
Adrenal tumors
Neuroblastoma
Pheochromocytoma
Adrenocortical carcinoma
Sympathetic tumors
Neuroblastoma
Ganglioneuroblastoma
Lymphomas
Malignant teratoma
Peritoneal space (including the liver)
Non-Hodgkin's lymphoma
Liver tumors
Hepatoblastoma
Hepatocarcinoma
Ovarian tumors
Malignant germ-cell tumors
Extraperitoneal pelvic space
Rhabdomyosarcoma
Sacrococcygeal teratoma
Neuroblastoma
Abdominal wall (bone and soft tissue)
Ewing's sarcoma
Mesenchymal tumors
Rhabdomyosarcoma
Fibrosarcoma
Non-Hodgkin's lymphoma

[a]Italics indicate the most common histologies.

The main types of malignant tumor found in the abdomen are summarized in Table 22.5. The tumor is sometimes too bulky to locate accurately by US, in which case CT can be carried out to help with identification.[7] Intravenous pyelography (IVP) is only rarely indicated, being used for kidney tumors (Diagram 22.3).

Table 22.6 Sites of primary neuroblastomas.[a]

Location	%
Cervical	5
Thoracic	17
Abdominal	70
Pelvic	2
Undetermined	5
Intraspinal	1

[a]Data for 173 cases, 1975–9.[11]

Neuroblastoma

This is the most common solid tumor in children: 10 cases per million children under 5 years old. Like ganglioneuroblastoma, it develops at the expense of the sympathetic nervous system. Along with the APUD (amine precursor uptake decarboxylation) system tumors, these tumors originate in cells of the neural crest, which are collectively known as cristopathies.[8,9] Their location is that of the sympathetic tissue, i.e. the medullo–surrenal, along the paravertebral sympathetic nerve with a possible 'hour-glass' intrarachidian extradural extension through the intervertebral foramina, and along the arterial vascular axes (Table 22.6).

Neuroblastomas have a lobulated structure composed of small embryonal cells which are sometimes grouped into pseudo-rosettes.[10] Amorphous calcifications are observed in 50–60% of cases. It is possible to observe cells at different stages of differentiation within the same tumor: the more differentiated the tumor, the richer the fibrillar substance and the larger the cells. Thus it is possible to observe cells with a ganglioneural appearance alongside embryonal cells in ganglioneuroblastomas. The majority of neuroblastomas occur in young children, 93% being less than 6 years of age at the time of diagnosis, and a third of these cases occurring in the first year.[11,12]

Symptoms leading to discovery are varied:[13] an abdominal mass, pain resulting from compression of an adjacent organ, symptoms resulting from metastatic diffusion, neurologic symptoms of spinal cord or radicular compression in laterovertebral tumors or in metastatic bone localizations of the vertebrae, a paraneoplasic syndrome such as diarrhea or polymyoclonia-opsoclonus.[14] Symptoms resulting from metastatic diffusion are frequent at the time of diagnosis and include pain in the bones or anemia resulting from osteomedullar metastases (50–70% of abdominal neuroblastomas are metastatic at the time of diagnosis, according to different series), and hepatomegaly (Pepper's syndrome in children under one year of age).

Imaging

Ultrasonography is the initial examination in the presence of an abdominal mass:[6,7,15] it identifies the retroperitoneal location of the tumor and its extrarenal nature, although the tumor can sometimes be bulky and therefore invade the suprainternal pole of the kidney. The lesion is heterogeneous in appearance, with calcified hyperechoic plaques, and infiltrates the prevertebral space with satellite adenopathies, which are often quite bulky and displace the large lumboaortic vessels. In 90–95% of cases, the diagnosis is established by assays of urinary catecholamines.[16,17] This should automatically be carried out in the presence of a retroperitoneal tumor in a child. Abdominal US examinations can also be useful in a systematic search for the primary tumor, when the neuroblastoma is discovered, because metastatic diffusion to the bones or liver does occur. For other locations, chest radiographs reveal neuroblastomas of the posterior mediastinum, US reveals primary pelvic tumors and CT reveals cervical neuroblastomas.

Neuroblastic lesions are staged on the basis of imaging data according to Evans' criteria (Table 22.7).[18,19] An example of the distribution of cases between clinical stages[21] is given in Table 22.8.

Assessment of extensions

Assessment of extensions takes into account the osteo- and lymphophilic character of the tumors and the therapeutic options, the two main choices being chemotherapy and surgery, in view of frequent bone and bone-marrow metastases at the time of diagnosis.[19–21] Medullograms and m-IBG scintigraphy show metastatic extensions and MR, when possible, tends to replace CT in locoregional tumor assessment (Diagram 22.4).[22–25]

Films of an unprepared abdomen and IVP are no longer considered useful, and films of the skeleton are only rarely indicated. If a child is in pain, CT may sometimes be more simple to carry out than MR in an emergency (see Figure 22.3).

Ultrasonography findings

The most typical form of tumor is lateral and prevertebral, situated above or within the kidney, with a solid heterogeneous echostructure including

Table 22.7 Clinical staging of neuroblastoma and 3-year disease-free survival.[11,18,20]

Stage	*Criterion*	*Survival (%)*
I	Tumor restricted to organ or structure of origin	95–100
II	Tumor extends in continuity beyond site of origin but not across midline; ipsilateral lymph nodes may be positive	85–95
III	Tumor extends in continuity across the midline; ipsilateral and controlateral lymph nodes may be positive	65–85
IV	Distant metastases to bone, liver, soft tissue, distant lymph nodes and brain	30–40
IVs	A stage I or II tumor with liver, skin and bone marrow metastases without radiological bony lesions	60–80

Figure 22.8 Distribution of clinical staging.[a]

Stage	%
I	4
II	23
III	16
IV	47
IVs	10

[a]Data for 135 cases, 1982–5.[21]

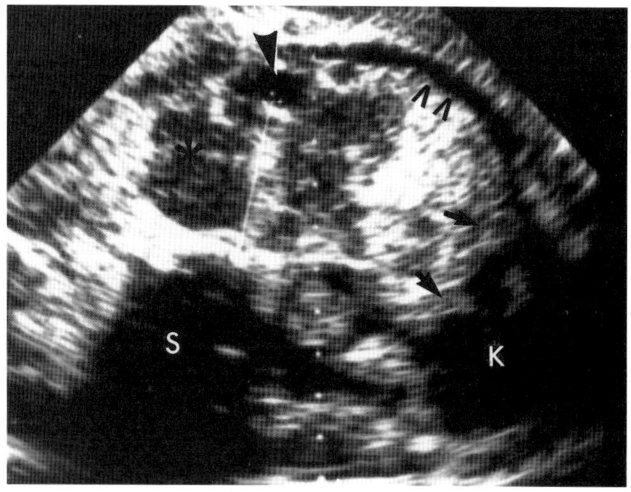

A

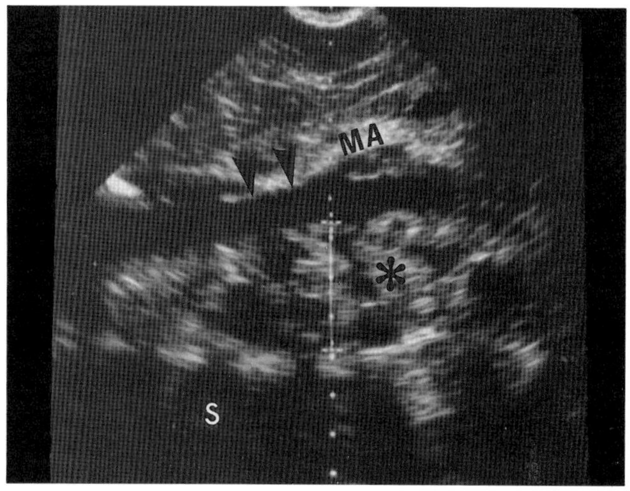

B

Figure 22.2

Paravertebral neuroblastoma (9-year-old): US axial view (**A**) and sagittal view (**B**). There is a laterovertebral mass (arrows) displacing the kidney (K) with prevertebral adenopathies (asterisk). S, lumbar spine; closed arrowhead, aorta; open arrowhead; splenic vein; MA, mesenteric artery.

highly echoic areas, of which certain have a posterior acoustic shadow that corresponds to calcifications; only rarely are there liquid plaques within the tumor. Higher up, the diaphragm is often involved and, within it, the tumor is badly defined and infiltrates the large vessels, often extending across the midline. It is often difficult to distinguish primary tumoral extension from adenopathies (Figure 22.2).[26]

Computed tomography findings

On a CT scan without injection of contrast material, the solid calcified mass infiltrates adjacent structures.[27,28] The tumor is rarely cystic.[29] It may be lateral in the case of primary surrenal involvement (Figure 22.3), laterorachidian in case of laterovertebral sympathetic involvement, or median, prevertebral and perivascular. Intrarachidian extradural extensions of laterovertebral tumors can also be partially calcified. With intravenous bolus injections of contrast material, the enhanced density of the tumor is usually heterogeneous, and this enhancement increases with the amount of contrast material injected and over time. It thus becomes possible to identify the vascular relations of the tumor, as well as relations with surrounding organs—the kidneys, the posterior surface of the liver to the right and the tail of the pancreas to the left, as well as the crura of the diaphragm (Figure 22.3). The CT scan also defines lymph-node extensions towards the posterior inframediastinal space (Figure 22.4) and lumboaortic and iliac chains. Intrarachidian extensions pass through the intravertebral foramina in an extradural situation and are caused by paravertebral tumors. This involvement is shown by CT after an intravenous injection of contrast material.[30] Intrarachidian tumoral extension appears dense in comparison with the meningeal sheaths (Figures 22.5 and 22.6).

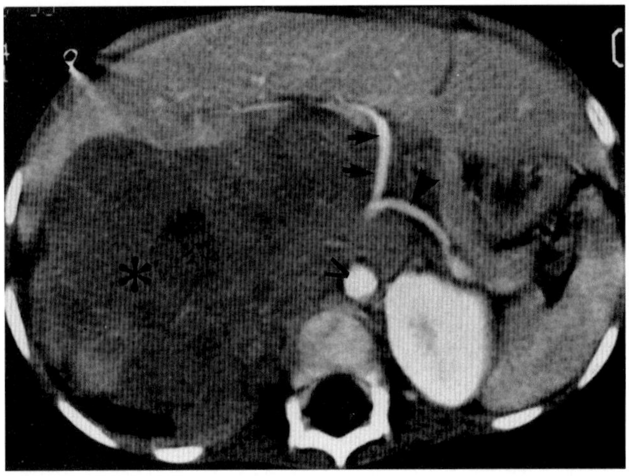

A

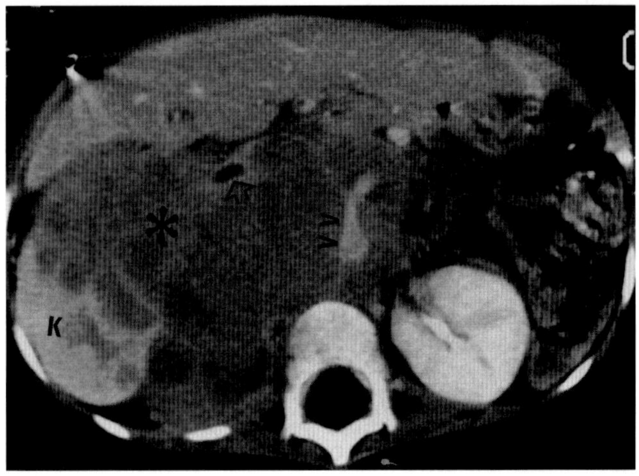

B

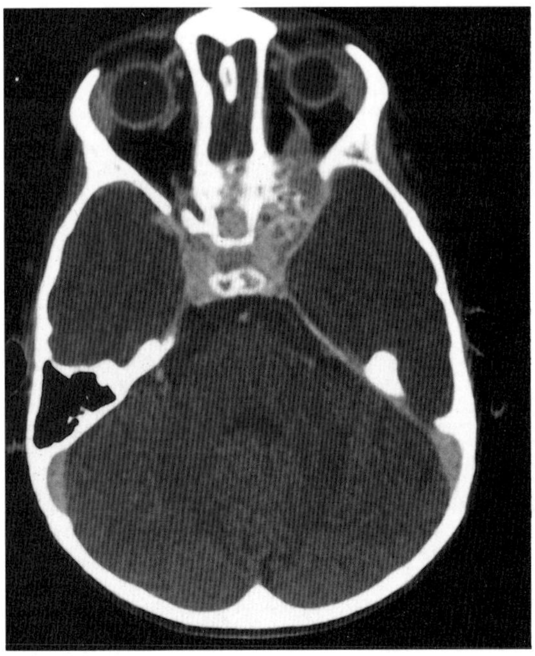

C

Figure 22.3

Right adrenal neuroblastoma (3-year-old): CT scan with iodine contrast bolus injection.

A Retrohepatic heterogeneous mass (asterisk) extended to the prevertebral space involving the celiac trunk and its collaterals.

B The upper pole of the right kidney (K) is invaded and there is thrombosis of the inferior vena cava (open arrow).

C At the level of the base of the skull bone metastases involve the left optic nerve.

Closed arrows, hepatic artery; closed arrowhead, splenic artery; open arrowheads, aorta and mesenteric artery.

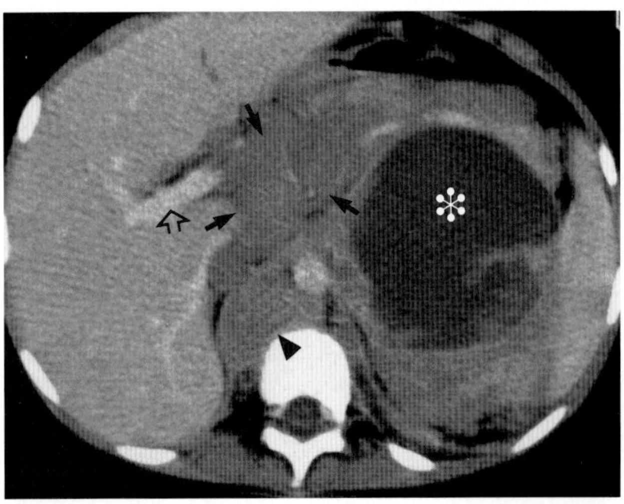

Figure 22.4

Left adrenal neuroblastoma (9-year-old): CT scan with iodine contrast bolus injection shows a cystic and solid mass (asterisk) with prevertebral (closed arrows) and retrocrural adenopathies (closed arrowhead). Open arrow, portal vein.

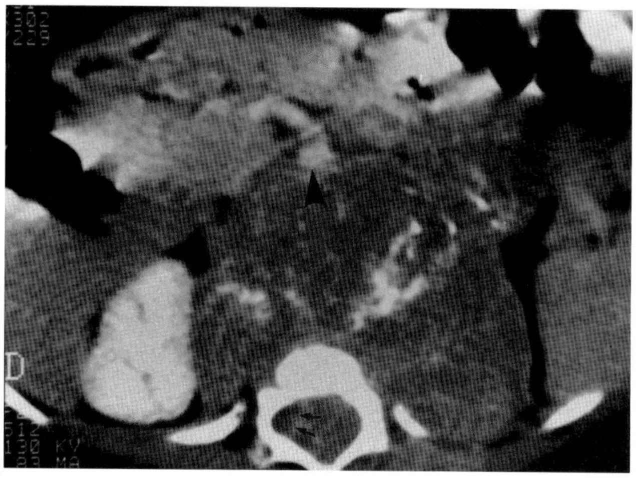

Figure 22.5

Neuroblastoma (2-year-old): CT scan with iodine contrast bolus injection shows a perivertebral calcified mass with compression of the dural sac by intraspinal spread (arrows). Arrowhead, abdominal aorta.

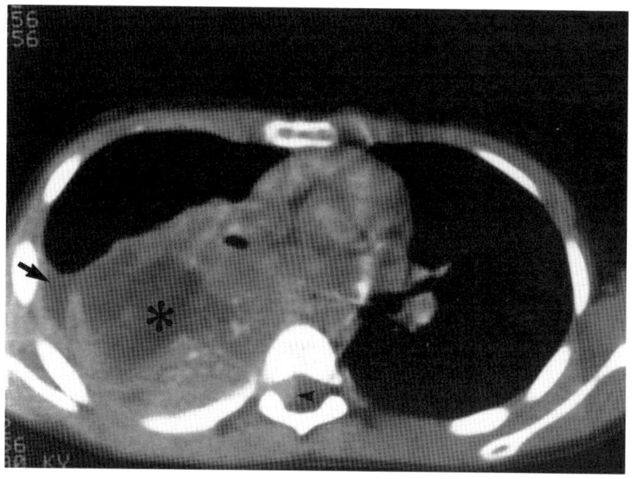

Figure 22.6

Thoracic neuroblastoma (10-year-old): CT scan after contrast injection shows a heterogeneous hypodense and calcified mediastinal mass (asterisk) with minimal pleural effusion (arrow) and hyperdense intraspinal extension (arrowhead).

Magnetic resonance imaging findings

Intraspinal extradural extensions are best studied with MR.[24,25] MR with spin echo in T1 allows an anatomic approach to tumoral relations and lymph-node extensions which is simpler and more exact than with CT,[31] as it does not require an intravenous injection of contrast material and facilitates a multidirectional study (Figure 22.7). Extradural extension is clearly visualized (Figure 22.8); this helps an understanding of why CT should be replaced by MR in the assessment of neuroblastomas.

The appearance is that of a tumoral mass with a heterogeneous hyposignal in T1-weighted sequences, due to calcifications, blood and tumoral tissue rich in cells (Figure 22.7). In T2-weighted sequences, the tumor signal is heterogeneously improved, whereas after an intravenous injection of gadolinium, the lesion has a relatively homogenous hypersignal which is sometimes difficult to distinguish from retroperitoneal fat. MR should be useful in detecting foci of bone and bone-marrow metastases; these require a specific treatment,[32,33] i.e. surgery for compressive vertebral bone metastases on the spinal cord (Figure 22.9), or radiotherapy to avoid blindness secondary to metastases of the base of the skull.

Scintigraphic findings

Scintigraphy with m-IBG (benzoguanidine labelled with iodine-123 or -131, which has a special affinity for neuroblastic tissue) gives an overall image of neuroblastic disease, depicting the primary tumor and metastatic diffusion.[26,34,35] Fixation of m-IGB takes place on the tumor and its metastatic extensions when the neuroblastoma secretes catecholamines. This examination has replaced both bone scintigraphy, which has less sensitivity, and bone radiography. It is useful in diagnosis, as well as in the assessment of metastatic extensions, along with medullograms and follow up during and after the termination of treatment (Figure 22.10).

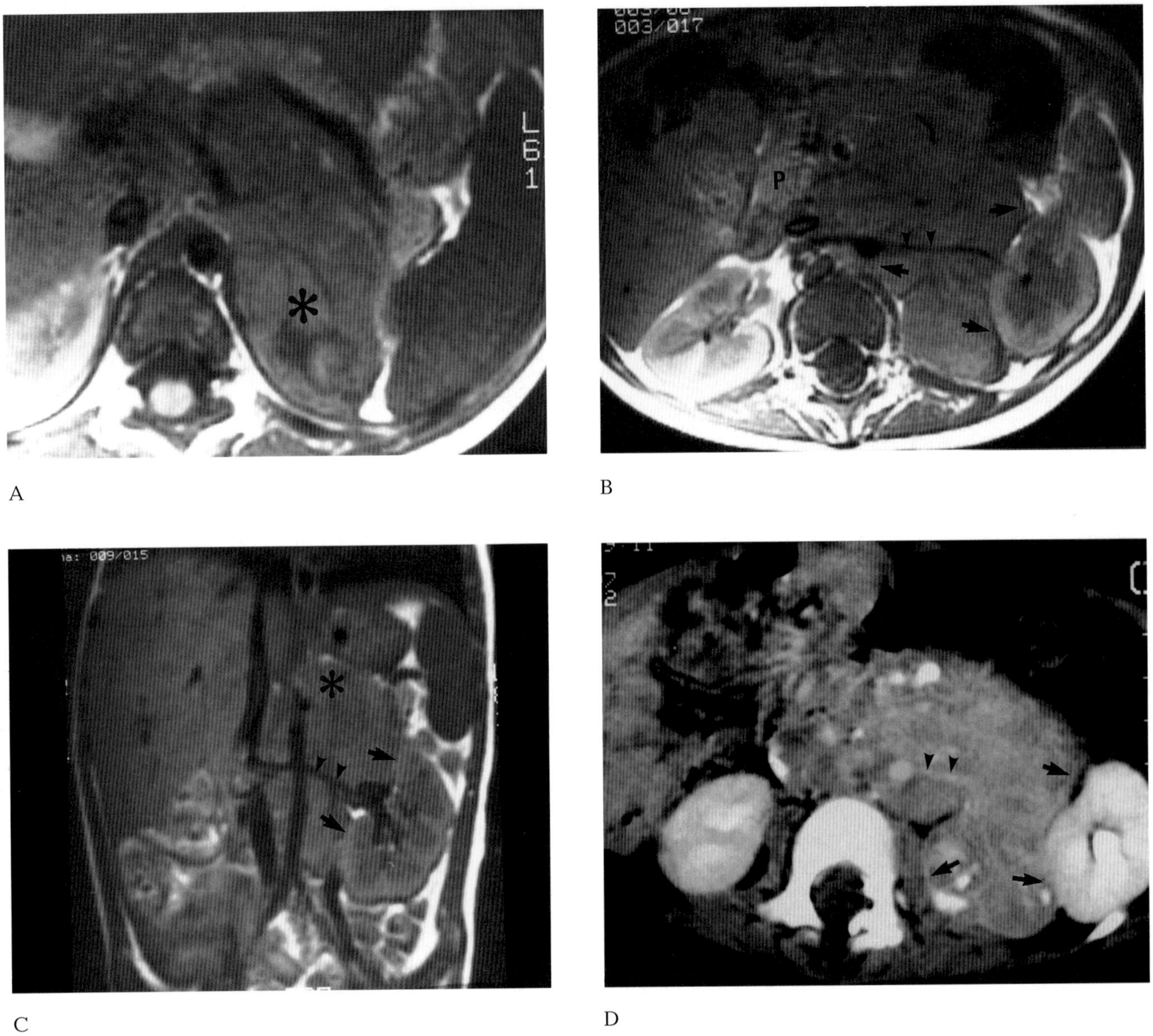

Figure 22.7

Neuroblastoma (2-year-old): (**A–C**) MR (600–800 ms, 20 ms) in axial (**A, B**) and coronal (**C**) view demonstrates a hypointense left adrenal mass (asterisk) with pararenal and periaortic adenopathies (arrows).

D In comparison, axial CT scan is less informative about the tumor's relationship with the vessels, but calcifications are better visualized.

P, head of the pancreas; arrowheads, left renal artery.

Follow up

Follow up during treatment is carried out with US examinations to verify the reduction in the size of the primary tumor by chemotherapy. Any decision to use extirpative surgery on the primary tumor after treatment should be preceded by CT or MR. A further post-operative CT scan should be carried out to check for persistent residual neuroblastic tissue,[26,36] in addition to m-IBG scintigraphy (Figure 22.11). At this stage, CT is sometimes preferable to MR, because of the better detection of calcified abdominal lesions. However, MR may be more precise for an uncalcified persistent mass (Figure 22.12). See Diagram 22.5.

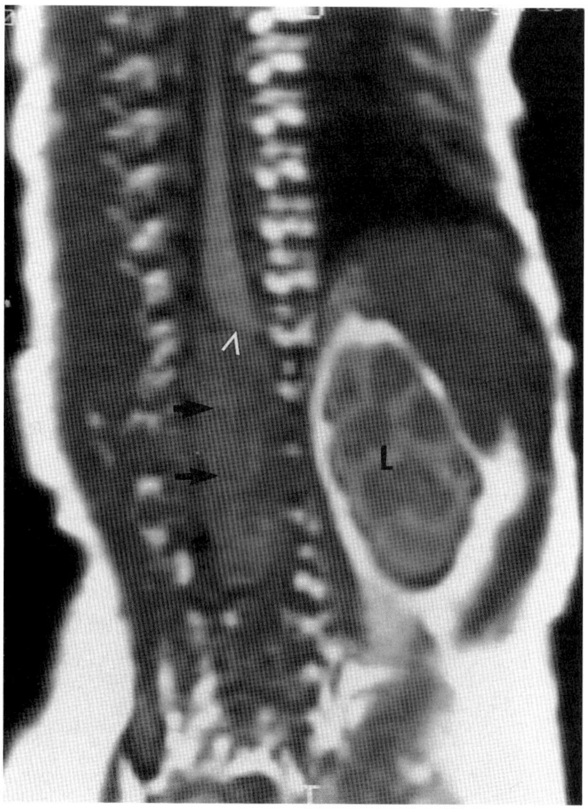

A

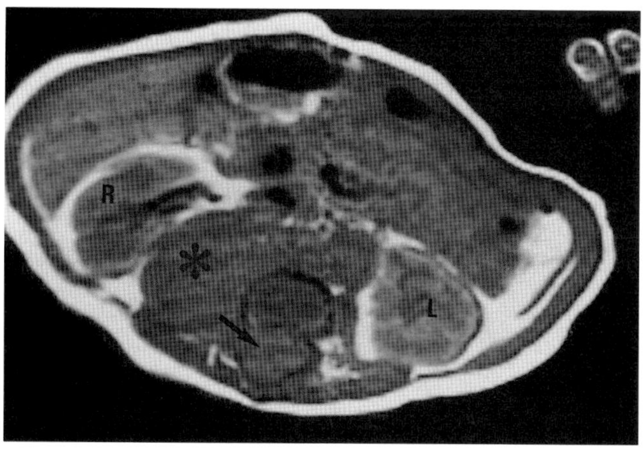

B

Figure 22.8

Paravertebral neuroblastoma (3-month-old): MR (600 ms, 20 ms) in coronal (**A**) and axial (**B**) views. There is a right paravertebral mass (asterisk) with intraspinal extension (arrows). Open arrowhead, spinal cord; R, right kidney; L, left kidney.

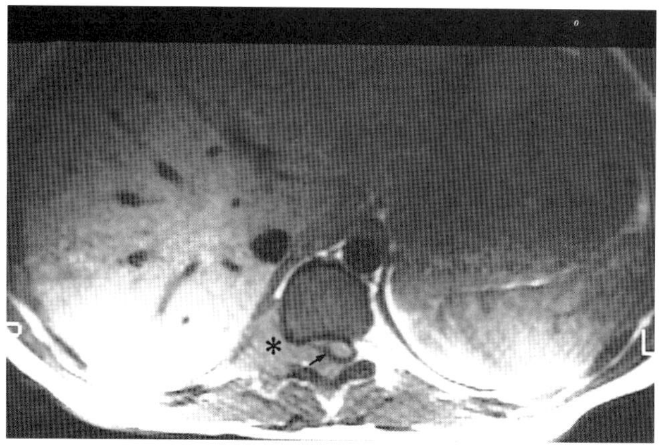

A

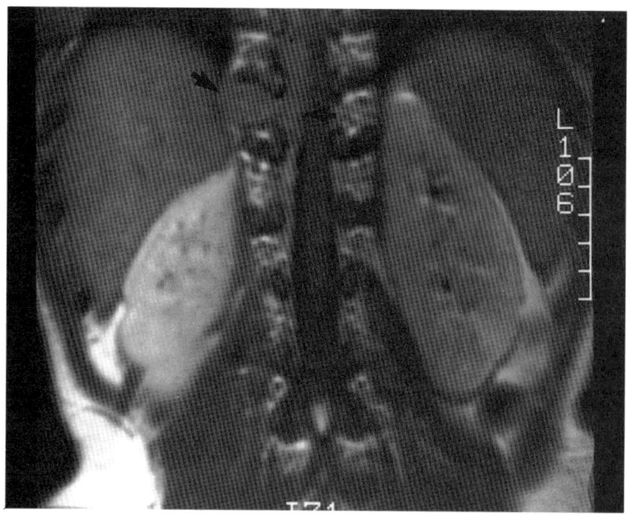

B

Figure 22.9

Pre-aortic neuroblastoma stage IV (10-year-old): MR (600–800 ms, 20 ms) of pyramidal syndrome.

A Axial view without gadolinium injection: there are bone metastases of the right dorsal pedicle with a hypointense soft tissue mass which fills in the foramen (asterisk) and displaces the spinal cord (arrow).

B Coronal view after gadolinium injection: there is moderate enhancement of the soft tissue mass which occupies the foramen (arrows).

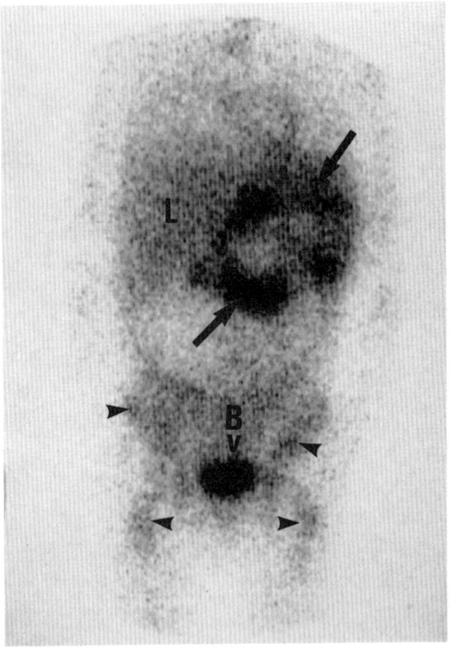

Figure 22.10

Left adrenal neuroblastoma (5-year-old), initial staging: m-IBG scintigraphy (coronal view) shows heterogeneous uptake of the primary tumor (arrows), diffuse uptake of the bone marrow (arrowheads): bone-marrow metastases. L, physiologic liver uptake; B, bladder.

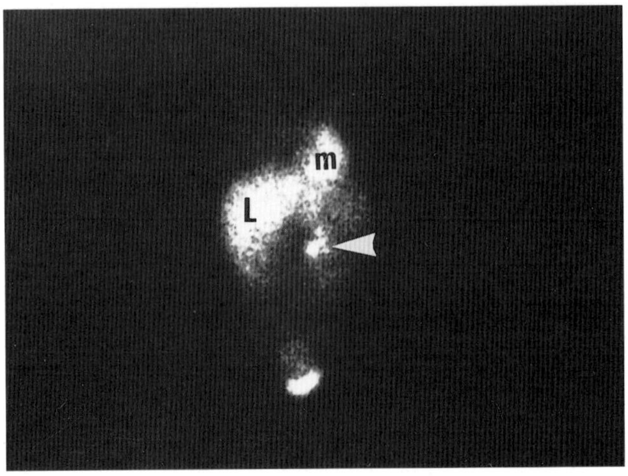

A

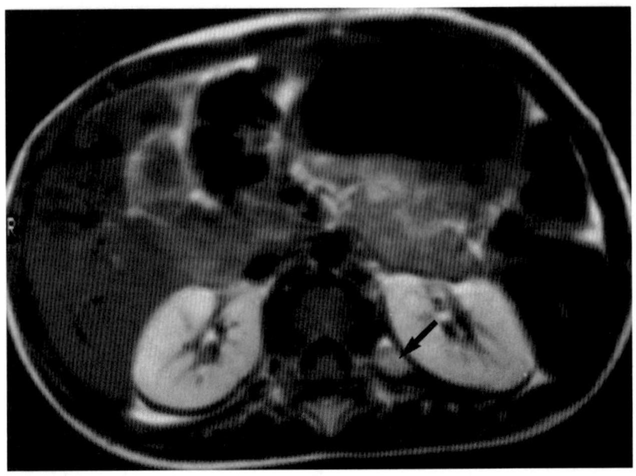

C

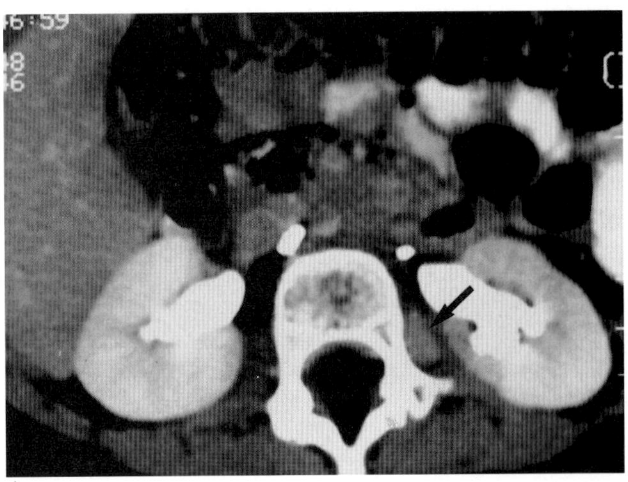

B

Figure 22.11

Post-surgical follow up of a laterovertebral neuroblastoma (4-year-old).

A m-IBG scintigraphy: left laterovertebral persistent uptake (arrowhead); L, physiologic liver uptake; m, myocardial uptake;

B CT scan with high-dose contrast injection (3–4 ml/kg of a hypo-osmolar iodinated contrast) shows a hyperdense residual mass (arrow) underlying at the psoas muscle.

C MR (700 ms, 30 ms) with gadolinium injection shows a hyperintense nodule close to the left kidney and vertebral pedicle (arrow).

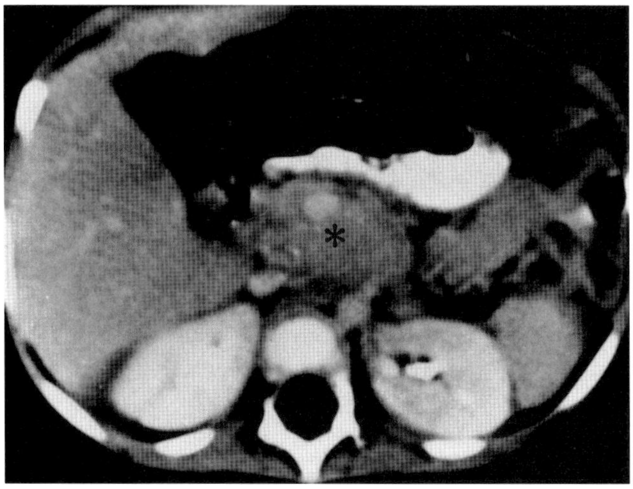

A

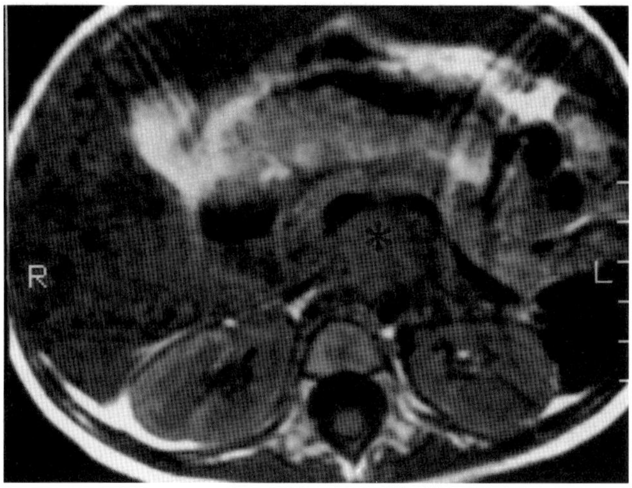

B

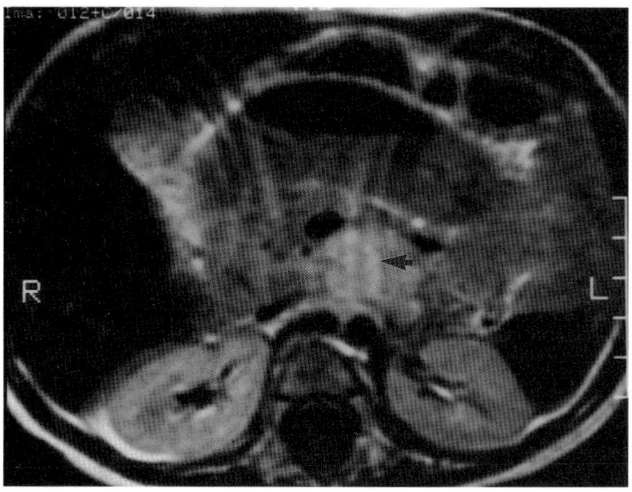

C

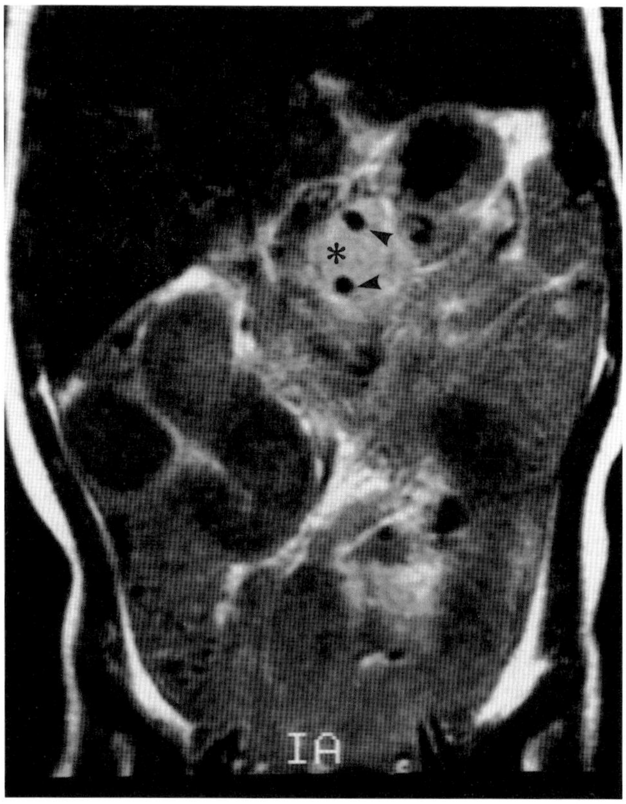

D

Figure 22.12

Post-operative follow up (3-year-old) for a stage III left adrenal neuroblastoma.

A Axial CT scan shows a persistent pre-aortic mass (asterisk).

B MR (600 ms, 20 ms) axial view without contrast material shows a hypointense persistent pre-aortic and retropancreatic mass (asterisk).

C,D Axial and coronal MR after gadolinium injection shows a hyperintense persistent tumor (arrow) with encasement (asterisk) of the superior mesenteric and celiac arteries (arrowheads).

Pepper's syndrome and neonatal forms

Pepper's syndrome: neuroblastomas in children in their first year have a better prognosis at all stages than in older children.[37] They are frequently revealed by a metastatic hypoechoic bulky hepatomegaly, which is more often infiltrating than nodular (stage IVs). CT shows a heterogeneous liver before injection of contrast material, with plaques of tumoral infiltration closely intermingled with healthy sections of the liver which has a higher density. This appearance is lost after the intravenous injection of contrast material (Figure 22.13). The main aim is to find the small primary adrenal tumor, which may be missed with US and require careful CT (Figures 22.13 and 22.14).

Neonatal tumors are often cystic and can be confused with adrenal hematoma.[38] The absence of tumoral regression or the presence of tumoral growth after two successive US examinations with 2-week interval between, or a rise in urinary catecholamines, leads to the diagnosis of the neuroblastoma.

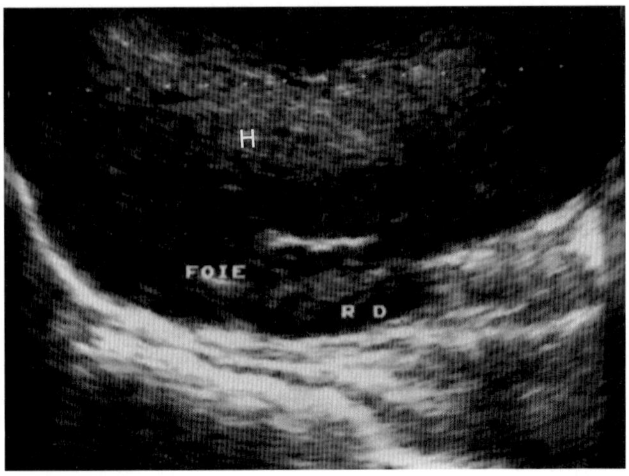

A

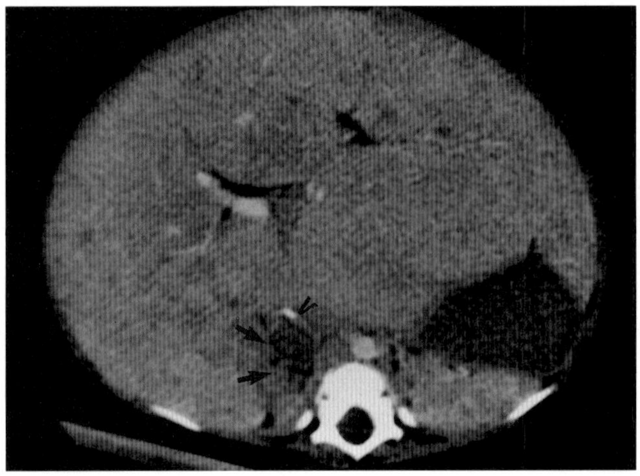

C

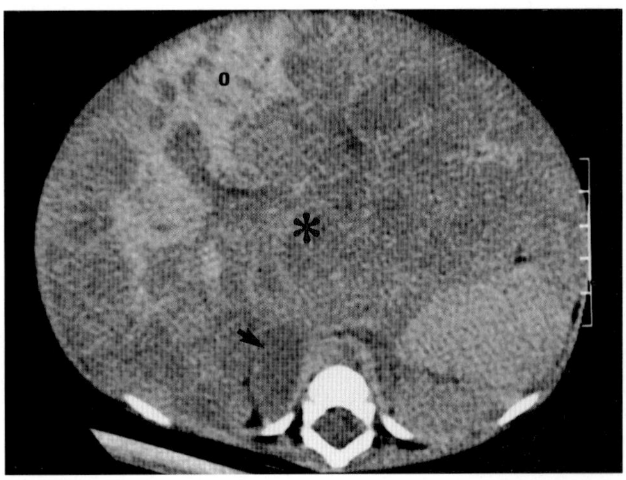

B

Figure 22.13

Pepper's syndrome (4-month-old).

A Longitudinal ultrasonography demonstrates bulky hepatomegaly (H); RD, right kidney.

B CT scan without contrast injection demonstrates heterogeneous hepatomegaly with mixed hypodense (asterisk) and isodense (open circle) liver; the arrow indicates a right adrenal mass.

C In a CT scan with contrast injection the liver abnormalities are obscured; closed arrow, hypodense right adrenal primary tumor; open arrowhead, inferior vena cava.

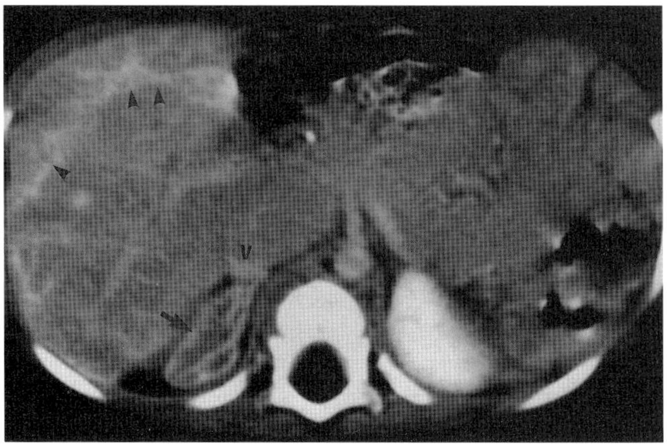

Figure 22.14

Pepper's syndrome, post-chemotherapeutic follow up (12-month-old). CT scan before surgery with bolus injection demonstrates heterogeneous liver with hyperdense bundles (closed arrowheads) corresponding to the fibrosis which replaces the metastatic neuroblastic infiltration; there is a right adrenal neuroblastoma (closed arrow). Open arrowhead, inferior vena cava.

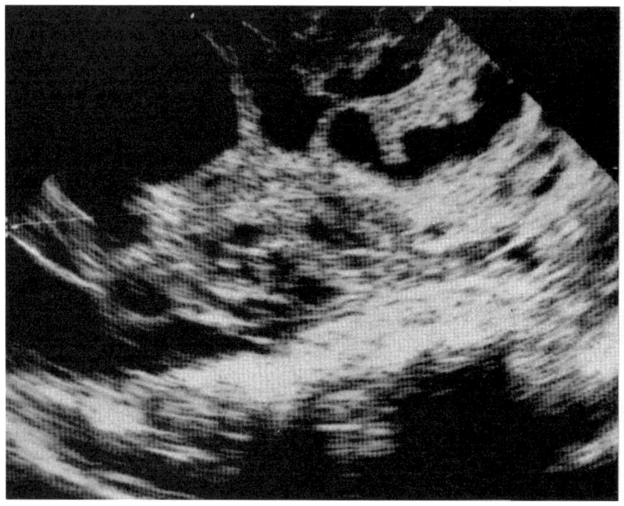

A

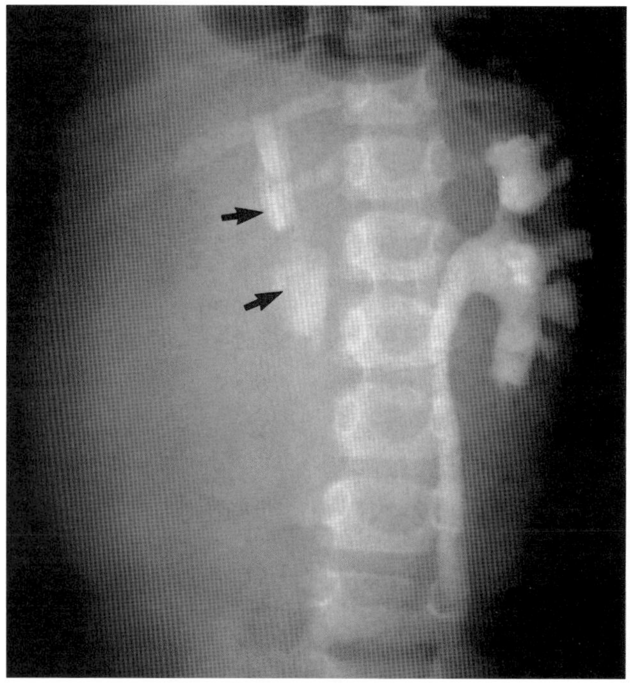

B

Figure 22.15

Abdominal mass (7-year-old).

A US (transverse view) shows a large cystic and solid mass.

B On IVP, a large space-occupying lesion compressing and distorting the calyces (arrows) is seen. It corresponds with a tumoral infiltration of the right kidney disordering the right excretory anatomy.

The diagnosis was a nephroblastoma; the left ureterohydronephrosis was due to an intraperitoneal extension of the tumor.

Tumors of the kidney

Nephroblastomas (Wilms' tumors) are the most common malignant tumors of the kidney. They occur as 5–7 cases per million children, and are the fourth most common tumor in children after tumors of the central nervous system, malignant lymphomas and neuroblastomas. They are highly chemo- and radiosensitive. Other types of malignant tumors of the kidney are rare in children. They are either anaplasic (Beckwith's tumor), sarcomatous or rhabdoid forms of nephroblastomas with unfavorable prognosis,[39] representing 10–12% of cases, or they are adult forms of carcinoma, such as Grawitz's tumor in older children. Histologically, nephroblastomas have three tissue components: undifferentiated blastomatous tissue, tissue with epithelial differentiation with glomerular or tubular rudiments, and tissue with mesenchymal fibroblastic and muscular differentiation.[10]

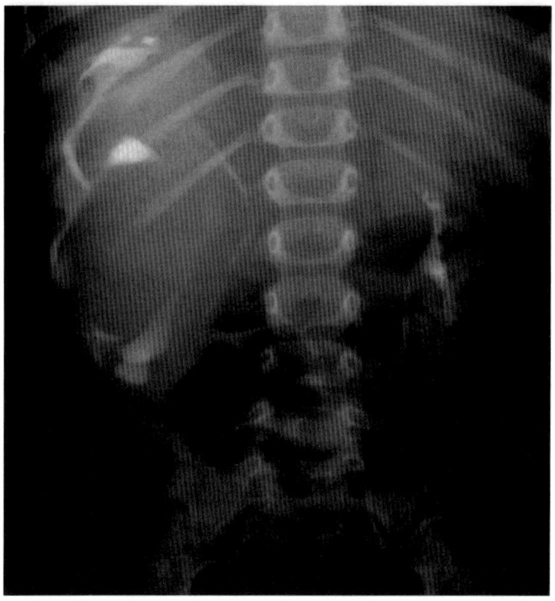

Figure 22.16

Wilms' tumor of the right kidney (3-year-old): IVP, anteroposterior view. There is distortion of right pelvis and calyces by a large tumor. The left kidney is normal.

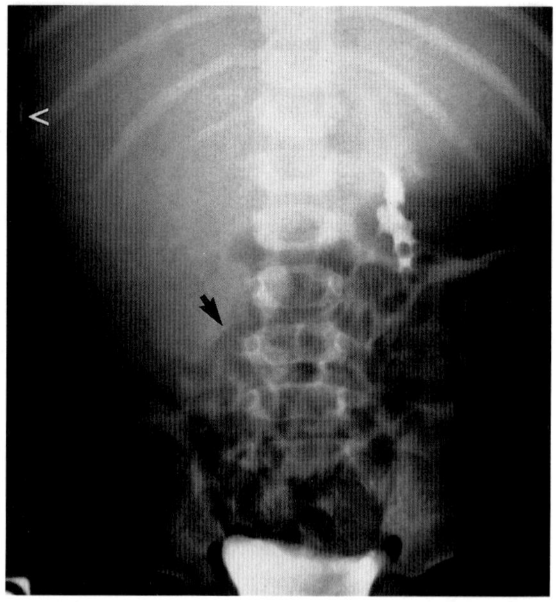

A

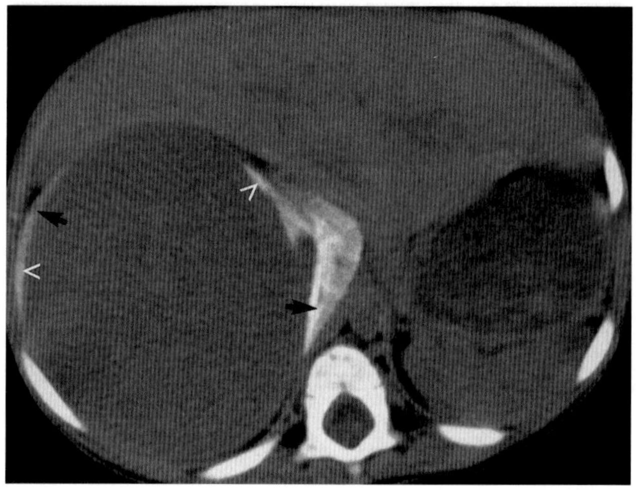

B

Figure 22.17

Right abdominal mass (17-month-old).

A IVP shows displacement of the digestive loops (closed arrow); there is minimal opacification of distorted calyces (open arrowhead).

B CT scan with contrast material demonstrates a large solid mass surrounded by residual renal parenchyma (closed arrows) with distorted opacified calyces (open arrowheads). No metastatic lymph nodes are present in the prevertebral space.

The diagnosis is nephroblastoma.

These tumors are observed mainly in children of 1–5 years of age. Discovery is usually linked to their size—a palpable mass is discovered by chance or during a physical examination—abdominal pain or, less often, hematuria.[21] They are often associated with certain congenital malformations such as aniridia, corporal hemihypertrophia, Wiedemann–Beckwith syndrome, etc.[4,5]

Imaging

US and IVP show a retroperitoneal intrarenal tumoral syndrome disorganizing the pyelocalycial cavities; it is often solid or a mixture of cystic and solid (Figures 22.15 and 22.16). The diagnosis of nephroblastoma is confirmed by CT and US.[40–44]

Bone metastases are among those nephroblastomas with a poor prognosis (sarcomatous or of anaplastic histology).

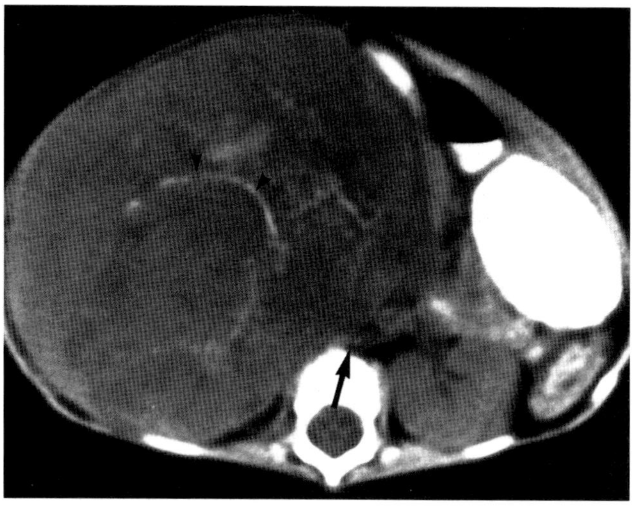

Figure 22.18

Right Wilms' tumor (16-month-old): CT scan without contrast material. There is a large solid mass with rounded calcifications (arrowheads) and no midline adenopathy (arrow).

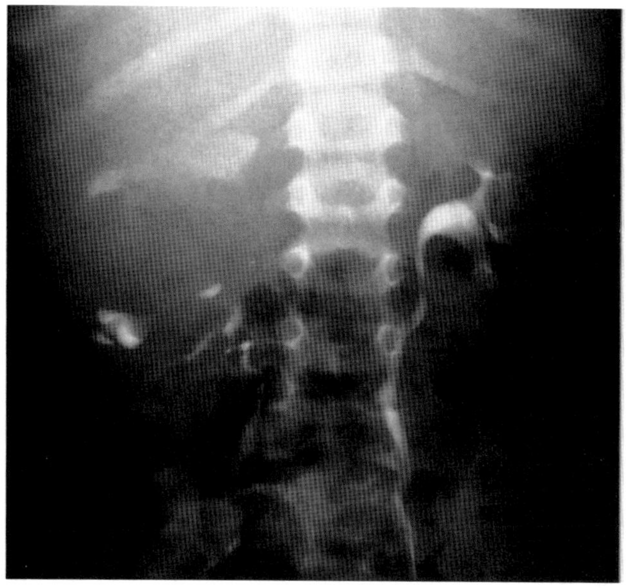

A

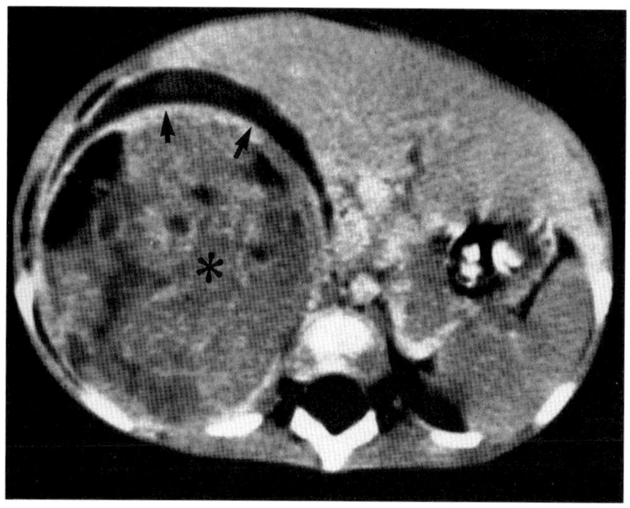

B

Figure 22.19

Right lumbar pain with abdominal mass (3-year-old).

A Excretory urogram shows right renal enlargement and disorganization of the calyces.

B CT scan with contrast material demonstrates a predominantly solid heterogeneous mass (asterisk), with an anterior hypodense crescent-shaped image (arrows) corresponding to a fissuring nephroblastoma.

Indications for CT

Sometimes CT is particularly indicated. In the case of bulky tumors which completely destroy the structure of the kidney and if the organ of origin is difficult to determine, CT will show discrete opacification of calycial cavities, renal parenchyma partially encircling the kidney denoting its rupture due to rapid development of a tumoral mass, and the absence of calcifications and of lymph-node extensions towards the midline, in contrast to neuroblastomas (Figure 22.17).[43,44] Rarely calcifications may be encountered in the nephroblastoma, typically curvilinear calcifications (Figure 22.18).

In these difficult cases without biological markers, it is possible to perform a safe percutaneous fine-needle biopsy to obtain a histologic specimen. This biopsy must be performed by a posterior translumbar route.

In cases of suspected fissures or tumoral rupture suggested by lumbar pains and acute anemia, CT may identify a crescent-shaped hypodensity around the tumor, fissures (Figure 22.19) (at a later stage with hematic accumulation in the

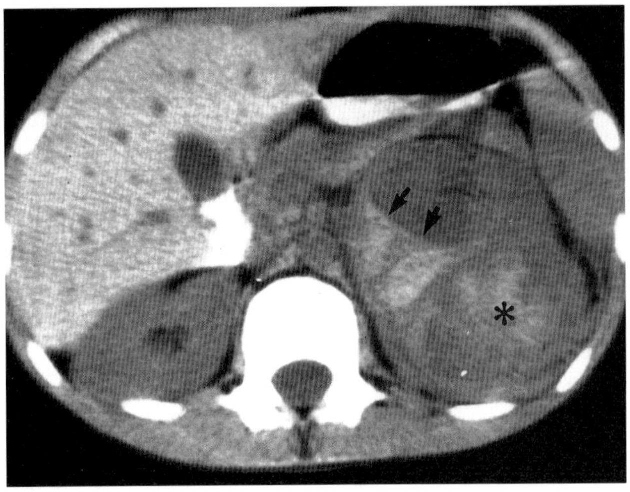

A

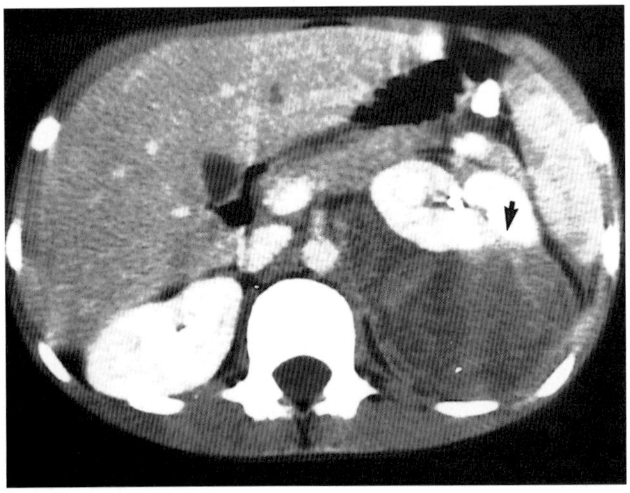

B

Figure 22.20

Left lumbar pain and anemia following a mild abdominal trauma (9-year-old).

A CT scan without contrast material shows a heterogeneous hyperdense retrorenal space-occupying lesion consisting of a hemorrhagic deposit (arrows) outlining the left kidney and a mass which occupies the perinephric space (asterisk).

B After contrast injection, note the rupture of the posterior cortical margin of the left kidney (arrow) by the tumoral process.

A surgical diagnosis of hemorrhagic nephroblastoma was made.

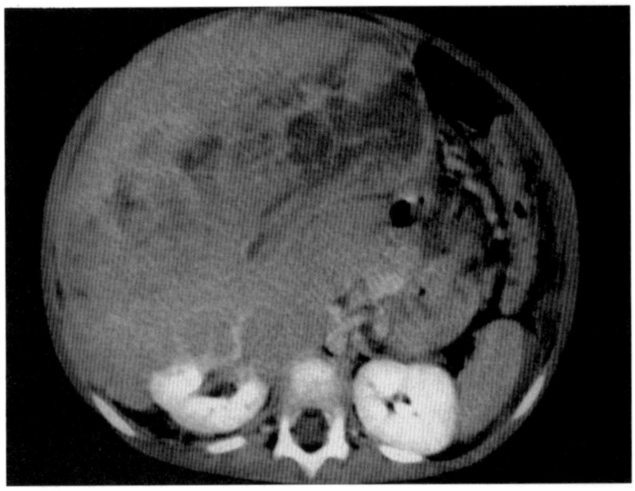

A

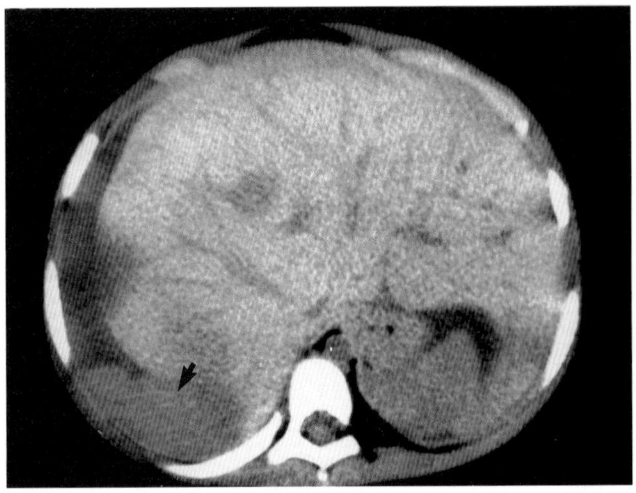

B

Figure 22.21

Right nephroblastoma (3-year-old): CT scan with contrast material.

A Destruction of the anterior part of the kidney, with a huge heterogeneous pseudocapsulated solid mass developing across the midline, without adenopathies.

B Ascites with a retrohepatic nodule (arrow), indicating a peritoneal diffusion.

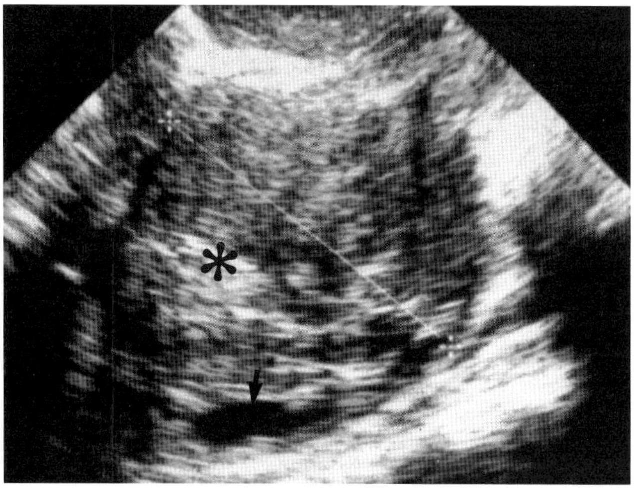

A

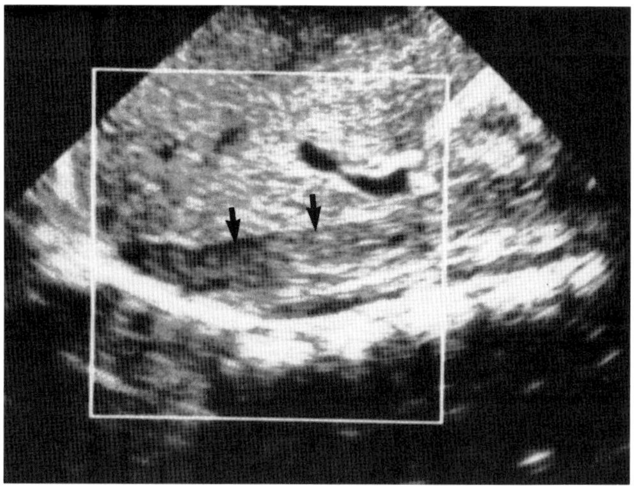

B

Figure 22.22

Nephroblastoma of the right kidney (6-year-old).

A US shows a heterogeneous hyper- and hypoechoic solid mass of the right kidney (asterisk), with distorted calyces (arrow).

B A longitudinal view through the inferior vena cava demonstrates enlargement and echoic lumen of the inferior vena cava (arrows); tumoral thrombosis was diagnosed.

perinephric space), retroperitoneal rupture (Figure 22.20) and intraperitoneal rupture (Figure 22.21). It is useful to bear in mind these latter complications, as nephroblastomas are fragile and rupture can occur after a slight trauma as a revealing factor of the disease, or during chemotherapy.[12,21] In all cases, it necessitates urgent surgical intervention and, if rupture is intraperitoneal, the stage of the disease is aggravated.

CT is also indicated in cases of suspected bilateral nephroblastoma.[44]

Assessment of extensions

Abdominal ultrasound examinations are required to measure the size of the primary tumor and to estimate the liberty of the inferior vena cava, which may be the location of tumoral thrombus[45] (increase in the calibre of venous lumen and central hyperechogenicity) (Figure 22.22). Observation of the contralateral kidney is made to eliminate the possibility of bilateral nephroblastoma. A liver study eliminates possible liver metastases. In doubtful cases, CT should be performed.

Chest radiographs can reveal pulmonary metastatic nodules or, in rare cases, mediastinal adenopathies. CT can be useful in doubtful cases.

Bone metastases should only be investigated if there are clinical signs—by radionuclide scintigraphy and radiographs of the skeleton—since metastases are lytic and more often without osteoblastic activity.

Follow up

Follow up after surgery is carried out with abdominal US and chest radiographs, supplemented by CT in cases in which suspected recurrences at the site of a nephrectomy or in an intraperitoneal location are suspected.[48] Recurrences may be solid or cystic, like the primary tumor (Figures 22.23 to 22.25). Bilateral nephroblastomas represent approximately 5–7% of cases and are most often detected during diagnosis by US of both kidneys (Figures 22.26 and 22.27). This is one of the rare indications of pre-surgical angiography, in order to anticipate partial nephrectomy, which is indispensable to conservation of sufficient renal function while carrying out surgery which is carcinologically adequate.

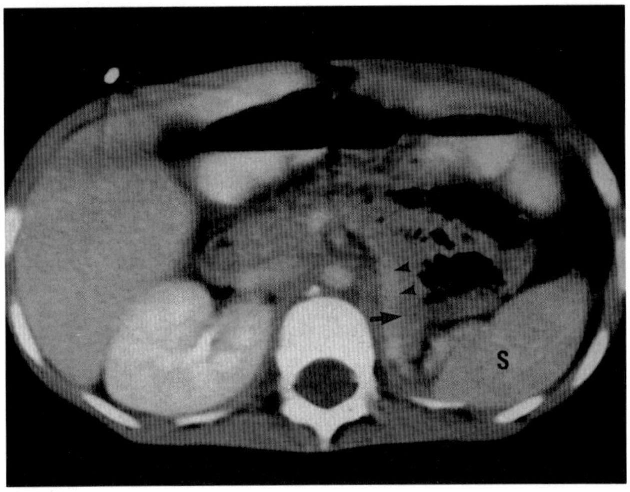

Figure 22.23

Left nephroblastoma, surgically resected (4-year-old): CT scan with contrast material. The renal fossae is occupied by the tail of the pancreas (arrow), splenic vessels (arrowheads) and digestive loops. S: spleen.

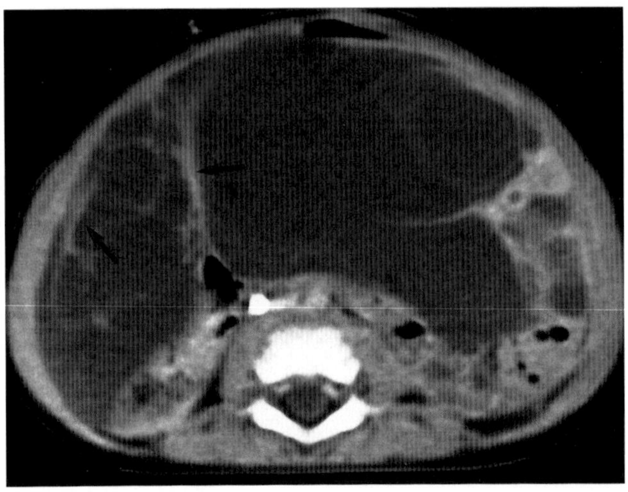

Figure 22.24

Intraperitoneal relapse of a left nephroblastoma (2-year-old): multiple cystic masses with thick edges (arrows) are seen.

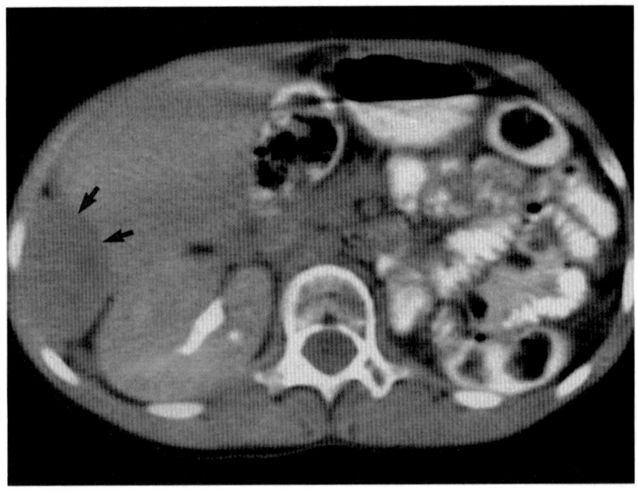

Figure 22.25

Intraperitoneal relapse of a surgically resected left Wilms' tumor (10-year-old). There is a solid mass close to the liver (arrows). The left lumbar fossae is occupied by digestive loops.

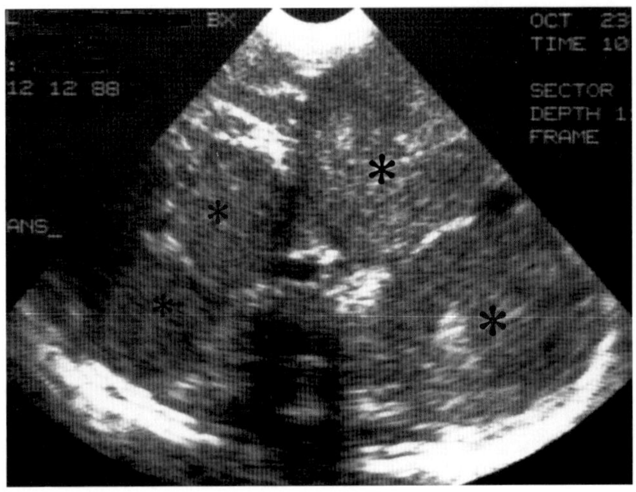

Figure 22.26

Bilateral nephroblastoma (10-month-old): US, transverse view. Multiple, solid space-occupying lesions distort both kidneys (asterisk). Courtesy of Professor F Diard, Bordeaux, France.

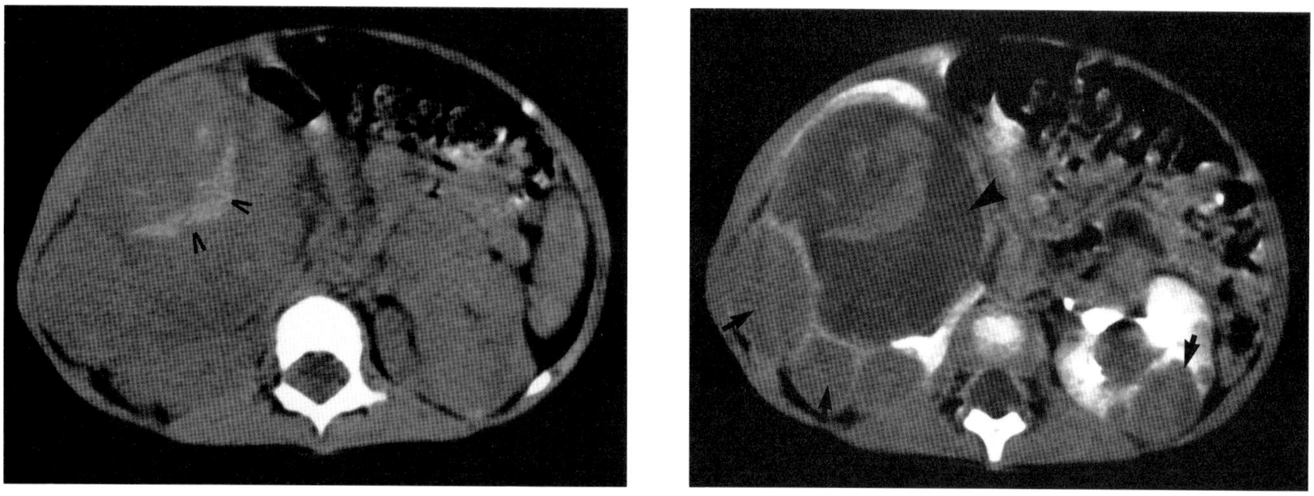

A B

Figure 22.27

Bilateral nephroblastoma (2.5-year-old).

A CT scan without contrast material shows enlarged kidneys with hyperdense hemorragic areas (open arrowheads) in the right side.

B After iodinated injection, multiple solid (arrows) and pseudo cystic (solid arrowhead) masses disorganizing the renal parenchyma and the calyces are seen.

Prognosis, staging and therapy

Prognostic factors are the stage (Table 22.9) and histology; the age of the patient and the size of the tumor were formerly considered to be prognostic factors but no longer appear significant in view of the efficiency of chemotherapy. Therapeutic decision trees (Diagram 22.6) are different in Europe and in the USA; children in the USA have initial surgery which establishes a histologic diagnosis, then polychemotherapy.[46] In Europe, chemotherapy is used first, to reduce the risk of tumoral rupture during surgery, which elevates the stage of the disease (Table 22.10), and surgery is

Table 22.9 Staging of nephroblastoma and 5-year disease-free survival.[a]

Stage	*Criterion*	*Survival (%)*
I	Tumor limited to kidney and completely excised without rupture of the renal capsule	86
II	Tumor extends beyond the kidney and completely excised: there is a local extension beyond the capsule into the perirenal soft tissues, or periaortic lymph node involvement; the renal vein is invaded outside the kidney	75
III	Incomplete excision: biopsy or ruptured tumor, or peritoneal implants or pathologic lymph nodes beyond the lumboaortic chains	66
IV	Hematogenous metastases (lung, liver, bone, brain)	48
V	Bilateral nephroblastoma	75

[a]Sixth study of International Society of Pediatric Oncology, 1980–7.[21]

Table 22.10 Tumoral rupture during surgery related to pre-surgical treatment.[21]

Pre-surgical treatment	*No. of cases*	*Percentage with rupture*	*P*
SIOP 1[a]			
20 Gy	73	4	0.01
None	63	32	
SIOP 2[a]			
20 Gy + actinomycin	85	5	0.0025
None	53	20	
SIOP 5[a]			
Chemotherapy	88	6	NS[b]
20 Gy + actinomycin	76	9	

[a]SIOP, International Society of Pediatric Oncology; first study, 1971–4; second study, 1974–6; fifth study, 1977–80.
[b]NS, not significant.

used after reduction by chemotherapy over 4–8 weeks. Children under 6 months of age undergo surgery immediately because of the higher frequency of mesoblastic nephroma, a benign tumor which cannot be differentiated from a nephroblastoma by imaging techniques,[47] at this age (33%). In all treatment plans, post-operative staging is fundamental and is based on the histologic analysis of the surgical sample, tumoral effraction of the renal capsule, invasion of perirenal fat, locoregional lymph-node involvement and the quality of surgical excision required to decide on the necessity of irradiation of the surgical site.

Nephroblastomatosis

Nephroblastomatosis is a nodular renal blastema, either subcapsular or a diffuse tumoral subcortical infiltrating mass which may be accompanied by a nephroblastoma, especially in bilateral forms. Histopathogenic relations between nephroblastomatosis and nephroblastoma are not yet clear; close, prolonged observation of the nephroblastomatosis is required to detect any eventual appearance of a nephroblastoma (Figure 22.28). CT is recommended. Experience with MR is limited to date but has given promising results.[49–51]

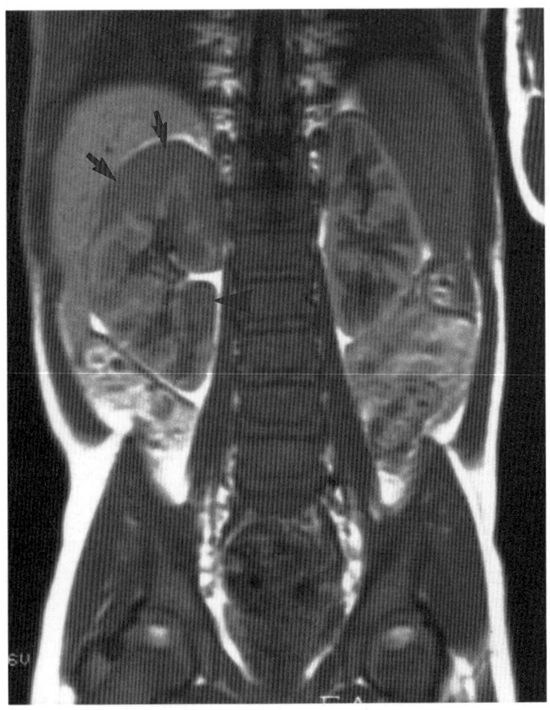

Figure 22.28

Nephroblastomatosis (2-year-old): MR, coronal view (380 ms, 25 ms). Cortical hypointense renal infiltration (arrows) is associated with a nodule (arrowhead). Courtesy of Dr S Neuenschwander, Paris, France.

Table 22.11 Clinical staging of non-Hodgkin's lymphoma (Murphy's classification), frequency and 5-year disease-free survival.[a]

Stage	*Criterion*	*Frequency (%)*	*Survival (%)*
I	One tumor or one lymph-node area (mediastinum or abdomen excluded)	8	100
II	One tumor with local lymph nodes Several lymph-node areas on the same side of diaphragm Resected intestinal tumor with one mesenteric lymph node	13	100
III	Tumor or lymph nodes on both sides of diaphragm Large thoracic tumor Large abdominal tumor Paraspinal tumor	48	75
IV	Any stage with cerebrospinal and/or bone marrow involvement	31	50

[a]Study, 1981–4.[21]

Adenocarcinoma of the kidney (hypernephroma, Grawitz's tumor)

In children adenocarcinoma of the kidney has the same histologic type as that in adults. Clinically, hematuria is more often observed. The child is usually older when the lesion is discovered, often in late childhood or adolescence, than in nephroblastoma. US shows a tumor that is often calcified and lumboaortic adenopathies. In the presence of one or several of these signs not corresponding to a nephroblastoma, CT is indispensable to assess lymph-node extension. Percutaneous fine-needle biopsy is carried out, either with ultrasound or with CT, using a translumbar approach, since the only possible treatment is surgery.

Non-Hodgkin's lymphomas

Malignant non-Hodgkin's lymphomas (NHL) in children can be differentiated histologically from those in adults because of the monomorphous nature of their cell proliferation: they are always diffuse and have a high grade of malignancy.[10] Clinically, they can be recognized because of the rapidity of tumoral growth, with early dissemination to the bone marrow and the central nervous system.[21,52] From an immunologic point of view, cell proliferation is either of the B-type (Burkitt's lymphomas) in an ENT or digestive location, or else of the T-type located in the mediastinum. Chemotherapy is the only possible treatment, with a global 5-year survival rate for all stages of 75%.[21,53] NHLs are rare before the age of 2 years and occur mainly towards 7 years. Discovery depends on their initial localization, but because of rapid tumoral growth, the mass is usually the revealing factor, accompanied by pain. A palpable abdominal mass or, less frequently, acute or subacute intestinal invagination in abdominal localizations, respiratory disorders in thoracic localizations, and cervical or jugal tumefaction and nasopharyngeal symptoms in ENT localizations, are the symptoms.

Medullar and neuromeningeal assessment is carried out by means of bone marrow aspirates and sampling of cerebrospinal fluid. Locoregional assessment with imaging remains simple, as prognosis depends on neuromeningeal and medullary involvement (Table 22.11) and the only possible treatment is chemotherapy; this should be instituted rapidly, as it is often urgent, especially in thoracic locations, because of the size of the tumoral mass and pericardial effusion.

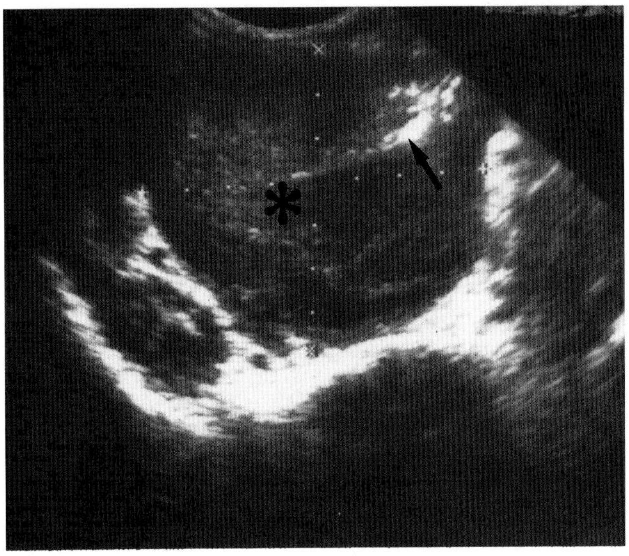

A

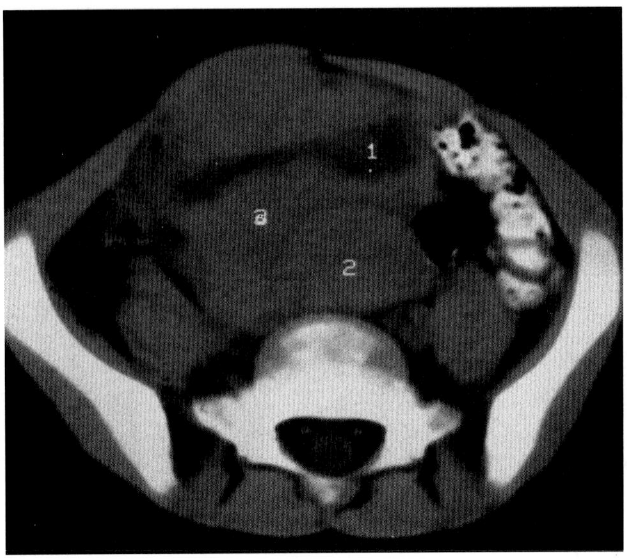

B

Figure 22.29

Large pelvic mass (6-year-old):

A US (transverse view) shows a hypoechoic mass (asterisk) targeted by a hyperechoic digestive loop (arrow).

B CT scan without contrast material shows the same lesion without any additional information.

A fine-needle biopsy demonstrated non-Hodgkin's lymphoma.

1, digestive loop; 2, lymphomatous lesion.

Imaging

In the most common abdominal forms (40%), abdominal US is usually used in order to detect lesions, guide percutaneous fine-needle biopsies and look for renal, hepatic and retroperitoneal lymph-node involvement.[54] Lymphomatous masses on US are characteristic, being solid and hypoechoic; target-like central hyperechogenicity is common and corresponds to the aerated intestinal lumen of these digestive lymphomas (Figure 22.29). They sometimes have an appearance of intestinal invagination, with multiconcentric hypoechoic rings surrounding a hyperechoic centre (Figure 22.30). Renal and hepatic lesions are also hypoechoic, nodular or infiltrating (Figures 22.31 and 22.32). CT is not considered useful except to investigate a bulky abdominal mass, which is difficult to study with US, or else to confirm renal involvement,[55] i.e. hypodense bilateral nodules, enlarged infiltrated kidney, adjacent involvement (Figures 22.33 and 22.34).

In the case of thoracic locations, plain chest radiography with films in different positions to detect pleural effusion, which is common, is carried out initially and guides the pleural puncture that leads to diagnosis (Figure 22.35). This is sufficient in most cases. US is used for bulky mediastinal masses to diagnose pericardial effusion. When there is no pleural effusion, CT is useful to guide a transthoracic fine-needle biopsy in order to obtain cytologic proof of the disease (Figure 22.36).

For cervical or ENT localizations, CT is useful to investigate any adjacent endocranial extensions and the consequences of the disease on the orbit, the cavum and the facial bones (Figures 22.36 and 22.37). (See Diagram 22.7.)

Follow up

Follow up during chemotherapy is undertaken with abdominal US and chest radiography. The regression of this tumor, which is extremely chemosensitive, can be spectacular, occurring even within a few days.

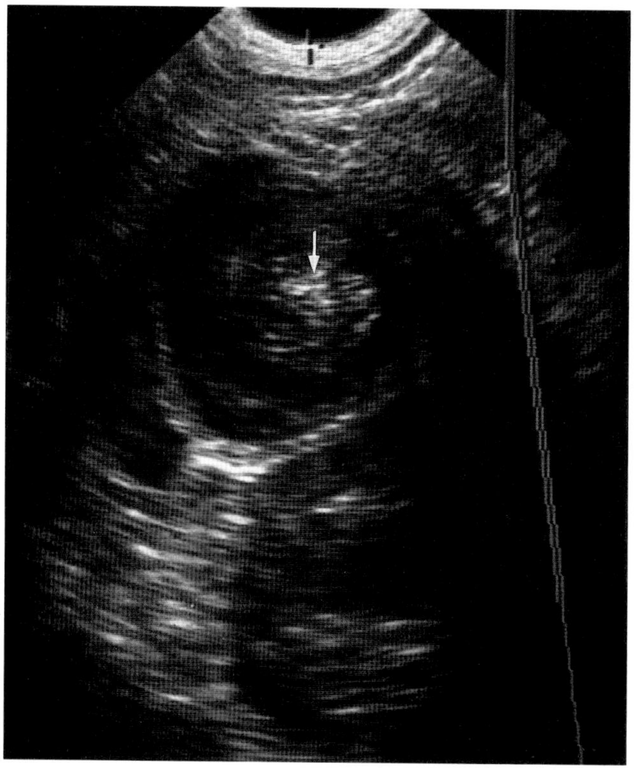

A

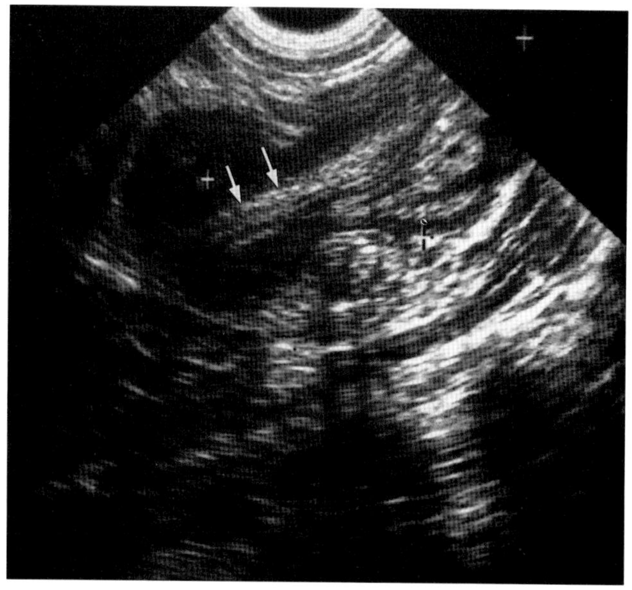

B

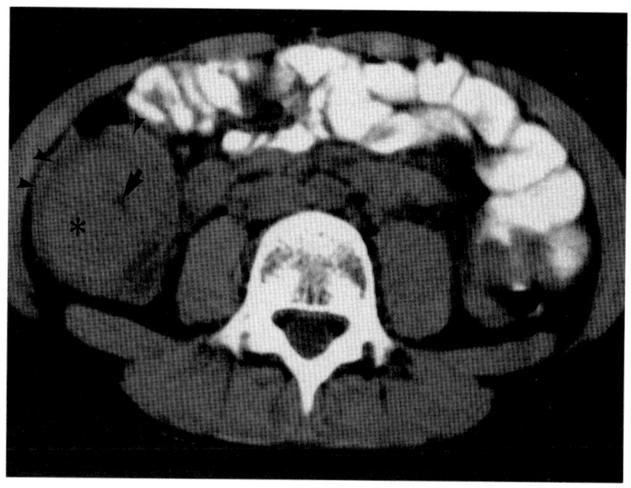

C

Figure 22.30

Subacute abdominal pain (13-year-old).

A,B US in transverse (**A**) and longitudinal (**B**) view: a hypoechogenic mass with multiconcentric rings is seen on the transverse view; the hyperechoic center corresponds to the digestive lumen (arrows): there is subacute intestinal invagination due to non-Hodgkin's lymphoma of the ileocecal junction.

C CT scan shows the invaginated digestive lumen (arrows) surrounded by lymphomatous infiltration (asterisk) and cecal wall (arrowheads).

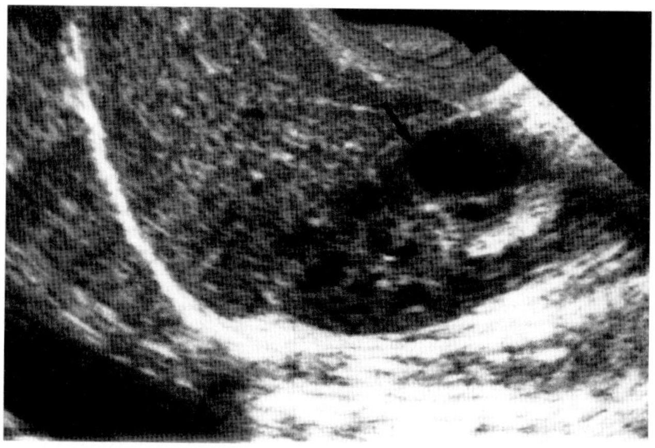

Figure 22.31

Abdominal non-Hodgkin's lymphoma (11-year-old): US, longitudinal view. There is a hypoechoic nodule in the right kidney (arrow).

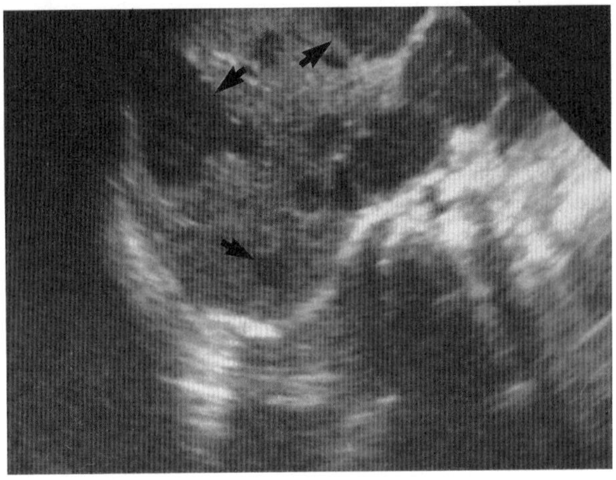

Figure 22.32

Abdominal non-Hodgkin's lymphoma stage IV (7-year-old): US, transverse view: multiple hypoechogenic nodules are seen in the liver (arrows).

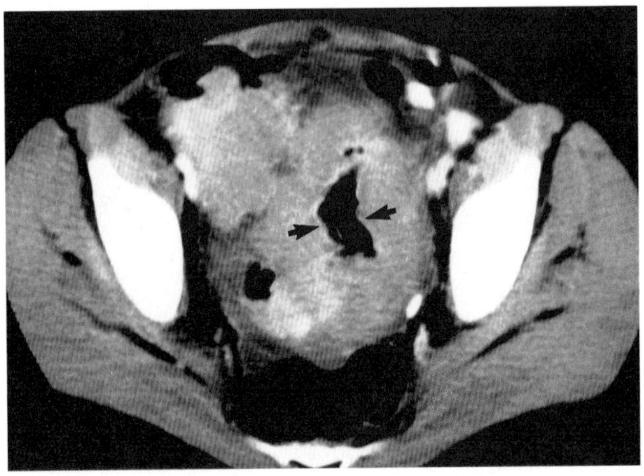

A

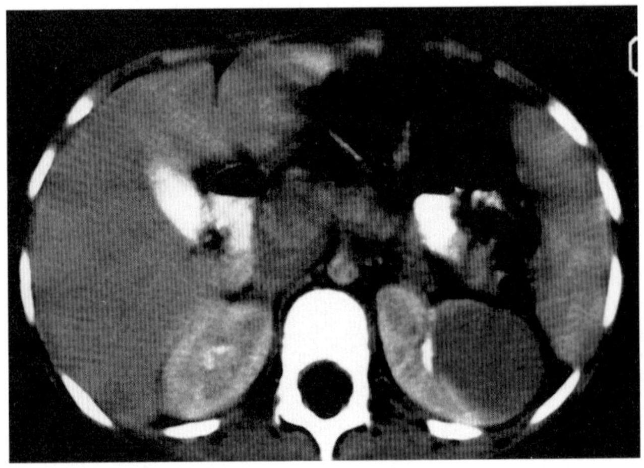

B

Figure 22.33

Abdominal non-Hodgkin's lymphoma (11-year-old): CT scan with iodine injection.

A A lymphomatous mass surrounds a digestive loop (arrows).

B There is a hypodense solid nodule of the left kidney.

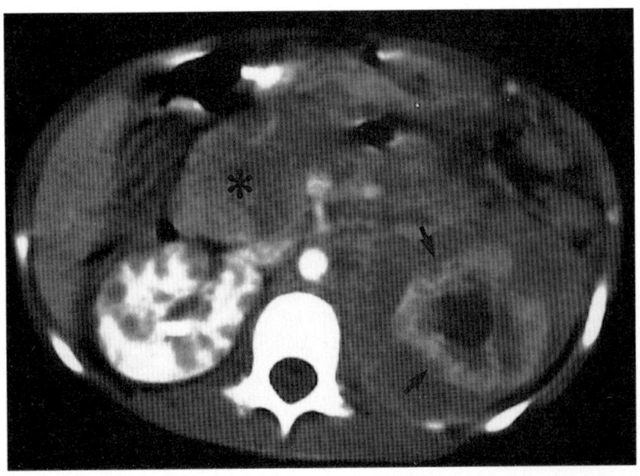

Figure 22.34

Abdominal non-Hodgkin's lymphoma, renal insufficiency (7-year-old): CT scan with contrast material. There is a mass infiltrating the head of the pancreas (asterisk), the left kidney (arrows) and the perinephric space. Multiple hypodense nodules are present in the right kidney which is obstructed.

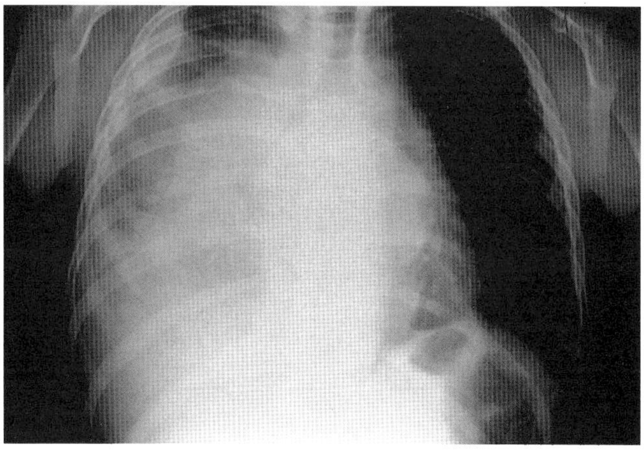

Figure 22.35

Enlarged mediastinum with right pleural effusion (12-year-old): chest radiograph. The diagnosis was established by pleural samplings as type-T non-Hodgkin's lymphoma.

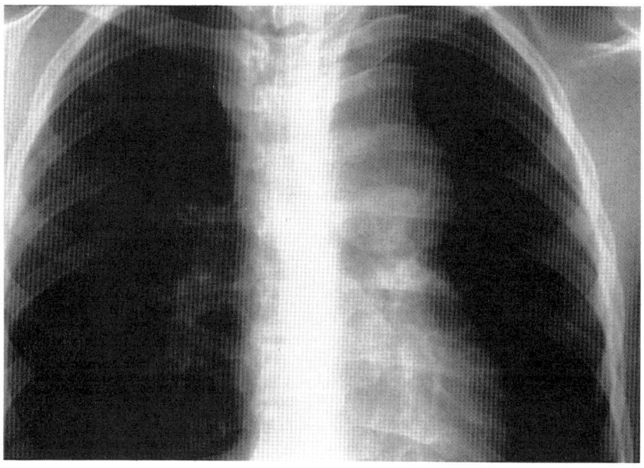

A

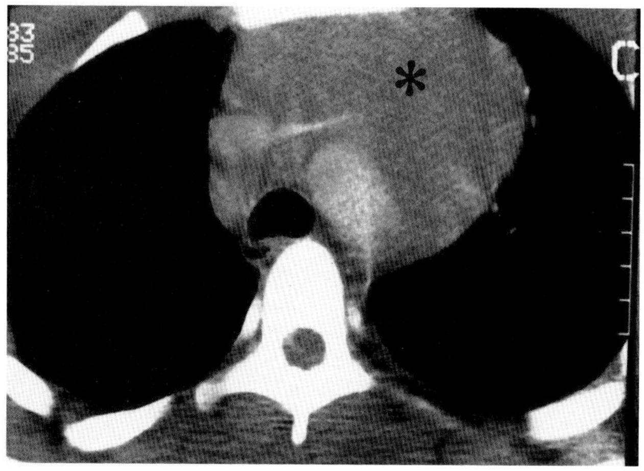

B

Figure 22.36

Type-T non-Hodgkin's lymphoma (15-year-old).

A Chest radiography demonstrates an enlarged mediastinum.

B CT scan with contrast material shows a solid mass occupying the thymic area (asterisk).

Fine-needle biopsy confirmed type-T non-Hodgkin's lymphoma.

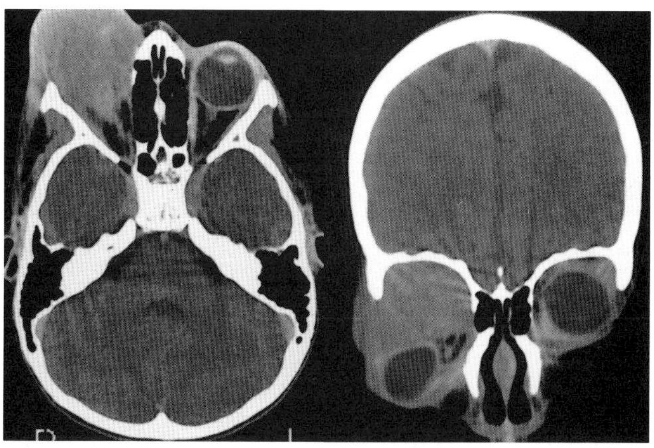

A B

Figure 22.37

Non-Hodgkin's lymphoma of the orbit (7-year-old): CT scan, axial (**A**) and coronal (**B**) views. There is a large space-occupying process displacing the eyeball downward, without endocranial extension.

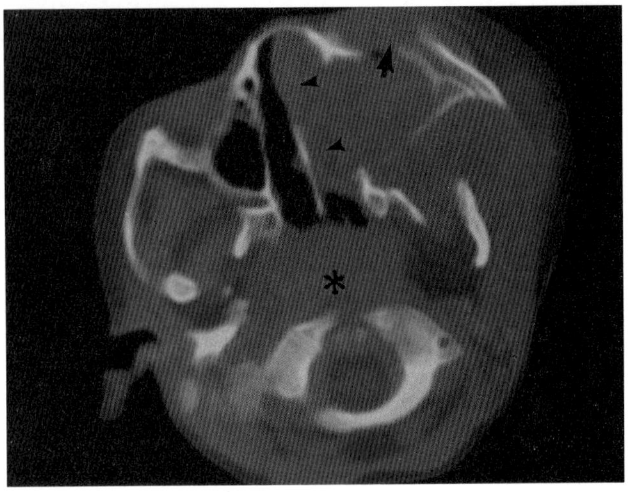

Figure 22.38

Facial non-Hodgkin's lymphoma (4-year-old): CT scan. A soft-tissue mass destroying the left facial bone is seen infiltrating the nasal fossae (arrowheads), and the cheek (arrow); there is adenoid hypertrophy (asterisk).

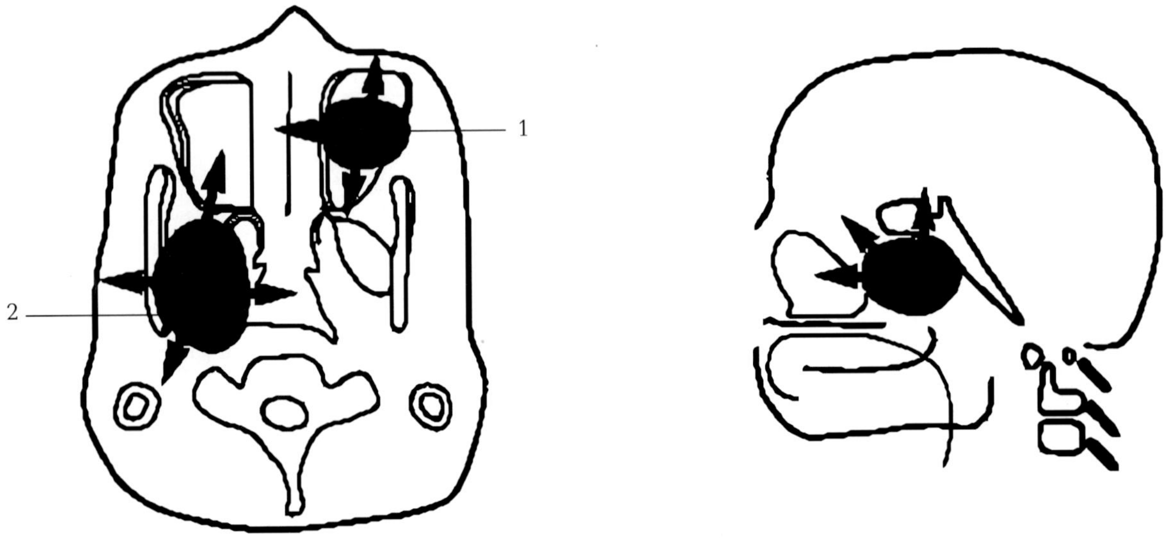

A

C

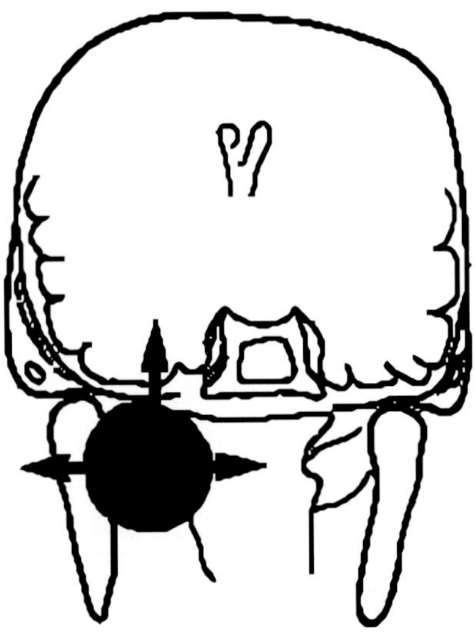

B

Figure 22.39

Rhabdomyosarcoma: pathways of extension in the head and neck.

A Axial view: 1, Paranasal rhabdomyosarcoma; involvement of the nasal fossae, pterygoid process and soft tissue of the cheek. 2, Nasopharyngeal rhabdomyosarcoma and the pterygomaxillary area: involvement of the nasopharyngeal lumen inwards, right mandible outwards, parotid area backwards and paranasal sinuses.

B Coronal view. Pterygomaxillary rhabdomyosarcoma: endocranial extension through the base of the skull.

C Sagittal view. Nasopharyngeal rhabdomyosarcoma; anterior extension towards choanae forwards and sphenoid area upwards.

Embryonal rhabdomyosarcoma

This is the most common of the malignant mesenchymal tumors in children, representing between 50 and 65% of them, according to the series. The average age at the time of diagnosis is between 3 and 5 years. Histologic diagnosis is based on two characteristics: myoid differentiation and structure. There are three different structural types: embryonal, alveolar and botryoid.[10] Revealing symptoms depend on the location of the primary tumor, about half occurring in the head and neck (Table 22.12).

Rhabdomyosarcomas of the head and neck originate essentially from the nasosinusal cavities or the rhinopharynx. Revealing symptoms result from the development of the tumoral mass: deformation of the face, unilateral nasal obstruction, persistent rhinorrhea, epistaxis, nasal voice tone, trismus. Auricular symptoms result from rhinopharyngeal tumors or those of the middle ear. Later on, radicular neurologic involvement may be observed, due to extensions towards the base of the skull. Satellite adenopathies, which are sometimes quite bulky, can lead to discovery. The mass is discovered after an ENT examination, followed by biopsies.

Table 22.12 Anatomic distribution of childhood rhabdomyosarcomas.[a]

Site	%
Head and neck	34
Orbit	10
Genitourinary	25
Limbs	14
Trunk	9
Retroperitoneal	8

[a]International Society of Pediatric Oncology Study, 1975–83.[21]

Imaging in diagnosis

CT scan is the first means of assessment, as it shows tumoral extensions (Figure 22.39).[56] But MR replaces CT for an accurate investigation of extensions towards the base of the skull (Figure 22.40).[57,58] Lateral and AP radiographs of the skull contribute little information.

Rhabdomyosarcomas of the orbit are revealed by exophthalmia and sometimes by tumefaction of the eyelid. A CT or, even better, an MR examination localizes the extraconical mass originating in the ocular muscles or from the eyelid invading intraorbital fat (Figure 22.41). A surgical biopsy is imperative.

Genitourinary rhabdomyosarcomas are usually discovered because of urinary disorders, such as dysuria or acute urine retention, or less frequently because of a polypoid mass of the vulva in small girls or an enlarged scrotum in small boys. The intrapelvic vesical or sub- and retrovesical mass can be detected with US (Figure 22.42), which shows the extent of obstruction of the urinary tract and can guide a percutaneous fine-needle biopsy. An IVP is not necessary. CT and/or MR will be performed to establish the staging of the tumor (Figures 22.42–22.44).[59]

Rhabdomyosarcomas of the limbs are characterized by the appearance of painless tumefaction within a muscle. Usually the diagnosis is obtained by means of an extirpative surgical biopsy, after pre-surgical US examinations, to eliminate the possibility of hematoma or lipoma. However, the best way to obtain an adequate diagnosis and treatment is to perform MR in order to determine the exact extension of the solid tumor (Figure 22.45) facilitating complete surgical excision. Staging of the disease differs in Europe and the USA (Table 22.13).

Prognosis, staging and therapy

Prognostic factors are localization (the best prognosis being for orbital, vaginal, vulvar and paratesticular locations), the parameningeal site, the stage and the sex of the child (evolution is less favorable in girls). The disease spreads to adjacent structures and to the lymph nodes. Metastases are uncommon at the time of diagnosis and can involve the lungs, the bone or bone marrow (Figure 22.46).

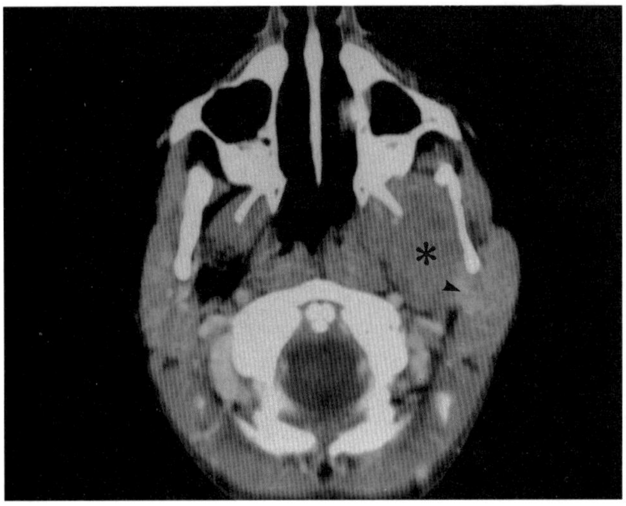

A

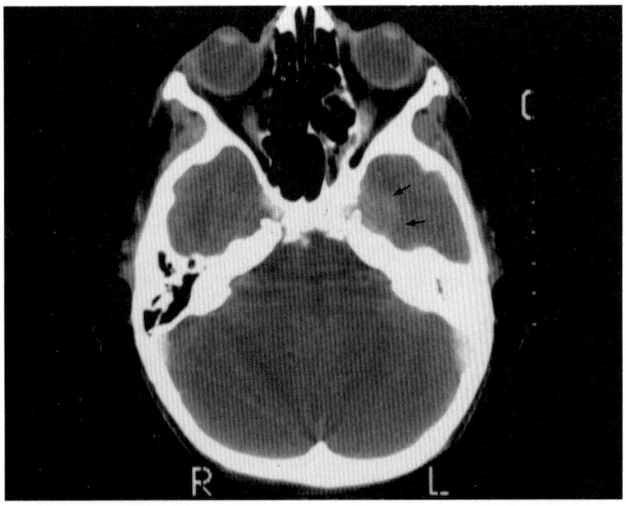

B

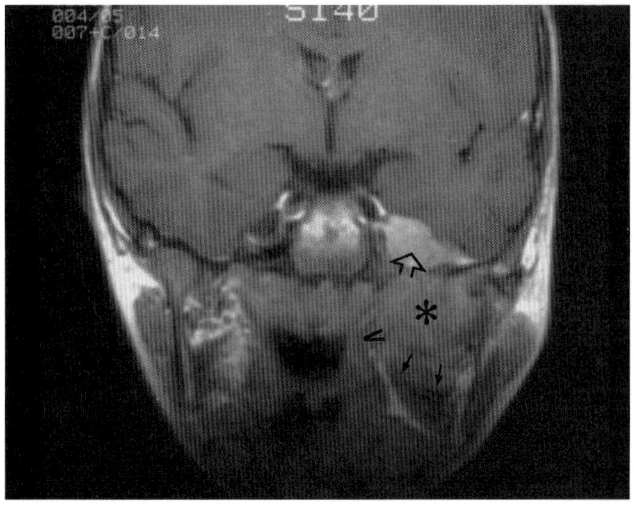

C

Figure 22.40

Infratemporal rhabdomyosarcoma (7-year-old).

A,B Axial CT scan with contrast material shows a space-occupying mass in the left pterygomaxillar area (asterisk) with parotidal extension outward (arrowhead) and endocranial spread in the temporal fossa through the foramen ovale (arrows).

C Coronal MR (600 ms, 20 ms) with gadolinium shows a hyperintense mass (asterisk) which is located in the left pterygomaxillar space, involving the pterygoid muscles (arrows) and the left lateral wall of the nasopharynx (open arrowhead); note the better evaluation of the hyperintense endocranial extension displacing the temporal lobe (open arrow), involving the cavernous sinus.

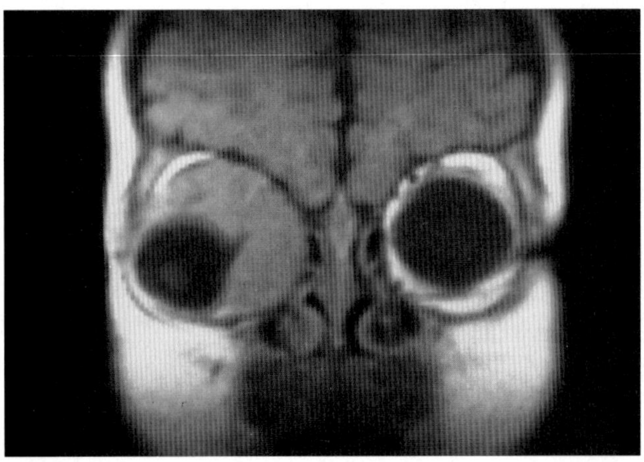

A

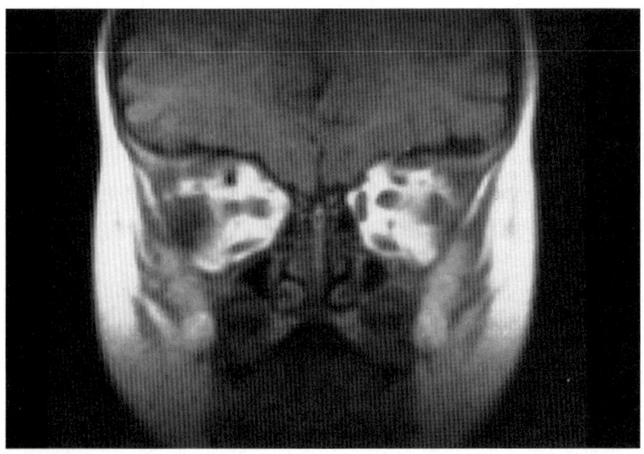

B

Figure 22.41

Rhabdomyosarcoma of the right eyelid (11-month-old): coronal MR (400 ms, 40 ms). There is a space-occupying mass in the right orbit which compresses and displaces the eyeball (**A**) without extension to the posterior aspect of the orbit (**B**).

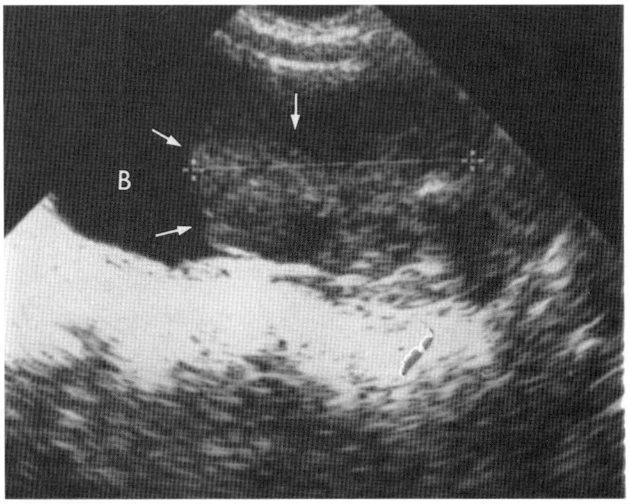

A

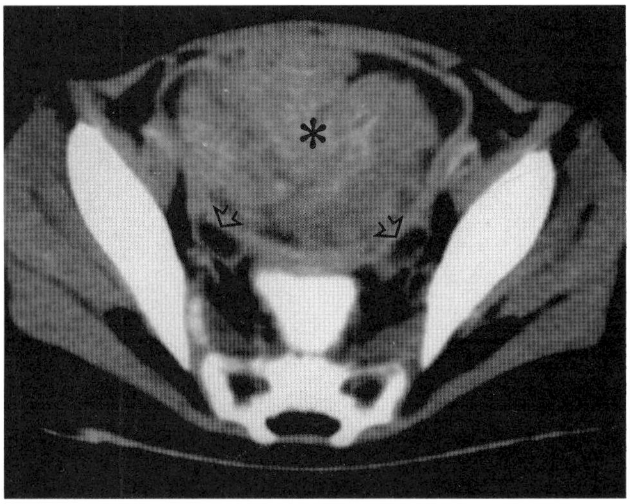

B

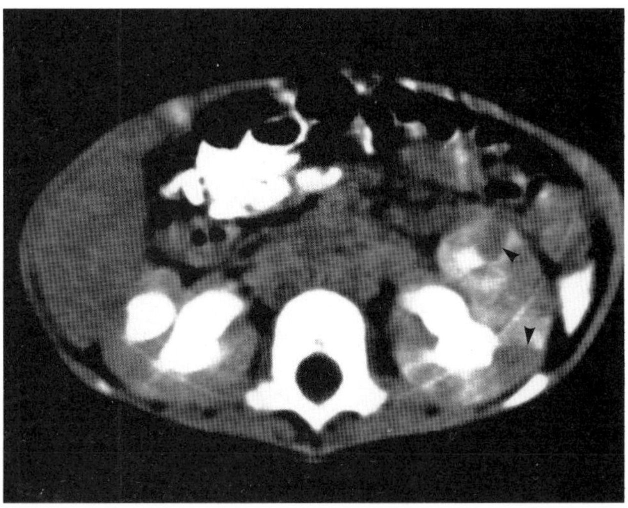

C

Figure 22.42

Prostatovesical rhabdomyosarcoma (3-year-old boy).

A US (longitudinal view) shows an echogenic mass (arrows) inside the bladder (B).

B CT scan with contrast material shows a lobulated hyperdense mass in the bladder (asterisk) and bilateral ureteral dilatations (open arrows).

C At the kidney's level, bilateral hydronephrosis with triangular cortical hypodensities due to an acute obstructive pyelonephritis (arrowheads) are seen.

Table 22.13 Clinical staging of rhabdomyosarcoma.

Group/ stage	*Criterion*
IRS group	
I	Localized disease, completely resected and normal regional lymph nodes: (a) Confined to muscle or organ of origin (b) Direct extension outside site of origin
II	(a) Grossly resected tumor with microscopic residual disease. (b) Regional disease completely resected but regional lymph nodes positive for tumor and/or extension of tumor into an adjacent organ. (c) Regional disease with involved lymph nodes grossly resected, but evidence of microscopic residual disease
III	Incomplete resection or biopsy with gross residual disease
IV	Metastatic tumor at clinical presentation
SIOP stage	
I	Tumor confined to organ of origin without clinical lymph nodes.
II	Tumor involving the contiguous tissues or with adjacent effusion, without clinical lymph nodes
III	Any tumor with regional lymph nodes
IV	Metastatic tumor

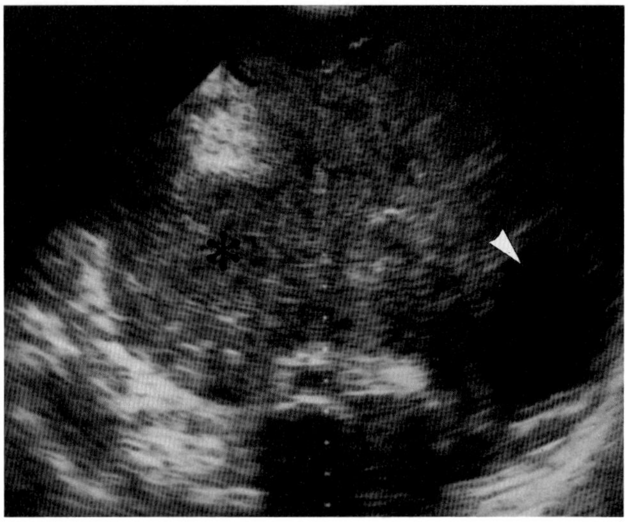

A

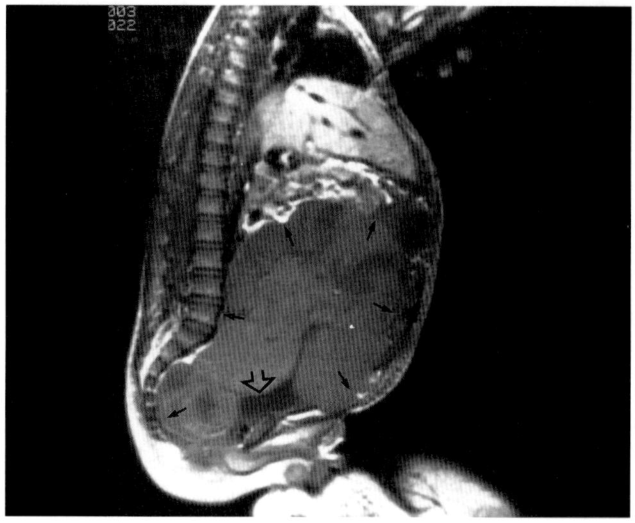

C

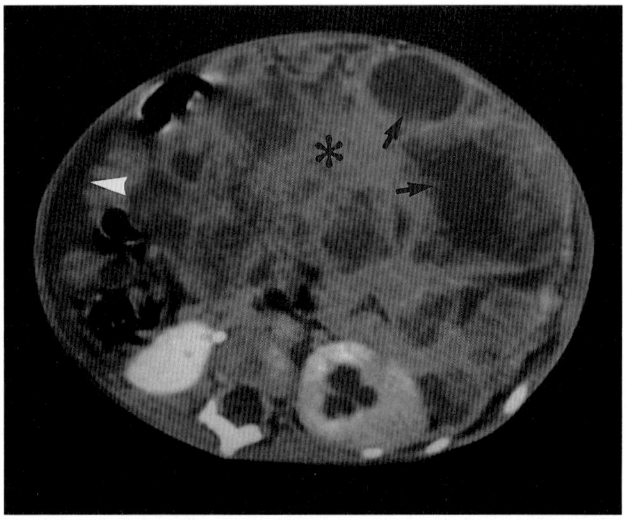

B

Figure 22.43

Pelvic rhabdomyosarcoma with a large intraperitoneal diffusion (4-year-old).

A US (transverse view) shows a large solid mass (asterisk) with cystic areas (arrowhead) which occupies the abdominopelvic cavity.

B CT scan with contrast material shows a mutilobulated heterogeneous solid (asterisk) and necrotic mass (arrows), with ascites (arrowhead) and dilated left kidney.

C MR (sagittal view, 900 ms, 25 ms) shows the bladder to be distorted (open arrow) by a large space-occupying mass which fills the entire pelvis and abdomen (closed arrows).

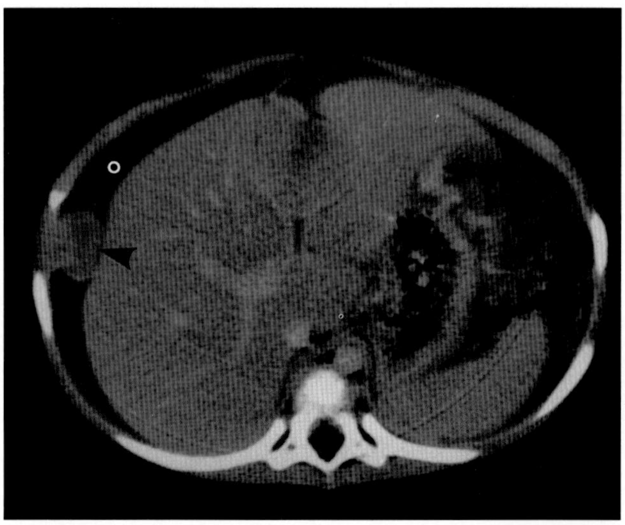

Figure 22.44

Pelvic rhabdomyosarcoma (3-year-old): CT scan with contrast material. There is a peritoneal metastatic nodule (arrowhead) and ascites (open circle).

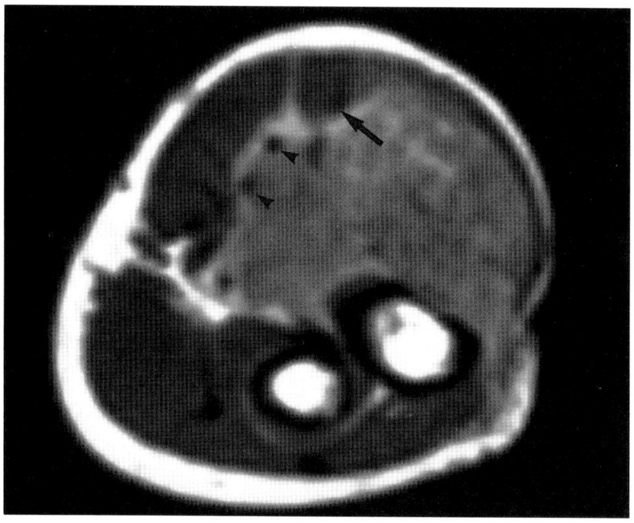

A

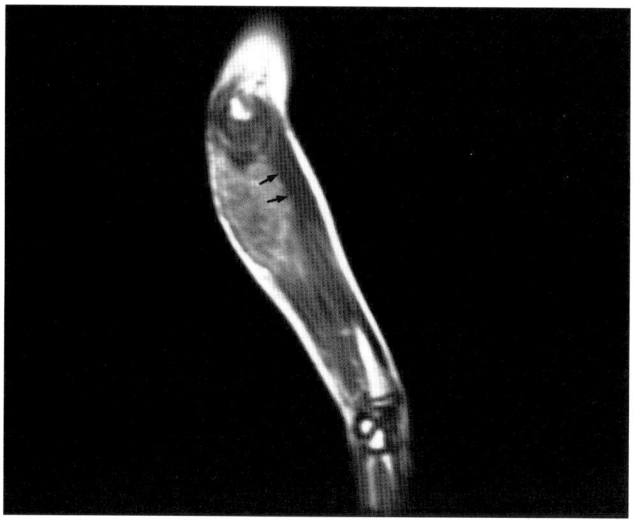

B

Figure 22.45

Rhabdomyosarcoma of the forearm (6-year-old): axial and coronal MR (500 ms, 20 ms) with gadolinium. Hyperintense soft tissue mass is clearly distinguished within the muscles (arrows); there is vascular encasement (arrowheads).

Pre-therapeutic imaging is carried out by different techniques, depending on the localization of the primary tumor (Diagram 22.8; Figures 22.41 to 21.46): for parameningeal sites, MR is more accurate than CT (Figures 22.40 and 22.47), but the age of the child should be taken into account for the practical execution of the examination. In investigation of the pelvic floor (Figure 22.43) or in the cases of tumors of the extremities or parietal tumors of the trunk, MR is useful, because of the possibility of multidirectional reconstruction. However, for abdominal lymphatic extensions, CT is preferable.

The treatment of rhabdomyosarcoma is based on the chemosensitivity of the tumors, with the possibility of complementary radiotherapy (Figures 22.48 and 22.49) and surgical extirpation. Local recurrences are a serious complication and are difficult to bring under control.

A special form of rhabdomyosarcoma occurs in older children or adolescents; it is revealed by diffuse bone metastases with deterioration of general health, anemia, fever and sometimes hypercalcemia.[60] The primary tumor is often small and difficult to locate, bone marrow is invaded by a proliferation of extrahemopoeitic myoblastic cells. In these rare forms, CT is used to locate the primary tumor and bone radiographs used, as lytic bone metastases do not absorb technetium, and bone scintigraphy is therefore not helpful.

The follow up of rhabdomyosarcoma is given in Diagram 22.9.

Malignant germ-cell tumors

These tumors are multipotential and result from cells derived from primary germ or gonocyte cells which migrate from the yolk sac to the sexual cords of the embryo. The cells may stop migrating and cause a benign or malignant tumor, originating either along the median line—from the sacrococcygeal region to the pineal gland, as in the case of a malignant extragonadal germ-cell tumor—or within the sex organs. The most frequent origin is the sacrococcygeal region, followed by the ovaries. The WHO classification subdivides the tumors into germ-cell seminomatous (dysgerminoma) or germ-cell non-seminomatous tumors,[10,21] the latter comprising diverse proportions of benign and malignant elements in children.

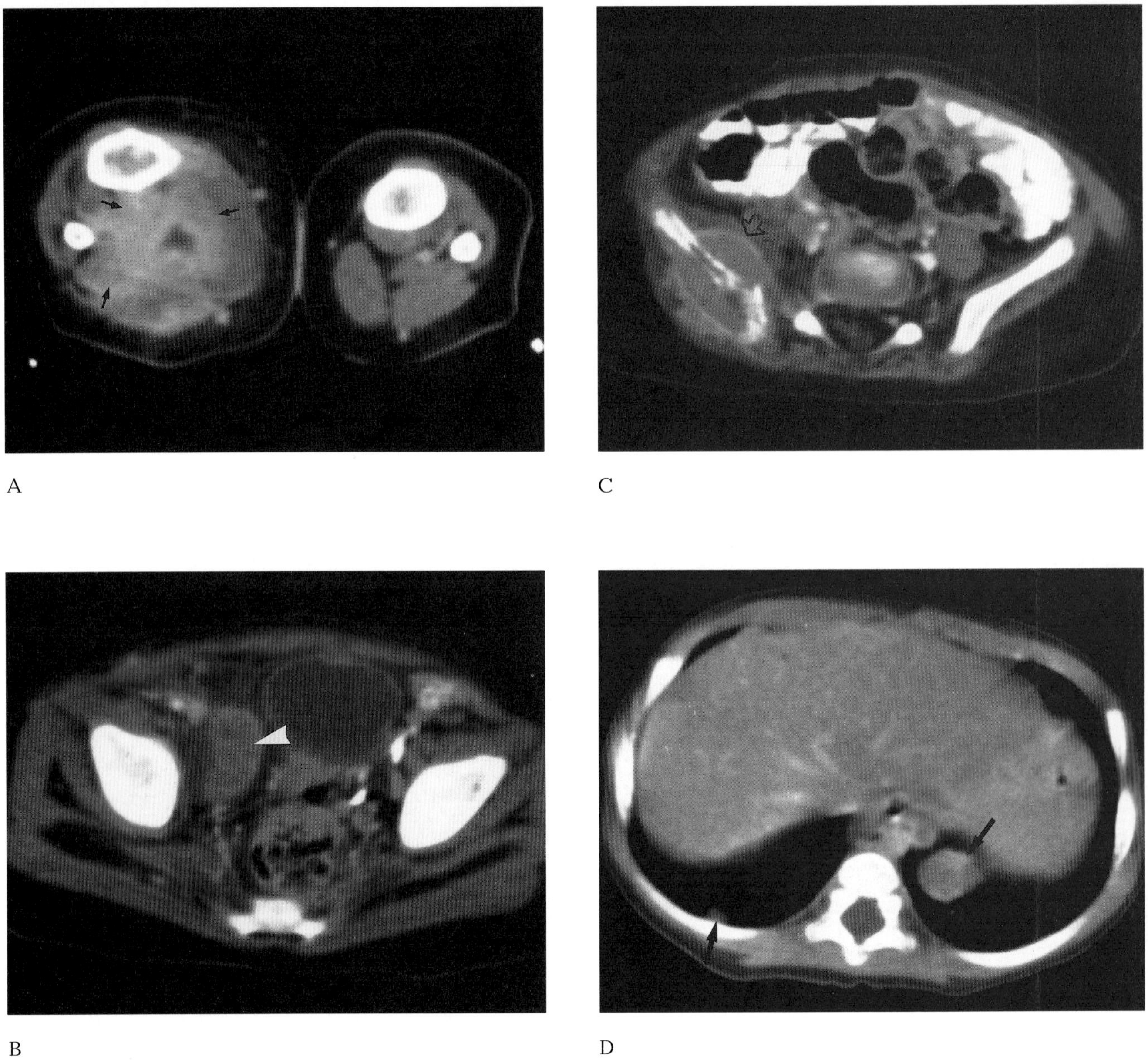

Figure 22.46

Stage IV rhabdomyosarcoma of the right calf (13-month-old): CT scan with contrast material.

A At the level of the lower limb, a hyperdense soft-tissue mass infiltrates the posterior muscles (arrows).

B At the level of the bladder, there is right iliac adenopathy (arrowhead).

C At the level of the iliac wing, there are bone metastases with a soft-tissue mass and cortical destruction (open arrow).

D At the thoracic level, pulmonary metastatic nodules (arrows) are seen.

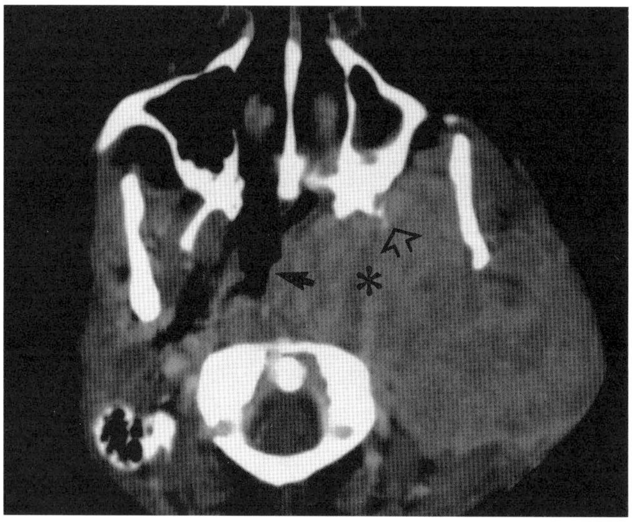

A

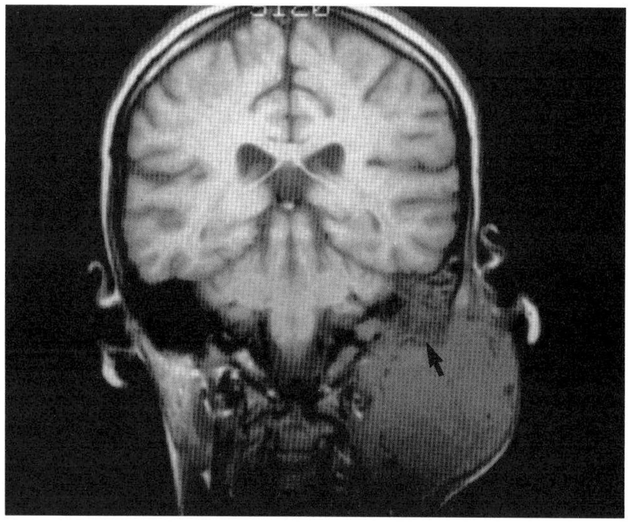

C

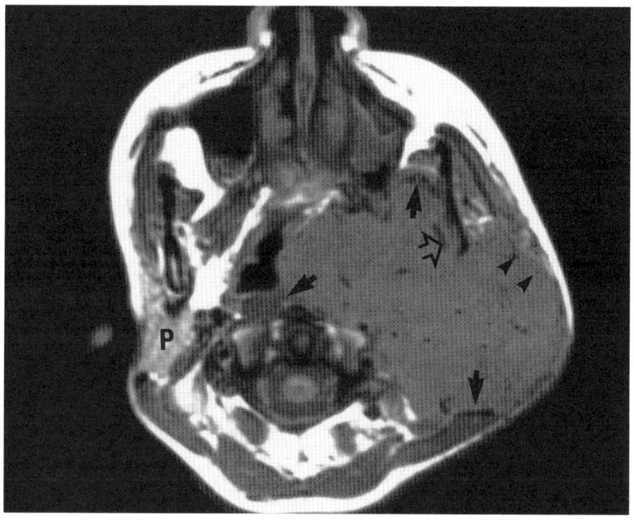

B

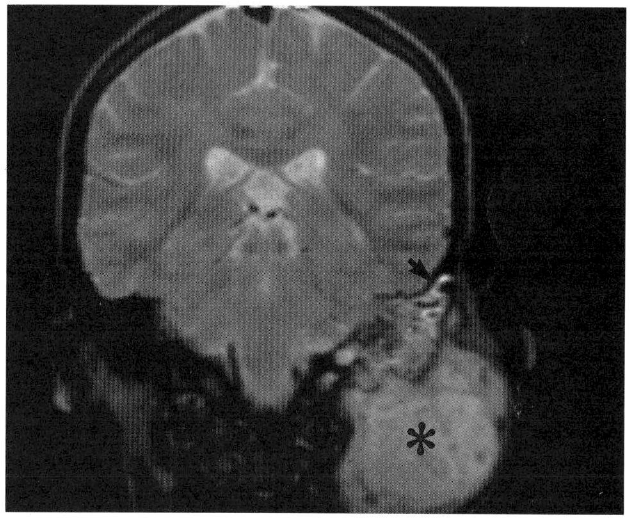

D

Figure 22.47

Parotidal rhabdomyosarcoma (14-year-old).

A Axial CT scan with contrast shows a large soft-tissue mass of the parotid extended to the infratemporal area (asterisk) and the nasopharynx (closed arrow) displacing the left mandible and destroying the pterygoid process (open arrow).

B Axial MR (600 ms, 20 ms): note the better estimation of tumoral extensions to the left mandible (open arrow), muscles (closed arrows) and destruction of the parotid gland (arrowheads); P, normal right parotid gland.

C On the coronal view, destruction of the petrous bone and involvement of the middle ear (arrow) are seen.

D On coronal MR (2000 ms, 90 ms) the tumor has a hyperintense signal on T2-weighted images (asterisk), but this is less than that of the inflammatory reaction in the mastoid (arrow). The coronal MR allows one to eliminate an endocranial spread of the tumor.

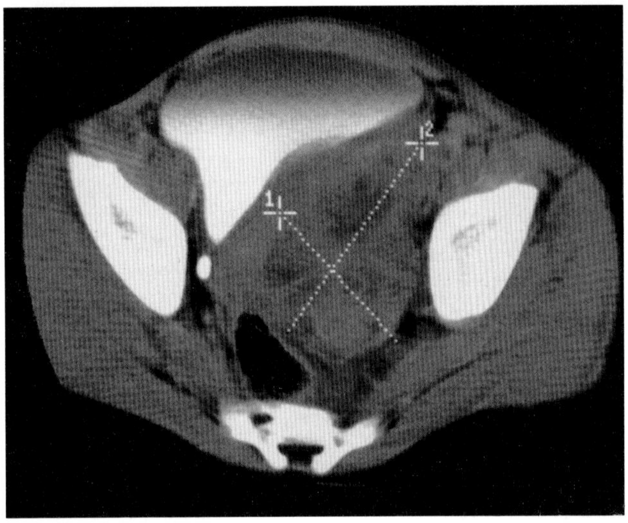

A

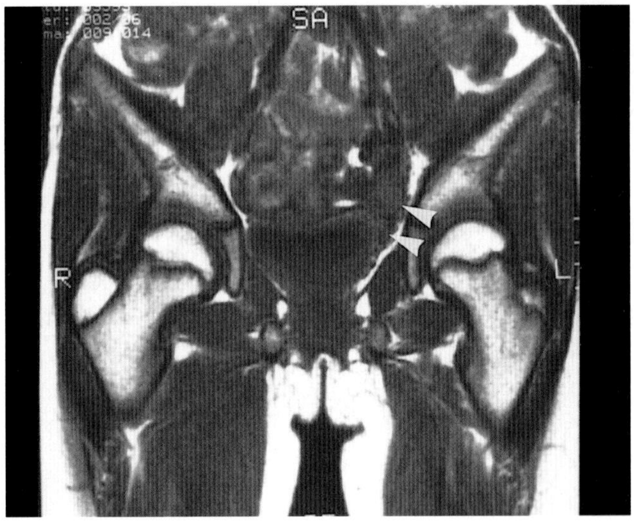

C

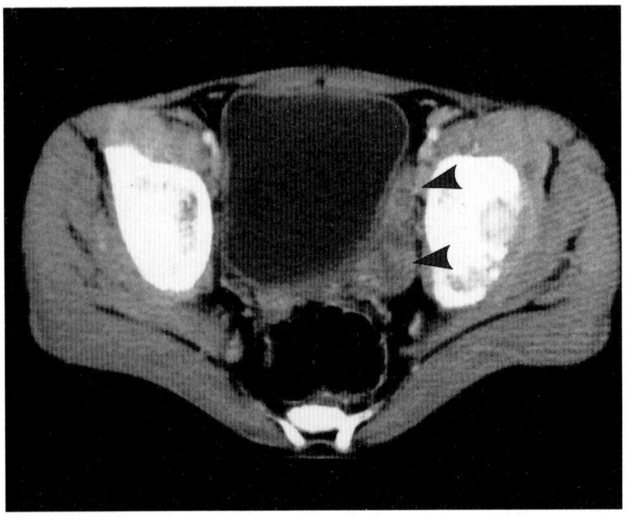

B

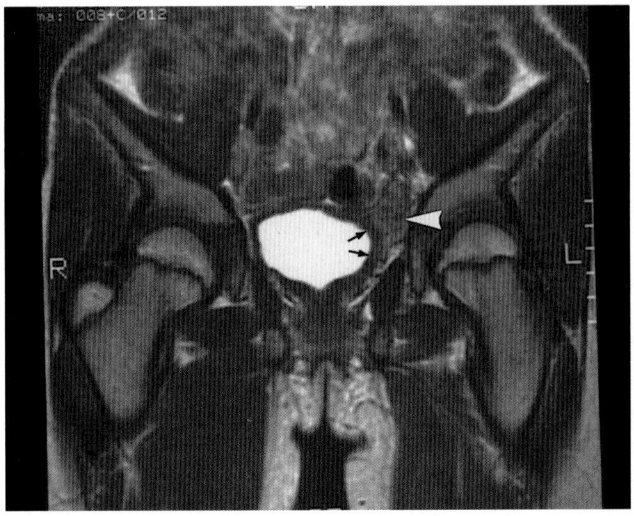

D

Figure 22.48

Pelvic rhabdomyosarcoma (10-year-old girl).

A CT scan with contrast material shows a heterogeneous solid mass located in the left pelvorectal area, compressing the bladder.

B Post-chemotherapeutic pre-surgical staging CT scan with contrast demonstrates heterogeneous residual lesion (arrowheads).

C MR coronal view (600 ms, 20 ms) demonstrates hypointense soft-tissue residual lesion (arrowheads).

D The lesion is enhanced after contrast injection close to the bladder wall (arrows).

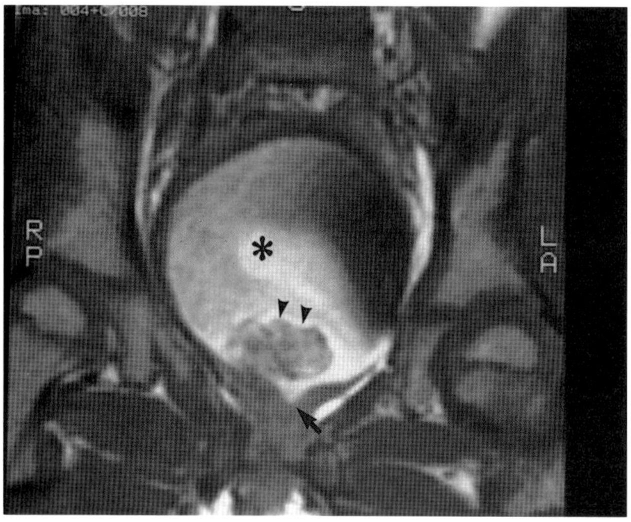

A

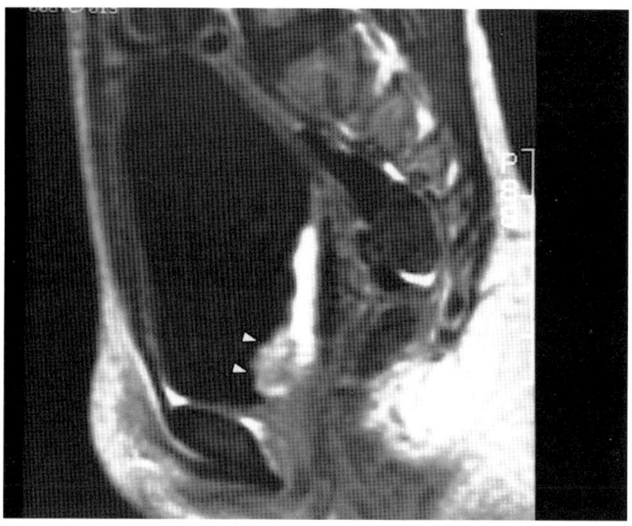

B

Figure 22.49

Vesical rhabdomyosarcoma (3-year-old girl): post-chemotherapeutic pre-surgical staging by gadolinium MR (600 ms, 20 ms) in coronal (**A**) and sagittal (**B**) views. Tumoral nodules (arrowheads) are surrounded by contrast material (asterisk) located above the cervix of the bladder (arrow).

These elements include:

- mature benign teratomas, consisting of well-differentiated tissue of various types such as cystic, fatty, nervous, mesenchymal or respiratory tissue,
- embryonal carcinoma,
- tumor of the endodermic sinus or yolk sac carcinoma, which secretes α_1-fetoprotein (AFP)
- choriocarcinoma (less often), secreting chorionic gonadotropins.

Prognosis depends on the most aggressive component of the tumor.

Extragonadal germ-cell tumors

These originate most often in the sacrococcygeal region and are discovered during the neonatal period.[21,61] It is important to recognize them as soon as possible, because under the age of 2 months more than 95% of these teratomas are benign, whereas after 1 year of age 50% are malignant. Although teratomas are clinically easily recognized at birth, later on recognition is due to palpation of a retrorectal pelvic mass following sphincter or intestinal disorders, which leads to investigation.

Imaging, therapy and follow up

US examinations and radiographs of the abdomen show a heterogeneous retrorectal presacral mass containing calcifications which may be organoid. Suspicion of teratoma leads to an assay of serous AFP and chorionic gonadotropins, and performance of either CT or preferably MR, in order to estimate any extension towards the sacral holes and the canal, the buttocks and the perineal area (Figures 22.50 and 22.51).[22]

Treatment is surgical if the lesion appears to be benign (age, absence of secretion of biologic markers) or chemotherapy then surgery if the lesion is malignant, bulky or metastatic (bone, lungs, liver).

Post-surgical follow up is biological using markers, with imaging for potential recurrence if there is sudden increase in the markers—either a CT scan or MR of the area where surgery was carried out. There is no special sign for a tumoral lesion in the surgical area, but a solid mass with increased density or signal after injection, which

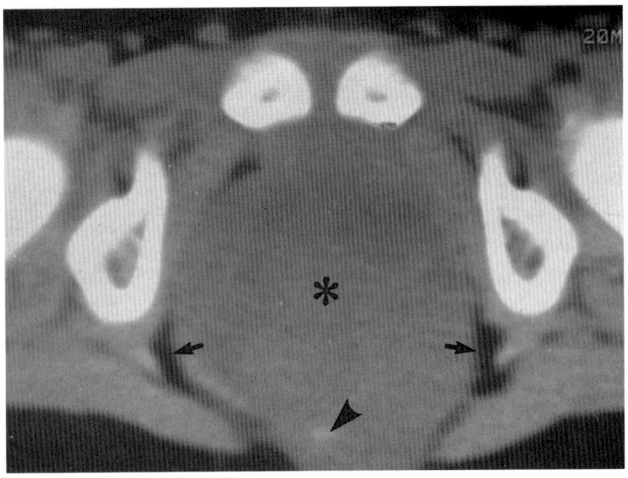

Figure 22.50

Paracoccygeal swelling which distorts the right buttock—malignant teratoma (3-year-old): CT scan without contrast material. There is a retrorectal calcified solid mass (asterisk) involving the coccyx (arrowhead) and the ischiorectal fossae (arrows).

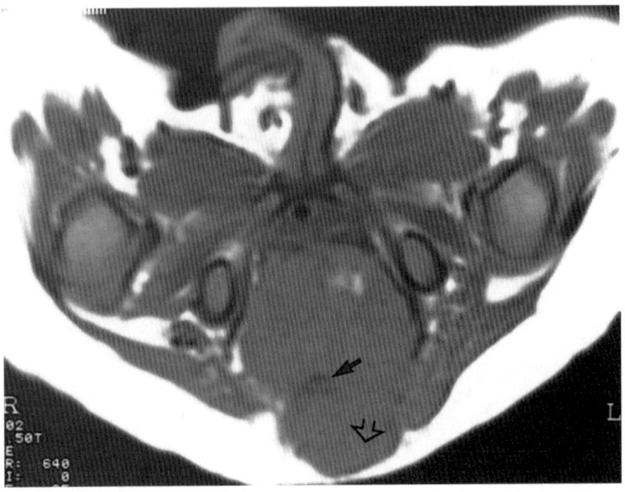

A

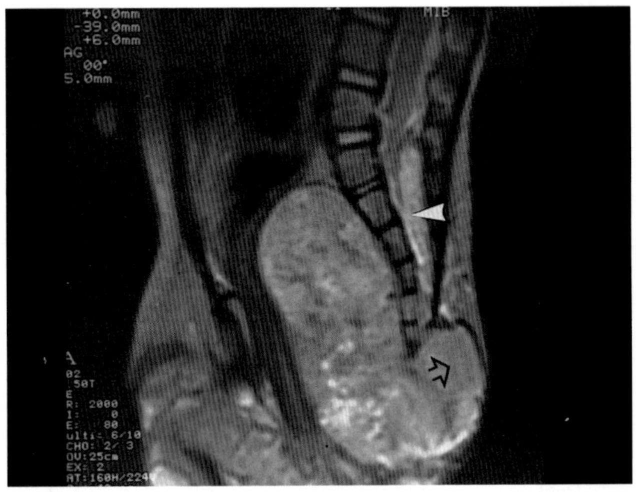

C

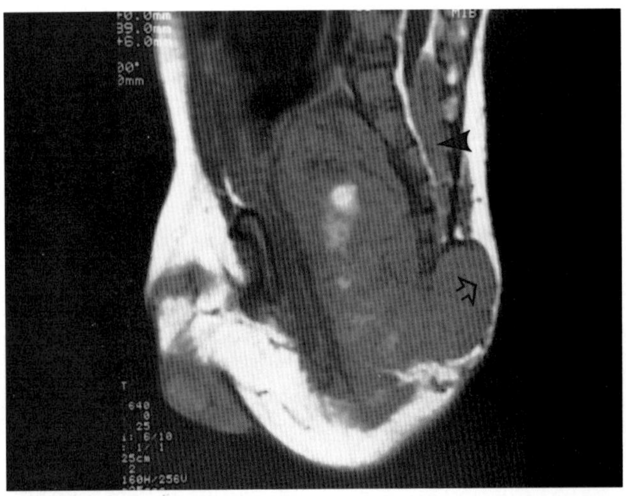

B

Figure 22.51

Malignant sacrococcygeal teratoma (1-year-old): MR. T1-weighted (640 ms, 25 ms), axial (**A**) and sagittal (**B**) views and a T2-weighted (2000 ms, 80 ms) image in a sagittal view (**C**) illustrate a large heterogeneous soft-tissue mass occupying the presacral space, including the coccyx (closed arrow) which extends towards the buttock and the retrosacral area (open arrow); intraspinal extension appears with a low signal on T1-weighted images and bright on T2 (arrowhead). (Courtesy of Dr Couture, Montpellier, France.)

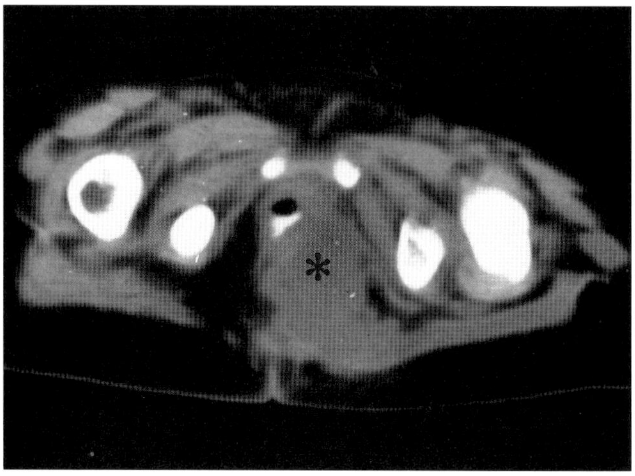

A

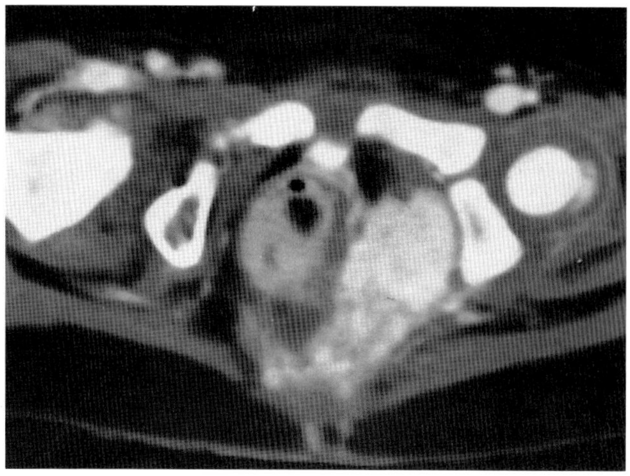

C

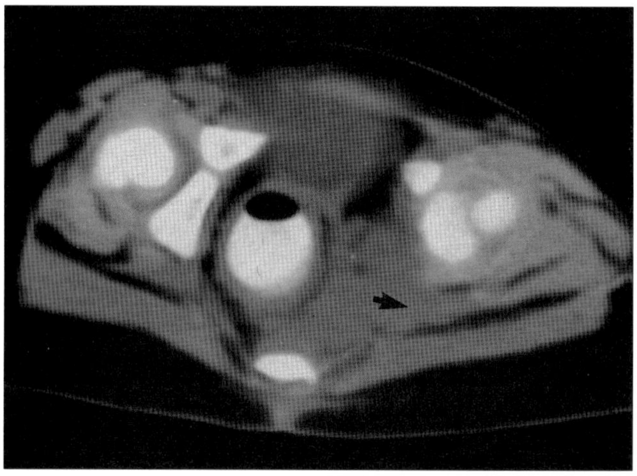

B

Figure 22.52

Malignant sacrococcygeal teratoma (2-year-old), increase of the serous AFP level after surgery:

A CT scan without contrast material: there is a solid space-occupying lesion (asterisk) in the left ischiorectal fossa, with an extension towards the buttock.

B At an upper level, extension towards the pelvorectal space and the ischiatic area is seen (arrow).

C CT scan with contrast material gives strong enhancement of the tumor.

shows some evolution after two successive examinations, confirms the relapse (Figure 22.52).

The uses of imaging in staging and follow up are outlined in Diagram 22.10.

Less frequent localizations for malignant teratomas are the retroperitoneum, the anterior and posterior mediastinum or the cervicofacial region. Diagnostic assessment and follow up are similar to that for other sites. Survival is affected by chemosensitivity of the tumor, operability and metastases.

Malignant germ-cell gonadal tumors

The ovary is the second site at which germ-cell tumors occur,[62] their histology being variable (Table 22.14). They are usually discovered because of the tumoral mass or endocrine secretions: palpable pelvic mass, abdominal pain, or less frequently precocious puberty, an acute abdominal syndrome due to torsion of the ovarian mass.

Table 22.14 Histologic type of gonadal tumors in childhood.

Ovarian tumors	*Testicular tumors*
Germ-cell tumor	Germ-cell tumor
Mature teratoma	Embryonal carcinoma
Dysgerminoma	Yolk-sac tumor
Embryonal carcinoma	Malignant teratoma
Yolk-sac tumor	Mature teratoma
Choriocarcinoma	Dysgerminoma
Malignant teratoma	Choriocarcinoma
Mixed germ-cell pattern	Mixed germ-cell pattern
Gonadoblastoma	Gonadoblastoma
Surface epithelium tumor	Sex-cord tumor
Sex-cord tumor	Malignant lymphoma
Miscellaneous	Para-testicular tumors
Malignant lymphoma	Rhabdomyosarcoma
	Metastatic tumor
	Neuroblastoma
	Wilms' tumor

Imaging and therapy

The pelvic mass is either solid or a mixture of solid and liquid, as seen with ultrasound, which shows it originates in the ovary. The discovery of a solid ovarian mass is usually suspicious and requires an assay of biological markers.

Assessment should include chest radiography to detect pulmonary metastases, followed by a thoracic CT scan in case of doubtful findings. Abdominal CT is performed to detect the lumbo-aortic adenopathies (the lymph-node relay of the ovary being laterocaval on the right, and latero-aortic on the left, under the renal pedicle (Figure 22.53), as well as to assess any eventual pelvic mass or those resulting from intraperitoneal diffusion, which are always difficult to distinguish from digestive loops, especially when small. The final assessment is bone scintigraphy. Initially, surgery is systematic if markers are negative, in order to make a diagnosis.

Chemotherapy is the complementary treatment for stages II, III and IV (see Table 22.15 for ovarian tumor stages). In the case of dysgerminomas, radiotherapy can be used, as these tumors are exceptionally radiosensitive.

Testicular tumors

These tumors are rare in children and are usually germ-cell tumors (Table 22.14). Testicular tumors which are revealed because of tumefaction of the testicle can usually be treated with surgery once US has shown a solid tumor located in the testis,[64] and analysis of the pathologic specimen has confirmed the diagnosis.

Assessment of extensions is made in the same way as for ovarian tumors, bearing in mind the fact that locoregional diffusion is usually seen in the lumbo-aortic lymph nodes and is not intraperitoneal, since the testicle is extraperitoneal (Figure 22.54).

Table 22.15 Clinical staging of ovarian tumors in childhood[63] and 3-year disease-free survival.

Stage	*Criterion*	*Survival (%)*
I	Tumor localized to one ovary without extracapsular spread	100
II	Bilateral ovarian tumor or lumboaortic lymph nodes	82
III	Pelvic or abdominal diffusion, tumoral ascites, rupture of the tumor	
IV	Metastases	75

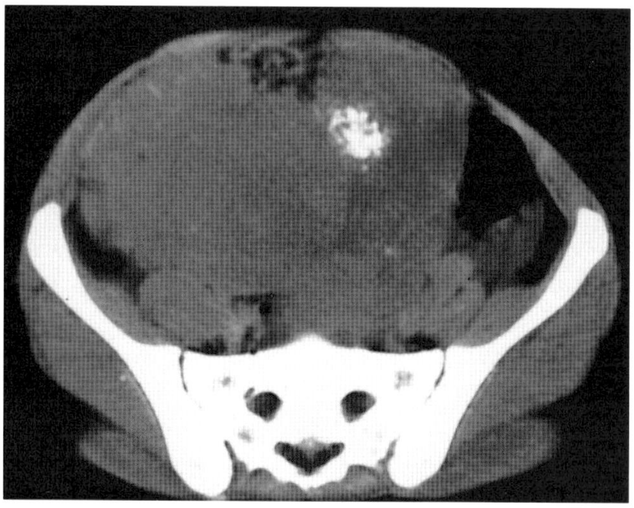

A

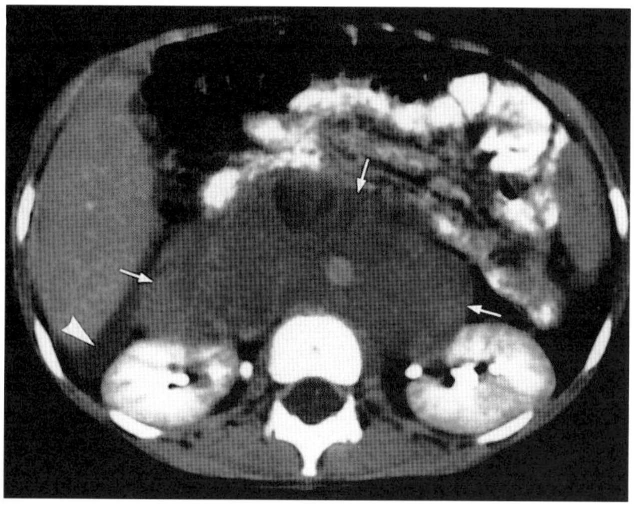

B

Figure 22.53

Ovarian germ-cell tumor (12-year-old girl): initial staging.

A Pelvic CT scan shows a large solid calcified mass.

B CT at the abdominal level shows lumboaortic adenopathies (arrows) and ascites (arrowhead).

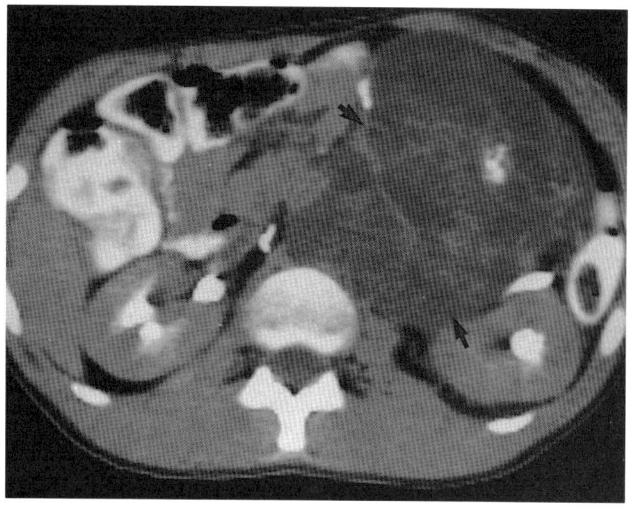

A

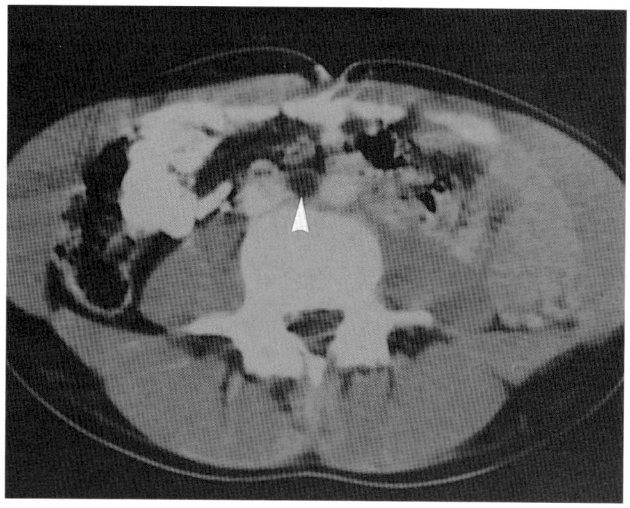

B

Figure 22.54

Germ-cell testicular tumor containing multiple histologic components (embryonal carcinoma, teratoma, choriocarcinoma and yolk-sac tumor) (15-year-old boy).

A CT in initial staging shows large heterogeneous calcified adenopathies (arrows) close to the aorta.

B Post-chemotherapeutic pre-surgical CT scan illustrates residual cystic adenopathy (arrowhead).

Histologic sampling confirmed mature teratoma.

Undifferentiated carcinoma of the cavum

This is the most frequent carcinoma in children. It has a special geographical distribution, around the Mediterranean and in South-East Asia. It has a double frequency peak: the second decade of life and the fifties. Infection by the Epstein–Barr virus is closely related to its distribution. The carcinoma is usually discovered in the same way as other tumors of the nasopharynx, i.e. due to progressive aggravation of nasal obstruction, with nasal tone, otitis and cervical adenopathies which are often rather bulky and sometimes misleading. The surgical biopsy of the primary tumor or the revealing adenopathies leads to a histologic investigation and diagnosis. The tumor is lymphophilic and may invade the cervical and mediastinal lymph-node chains. Distant bone metastases may be observed or, more rarely, metastases in the lungs.

Imaging and therapy

Locoregional assessment is carried out by CT or preferably MR (Figure 22.55),[65] which can be used to direct the biopsy and assess extensions towards the base of the skull or the dura mater, which is the major local risk with this disease (Figure 22.56). Chest radiographs are used to search for

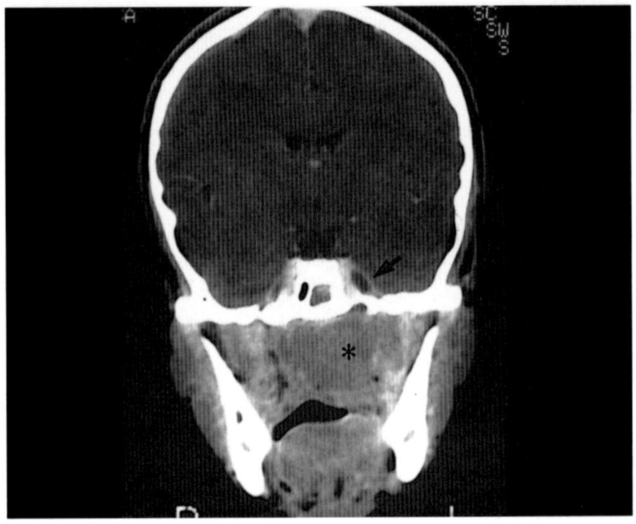

A

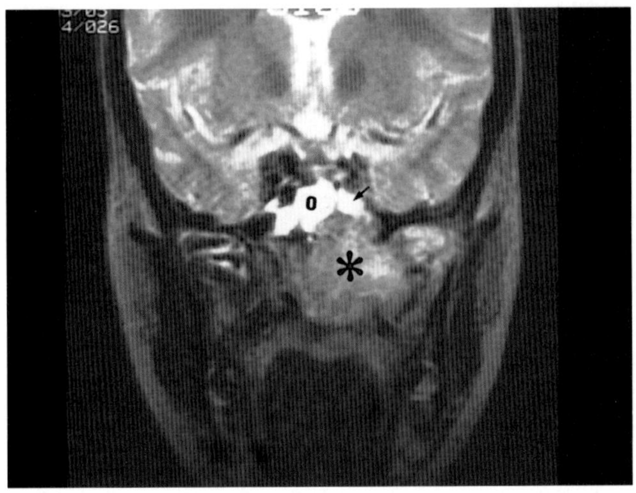

B

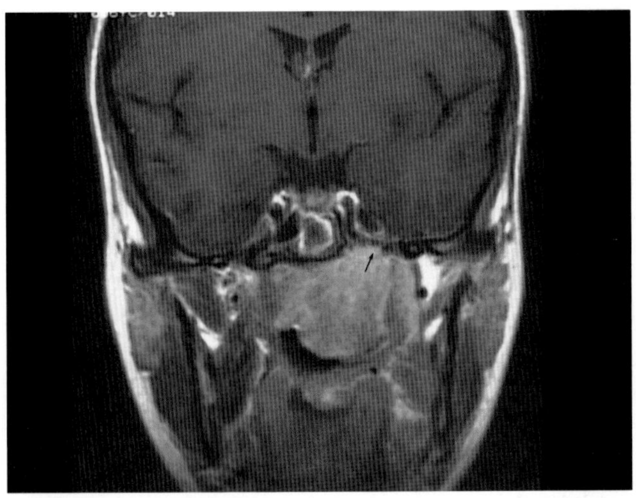

C

Figure 22.55

Undifferentiated carcinoma of the cavum (14-year-old): initial staging.

A Coronal CT scan with contrast material shows a space-occupying lesion in the nasopharyngeal lumen (asterisk), mild asymmetry of the left sinus cavernous and the trigeminal ganglion (arrow).

B Coronal MR (2000 ms, 100 ms) gives a clear distinction between the hypointense signal of the tumor (asterisk) compared to the hyperintense inflammatory reaction (open circle) in the partially invaded sphenoidal sinus (arrow).

C Coronal MR (600 ms, 20 ms) with gadolinium shows tumoral extensions near to the internal carotid artery through the foramen lacerum (arrow), which mildly displaces the trigeminal ganglion.

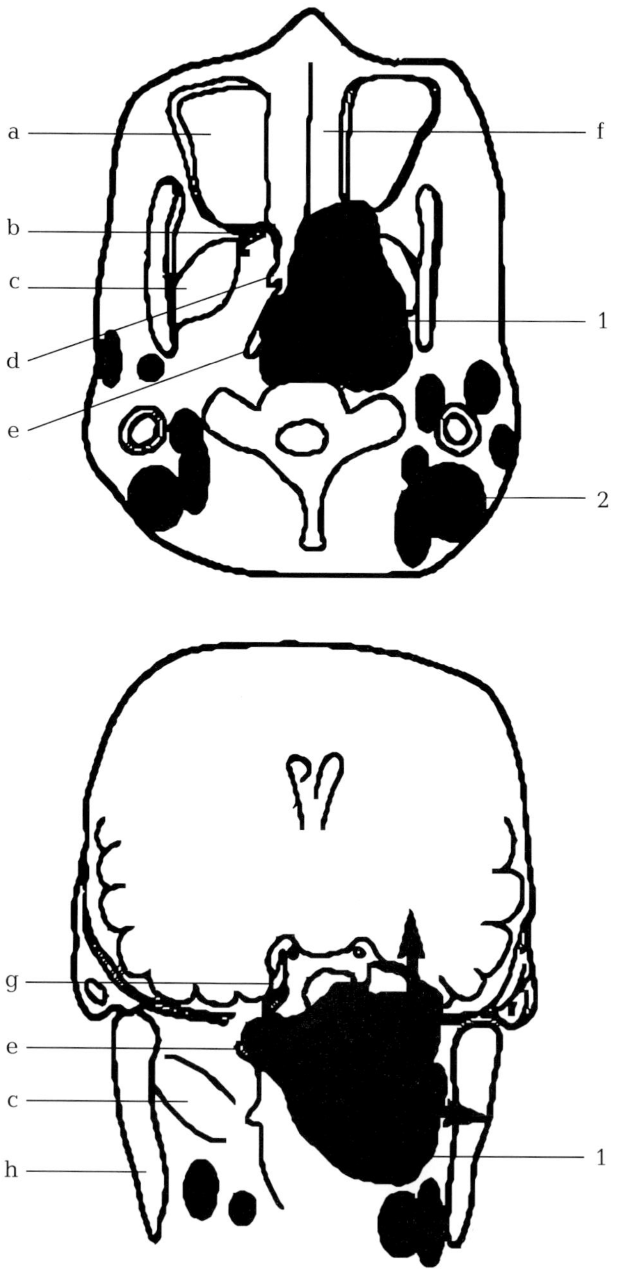

Figure 22.56

Undifferentiated carcinoma of the cavum: axial and coronal views of local and regional extent.

a, paranasal sinuses; b, pterygoid process; c, pterygomaxillary area; d, tubar orifice; e, Rosenmüller fossae; f, nasal fossae; g, cavernous sinus; h, mandible; 1, primary UCNT; 2, regional lymph nodes.

pulmonary and mediastinal lymph-node metastases, aided by a thoracic CT scan, and bone scintigraphy for bone metastases.

Treatment consists of chemotherapy, followed by radiotherapy of the nasopharynx and cervical lymph-node chains, the volume of which being estimated by post-chemotherapeutic CT.

Retinoblastoma

This malignant tumor of the retina is sporadic or hereditary,[66] and is of neuroectodermic origin. Bilateral or multifocal forms are more frequent in hereditary cases. The average age at the time of diagnosis is 2 years for unilateral forms and less for bilateral forms (1 year). The revealing symptom is usually a whitish reflection seen in the pupil. An ophthalmological examination under general anesthesia reveals the tumor and assesses extensions to the retina, determining the extent of involvement.

Imaging and therapy

Orbital US can help reveal a solid mass that may be obscured by detachment of the retina or reveal hemorrhaging. It can also reveal echoic calcifications in the midst of the mass. From a retinal tumor, the retinoblastoma can extend locally to the choroid, with a risk of hematogenous dissemination to the bone or the lungs, because of the rich vascularity, towards the optic nerve with a risk of meningeal diffusion, either through the invasion of the meningeal nerve sheath or by direct extension via the optic foramen, and finally towards the sclera and the orbital fat, with the risk of lymph-node dissemination and local recurrence after exenteration.

Assessment of extensions should include a CT or MR of the orbital region and the subarachnoidal spaces (Figure 22.57).[67,68] This may necessitate general anesthesia in these very young children, to avoid any artifacts due to motion of the eyeball. The presence of tumoral cells in the cerebrospinal fluid should be sought by lumbar puncture and chest radiography to detect pulmonary metastases. Finally, depending on clinical symptoms (pain in the bones), bone scintigraphy and bone-marrow aspirates should be undertaken.

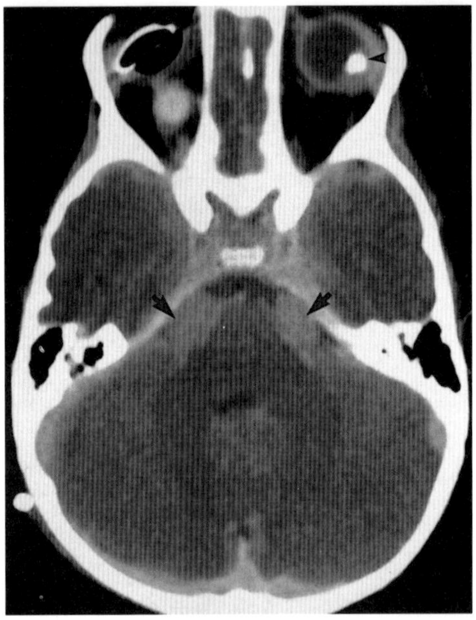

A

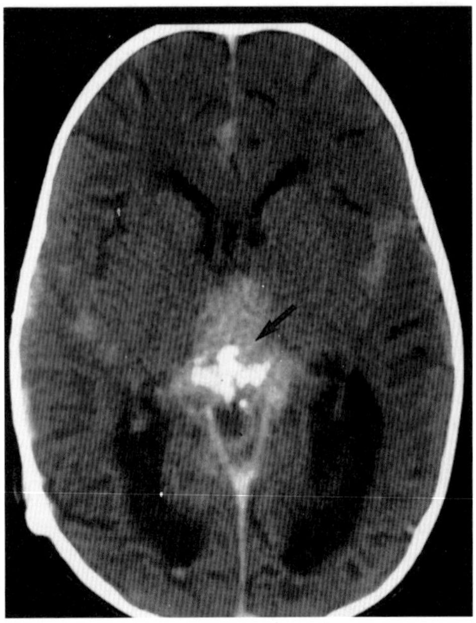

B

Figure 22.57

Bilateral retinoblastoma with pinealoblastoma—trilateral retinoblastoma syndrome (2-year-old): CT scan with contrast material.

A Prosthesis of the right orbit, calcified retinoblastoma of the left eyeball (arrowhead) and meningeal tumoral extension in the peripontic cisterna (arrows).

B A hyperdense and calcified space-occupying lesion located at the pineal gland (arrow) with ventricular dilatation.

Table 22.16 Unfavorable prognostic factors in retinoblastoma.

Delay at diagnosis
Unilateral tumor in a child over 3–4 years old
Extraretinal spread: choroid, optic nerve, orbit
Undifferentiated type
CNS or hematogenous metastases

Treatment is enucleation, which allows the staging of the tumor from the surgical specimen, and the observation of unfavorable prognostic factors (Table 22.16).

Hepatic tumors

These tumors are rare in children and are represented by the hepatoblastoma in children of 3 years and under, and hepatocarcinoma in older children or adolescents. They have the peculiarity of secreting AFP which facilitates diagnosis.

Hepatoblastoma

Histologically, the hepatoblastoma is hypervascularized, necrotic and sometimes calcified; it has an epithelial component associated with a mesenchymal component derived from the blastema. The revealing symptom is usually an abdominal mass, which is shown by US to originate in the liver. This mass is uni- or plurinodular, polylobed, with a variable echogenicity: hyper-, iso- or hypoechoic (Figure 22.58). The tumor is sometimes so bulky and badly defined that it is difficult to determine from which organ it originates; it is then necessary to try to detect occlusion of the segmentary or lobar portal branches, or invasion of a subhepatic vein, which is highly suggestive of a malignant hepatic tumor.[69,70] An abdominal plain film can show calcifications in the hepatic area without specificity. Diagnosis is based on serous AFP assays. If negative, a fine-needle biopsy should be carried out under general anesthesia (in view of the age of the patient) and directed by US.

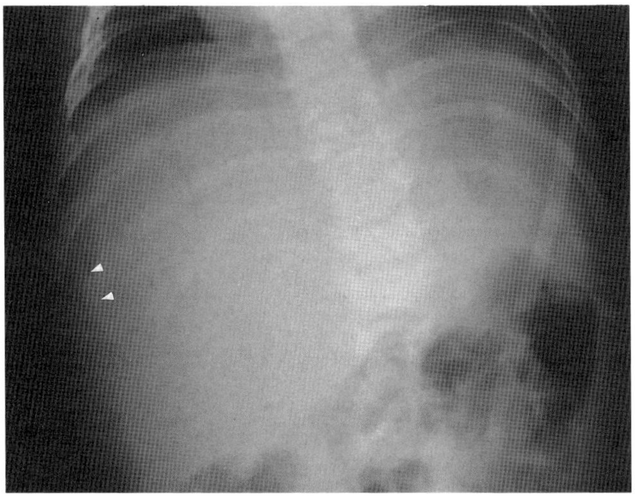

A

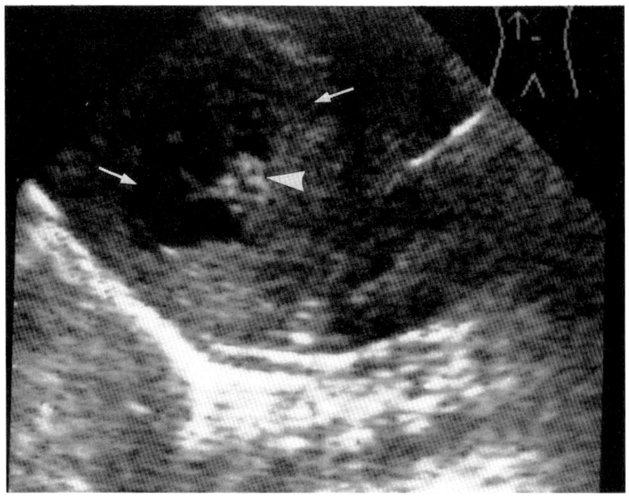

C

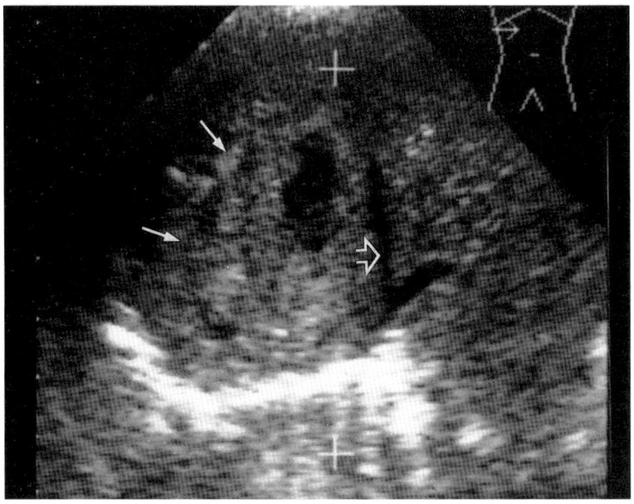

B

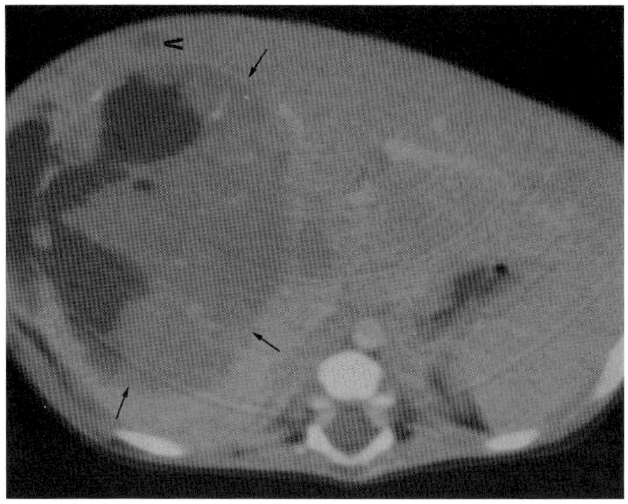

D

Figure 22.58

Hepatoblastoma of the right lobe (2-month-old).

A Plain abdominal radiograph shows hepatomegaly with discrete calcifications (arrowheads).

B,C US, transverse (**B**) and longitudinal (**C**): hyper- and hypoechoic mass (closed arrows) contains calcifications (arrowhead) close to the sagittal subhepatic vein (open arrow).

D CT scan with contrast injection shows a large heterogeneous pseudocapsulated mass (arrows) with accessory nodule (open arrowhead).

Imaging, therapy and follow up

Assessment should include, in addition to US examination, a hepatic CT scan or, preferably, MR.[71] The CT scan often shows a pseudoencapsulated tumor which is hypodense before injection, and heterogeneous and often hypodense, compared with a healthy liver, after an intravenous injection of contrast material (Figure 22.58). Distant nodules are frequent. As with US, on CT the lobular or segmentary localization of the tumor should be defined, as well as occlusions of the portal or subhepatic veins and any extensions towards the portal bifurcation, the hepatic pedicle

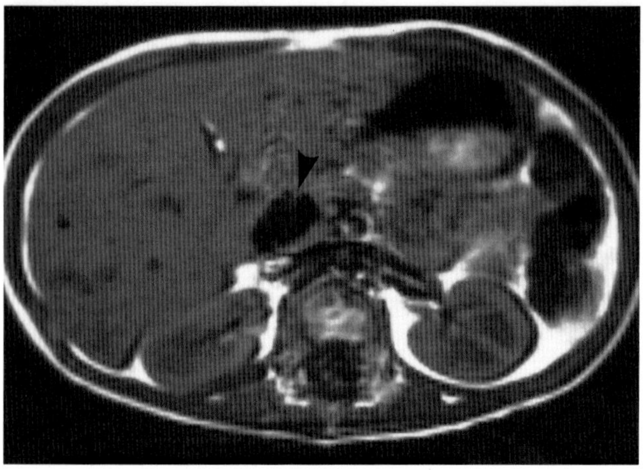

A

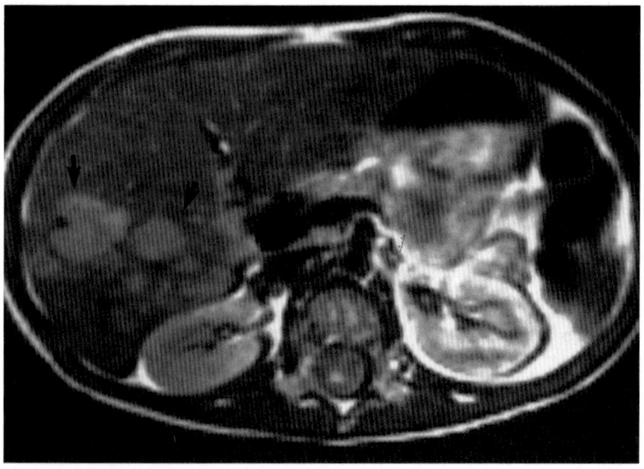

B

Figure 22.59

Post-chemotherapeutic pre-surgical staging for a hepatoblastoma of the right lobe (4-year-old).

A Axial MR (600 ms, 20 ms) shows cavernoma of the portal vein (arrowhead).

B Axial MR (2000 ms, 40 ms) shows a multilobulated hyperintense mass of the right lobe (arrows); note the better delineation of the tumor in this long TR sequence.

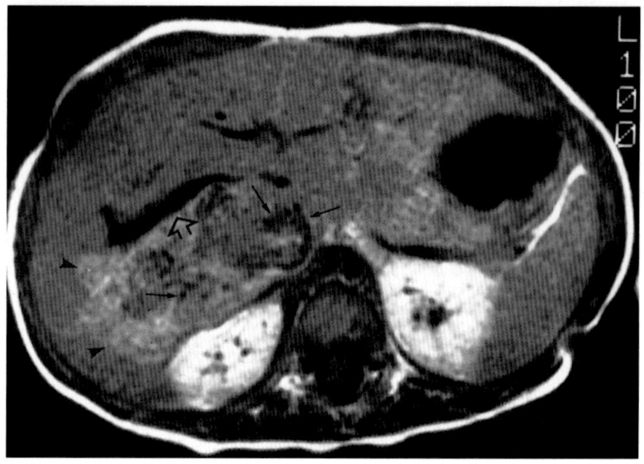

Figure 22.60

Pre-surgical staging for a hepatoblastoma of the caudate lobe (1-year-old): Axial MR (600 ms, 20 ms) with gadolinium injection. There is a heterogeneous hypo- and hyperintense mass (arrowheads) close to the right portal vein (open arrow); the hypointense areas are due to foci of calcifications (closed arrows).

or the retrohepatic inferior vena cava. But it is with MR that the tumor and its extensions are best shown, especially on sequences with a long repetition time (1500–2000 ms), with an echo time of 40 ms (Figure 22.59), or after the injection of contrast medium (gadolinium) on a sequence with a short repetition time of 500–600 ms (Figure 22.60).

Arteriography is not advisable at the assessment stage, as initial treatment is chemotherapy in order to facilitate the use of surgery.[21] It is only if the tumor is small and does not secrete biological markers that surgery may be used in the first instance after hepatic arteriography. In other cases, it is only after reduction of the tumor by chemotherapy that surgery is considered, and MR shows the tumoral residue much more accurately, especially in view of the fact that modifications resulting from treatment make the tumor difficult to differentiate from the healthy liver by US or CT. Involvement of the hepatic pedicle or portal cavernoma (a portal thrombosis with collateral blood supply) due to tumoral infiltration are extensions which are unfavorable for successful surgery. If surgery is considered, pre-operative arteriography gives the surgeon an idea of the vascular outline which helps plan hepatic excision.

Investigation of the presence of metastases (in the lungs or less frequently in the bone) includes chest radiography, supplemented if necessary with

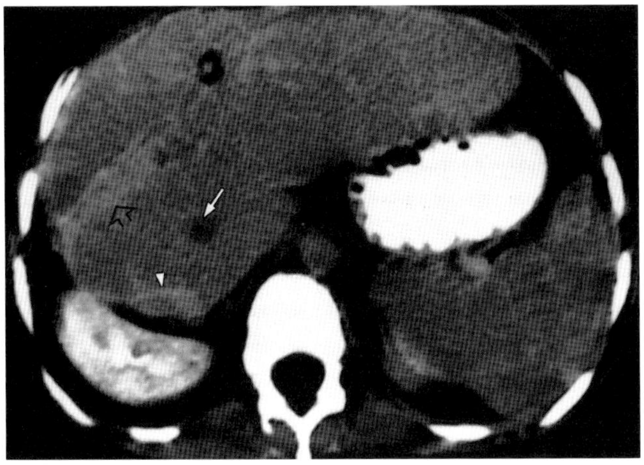

A

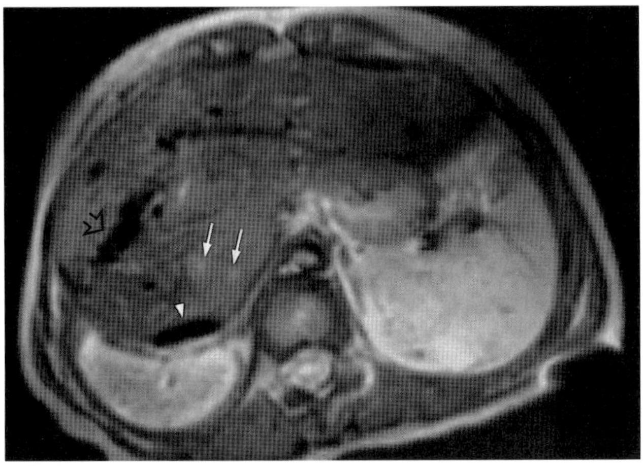

B

Figure 22.61

Right hepatectomy because of hepatoblastoma (16-year-old): post-surgical follow up with increase of the serous α-fetoprotein level.

A CT scan with contrast material shows a hypodense nodule located in the quadrate lobe (arrow).

B Axial MR (2000 ms, 40 ms) demonstrates two hyperintense nodules in the quadrate lobe (arrows).

Arrowhead, inferior vena cava; open arrow, portal vein.

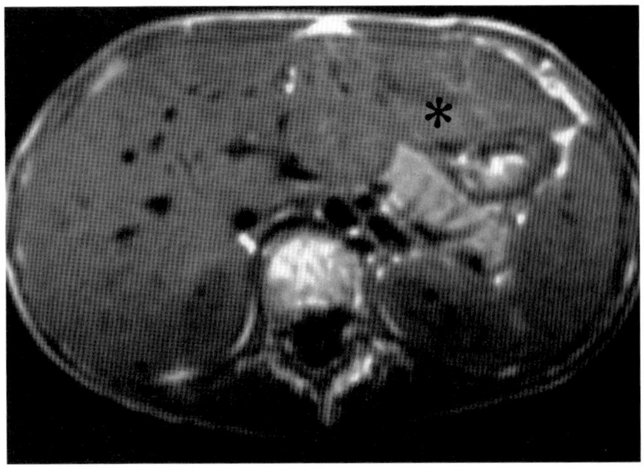

A

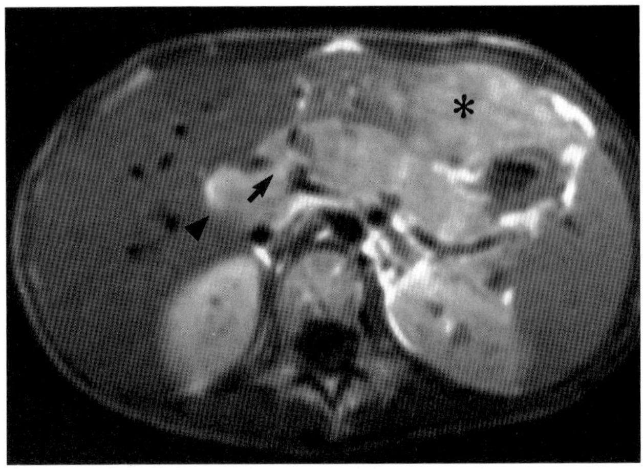

B

Figure 22.62

Hepatocarcinoma of the left lobe (13-year-old).

A Axial MR (700 ms, 20 ms) shows a discrete hyperintense signal of the left lobe (asterisk) compared to the right lobe.

B MR (700 ms, 20 ms) with bolus injection of gadolinium enhances the hepatic tumor, which includes the left lobe (asterisk) and the caudate lobe (arrowhead). There is encasement of the portal pedicle (arrow).

a thoracic CT scan in doubtful cases, bone scintigraphy being of no value in the absence of clinical symptoms.

Post-surgical follow up will make use of serous AFP samples and MR (Figure 22.61) only if the level of biological markers becomes abnormal.

An imaging strategy is given in Diagram 22.11.

Hepatocarcinoma

Histologically, hepatocarcinoma has a more marked epithelial differentiation, without blastomatous components. The difference from hepatoblastoma lies in its low chemosensitivity and, as in adults, prognosis is unfavorable if surgery cannot be used initially, especially if hepatocarcinoma occurs in addition to an existing hepatic disorder. Assessment of extensions is identical to that for hepatoblastomas (Figure 22.62).

Hodgkin's disease

In children Hodgkin's disease is rare and is no different from that observed in adults except for the consequences of radiotherapy on growth. Prognosis is extremely favorable—88% survival without recurrence after 4 years—the incidence of localized stages at the time of diagnosis (Table 22.17) justifying a reduction in the aggressiveness of treatment in cases with favorable prognosis, especially where radiotherapy is concerned. Discovery (cervical or mediastinal adenopathies), assessment of extension and follow up during treatment are similar to those for Hodgkin's disease in adults[55] and are therefore not described here.

Table 22.17 Distribution and 5-year disease-free survival in childhood Hodgkin's disease.[a]

Stage	*Frequency*		*Survival (%)*
	No. of cases	*%*	
IA+IIA	104	57	
IB+IIB	24	13	95
III	31	17	
IV	25	13	44

Leukemia

The most frequent form of leukemia in children is acute lymphoblastic leukemia. This is a curable disease; its prognosis has been modified with aggressive chemotherapy and autologous or donor bone-marrow transplants. At present, the overall survival rate is 60–70%.[21]

Although oncologic imaging plays only a small part in the diagnosis and assessment of various forms of leukemia, there are certain pseudo-tumoral forms of acute lymphoblastic leukemia which are identical to NHLs, especially if a bulky mediastinal mass with pleural and/or pericardial effusion is discovered on chest radiographs. Diagnosis is based on the presence of blasts circulating in the peripheral blood. In cases of considerable hyperleukocytosis in infants, chest radiographs may reveal a mixed alveolar and interstitial syndrome of leukemic origin affecting cardiorespiratory functions and thus necessitating prompt treatment.

Imaging of the post-immunosuppressive disorders

Follow up during treatment should include vigilance for immunosuppression or drug toxicity, with chest radiographs. In case of superinfection, the infections observed vary from the common to the opportunist, including viral infections. In all cases, chest radiographs do not diagnose the infection. Diagnosis has to be by alveolar irrigation or even a pulmonary biopsy, though certain radiographic signs can be evocative: excavated parenchymal pulmonary lesions suggest necrosing infections (staphylococci, Klebs–Löffler bacilli or pyocyanic bacilli) or opportunist fungal infections such as aspergillosis. During periods of aplasia, the absence of polymorphonuclear leukocytes prevents the formation of the inflammatory reaction that would appear as radiological opacities, which are observed only after aplasia. Thoracic radiographs also help to judge the diffusion or localization of the infection. It can be useful to supplement these with a pulmonary CT scan, if the state of the child permits this, in order to detect any pulmonary lesions which are difficult to visualize by chest radiography or to assess the extent of parenchymal lesions. In these cases, fine sections are necessary (1–2 mm) with a short scan-time of 0.5–1.0 s (Figure 22.63).

In *Candida* infections in transplant patients, hepatosplenic, pulmonary and cerebral localizations should be investigated, first by US and then by CT if necessary.[72] These take the form of

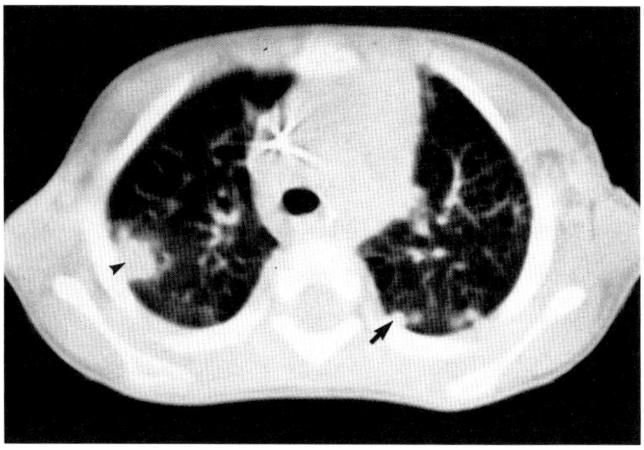

Figure 22.63

Abdominal neuroblastoma, *Candida albicans* septicemia (2-year-old): CT scan (2.5 mm slice thickness). A mixed nodular (arrow) and poor delineated alveolar pattern (arrowhead) is disseminated in both lungs. The diagnosis was pulmonary candidosis.

microabscesses in the liver and spleen and are often more easy to detect without an injection of contrast medium (Figure 22.64).

The neurologic toxicity of drugs or infectious encephalic complications can be established either by an encephalic CT scan or, preferably, MR. Methotrexate can be responsible for lesions of the white matter (Figure 22.65). This toxicity may be potentialized by encephalic radiotherapy, resulting in acute, subacute or chronic demyelizing leukoencephalopathies. Chemotherapy (vincristine) may also lead to coagulation disorders responsible for thrombosis of the endocranial venous sinuses, leading to convulsions or motor defiency.

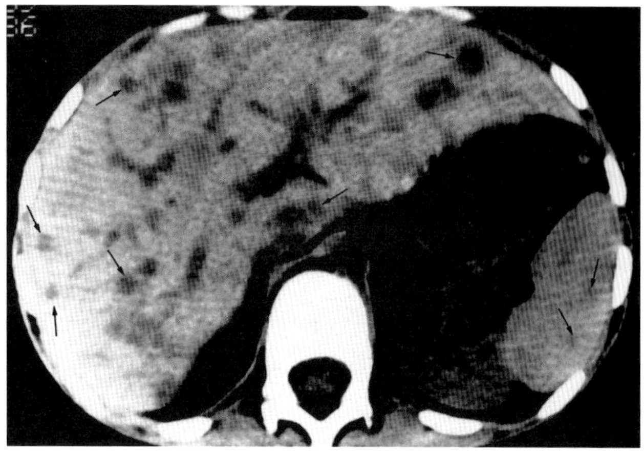

A

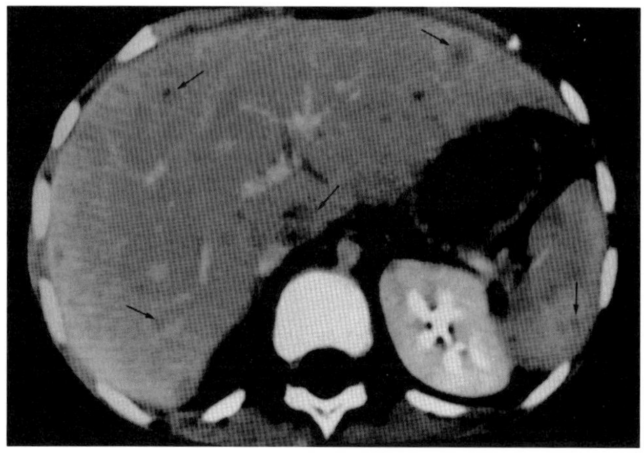

B

Figure 22.64

Abdominal non-Hodgkin's lymphoma, *Candida albicans* septicemia (9-year-old): CT scan without (**A**) and with contrast material (**B**). Multiple splenic and hepatic microabscesses secondary to fungal infection are present (arrows); note the better visualization of the abscesses before contrast injection.

Secondary malignant tumors

Although rare, the observation of a secondary malignant pathology is an unfavorable complication,[73] as it most often resists standard treatment. The most common secondary malignancies are acute non-lymphocytic leukemias, which appear within a period of 5 years. Secondary solid tumors appear later, within an average of 8–10 years. These consist mainly of sarcomas of the bone, such as osteosarcomas or chondrosarcomas, for which surgery is the only cure, since these are resistant to chemotherapy. Even later, cancers of the thyroid

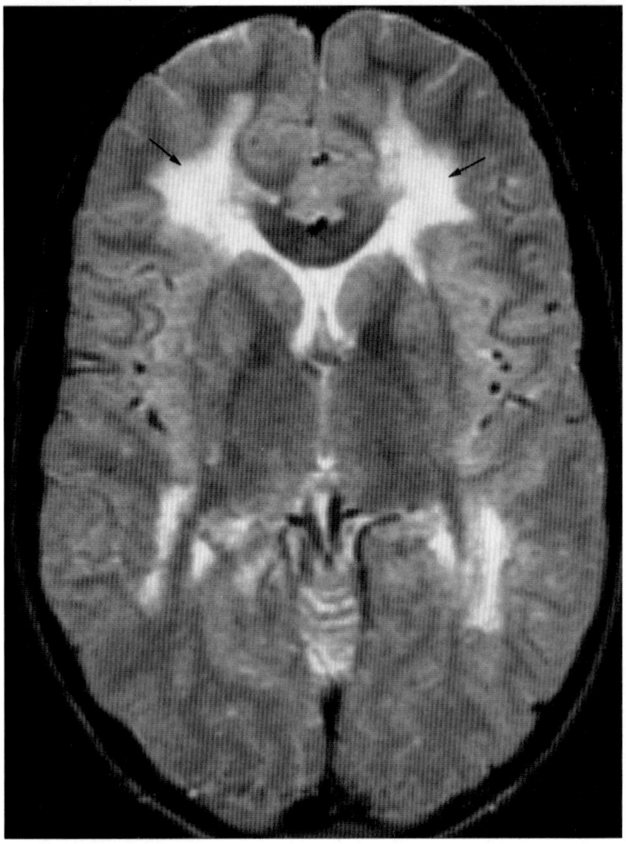

Figure 22.65

Epileptic crisis after high-dose methotrexate therapy (11-year-old). Axial MR (2000 ms, 90 ms) shows a hyperintense signal of the white matter due to the methotrexate toxicity (arrows).

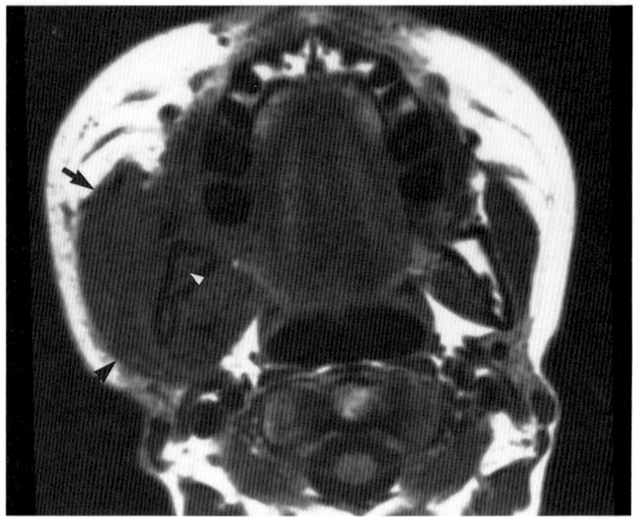

A

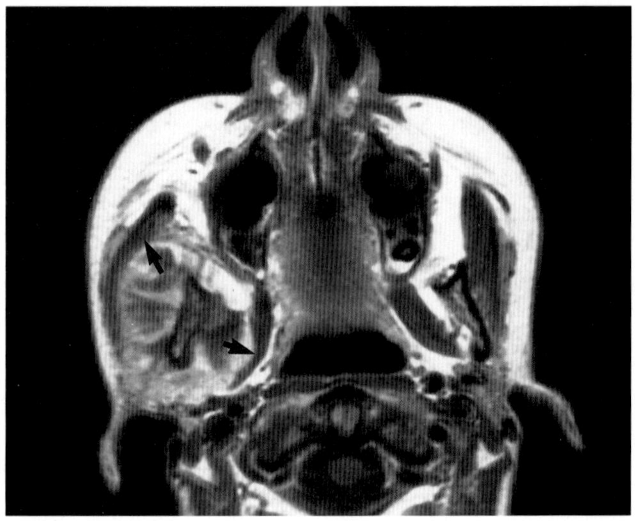

B

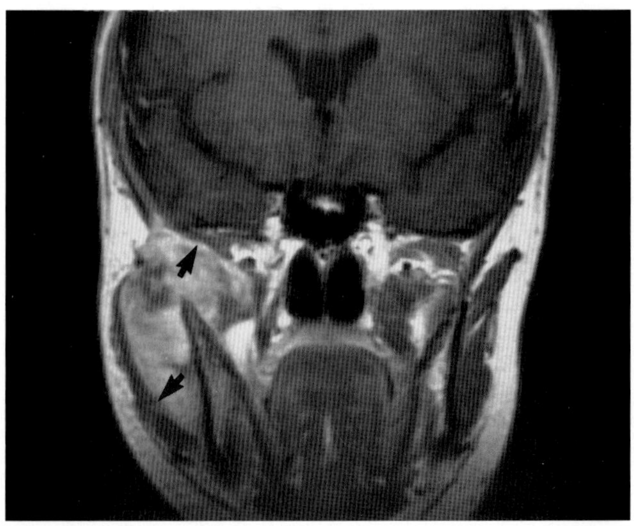

C

Figure 22.66

Radio-induced sarcoma of the right mandible (20-year-old) following head and neck rhabdomyosarcoma treated by radiation therapy 14 years ago.

A Axial MR (600 ms, 20 ms) shows a hypointense mass around the mandible (arrows); note the hypointense signal of the involved bone-marrow (arrowhead) in comparison with the left normal mandible.

B,C Axial (**B**) and coronal (**C**) MR (600 ms, 20 ms) with gadolinium gives heterogeneous enhancement of the tumor, which is sharply delineated from the surrounding muscles (arrows).

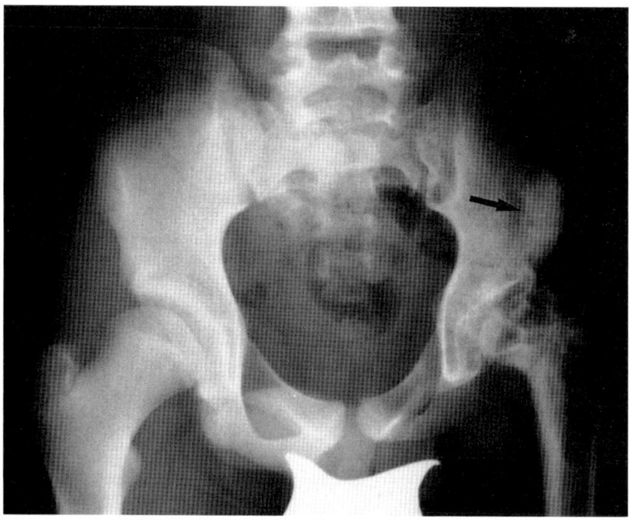

A

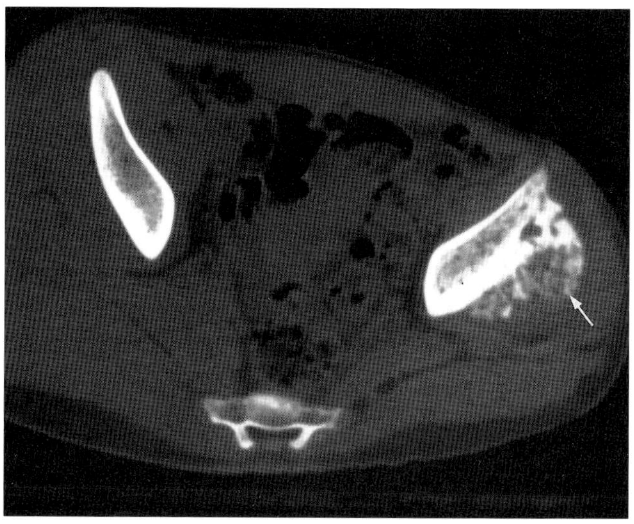

B

Figure 22.67

Rhabdomyosarcoma of the pelvis treated 7 years ago by radiation (45 Gy) (16-year-old).

A Standard plain film demonstrates hemiatrophy of the left iliac bone with osteonecrosis of the femoral head and an osteoblastic iliac area (arrow).

B CT scan shows an osseous lesion of the left ilium with osteogenesis in the soft tissue (arrow). The diagnosis was radio-induced osteosarcoma.

can occur (around 17 years later, on average). These secondary solid tumors may also occur in previously irradiated areas. Diagnostic and pre-therapeutic assessment depends on the examination best adapted to the localization of the lesion: CT or MR to establish tumoral extensions (Figures 22.66 and 22.67).

Imaging of sequelae

The long-term consequences of treatment have a considerable effect on functional prognosis. The direct toxicity of chemical drugs on the parenchyma, the effect of radiotherapy on growth, static disorders following surgery, all accumulate and may potentialize each other.

Bone sequelae

Radiotherapy arrests growth in the bone by sterilizing the growth cartilage.[74,75] This leads to two types of consequence:

- Morphological and esthetic sequelae, such as shortening of the trunk or of a limb or facial deformity, may arise.
- Functional or orthopedic after-effects, such as static spinal disorders (e.g. scoliosis); these are aggravated by surgery. Radiographs of the spine show scoliotic deformation (Figure 22.68), with partial or total atrophy of the irradiated vertebrae, and indicate whether it can be corrected by an appropriate brace. If MR is used, it shows the fatty involution of the hemopoietic marrow, the margins of which are geometrically defined by the radiation field (Figure 22.69).

Pulmonary sequelae

Certain drugs, for example actinomycin D and bleomycin, have a possible pulmonary toxicity which may be potentialized by radiotherapy. They are responsible for pulmonary fibrosis (Figure 22.70) and radiological interstitial involvement of different degrees of gravity. Radiotherapy can have two types of effect on the thorax.[76]

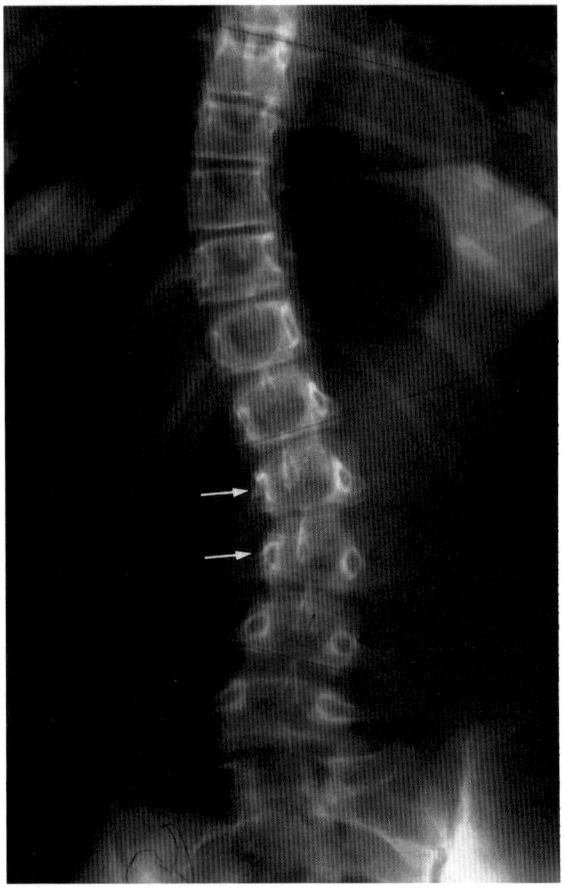

Figure 22.68

Radiation therapy (30 Gy) 9 years previously for a right nephroblastoma. Stand-up abdominal plain film shows lumbar scoliosis due to insufficient growth of the right aspect of the vertebral bodies (arrows) secondary to the radiation therapy.

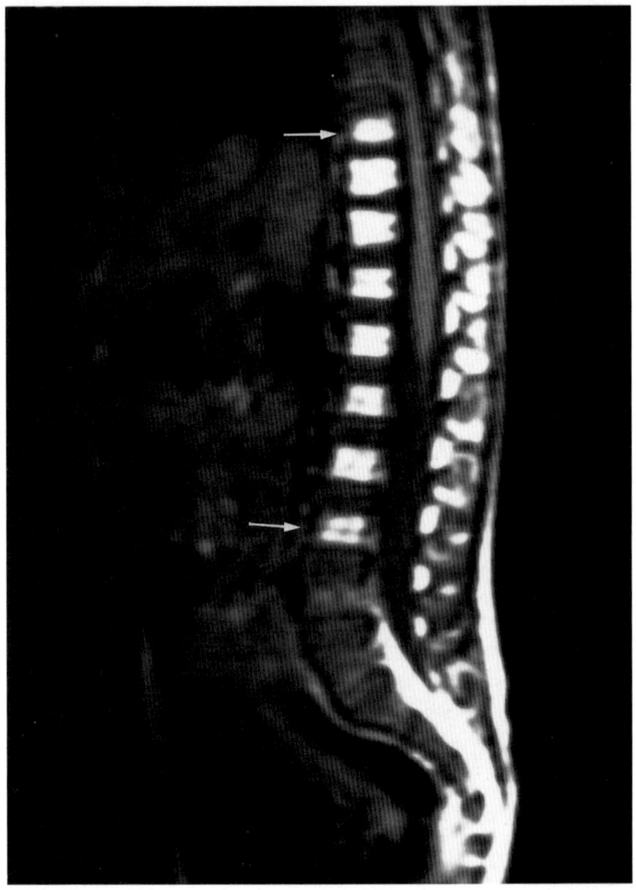

Figure 22.69

Abdominal neuroblastoma treated by surgery and radiation therapy (35 Gy) (5-year-old). Sagittal MR (500 ms, 25 ms) shows a sharply delineated hyperintense signal from the vertebral body (arrows) due to the post-radiotherapeutic lipomatous involution of the hematopoietic bone marrow.

- Progressive retractile fibrosis of the pulmonary parenchyma with bronchiectasis can occur in the year following the termination of radiotherapy. It is preceded by a subacute alveolar stage 2–6 months after the completion of treatment and may be associated with pleural and/or pericardial effusion. Pulmonary fibrosis is accompanied by fibrous mediastinal modifications and depends on the radiation dose received, abnormalities occurring from a dose of 40 Gy upwards (Figures 22.71 and 22.72); more than a year after the termination of treatment, it becomes stable.
- Growth disorders brought about within the rib cage may aggravate respiratory deficiency.

Cardiovascular sequelae

Anthracyclins are toxic to the myocardium. US is the easiest way of judging the extent of myocardial modifications. Here again, the association of cardiotoxic drugs and thoracic radiotherapy increases the gravity of the medium and long-term consequences of treatment, such as pericarditis or myocarditis. Radiotherapy can also be responsible for arterial stenosis, which leads to delayed progressive, disabling clinical symptoms. Angiography is used in assessment (Figure 22.73).

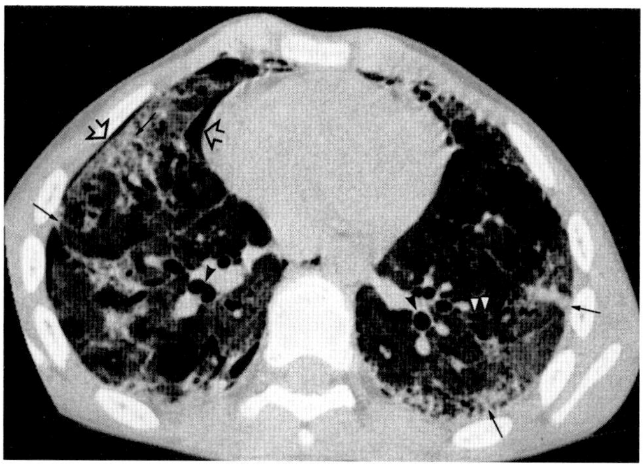

Figure 22.70

Undifferentiated carcinoma of the cavum (13-year-old): post-bleomycin pulmonary fibrosis. CT scan (1 mm thickness) shows retractile interstitial lesions (closed arrows) which create dilatations of the bronchi (arrowhead) and mild pneumothorax (open arrows); note the thickening of the minor fissure.

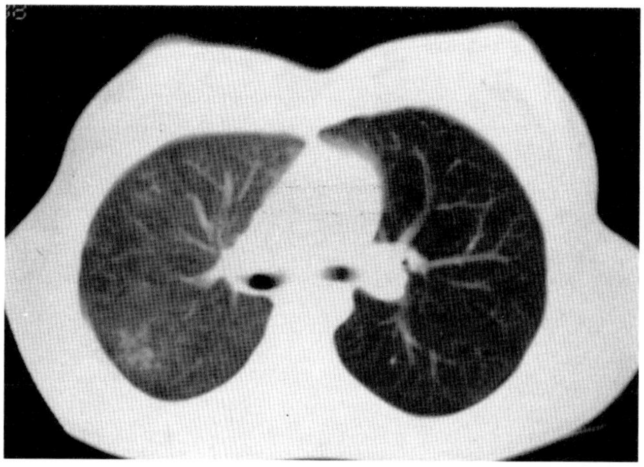

A

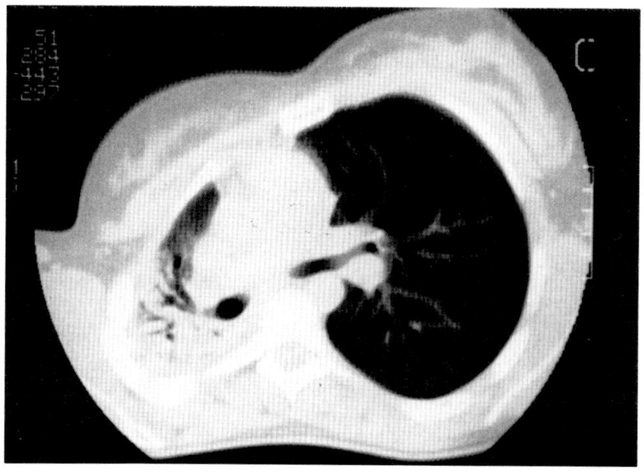

C

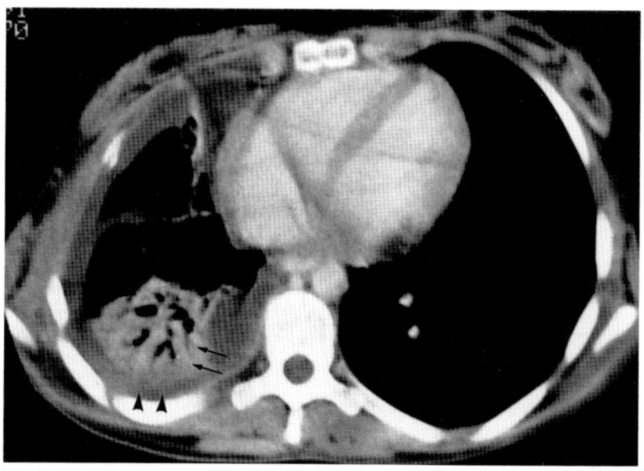

B

Figure 22.71

Rhabdomyosarcoma of the right chest wall (16-year-old).

A CT scan 2 months post-radiotherapy (50 Gy on chest wall, 40 Gy on right lung and pleura) shows mild alveolar opacity of the right lung.

B One month later, CT shows a clearly alveolar opacity (arrows) with pleural effusion (arrowheads); there is subacute post-radiation pneumonia.

C One year later, significant retractile fibrosis of the right lung has occurred.

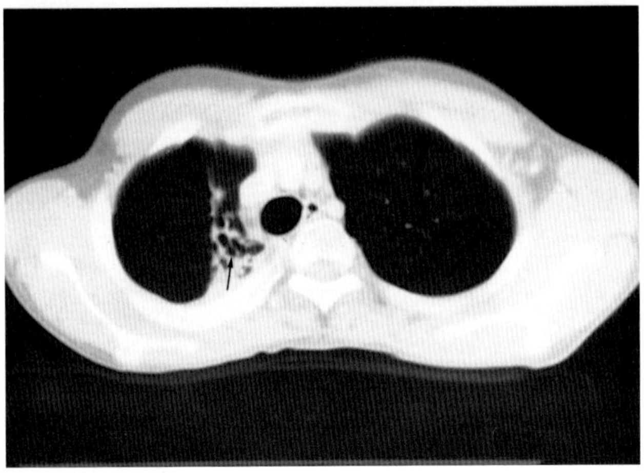

Figure 22.72

Malignant mesenchymal tumor of the right apical chest wall treated by radiation therapy (45 Gy) 2 years previously (13-year-old). CT scan shows sharply delineated retractile fibrosis containing bronchiectasis (arrow).

Digestive sequelae

Digestive sequelae consist mainly of digestive post-radiotherapeutic stenosis which is best studied with upper gastrointestinal series and small bowel series of examinations with contrast material (barium oral opacification). They are uncommon nowadays, because of the avoidance of wide abdominal irradiation in children. In the case of the liver, if irradiation of a perinephric space for the treatment of a right nephroblastoma, for example, is widespread, or if an adjuvant treatment with drugs potentializing the effects of radiotherapy (such as actinomycin D) is used, this may result in the appearance of veno-occlusive disease. US shows hepatomegaly, with subhepatic veins disappearing or being difficult to visualize and ascites. If the radiation field was limited, focal modifications are observed in the density or signal from the liver on CT or MR, which have the peculiarity of having well-defined margins according to the geometric fields and dose of radiotherapy received.

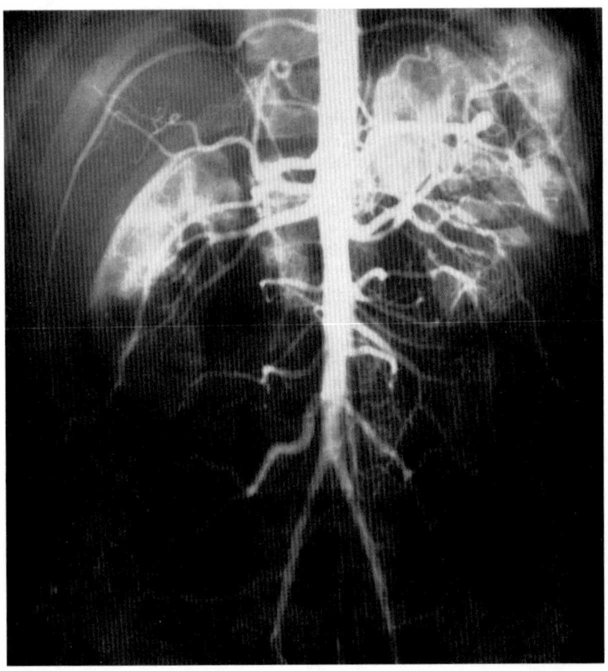

Figure 22.73

Malignant teratoma treated by pelvic radiotherapy (30 Gy) at 1 year of age (10-year-old). Abdominal angiography shows strong stenosis of the iliac vessels; there is insufficient growth of the iliac bones.

Urinary sequelae

Uniform atrophy of the kidney (Figure 22.74), which may be partial or total, ureteral stenosis and a reduction in the size of the bladder, which has thickened walls, are the sequelae of irradiation of the urinary tract.[77]

Encephalic sequelae

Certain drugs, such as methotrexate and vincristine, are neurologically toxic (necrotizing leukoencephalopathy and peripheral neuropathy, respectively) and radiotherapy potentializes their effects, especially on the central nervous system, where they are indicated in the prevention of cerebromeningeal recurrences. It can be useful to provide proof of this toxicity with imaging. MR is the most sensitive technique: plaques of demyelization of the white matter, which has a hypersignal on T2-weighted sequences, and cortical atrophy with widening of sulcus and ventricles are seen, but the calcifications of central gray nuclei are better seen on a CT scan.

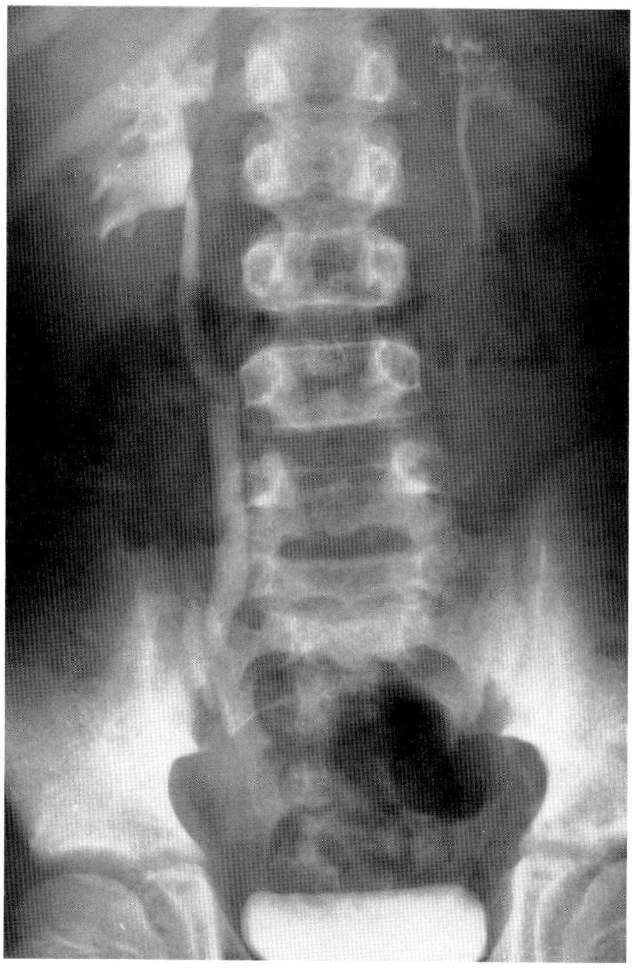

A

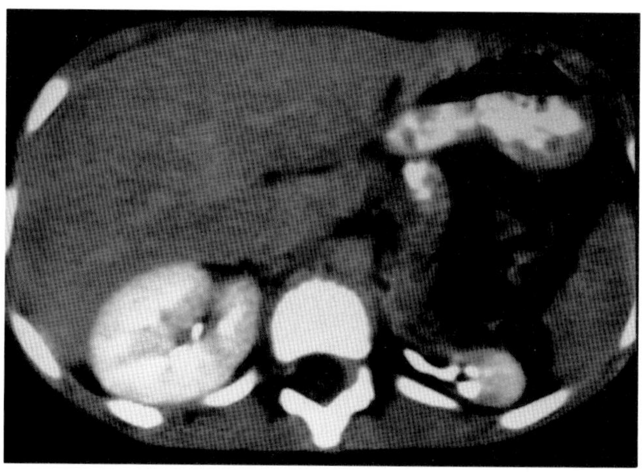

B

Figure 22.74

Radiation therapy (35 Gy) 2 years ago for a left adrenal neuroblastoma. IVP (**A**) and CT with contrast injection (**B**) show atrophy of the left kidney which keeps a uniform anatomy of the calyces.

References

1. Schatz CJ, Becker TS, Normal CT anatomy of the paranasal sinuses, *Radiol Clin N Am* (1984) **22**:107–18.
2. Smoker WRK, Gentry LR, Computed tomography of the nasopharynx and related spaces, *Semin Ultrasound CT MR* (1986) **7**:107–30.
3. Siegel MJ, Nadel SN, Glazer HS, et al, Mediastinal lesions in children: comparison of CT and MR, *Radiology* (1986) **160**:241–4.
4. Fraumeni JF Jr, Geiser CF, Manning MD, Wilms' tumor and congenital hemihypertrophy: report of five new cases and review of the literature, *Pediatrics* (1967) **40**:886–99.
5. Pendergrass TW, Congenital anomalies in children with Wilms' tumor: a new survey, *Cancer* (1976) **37**:403–8.
6. Hayden KC Jr, Swischuk LE, *Pediatric ultrasonography* (Williams and Wilkins: Baltimore 1987).
7. Brasch RC, Abols IB, Gooding CA, et al, Abdominal disease in children: a comparison of computed tomography and ultrasound, *AJR* (1980) **134**: 153–8.
8. Bolande RP, The neurocristopathies. A unifying concept of disease arising in neural crest maldevelopment, *Human Pathol* (1974) **5**:409–29.
9. Kissel P, André JM, Jacquier A, *The neurocristopathies* (Masson: New York 1981).
10. Dehner LP, *Pediatric surgical pathology* (Williams and Wilkins: Baltimore 1987).
11. Hartmann O, Scopinaro M, Tournade MF, et al, Neuroblastomes traités à l'Institut Gustave Roussy de 1975 à 1979. Cent soixante treize cas, *Arch Fr Pediatr* (1983) **40**:15–21.
12. Schweisguth O, *Tumeurs solides de l'enfant* (Flammarion Médecine-Sciences: Paris 1979).
13. Evans AE, Natural history of neuroblastoma. In: Evans AE, ed, *Advances in neuroblastoma research* (Raven Press: New York 1980) 3–12.
14. Kaplan SJ, Holbrook CT, McDaniel HG, et al, Vasoactive intestinal peptides secreting tumors of childhood, *Am J Dis Child* (1980) **134**:21–4.
15. Kirks DR, Merten DF, Grossman H, et al, Diagnostic imaging of pediatric abdominal masses: an overview, *Radiol Clin North Am* (1981) **19**:527–45.
16. Gitlow SE, Bertani LM, Rausen A, et al Diagnosis of neuroblastoma by quantitative and qualitative determination of catecholamine metabolites in urine, *Cancer* (1970) **5**:1377–83.
17. Labrosse EH, Com-Nougue C, Zucker JM, et al, Urinary excretion of 3-methoxy-4-hydroxymandelic acid and 3-methoxy-4-hydroxyphenylacetic acid by 288 patients with neuroblastoma and related neural crest tumors, *Cancer Res* (1980) **40**:1995–2001.
18. Evans AE, d'Angio GJ, Randolph J, A proposed staging for children with neuroblastoma, *Cancer* (1971) **27**:374–9.
19. Evans AE, Staging and treatment of neuroblastoma, *Cancer* (1980) **45**:1799–802.

20. Hartmann O, Benhamou E, Beaujean F, et al, Repeated high dose chemotherapy followed by purged autologous bone marrow transplantation as consolidation therapy in metastatic neuroblastoma, *J Clin Oncol* (1987) **5**:1205–11.

21. Lemerle J, *Cancers de l'enfant* (Flammarion Médecine-Sciences: Paris 1989).

22. Harris TM, Cohen MD, Abdominal magnetic resonance imaging, *Pediatr Radiol* (1989) **20**:10–19.

23. Dietrich RB, Kangarloo H, Lenarsky C, et al, Neuroblastoma: the role of MR imaging, *AJR* (1987) **148**:937–42.

24. Kagan AR, Steckel RJ, Dietrich RB, et al, Retroperitoneal mass with intra-dural extension: value of MRI in neuroblastoma, *AJR* (1986) **146**:251–4.

25. Siegel MJ, Jamroz GA, Glazer HS, et al, MR imaging of intraspinal extension of neuroblastoma, *J Comput Assist Tomogr* (1986) **10**:593–5.

26. Neuenschwander S, Ollivier L, Toubeau M, et al, Local evaluation of abdominal neuroblastoma stage III and IV: use of US, CT and ^{123}I-metaiodobenzylguanidine (MIBG) scintigraphy, *Ann Radiol* (1987) **30**:491–6.

27. Stark DD, Brasch RC, Moss AA, et al, Neuroblastoma: diagnostic imaging and staging, *Radiology* (1983) **148**:101–6.

28. Armstrong AE, Harwood-Nash DCF, Ritz CR, et al, CT of neuroblastomas and ganglioneuromas in children, *AJR* (1982) **139**:571–5.

29. Atkinson GO Jr, Zaatari GS, Lorenzo RL, et al, Cystic neuroblastoma in infants: radiographic and pathologic features, *AJR* (1986) **146**:113–17.

30. Geoffray A, Couanet D, Neuenschwander S, et al, Computed tomography diagnosis of extradural involvement of paraspinal tumors in children, *Ann Radiol* (1986) **29**:333–8.

31. Cohen MD, Smith JA, Cory DA, et al, The visualization of major blood vessels by magnetic resonance in children with malignant tumors, *Radiographics* (1985) **5**:441–55.

32. Couanet D, Geoffray A, Hartmann O, et al, Bone marrow metastases in children's neuroblastoma studied by magnetic resonance imaging. In: Evans AE, d'Angio JG, Knudson AG, et al, eds, *Advances in neuroblastoma research*, vol 2 (Alan R Liss: New York 1988) 547–55.

33. Carmody RF, Yang PJ, Seeley GW et al, Spinal cord compression due to metastatic disease: diagnosis with MR imaging versus myelography, *Radiology* (1989) **173**:225–9.

34. Bomanji J, Levison DA, Flatman WD, et al, Uptake of iodine-123 MIBG by pheochromocytomas, paragangliomas and neuroblastomas: a histopathological comparison, *J Nucl Med* (1987) **28**:973–8.

35. Lumbroso JD, Guermazi F, Hartmann O, et al, Metaiodobenzylguanidine (mIBG) scans in neuroblastoma: sensitivity and specificity, a review of 115 scans. In: Evans AE, d'Angio JG, Knudson AG, et al, eds, *Advances in neuroblastoma research,* vol 2 (Alan R Liss: New York 1988) 689–705.

36. Stark DD, Brasch RC, Moss AA, et al, Recurrent neuroblastoma: the role of CT alternative imaging tests, *Radiology* (1983) **148**:107–12.

37. Labreveux de Cervens, C, Hartmann O, Valteau D, et al, Syndrome de Pepper néo-natal. A propos d'une série de 22 cas, *Arch Fr Pédiatr* (1990) **47**:91–6.

38. Forman HP, Leonidas JC, Berdon WE, et al, Congenital neuroblastoma: evaluation with multimodality imaging, *Radiology* (1990) **175**:365–8.

39. Becwith JB, Palmer NF, Histopathology and prognosis of Wilm's tumor. Results from the First National Wilm's Tumor Study Pathology, *Cancer* (1978) **41**:1937–48.

40. Jaffe MH, White SJ, Silver TM, et al, Wilms' tumor: ultrasonic features, pathologic correlation, and the diagnostic pitfalls, *Radiology* (1981) **140**:147–52.

41. Cohen MD, Siddiqui A, Weetman R, et al, A rational approach to the radiologic evaluation of children with Wilms' tumor, *Cancer* (1982) **50**:887–92.

42. Hartman DS, Sanders RC, Wilms' tumor versus neuroblastoma: usefulness of ultrasound in differentiation, *J Ultrasound Med* (1982) **1**:117–22.

43. Miller HJ, *Imaging in pediatric oncology* (Williams and Wilkins: Baltimore 1985).

44. White KS, Grossman H, Wilms' and associated renal tumors of childhood, *Pediatr Radiol* (1991) **21**:81–8.

45. Slovis TL, Philippart AI, Cushing B, et al, Evaluation of the inferior vena cava by sonography and venography in children with renal and hepatic tumors, *Radiology* (1981) **140**:767–72.

46. d'Angio GJ, Breslow N, Beckwith JB, et al, Treatment of Wilms' tumor, *Cancer* (1989) **64**:349–60.

47. Bolande RP, Brough AJ, Izant RJ, Congenital mesoblastic nephroma of infancy. A report of eight cases and the relationship to Wilm's tumor, *Pediatrics* (1967) **40**:272–8.

48. Brasch RC, Randel SB, Gould RC, Wilms' tumor follow-up evaluation: comparison of computed tomography and non-CT imaging. Consideration of accuracy, expense, and radiation exposure, *AJR* (1981) **137**:1005–8.

49. Bove KE, McAdams AJ, The nephroblastomatosis complex and its relationship to Wilms' tumor, a clinicopathologic treatise, *Perspect Pediatr Pathol* (1976) **3**:185–223.

50. Rosenfield NS, Shimkin P, Berdon W, et al, Wilms' tumor arising from spontaneously regressing nephroblastomatosis, *AJR* (1980) **135**:381–4.

51. Fernback SK, Feinstein KA, Donaldson JS, et al, Nephroblastomatosis: comparison of CT with US and urography, *Radiology* (1988) **166**:153–6.

52. Willoughby M, Bone marrow and CNS involvement in non-Hodgkin's lymphoma. In: Graham-Pole J, ed, *Non Hodgkin's lymphoma in children. Masson monographs in pediatric hematology/oncology* (Masson: New York 1980) 147–63.

53. Wollner N, Exelby PR, Lieberman PH, Non Hodgkin's lymphoma in children. A progress report on the original patients treated with the LSA_2L_2 protocol, *Cancer* (1979) **44**:1990–9.

54. Miller JH, Hindman BW, Lam AHK, Ultrasound in the

evaluation of small bowel lymphoma in children, *Radiology* (1980) **135**:409–14.

55. Cohen MD, Siddiqui AR, Weetman RM, et al, Hodgkin disease and non-Hodgkin lymphomas in children: utilization of radiological modalities, *Radiology* (1986) **158**:499–505.

56. Geoffray A, Vanel D, Masselot J, et al, Contribution of computed tomography (CT) in the study of 24 head and neck embryonic rhabdomyosarcomas in children, *Eur J Radiol* (1984) **4**:177–80.

57. Dietrich RB, Lufkin RB, Kangarloo H, et al, Head and neck MR imaging in the pediatric patient, *Radiology* (1986) **159**:769–76.

58. Youdem DM, Lexa FJ, Bilaniuk LT, et al, Rhabdomyosarcomas in the head and neck: MR imaging evaluation, *Radiology* (1990) **177**:683–6.

59. Tannous WN, Azouz EM, Homsy YL, et al, CT and ultrasound imaging of pelvic rhabdomyosarcoma in children. A review of 56 patients, *Pediatr Radiol* (1989) **19**:530–4.

60. Ruyman FB, Newton WA, Ragab AH, et al, For IRS: bone marrow metastases at diagnosis in children and adolescents with rhabdomyosarcoma, *Cancer* (1984) **53**:368–73.

61. Shapiro SA, Malignant sacrococcygeal teratoma, *Med Pediatr Oncol* (1980) **8**:171–5.

62. Brodeur GM, Howarth CB, Pratt CB, et al, Malignant germ cell tumors in 57 children and adolescents, *Cancer* (1981) **48**:1890–8.

63. Wollner N, Exelby PR, Woodruff JM, et al, Malignant ovarian tumors in childhood. Prognosis in relation to initial therapy, *Cancer* (1976) **37**:1953–64.

64. Arger PH, Mulhern CB Jr, Coleman BG, et al, Prospective analysis of the value of scrotal ultrasound, *Radiology* (1981) **141**:763–6.

65. Braun IF, MRI of the nasopharynx, *Radiol Clin North Am* (1989) **27**:315–30.

66. Knudson AG Jr, Retinoblastoma: a prototypic hereditary neoplasm, *Semin Oncol* (1978) **5**:57–60.

67. Lallemand D, Brasch RC, Char DH, Orbital tumors in children: characterization by computed tomography, *Radiology* (1984) **151**:85–8.

68. Mafee MF, Goldberg MF, Greenwald MJ, et al, Retinoblastoma and simulating lesions: role of CT and MR imaging. *Radiol Clin North Am* (1987) **25**:667–82.

69. Brunelle F, Chaumont P, Hepatic tumours in children: ultrasonic differentiation of malignant from benign lesions, *Radiology* (1984) **150**:695–9.

70. de Campo M, de Campo JF, Ultrasound of primary hepatic tumours in childhood, *Pediatr Radiol* (1988) **19**:19–24.

71. Finn JP, Hall-Craggs MA, Dicks-Mireaux C, et al, Primary malignant liver tumors in childhood: assessment of resectability with high-field MR and comparison with CT, *Pediatr Radiol* (1990) **21**: 34–8.

72. Miller JH, Greenfield, LD, Wald BR, Candidiasis of the liver and spleen in childhood, *Radiology* (1982) **142**:375–80.

73. Meadows AT, Patterns of second malignant neoplasms in children, *Cancer* (1977) **40**:1903–11.

74. Smith R, Davidson JK, Flatman GE, Skeletal effects of orthovoltage and megavoltage therapy following treatment of nephroblastoma, *Clin Radiol* (1982) **33**:601–13.

75. Probert JC, Parker BR, The effect of radiation therapy on bone growth, *Radiology* (1975) **114**:155–62.

76. Libshitz HI, *Diagnostic roentgenology of radiotherapy change* (Williams and Wilkins: Baltimore 1979).

77. Andersen BL, Lauver JW, Ross P, et al, Demonstration of radiation nephritis by computed tomography, *Comput Radiol* (1982) **6**:187–91.

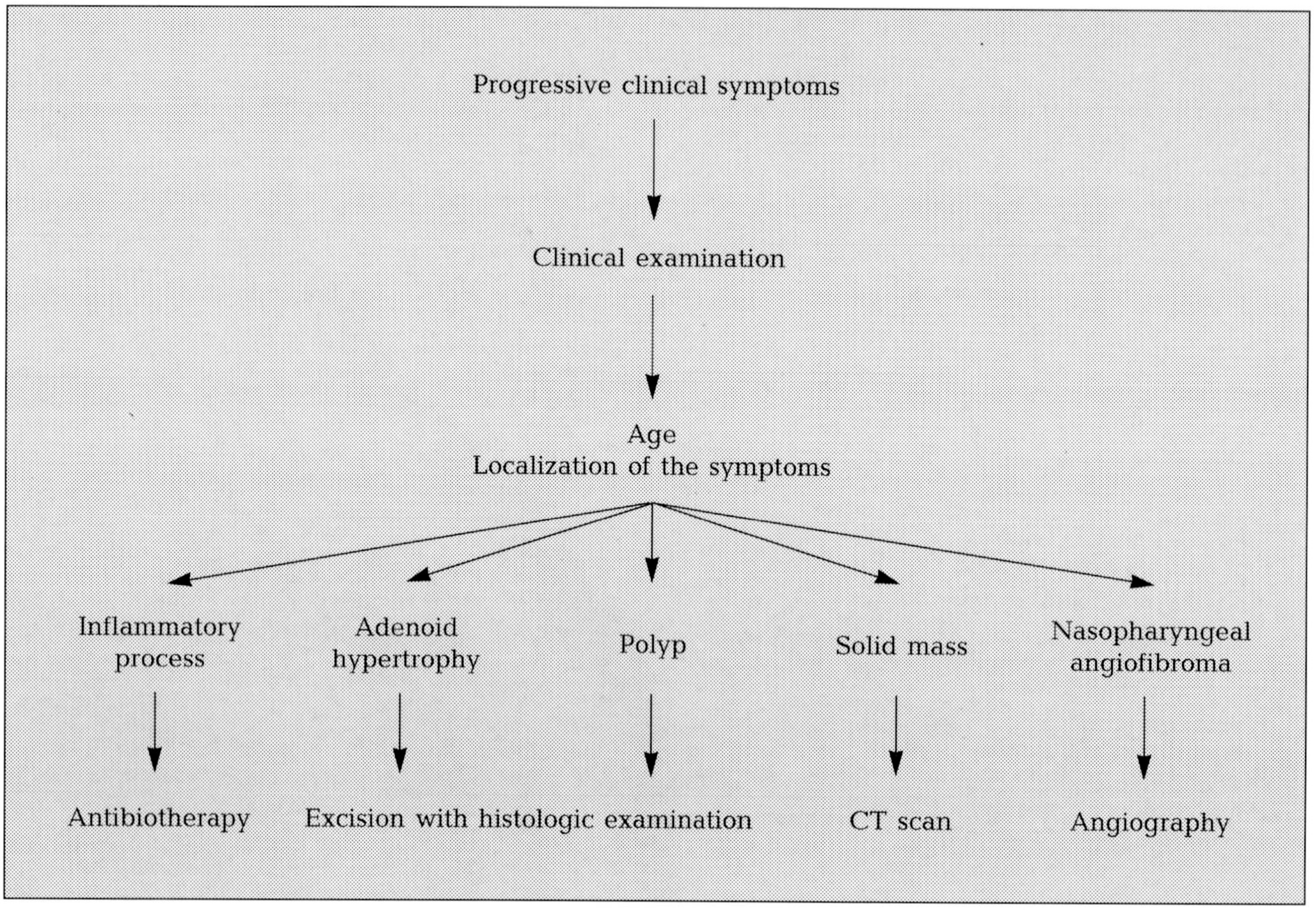

Diagram 22.1

Clinical practice and imaging strategy in pediatric head and neck pathology.

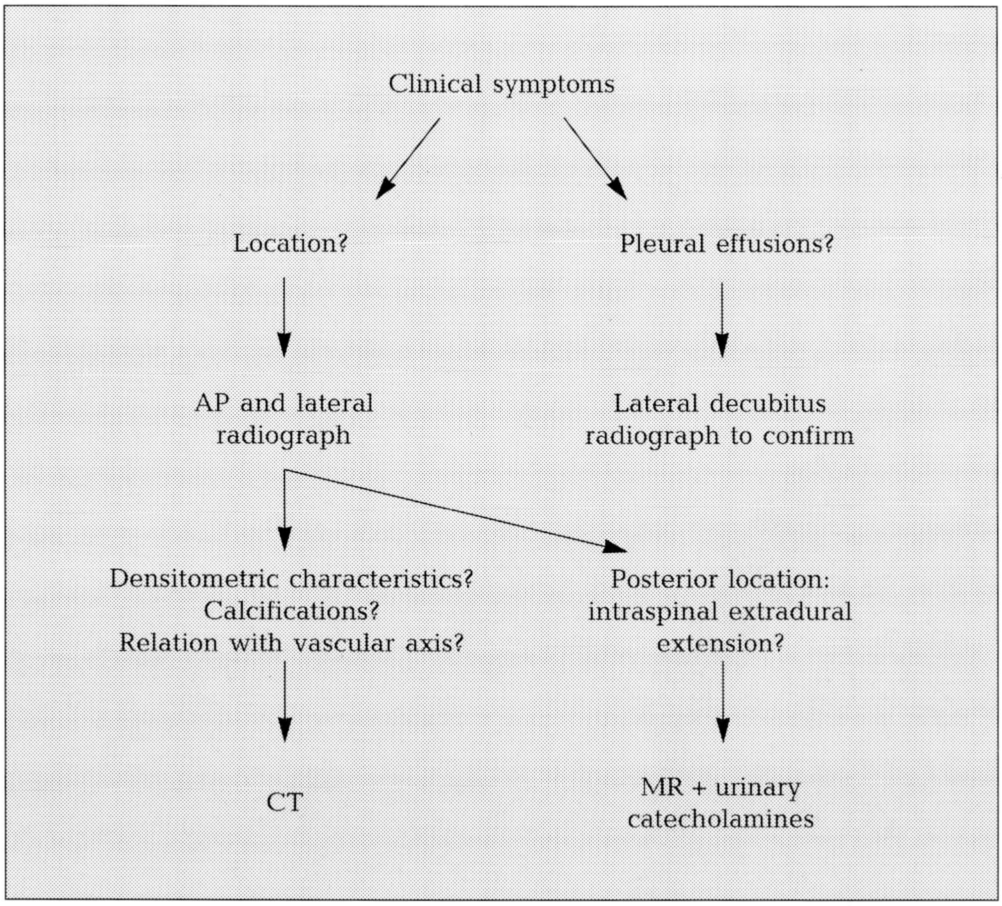

Diagram 22.2

Imaging strategy in pediatric thoracic pathology.

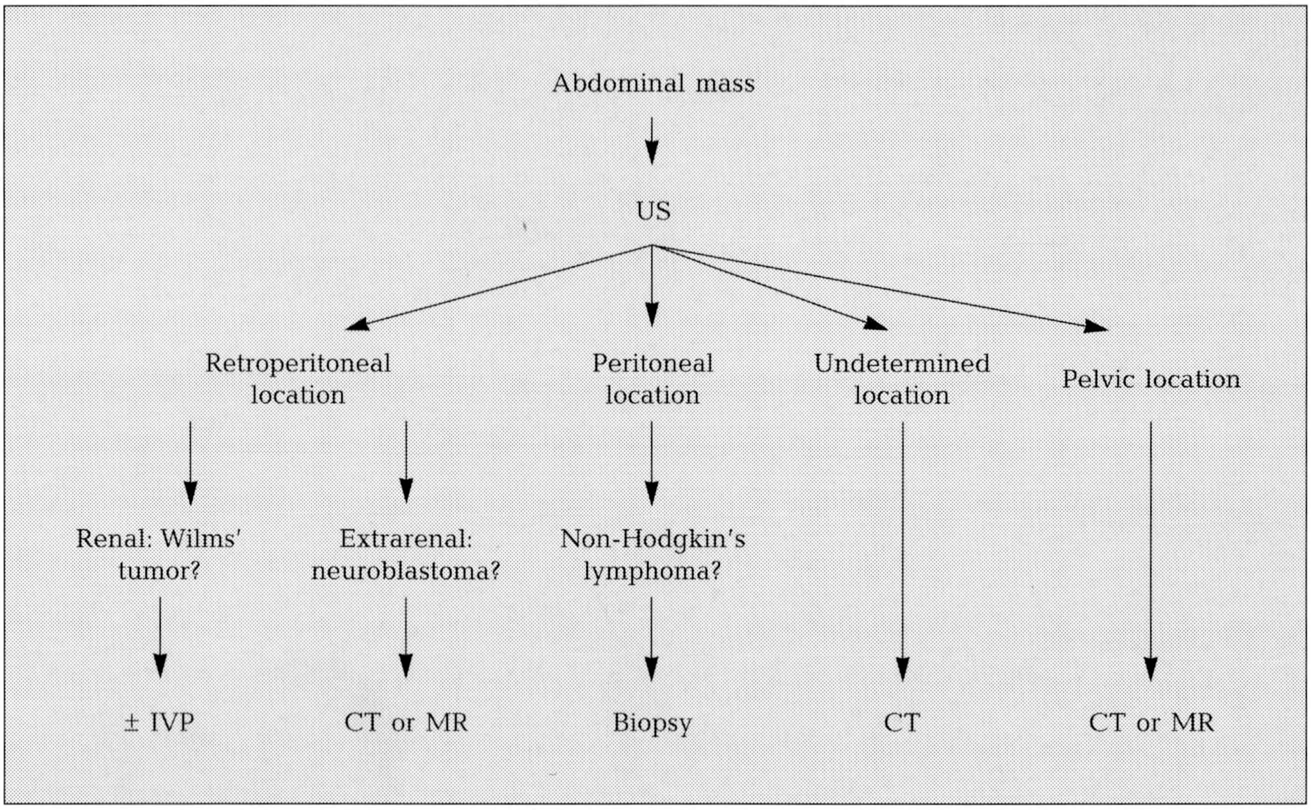

Diagram 22.3 Imaging strategy for an abdominal mass in childhood.

Diagram 22.4 Pre-therapeutic staging of neuroblastoma.

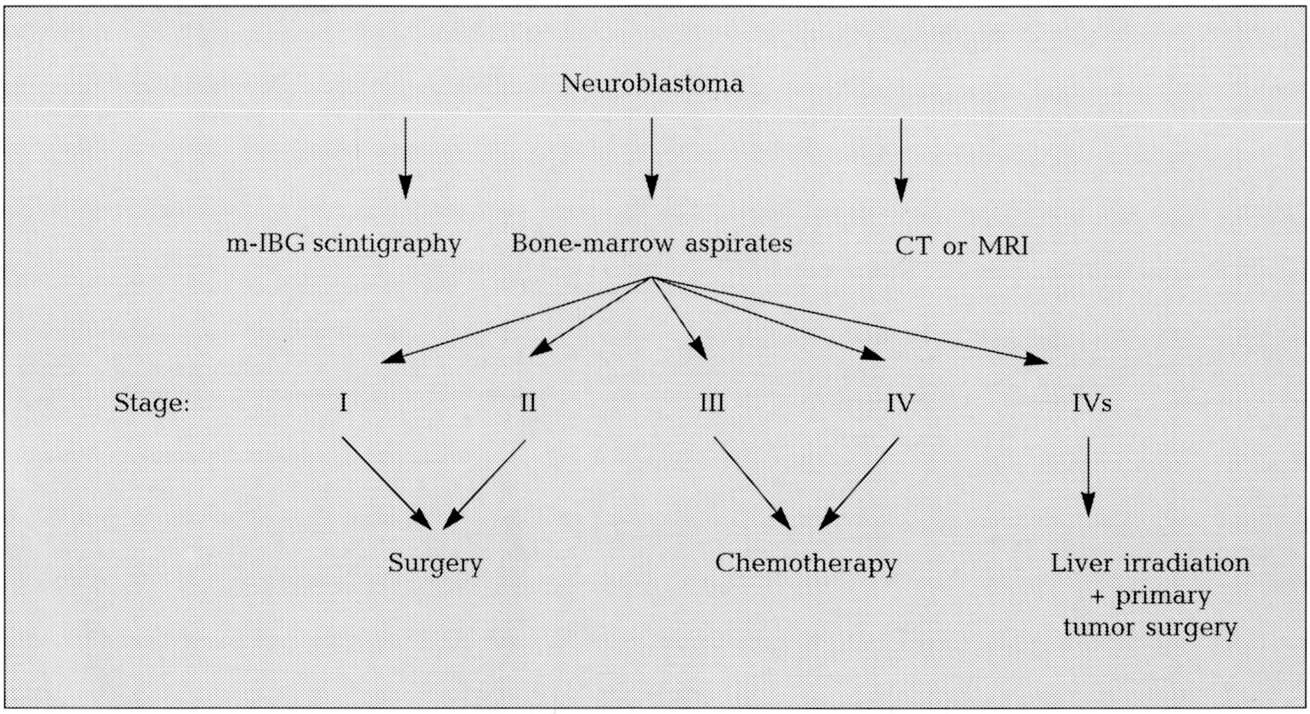

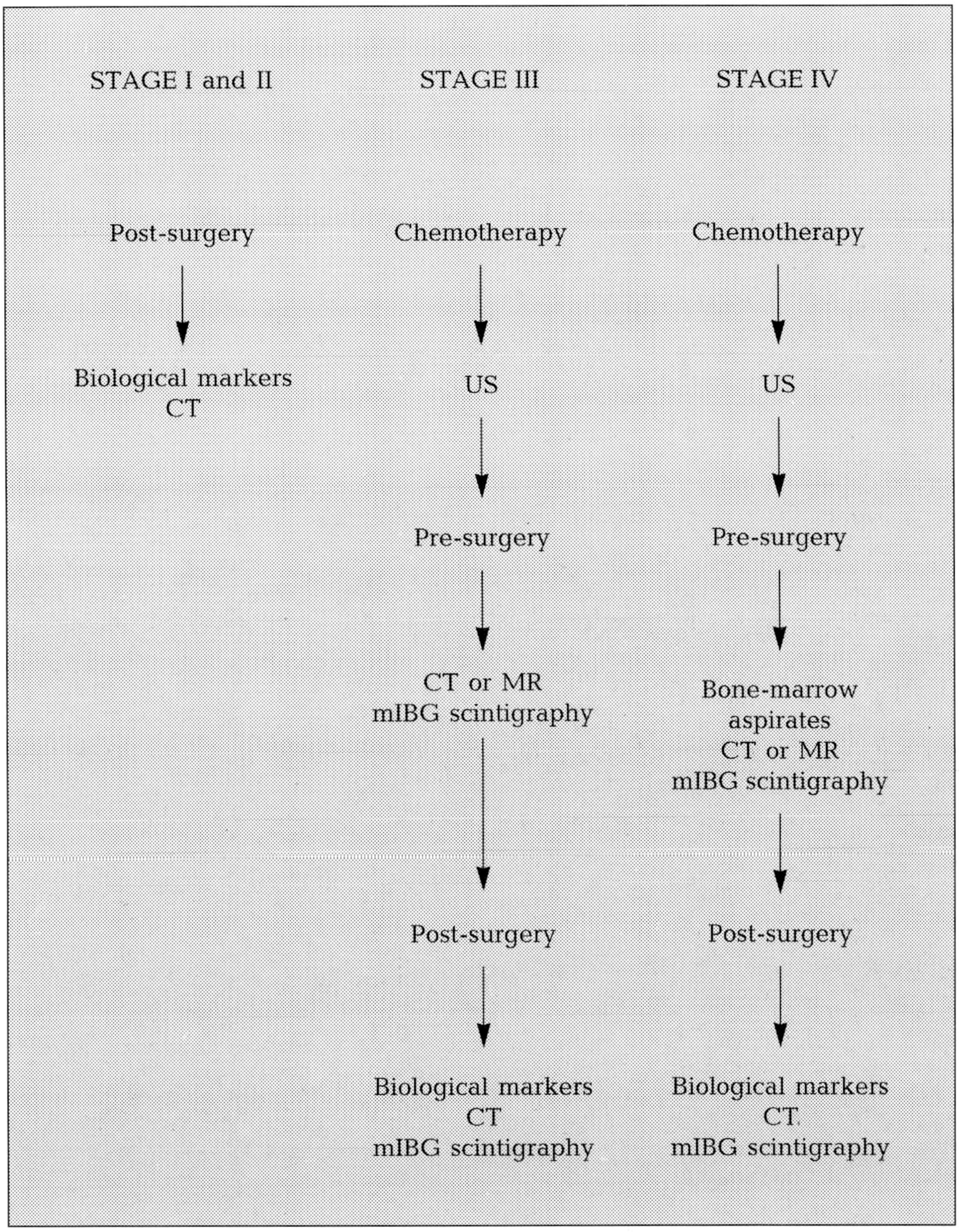

Diagram 22.5

Imaging strategy for follow up in neuroblastoma.

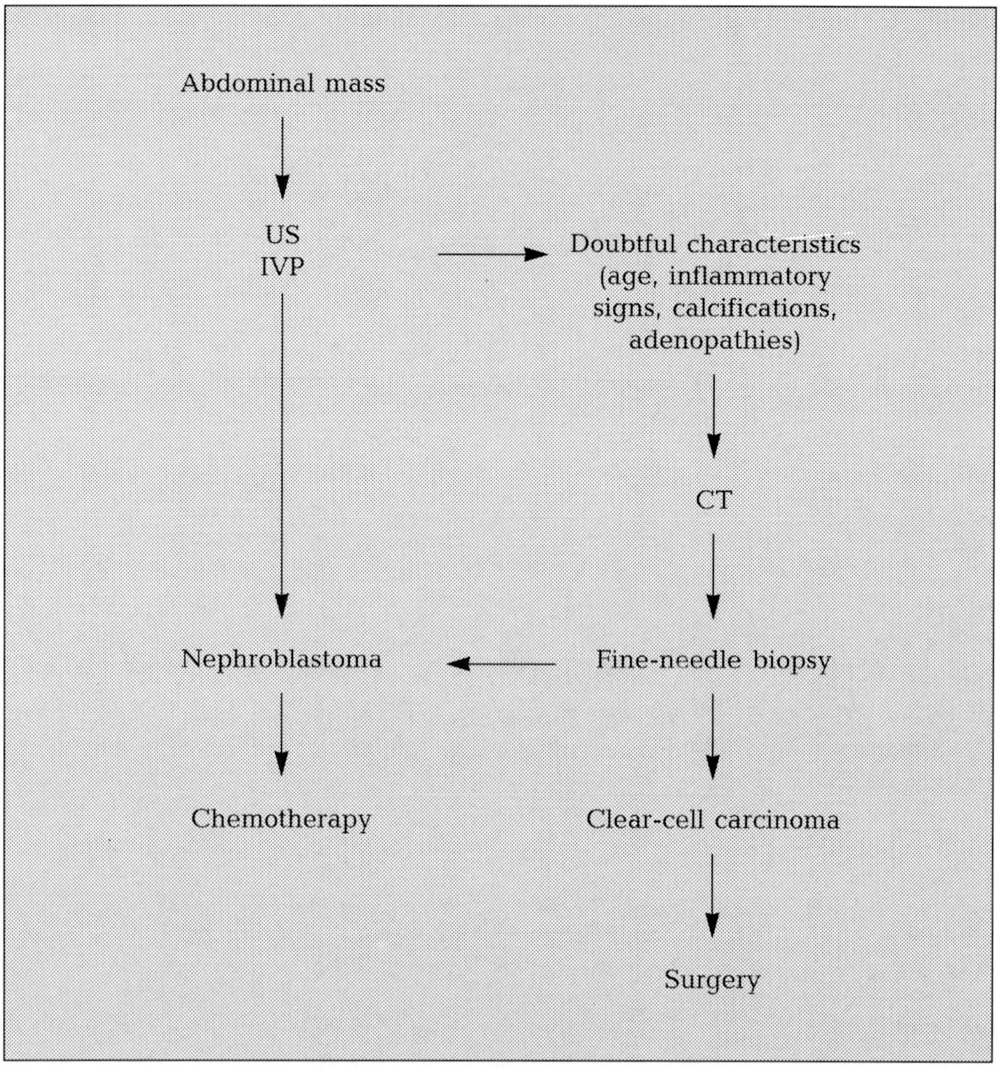

Diagram 22.6

Imaging strategy for tumors of the kidney.

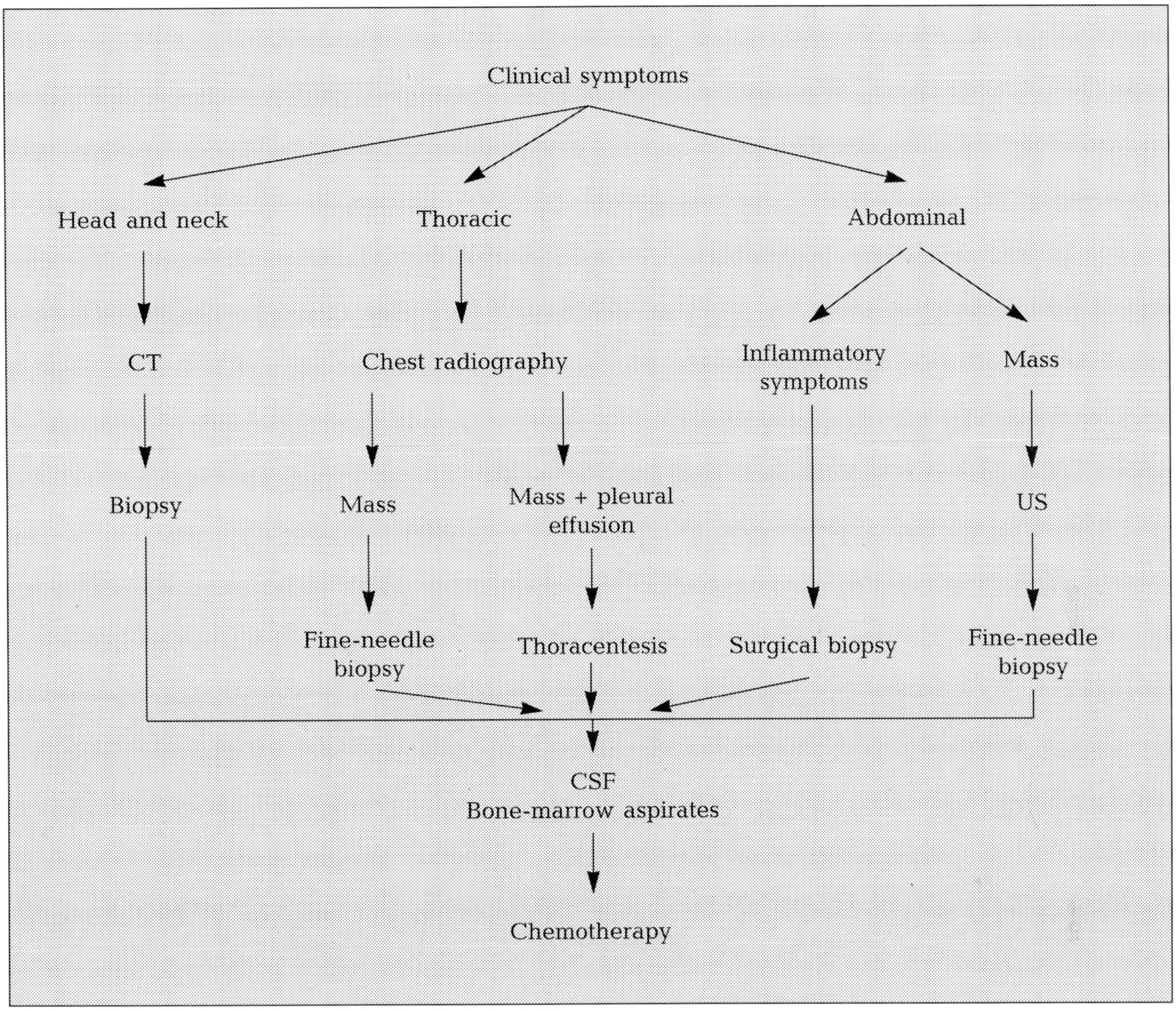

Diagram 22.7

Imaging strategy in non-Hodgkin's lymphoma.

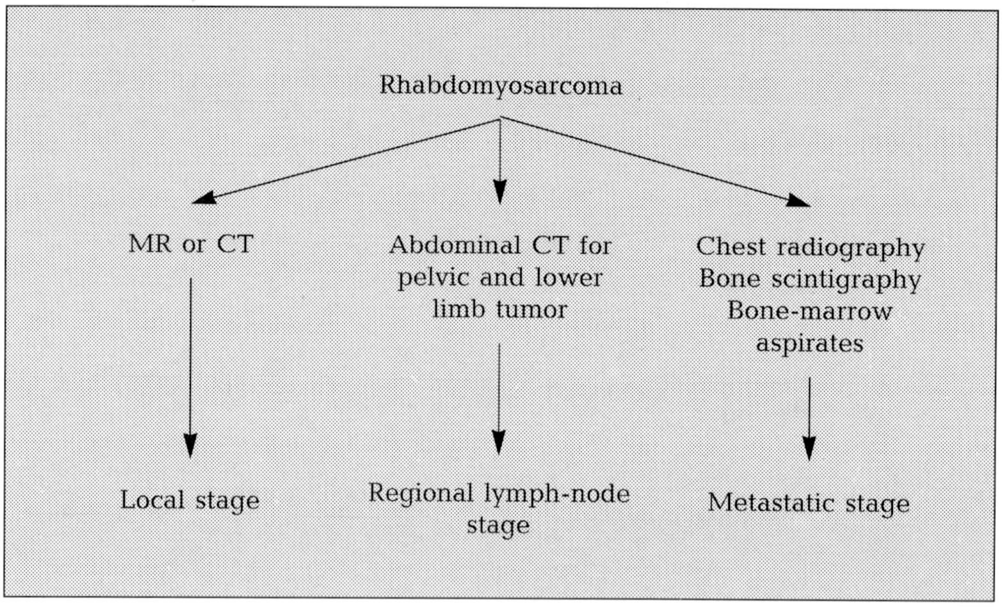

Diagram 22.8

Initial staging of rhabdomyosarcoma.

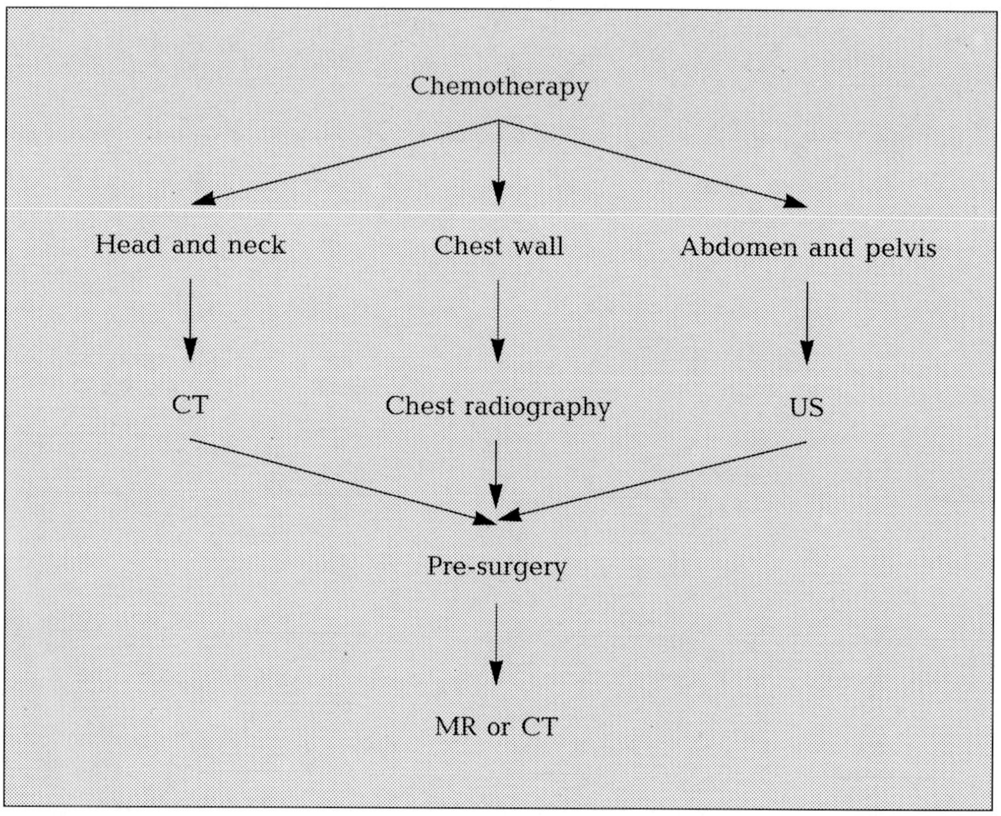

Diagram 22.9

Follow up of rhabdomyosarcoma.

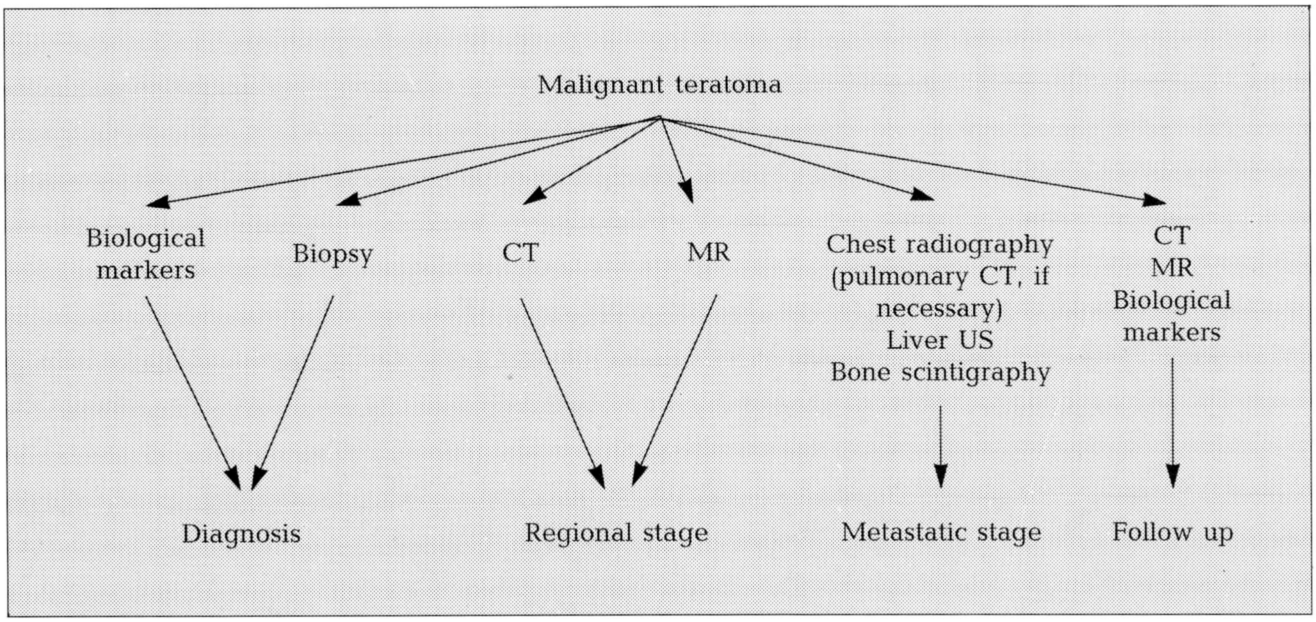

Diagram 22.10

Staging of malignant teratoma.

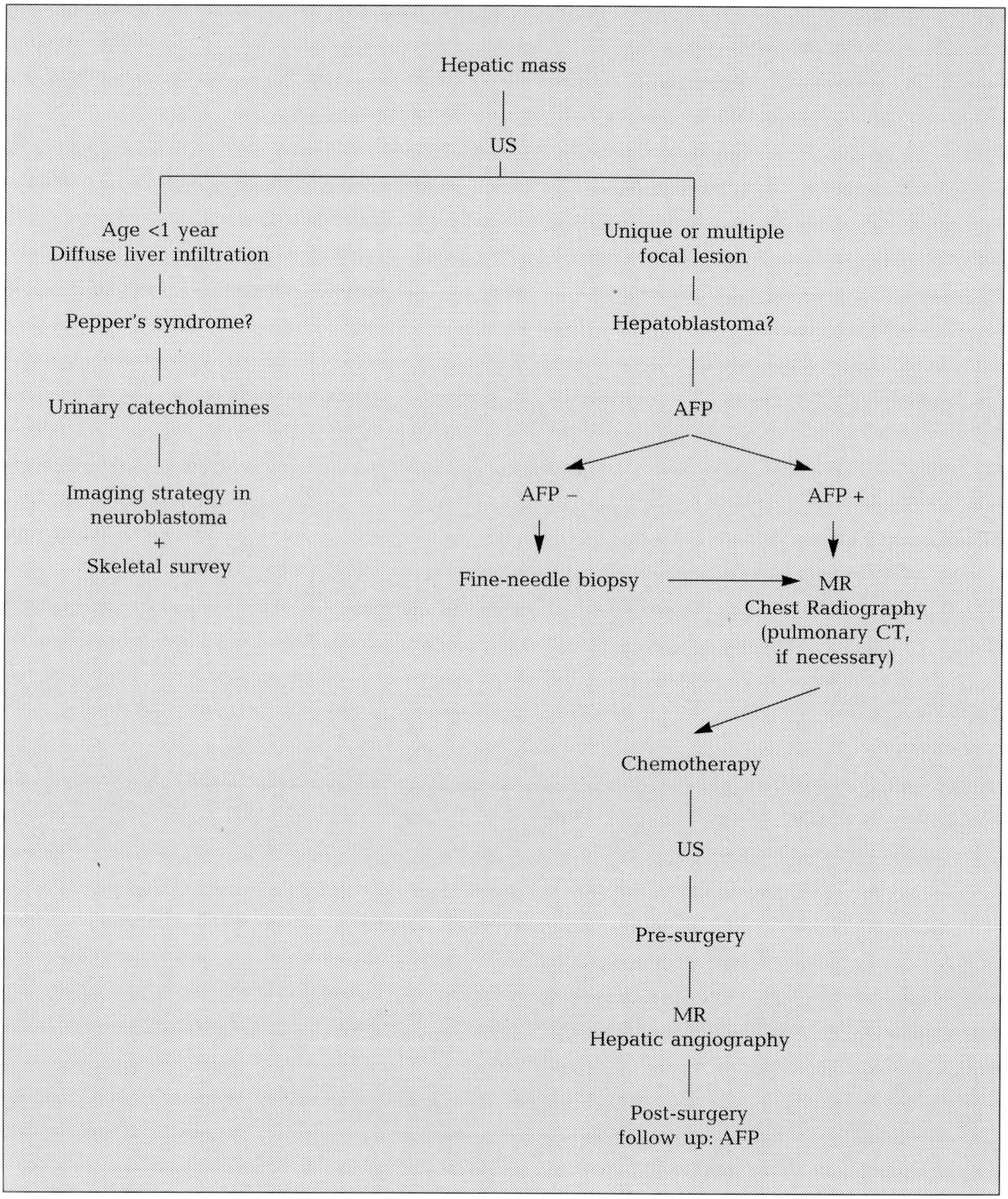

Diagram 22.11

Imaging strategy in malignant hepatic tumors.

Index